LABORATORY DIAGNOSIS
OF DISEASES CAUSED BY
TOXIC AGENTS

LABORATORY DIAGNOSIS OF DISEASES CAUSED BY TOXIC AGENTS

Compiled and Edited by

F. WILLIAM SUNDERMAN, M.D., Ph.D., Sc.D.

Director, Institute for Clinical Science
Director of Education, Association of Clinical Scientists
Clinical Professor of Medicine, Jefferson Medical College
Medical Advisor, Rohm and Haas Company
Philadelphia, Pennsylvania

and

F. WILLIAM SUNDERMAN, JR., M.D.

Professor and Head
Department of Laboratory Medicine
McCook Teaching Hospital
University of Connecticut School of Medicine
Hartford, Connecticut 06112

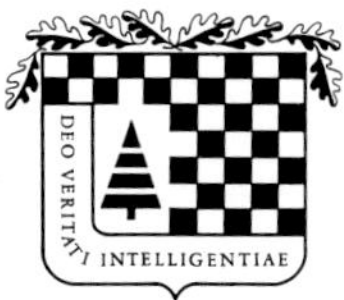

WARREN H. GREEN, INC.

St. Louis, Missouri, U.S.A.

Published by

WARREN H. GREEN, INC.
10 South Brentwood Blvd.
St. Louis, Missouri 63105, U.S.A.

Library of Congress Catalog Card No. 77-96992

Printed in the United States of America
4-A (167)

Preface

This book contains the edited proceedings of an Applied Seminar on the Laboratory Diagnosis of Diseases Caused by Toxic Agents, held in Washington, D.C., under the auspices of the Association of Clinical Scientists. In organization and format, this volume is similar to the published proceedings of nine previous seminars. The topic for this year's seminar was selected in order to acquaint scientists with the recent acquisition of knowledge of diseases caused by toxic agents. It is our feeling that this topic is timely since our present era is one in which there is unusual concern about air and water pollution, exposure to drugs and toxic agents and their relation to disease.

The rapid advances in technological operations and the unprecedented complexities of industrial processes in recent years have enormously increased the hazards to which people are being exposed in their daily lives. Newer types of clothing, food, drugs, chemicals, and electrical and mechanical devices are replacing older types of products. Many of these newer developments are creating special hazards of exposure. In the evaluation and diagnosis of pathological states caused by exposure to toxic agents, the clinical laboratory is being called upon to assume an increasingly important role.

This book has been divided into four parts: General Toxicologic Considerations; General Methodologic Considerations; Specific Toxic Agents; and Clinicopathologic Considerations. It is our fervent hope that workers in clinical laboratories will find the book especially useful in the newer field of clinical toxicology.

Our grateful appreciation is expressed to the lecturers who have generously contributed their time and energies to the success of the Applied Seminar and to Mr. Warren H. Green, and his staff for their gracious cooperation.

F. William Sunderman, M.D.

Institute for Clinical Science
1833 Delancey Place
Philadelphia, Pennsylvania 19103

March 4, 1970

Seminar Faculty

DIRECTOR OF SEMINAR
F. WILLIAM SUNDERMAN, M.D., PhD., Sc.D.
Institute for Clinical Science
Philadelphia, Pennsylvania

GONZALO E. APONTE, M.D.
Jefferson Medical College
Philadelphia, Pennsylvania

HALLA BROWN, M.D.
George Washington University
Washington, D.C.

RODNEY F. CARLTON, M.D.
University of Arkansas
School of Medicine
Little Rock, Arkansas

E. P. CASMAN, Ph.D.
Food & Drug Administration
Washington, D.C.

JACOB CHURG, M.D.
Barnert Memorial Hospital
Paterson, New Jersey

J. WESLEY CLAYTON, JR., Ph.D.
Hazelton Labs., Inc.
Falls Church, Virginia

HERBERT DERMAN, M.D.
City of Kingston Laboratory
Kingston, New York

KENNETH P. DuBOIS, Ph.D.
Univ. of Chicago Medical School
Chicago, Illinois

KURT M. DUBOWSKI, Ph.D.
Univ. of Okla. Medical Center
Oklahoma City, Oklahoma

RUSSELL S. FISHER, M.D.
Medical Examiner's Office
Baltimore, Maryland

MARVIN FORLAND, M.D.
Univ. of Texas Medical School
San Antonio, Texas

ALFRED H. FREE, Ph.D.
Ames Company
Elkhart, Indiana

HELEN M. FREE, B.S.
Ames Company
Elkhart, Indiana

HENRY C. FREIMUTH, Ph.D.
Medical Examiner's Office
Baltimore, Maryland

LEON GOLBERG, D.Sc., D.Phil., M.B.
Albany Med. College of Union U.
Albany, New York

LEO R. GOLDBAUM, Ph.D.
Armed Forces Institute of Pathology
Washington, D.C.

ERVIN A. GOMBOS, M.D.
New York University
School of Medicine
New York, New York

HARRY W. HAYS, Ph.D.
Agric. Research Service
U.S. Dept. of Agriculture
Washington, D.C.

PETER B. HERDSON, Ph.D., M.B.
University of Auckland
Medical School
Auckland, New Zealand

PETER N. HORVATH, M.D.
Georgetown University
School of Medicine
Washington, D.C.

J. DE LA HUERGA, M.D., Ph.D.
Grant Hospital
Northwestern Univ. Medical School
Chicago, Illinois

JAMES J. HUMES, M.D.
St. John Hospital
Detroit, Michigan

CECIL B. JACOBSON, M.D.
George Washington University
School of Medicine
Washington, D.C.

JOHN H. JONES, M.S.
Food & Drug Administration
Washington, D.C.

ROBERT E. JONES, JR., M.D.
Anderson Memorial Hospital
Anderson, South Carolina
KENDALL K. KANE, M.D.
St. Luke's Hospital
New York, New York
JOHN E. KASIK, M.D., Ph.D.
University of Chicago
School of Medicine
Chicago, Illinois
GEOFFREY KENT, M.D., Ph.D.
Chicago Wesley Memorial Hospital
Chicago, Illinois
ROBERT A. KYLE, M.D.
Mayo Clinic
Rochester, Minnesota
ARTHUR M. LANGER, Ph.D.
Mt. Sinai School of Medicine
New York, New York
MARVIN LEGATOR, Ph.D.
Food & Drug Administration
Washington, D.C.
M. LUBRAN, M.D.
University of Chicago
College of Medicine
Chicago, Illinois
E. W. MAYNERT, M.D., Ph.D.
University of Illinois
College of Medicine
Chicago, Illinois
E. W. MAYNERT, M.D., Ph.D.
University of Illinois
College of Medicine
Chicago, Illinois
PAUL N. MORGAN, Ph.D.
V. A. Hospital
Little Rock, Arkansas
ROBERT C. MUEHRCKE, M.D.
West Suburban Hospital
Oak Park, Illinois
JOSEPH C. OLSON, JR., Ph.D.
Food & Drug Administration
Washington, D.C.
W. WALTER OPPELT, M.D.
University of Florida
School of Medicine
Gainesville, Florida
HERBERT S. POSNER, Ph.D.
National Environ. Health
Sciences Center
Research Triangle Park, North Carolina
WILLIAM C. PURDY, Ph.D.
University of Maryland
College Park, Maryland
HOWARD QUITTNER, M.D.
University of Arkansas
School of Medicine
Little Rock, Arkansas
JOHN W. REBUCK, M.D., Ph.D.
Henry Ford Hospital
Detroit, Michigan
F. LEE RODKEY, Ph.D.
U. S. Naval Med. Res. Institute
National Naval Medical Center
Bethesda, Maryland
IRENE E. ROECKEL, M.D.
University of Kentucky
School of Medicine
Lexington, Kentucky
JOSEPH F. SADUSK, JR., M.D.
Parke, Davis and Company
Detroit, Michigan
JOHN SAVORY, Ph.D.
University of Florida
College of Medicine
Gainesville, Florida
JOSEPH C. SHERRICK, M.D.
Northwestern University Medical School
Passavant Memorial Hospital
Chicago, Illinois
RALPH G. SMITH, Ph.D.
Wayne State University
Detroit, Michigan
BENJAMIN H. SPARGO, M.D.
University of Chicago
College of Medicine
Chicago, Illinois
WERNER U. SPITZ, M.D.
Medical Examiner's Office
Baltimore, Maryland
HAROLD STEVENS, M.D.
George Washington University
School of Medicine
Washington, D.C.
ABRAHAM STOLMAN, Ph. D.
Conn. State Dept. of Health
Hartford, Connecticut
F. WILLIAM SUNDERMAN, M.D., Ph.D.
Institute for Clinical Science
Philadelphia, Pennsylvania
F. WILLIAM SUNDERMAN, JR., M.D.
University of Connecticut
School of Medicine
Hartford, Connecticut
CHARLES J. UMBERGER, Ph.D.
Office of Chief Med. Examiner
New York, New York

FREDERICK I. VOLINI, M.D.
West Suburban Hospital
Oak Park, Illinois

EARL B. WERT, M.D.
Mobile Infirmary
Mobile, Alabama

MORRIS F. WIENER, M.D.
State University of New York
Syosset Hospital
Manhasset, New York

J. H. WILKINSON, Ph.D., D.Sc.
Charing Cross Hospital
University of London
London, England

BENNIE ZAK, Ph.D.
Wayne State University
Detroit, Michigan

Contributors

KATHLEEN AHEARN, B.A.
Washington, D.C.
LUIS ARIAS-BERNAL, M.D.
Washington, D.C.
JOHN R. BARNES, Ph.D.
Newark, Delaware
JOSEPH M. BEALS, M.D.
Detroit, Michigan
JAMES W. BUTLER
Detroit, Michigan
PARITOSH K. DE, Ph.D.
New York, New York
ANA DEL RIEGO, D.Pharm.
Washington, D.C.
FRANKLIN D. GRIFFITH, Ph.D.
Newark, Delaware
WILLIAM J. HERMANN, JR., B.S.
Detroit, Michigan
J. M. KAUFFMAN, M.S.
Myerstown, Pennsylvania
SHELDON E. KRASNOW, M.D.
Oak Park, Illinois
DEAN A. LeSHER, M.D., Ph.D.
Detroit, Michigan
VALERIE MAGYAR, B.A.
Washington, D.C.
EMILIO ORFEI, M.D.
Chicago, Illinois
E. A. PETRUS, M.D.
Chicago, Illinois
DAVID RESK, M.D.
Oak Park, Illinois
NORRIS O. ROSZEL
Gainesville, Florida
F. SPERLING, Ph.D.
Washington, D.C.
R. DONALD STRAHM
Huntsville, Alabama
WILMIER M. TALBERT, JR., M.D.
Lexington, Kentucky
ELIZABETH VOSBECK, M.A.
Washington, D.C.
LOUIS A. WILLIAMS, B.S.
Detroit, Michigan

Contents

LABORATORY DIAGNOSIS OF DISEASES CAUSED BY TOXIC AGENTS

PART I

GENERAL TOXICOLOGIC CONSIDERATIONS

Chapter 1

Modes of Action of Toxic Agents

LEON GOLBERG, D.Sc., D.Phil., M.B.

To-day, the powerful tools at our disposal enable us to analyze toxic effects in terms of attack on particular molecules, or groups within those molecules. In fact, the point has been reached when the plethora of observed effects on biochemical or biological systems presents difficulties in sifting out those actions that are relevant under the conditions of exposure with which we are concerned. Compounds that alkylate or acylate nucleic acids or proteins, that react with sulfhydryl groups, chelate metals, inhibit enzymes, or uncouple oxidative phosphorylation do not necessarily thereby cause toxic effects in the intact animal or in man. The capacity for metabolic adjustment and other available adaptive and repair mechanisms often decide the issue.

In a few classical instances, such as fluoroacetate, trivalent arsenic and 2, 4-dinitrophenol, the biochemical mechanisms of toxic action have been elucidated (Barnes and Paget, 1965). For the most part, however, the state of the art is not yet such that we can achieve those neatly-packaged classifications of primary actions and secondary effects favored by the pathologist. In what must inevitably be a personal selection, some current problems are presented to illustrate the shift of emphasis in modern Toxicology from the study of acute poisoning involving massive doses to consideration of long-term hazards, necessitating the elaboration of more fundamental approaches and sensitive tests for actions exercised under ordinary conditions of exposure.

Some Actions Manifested at the Subcellular Level

The majority of long-term effects brought about by low doses of chemical agent are primarily actions exercised on one or other of the processes that maintain function, growth or replication of cells. Such actions may originate in effects on any of the steps involved in DNA synthesis, transcription or translation of the genetic message; or they may be attacks on subcellular integrity as expressed in polysome-ribosome relationship, rough and smooth endoplasmic reticulum, mitochondria, lysosomes or microbodies. Membrane effects may be involved. Finally, toxic action may result from interaction with proteins, particularly enzymes, the attack being directed at active or allosteric sites, or at metals that are essential for their catalytic function.

The biochemical manifestations of hepatotoxic action at the molecular level show many similarities and subtle differences. In the cytoplasm, direct actions on the rough endoplasmic reticulum (RER), for instance by hepatotoxic agents such as carbon tetrachloride (Smuckler and Benditt, 1963, 1965) and dimethylnitrosamine (Villa-Trevino, 1967), result in detachment and partial disruption of protein-synthesizing polysomal units, with increase of the number of free ribosomes. In consequence the rate of endogenous protein synthesis is decreased but the response to stimulation by an external coding agent, polyuridylic acid (poly-U), is enhanced owing to the increased availability of ribosomal surface on the free ribosomes for interaction with messenger (Smuckler, Parthier and Hultin, 1968). Not all hepatotoxic agents that affect RER show the same results. Many induce hepatomegaly, an effect discussed further below. At high doses, coumarin enhances both endogenous and poly U-stimulated amino-acid incorporation into protein; it also influences the "pH 5 enzyme" in the microsomal supernatant (Nievel and Golberg, 1967). Repeated low doses of coumarin leave endogenous protein synthesis unchanged but still increase the response to stimulation by the synthetic messenger (Nievel and Golberg, 1968).

The aflatoxins and pyrrolizidine alkaloids (retrorsine and lasiocarpine) also inhibit the incorporation of labelled amino acids into protein *in vivo* and *in vitro,* associated with disruption of polysomes (Villa-Trevino and Leaver, 1968). Yet, their pathological manifestations in the rat liver are very different. Retrorsine, like dimethylnitrosamine, produces centrilobular necrosis and hemorrhage; aflatoxin B_1 induces acute periportal necrosis. Thus, the common effect on protein synthesis demands more detailed investigation: is the mRNA produced inadequate or defective, or does it suffer damage? Long-term administration of low doses of a variety of chemical carcinogens of this sort elicits only slight or reversible cytoplasmic alterations. Hence, Svoboda and Higginson (1968) conclude that such changes are consequences of events initiated in the nucleus.

Villa-Trevino (1967) has furnished suggestive evidence that dimethylnitrosamine methylates mRNA. Aflatoxin B_1 and retrorsine inhibit the incorporation of orotate into liver nuclear RNA 1 hour after administration (Villa-Trevino and Leaver, 1968). The aflatoxins probably interact with DNA and prevent transcription by DNA polymerase (Clifford and Rees, 1967; Clifford, Rees and Stevens, 1967). According to Moulé and Fraysinnet (1968), the inhibition of transcription by aflatoxin preferentially involves nucleolar RNA, since within 15 min of administration newly-synthesized 45S RNA disappears and segregation occurs of the morphological components of the nucleolus (Svoboda, Racela and Higginson, 1967). Also, with 3′-methyl-4-dimethylaminoazobenzene and 4- nitroquinoline-N-oxide, there is a general inhibition of nucleolar biosynthetic reactions involving DNA-dependent RNA polymerase (Paul, Reynolds and Montgomery, 1967) especially synthesis of 45S and 55S nucleolar RNA (Floyd, Unuma and Busch, 1968).

The emphasis on primary nuclear events draws attention to the nuclear histones, which are perhaps the most important of the various protein fractions in the cell capable of binding foreign compounds or their metabolites. The capacity of these histones to repress DNA-dependent DNA and RNA synthesis suggests that control may be impaired by seemingly unimportant structural modifications consequent upon such binding. Reese and Varcoe (1967) showed that p-dimethylaminoazobenzene was bound to a relatively small extent by histones of rat liver cell nuclei. More recently, binding of 2-acetylaminofluorene to arginine-rich histones and, to a lesser degree, to other basic nuclear proteins, was reported by Barry, Ovechka and Gutmann (1968).

The earlier interest in binding of foreign compounds by fractions of soluble cytoplasmic liver proteins has given place to a preoccupation with binding to various forms of RNA and to DNA (for examples, see Table in Farber, 1968). Farber (1968) has even reported binding to what seems to be an abnormal form of glycogen in nodules of hyperplastic liver cells. What is important to note is the suggestion that traces of compounds like p-dimethylaminoazobenzene and 2-acetylaminofluorene persist in bound form for long periods of time.

The nitrosamines and pyrrolizidine alkaloids represent examples of a class of toxic agent to which Barnes (1968) has applied the title of "hit and run" poisons. Under appropriate conditions, no immediate effect is seen; the delay in appearance of toxic manifestations provides ample time for removal of the toxicant from the body. In the case of nitrosamines, despite the evidence of alkylation of guanine in nucleic acids, no proof of a persistent residuum is yet forthcoming (Magee and Barnes, 1967). The pyrrolizidine alkaloids have recently been shown to give rise to a new class of pyrrole metabolites (Mattocks, 1968), with capacity to reproduce the pulmonary edema and pleural effusion that develop in rats 4-5 weeks after a single dose of monocrotaline or fulvine. The suggestion is that during the phase of initial liver damage the metabolites are liberated, act on the lungs and set in train the lethal delayed effects that are revealed long after the toxin and its metabolites have left the body. Again, one wonders whether some form of residual toxicant persists, bound in the lungs, to exercise its evil influence.

Effects on Systems Studied *in vitro*

The smectic mesophase or liquid crystal form of cholesterol-lecithin affords a remarkably useful *in vitro* model for the study of physico-chemical influences exercised by toxic agents. Sessa and Weissmann (1968a) have stressed the similarity between the properties of such phospholipid "spherules" and those of biological membranes in respect of their lipid components. Thus the actions of ionic and non-ionic surfactants reflect their behavior when interacting with natural membranes such as erythrocyte ghosts. In particular, the amphipathic agents lysolecithin or saponin mimic the effect of bacterial hemolysins such as streptolysin S and staphylococcal α-toxin. The polyene antibiotics nystatin, amphotericin B and filipin also disrupt spherules. Stabilization of spherules is achieved with cortisone and cortisol, as in the case of lysosomes. Studies of the mechanism of hemolytic action of filipin by Sessa and Weissmann (1968b) have demonstrated the versatility of spherules, in which composition can be varied at will, in comparison with erythrocyte and other naturally-derived membranes.

A most important instance of phospholipid micelles is the pulmonary lipoprotein surfactant, whose presence is demonstrable *in vitro*. Manktelow (1967) observed severe depletion or absence of pulmonary surfactant in mice treated intravenously with paraquat (1,1′-dimethyl - 4,4′ - dipyridilium dichloride). Characteristic pulmonary congestion, alveolar collapse, dilated alveolar ducts and bronchioles and occasional hyaline membranes were seen, suggesting a similarity to respiratory distress syndrome in human neonates. The irreversible proliferative alveolitis, presumably secondary to loss of surfactant, develops in man after an interval during which most, if not all, of the paraquat is excreted from the body. Despite the close similarity of the effects in animals (Clark, McElligott and Hurst, 1966) to those in man, no suggestion has yet been put forward concerning the primary event in this syndrome. Paraquat itself has apparently no direct effect on pulmonary surfactant.

A further step in the study of what may be termed the "intrinsic" toxic potential of a compound, namely its effect in the absence of hormonal and other metabolic regulation factors of the whole animal, is the use of cell cultures. The advantages and limitations of cell and organ cultures have been set out by Dawson and Dryden (1967), who emphasize the surprising reluctance on the part of investigators to use human material; yet, this would appear to be one of the principal benefits to be gained in the study of toxic action. Not only normal cell lines but also those reflecting metabolic defects of the whole individual are available (Priest, 1968). One of the most striking applications has been the use of lymphoblast transformation as an *in vitro* test in the diagnosis of human sensitization by drugs and other chemicals (Halpern, Ky, Amache, Lagrue and Hazard, 1967). It is also possible to distinguish metabolic blocks, as demonstrated in studies on the mode of toxic action of 2,2-bis (p-chlorophenyl) acetic acid (DDA), the principal urinary metabolite of DDT. Johnson and Weiss (1967) demonstrated that mevalonic acid, but not acetate, completely protects against the cytotoxicity of DDA in cultured KB and HeLa cells, thus suggesting an effect in the pathway of biosynthesis of sterols and ubiquinones.

The fact that human liver cells can be cultured under conditions permitting selective changes in nutrient environment has facilitated the study of cytotoxicity on exposure to vapors of halogenated anesthetics. Whereas differentiated human embryo liver cell cultures degenerated rapidly under chloroform, they showed no effect of halothane (Rees and Zuckerman, 1967). Using Chang cultured human liver cells, Corssen, Sweet and Chenoweth (1966) and Corssen (1968) found that chloroform, halothane and methoxyflurane, at representative clinical concentrations, had only minimal effects as long as the cells were amply supplied with essential nutrients. Nutritional deprivation enhanced hepatotoxicity (Corssen and Sweet, 1967).

Perfused Organs

Among human and animal organs perfused *in vitro,* the most common are liver, kidney, heart, lung, pancreas, small intestine and placenta. For the study of toxic action, these preparations have the advantage of complete control of the conditions of exposure of the individual organ, thus permitting the study of a single chemical and only those metabolites formed by the organ. A further refinement is the use of the regenerating liver for purposes of perfusion (Mutschler and Gordon, 1966) ; in addition to the sensitivity of this preparation to toxic action, the fact that the activity of drug-metabolizing enzymes is at a low ebb may be expected to preserve the test compound in unchanged form. The perfused organ makes it possible to circumvent the difficulty of achieving effective concentrations of inhibitors at metabolic sites, for instance in the liver (Stitzel, Tephly and Mannering, 1968) and thus to study such mechanisms of toxic action *in vivo.*

The perfused rat liver permits the detection of early changes brought about by acute poisons such as phalloidin (Miller and Wieland, 1967) and by relatively mild hyperoxia. Although with a pO_2 of 200 mm Hg the organ appears normal in most respects for some hours, lysosomal changes are detectable by histochemical means and ultrastructurally within 35-40 minutes (Abraham, Dawson, Grasso and Golberg, 1968) . The effect of hypothermia on uptake, biotransformation and excretion of compounds can also be followed (Kalser, Kelvington and Randolph, 1968) · Because drug metabolizing enzyme activity may be varied at will, the modification of toxic effects of a compound on the liver may be studied in relation to its state of metabolism. Such modifications were brought about in the case of a methylhydrazine derivative and monomethylhydrazine itself by Baggiolini and Dewald (1968) , the rats being pretreated with 20-methylcholanthrene or SKF 525-A.

The isolated perfused calf liver provides a unique example of the usefulness of such preparations for study of the hepatotoxicity of anesthetics. The intact animal exposed to halothane becomes anesthetized and dies from respiratory depression before an effect on the liver can be manifested. Middleton, Roth, Smuckler and Nyhus (1966) and Smuckler, Bombeck and Nyhus (1968) perfused calf liver *in vitro* with 3% halothane in the aerating gas. No effect on structure or function was observed; but when the calf had been anesthetized with halothane 1 week before, the perfusion with 3% halothane produced distinctly adverse changes, including decreased oxygen utilization, decreased BSP excretion and increased rate of SGOT release.

Regenerating Liver

After partial hepatectomy the regenerating liver provides an opportunity to study controlled compensatory growth associated with metabolic events whose peaks of activity are arranged according to a strict timetable. The advantages that flow from the use of such a system are illustrated by the findings of Witschi

(1968) regarding the action of parenterally administered beryllium. This toxicant localizes in nuclei of regenerating liver, where it prevents DNA synthesis without influencing the incorporation of precursors into RNA or nuclear protein, without hindering restoration of gross liver mass, nor producing liver necrosis up to the time of sacrifice, 28 hours.

Partial hepatectomy also serves to produce chromosomal injury in irradiated rats, with delay in onset of DNA synthesis and mitosis, as well as abnormalities in cell population kinetics (Fabrikant, 1968). Although damaged chromosomes are no longer seen after a year (Curtis, Tilley and Crowley, 1964), a latent carcinogenic state may be revealed up to 9 months or more after irradiation by administering carbon tetrachloride (Curtis, Czernik and Tilley, 1968), which presumably acts by inducing a wave of mitosis.

Metabolic Effects Expressed in the Whole Animal

The development of enlarged but otherwise apparently normal organs is a frequent observation in the course of toxicity tests in animals (Smyth, Weil, Adams and Hollingsworth, 1952). The liver is the most common of these indicators of metabolic stress and on many occasions is the sole positive finding in toxicity tests (Weil and McCollister, 1963) in several common species of laboratory animal. The increase in relative liver weight (RLW) is attributed to one of three causes: functional enlargement, i.e., physiologic response to an increased workload; toxic enlargement, indicative of pathological effects; and thirdly, an effect mediated through endocrine regulators such as thyroid hormone or glucocorticoids (Golberg, 1966; Barka and Popper, 1967). These mechanisms are not necessarily mutually exclusive. Liver enlargement that begins in response to a stimulus causing a proliferation of smooth endoplasmic reticulum (SER) with increased activity of drug-metabolizing enzymes, may progress, as administration of the test material continues, to a state where hepatotoxicity is manifest. A situation of this sort has recently been described in the case of dieldrin (Hutterer, Schaffner, Klion and Popper, 1968). After attainment of the "new steady state" at 14 days, a stage of decompensation is reached at 52 days, marked by a return of drug-metabolizing enzyme activity to normal (despite the maintenance of a proliferated state of the SER), coincident with commencing impairment of mitochondrial function. This observation of hypertrophic, hypoactive SER may explain the failure to find a no-effect level for increased RLW produced by long-term administration of aldrin and dieldrin, even at 2.5 ppm in rats and 1 ppm in dogs (Hodge, Boyce, Deichmann and Kraybill, 1967).

Instead of demonstrating the transition from physiologic to pathologic liver enlargement on a temporal basis, the changeover can be revealed by a study of the relative threshold doses, given daily over a fixed period, that bring about stimulation of drug-metabolizing enzymes, increase in RLW, fall in glucose 6-phosphatase (as an index of hepatotoxicity) and, finally, frank histopathologic changes (Golberg, Grasso, Feuer and Gilbert, 1967). Penetrating light was thrown on this sequence of effects by measuring the level of test compound present in the liver under these conditions. Whereas the level in the liver remained low and almost constant over the dose range 0.5-50 mg/kg, there was a sharp rise in liver concentration at 75 mg/kg, with considerable animal-to-animal variation within the group, and fatty change made its appearance for the first time (Goldberg, 1967). These findings suggest that, at low doses of some hepatotoxic compounds, the initial physiologic response of SER and RLW succeeds in maintaining a low level of toxicant in the liver; but that, when the liver's capacity in this respect is exceeded, pathologic change is associated with "flooding" of the liver by the compound. The need for measurement of tissue concentrations of toxicants at the site of action, stressed by Brodie, Cosmides and Rall (1965), remains as great as ever.

Returning to the question of liver enlargement, the sequence of hyperplasia and hypertrophy, with increase in degree of polyploidy, seems to be followed in the course of functional enlargement as it is during normal growth of the rat (Schlicht, Koransky, Magour and Schulte-Hermann, 1968; Schulte-Hermann, Thom, Schlicht and Koransky, 1968). Whether toxic enlargement follows this path is uncertain. In the case of increase in RLW brought about by endocrine intervention, the magnitude of the increase is limited and the attribution of an observed effect to this cause is difficult to establish. In fact, the borderline between the functional form of liver enlargement and the endocrine type has become blurred by the observation that phenobarbital and chlordane, both powerful inducers of drug-metabolizing enzymes, produce a striking increase in hepatocellular binding of thyroxine (T_4) (Bernstein, Artz, Hasen and Oppenheimer, 1968). This effect is not a displacement of T_4 from plasma proteins. The increased accumulation of T_4 by the liver results in increased hormonal turnover (Oppenheimer, Bernstein and Surks, 1968). 3,4-Benzpyrene does not affect T_4 binding in the liver. It is not yet clear whether these and possibly other changes in hormonal equilibria are responsible for the mitochondrial actions of phenobarbital, especially its effect on glucuronylating enzymes (Zeidenberg, Orrenius and Ernster, 1967.)

It now appears that there are two general ways in which hepatic drug-metabolizing enzymes (DME) may be induced: preferential synthesis of cytochrome P-450, with quantitative increase in amount of mixed function oxidases, result from the action of phenobarbital and other even more powerful inducers; and synthesis of cytochrome P-446, coupled with development of greater substrate affinity by DME, develops in response to 3-methylcholanthrene (Hildebrandt, Remmer and Estabrook, 1968; Alvares, Schilling and Kuntzman, 1968).

Two types of functional liver response may hence be distinguished. The first, elicited by the powerful stimulators of drug-metabolizing enzymes (DME), involves a large increase in RLW, the appearance of increased numbers of profiles of SER, increased activity in a wide range of DME and increased hepatocellular binding of T_4 which may perhaps be localized on the SER and act as the mediator to increase protein synthesis. The second type of liver response, brought about by polycyclic aromatic hydrocarbons or lipid-soluble azo dyes as 3′-methyl-4-dimethylaminoazobenzene (Arcasoy, Smuckler and Benditt, 1968) involves a small increase in RLW, in some instances a loss of RNA and liver protein, an increase in SER but a decrease of some DME with interruption of microsomal electron transport, associated with a reduced content of cytochrome P-450 and an enhanced activity in a distinct range of DME. Here, there is no increased hepatocellular binding of T_4. Moreover, at sufficient exposures mitochondrial changes are seen, indicating toxic action, possibly as a prelude to carcinogenesis. In other cases, toxins and carcinogens not only reduce the activity of liver DME and the concentration of cytochrome P-450 but also block phenobarbital stimulation of liver enlargement (Sunderman, 1968).

The drug clofibrate (ethyl p-chlorophenoxyisobutyrate, CPIB) offers a practical illustration of the difficulty experienced in drawing conclusions regarding hepatotoxicity. Clofibrate causes an increase in RLW in mice, hamsters, rats, dogs, and monkeys (Best and Duncan, 1964; Azarnoff, Tucker and Barr, 1965; Gould, Swyryd, Coan and Avoy, 1966; Platt and Thorp, 1966). In the monkey, a rise in SGOT was noted (Thorp, 1962, 1963b) and was considered to reflect an increased concentration of the enzyme in liver cells. The enlarged livers of rats fed CPIB accumulate ubiquinone (Lakshmanan, Phillips and Brien, 1968) and have higher levels of pyridine nucleotides but lower tryptophan pyrrolase activity (Platt and Cockrill, 1966). The pattern of changes in the activities of rat liver oxidoreductases suggested that the increase in RLW was functional in type (Platt and Cockrill, 1967). Although Thorp (1962, 1963b) reported that the microscopic appearance of the liver was normal, striking hepatic ultrastructural changes have been described in rats and mice (Paget, 1963; Hess, Staubli and Riess, 1965; Svoboda and Azarnoff, 1966). The most notable effect was the tenfold increase in microbodies, but proliferation of SER and mitochondrial changes were also present. Two weeks after withdrawal of the drug, the RLW returned to normal but the microbodies and mitochondrial changes persisted. After 2 years' administration of CPIB, the RLW in some experimental groups was the same as in controls (Platt and Thorp, 1966) but no statement on ultrastructural changes has been made.

Thorp (1962, 1963a) postulated that clofibrate acts like 2,4-dichlorophenoxyacetic acid (2,4-D) in displacing thyroxine (T_4) from its plasma binding sites into the liver (Florsheim, Velcoff and Williams, 1963). There is no record whether 2,4-D causes proliferation of SER or increase in RLW; increased availability of hepatocellular SER-binding sites for T_4 would serve to explain why T_4 is displaced into the liver and not into other organs. Florsheim *et al.* (1963) sought evidence for increased hepatic binding but their results were inconclusive. Platt and Thorp (1966) attributed the changes in liver weight, as well as protein and glycogen contents, to a hyperthyroid effect on the liver due to displacement of T_4 from the plasma. However, Osorio, Walton, Browne, West and Whystock (1965) found that clofibrate enhances liver retention of T_4 by a primary effect on the liver. Westerfield, Richert and Ruegamer (1968) studied the prolonged elevation of mitochondrial α-glycerophosphate dehydrogenase in liver and kidney and concluded that simple displacement of T_4 from plasma was an inadequate explanation; nor could it account for the large increases in RLW.

In man, this mechanism fails to explain the clofibrate effect on catecholamine-induced metabolic changes (Hunninghake and Azarnoff, 1968). Subjects given CPIB had *lowered* hepatic T_4 distribution space and hepatic T_4 content (Musa, Ogilvie and Dowling, 1968). A recent report of human experience with the compound describes reversible elevations of serum transaminases which, in the context of hepatic and muscular tenderness as well as abnormally high serum creatine phosphokinase, suggests a primary acute muscular syndrome (Langer and Levy, 1968).

Interpretation of the increase in RLW brought about by halothane, 2-bromo-2-chloro-1,1,1-trifluoroethane (Kunz, Schaude, Schmid and Siess, 1966; Kunz, Schaude, Schimassek, Schmid and Siess, 1966) presents a related problem. According to Van Dyke and Chenoweth (1965) the formation of trifluoroethanol glucuronide and trifluoroacetate in man and animals is the consequence of the action of microsomal enzymes requiring NADPH, and pretreatment with phenobarbital greatly increases the degree of biotransformation. Fluroxene, 2,2,2-trifluoroethyl vinyl ether, is metabolized to the same products in the mouse and dog; again pretreatment with phenobarbital or polycyclic hydrocarbons stimulates metabolism while actinomycin D blocks it (Blake, Rozman, Cascorbi and Krantz, 1967). According to Stier (1968), trifluoroacetate is the main metabolite of halothane and is responsible both for the increase in RLW and the distinct alterations in enzyme pattern. The results of Schimassek, Kunz and Gallwitz (1966), like those of Smuckler *et al.* (1968) referred to earlier, point to predominant mitochondrial involvement. The most striking change is the enhanced activity of α-glycerophosphate dehydrogenase, suggesting a thyroidal effect, as in the case of CPIB above. Authors have stressed how much less acutely toxic trifluoroacetate is than monofluoroacetate; but it may be that trifluoroacetate acts like 2,4-D in some respects, and that the effects of halothane *in vitro* on mitochondrial electron transport mechanisms and respiratory control (Cohen and Marshall, 1968) are only a part of the hepatic changes occurring in the intact animal.

Envoi

An attempt has been made to avoid compiling yet another catalog of toxic actions, starting with inorganic poisons, progressing to metal-organic compounds and finally traversing from abietic acid all the weary way to zoalene. Safety evaluation necessitates exploration of the modes of action of compounds by every approach that will yield relevant information. The road to complete understanding is usually long and arduous but there is no alternative if health and well-being are to be safeguarded and the integrity of man's environment preserved.

BIBLIOGRAPHY

ABRAHAM, R., DAWSON, W., GRASSO, P., and GOLBERG, L.: Lysosomal changes associated with hyperoxia in the isolated perfused rat liver. Exper. Molec. Pathol, *8*:370-387, 1968.

ALVARES, A. P., SCHILLING, G. R., and KUNTZMAN,

R.: Differences in the kinetics of benzpyrene hydroxylation by hepatic drug-metabolizing enzymes from phenobarbital and 3-methylcholanthrene-treated rats. Biochem. Biophys. Res. Commun., *30*:588-593, 1968.

Arcasoy, M., Smuckler, E. A., and Benditt, E. P.: Acute effects of 3′-methyl-4-dimethylaminoazobenzene intoxication on rat liver. Amer. J. Pathol., *52*:841-867, 1968.

Azarnoff, D. L., Tucker, D. R., and Barr, G. A.: Studies with ethyl chlorophenoxyisobutyrate (clofibrate). Metabolism, *14*:959-965, 1965.

Baggiolini, M., and Dewald, B.: Stoffwechsel von Pharmaka in der isoliert perfundierten Rattenleber. Untersuchungen über das Methylhydrazinderivat, Ibenzmethyzin. *In,* "Stoffwechsel der isoliert perfundierten Leber," Ed. W. Staib and R. Scholz. Springer-Verlag, Berlin, 1968 pp. 200-207.

Barka, T., and Popper, H.: Liver enlargement and drug toxicity. Medicine, *46*:103-117, 1967.

Barnes, J. M.: Poisons that hit and run. New Scientist, *38*:619-620, 1968.

Barnes, J. M., and Paget, G. E.: Mechanisms of toxic action. Progress in Med. Chem., *4*:18-38, 1965.

Barry, E. J., Ovechka, C. A., and Gutmann, H. R.: Interaction of aromatic amines with rat liver proteins *in vivo* II. Binding of N-2-fluorenylacetamide-9-^{14}C to nuclear proteins. J. Biol. Chem,. *243*:51-60, 1968.

Bernstein, G., Artz, S. A., Hasen, J., and Oppenheimer, J. H.: Hepatic accumulation of ^{125}I-thyroxine in the rat: augmentation by phenobarbital and chlordane. Endocrinology, *82*:406-409, 1968.

Best, M. M., and Duncan, C. H.: Hypolipemia and hepatomegaly from ethyl chlorophenoxyisobutyrate (CPIB) in rat. J. Lab. Clin. Med., *64*:634-642, 1964.

Blake, D. A., Rozman, R. S., Cascorbi, H. F., and Krantz, J. C. Jr.: Anesthesia LXXIV: Biotransformation of fluroxene — I. Metabolism in mice and dogs *in vivo*. Biochem. Pharmacol., *16*:1237-1248, 1967.

Brodie, B. B., Cosmides, G. J., and Rall, D. P.: Toxicology and the biomedical sciences. Science, *148*:1547-1554, 1965.

Clark, D.G.,McElligott, T. F., and Hurst, E.W.: The toxicity of paraquat. Brit. J. Indust. Med., *23*:126-132, 1966.

Clifford, J. I., and Rees, K. R.: The action of aflatoxin B_1 on the rat liver. Biochem. J., *102*:65-75, 1967.

Clifford, J. I., Rees, K. R., and Stevens, M. E. M.: The effect of aflatoxins B_1, G_1 and G_2 on protein and nucleic acid synthesis in rat liver. Biochem. J., *103*:258-261, 1967.

Cohen, P. J., and Marshall, B. E.: Effects of halothane on respiratory control and oxygen consumption of rat liver mitochondria. *In Toxicity of Anesthetics,* Ed. B. R. Fink. The Williams & Wilkins Co., Baltimore, 1968, pp. 24-34.

Corssen, G.: Cytotoxic Effects of halogenated anesthetics. *In, Toxicity of Anesthetics,* Ed. B. R. Fink. The Williams & Wilkins Co., Baltimore, 1968, pp. 50-58.

Corssen, G., and Sweet, R B.: Effects of halogenated anesthetic agents on selectively starved cultured human liver cells. Anesth. Analgesia, *46*:575-588, 1967.

Corssen, G., Sweet, R. B., and Chenoweth, M. B.: Effects of chloroform, halothane and methoxyflurane on human liver cells in vitro. Anesthesiology, *27*:155-162, 1966.

Curtis, H. J., Czernik, Carol, and Tilley, John: Tumor induction as a measure of genetic damage and repair in somatic cells of mice. Radiation Res., *34*:315-319, 1968.

Curtis, H. J., Tilley, J., and Crowley, C.: Elimination of chromosome aberrations in liver cells by cell division. Radiation Res., *22*:730-734, 1964.

Dawson, M., and Dryden, W. F.: Tissue culture in the study of the effects of drugs. J. Pharm. Sci., *56*:545-561, 1967.

Fabrikant, J. I.: Radiation effects on a conditional cell renewal system under continuous low doserate exposure. Amer. J. Roentgenol., *102*:811-821, 1968.

Farber, E.: Biochemistry of carcinogenesis. Cancer Res., *28*:1859-1869, 1968.

Florsheim, W. H., Velcoff, S. M., and Williams, A. D.: Some effects of 2,4-dichlorophenoxyacetic acid on thyroid function in the rat: effects on peripheral thyroxine. Endocrinology, *72*:327-333, 1963.

Floyd, L. R., Unuma, T., and Busch, H.: Effects of aflatoxin B_1 and other carcinogens upon nucleolar RNA of various tissues in the rat. Exper. Cell. Res., *51*:423-438, 1968.

Golberg, L.: Liver enlargement produced by drugs: its significance. Proc. Eur. Soc. Study Drug Toxicity, *7*:171-184, 1966.

Golberg, L.: The amelioration of food. The Milroy Lectures. J. Roy. Coll. Phycns. Lond., *1*:385-426, 1967.

Golberg, L., Grasso, P., Feuer, G., and Gilbert, D.: Activities of microsomal enzymes in relation to liver enlargement. Biochem. J., *103*:12P, 1967.

Gould, R. G., Swyryd, E. A., Coan, B. J., and Avoy, D. R.: Effects of chlorophenoxyisobutyrate (CPIB) on liver composition and triglyceride synthesis in rats. J. Atheroscler. Res, *6*:555-564, 1966.

Halpern, B., Ky, N T., Amache, N., Lagrue, G., and Hazard, J.: Diagnostic de l'allergie medicamenteuse "in vitro" par l'utilisation du test de transformation lymphoblastique (T.T.L.). Presse médicale, *75*:461-465, 1967.

Hess, R., Stäubli, W., and Riess, W.: Nature of the hepatomegalic effect produced by ethyl-chlorophenoxyisobutyrate in the rat Nature, *208*:856-858, 1965.

Hildebrandt, A., Remmer, H., and Estabrook, R. W.: Cytochrome P-450 of liver microsomes — one pigment or many. Biochem. Biophys. Res. Commun., *30*:607-612, 1968.

Hodge, H. C., Boyce, A. M., Deichmann, W. B., and Kraybill, H. F.: Toxicology and no-effect levels of aldrin and dieldrin. Toxicol Applied Pharmacol., *10*:613-675, 1967.

Hunninghake, D. B., and Azarnoff, D. L.: Clofibrate effect on catecholamine-induced metabolic changes in humans. Metabolism, *17*:588-595, 1968.

Hutterer, F., Schaffner, F., Klion, F. M., and Popper, H.: Hypertrophic, hypoactive smooth endoplasmic reticulum: a sensitive indicator of hepatotoxicity exemplified by dieldrin. Science, *161*:1017-1019, 1968.

Johnson, W. J., and Weiss, S. A.: Cytotoxicity of dichlorophenylacetic acid (DDA) upon cultured KB and HeLa cells, and its reversal by mevalonic acid. Proc Soc. Exp. Biol. Med., *124*:1005-1008, 1967.

Kalser, S. C., Kelvington, E. J., and Randolph, M. M.: Drug metabolism in hypothermia. Uptake, metabolism and excretion of S^{35}-sulfanilamide by the isolated, perfused rat liver. J. Pharmacol. Exp. Therap., *159*:389-398, 1968.

Kunz, W., Schaude, G, Schimassek, H., Schmid, W., and Siess, M.: Stimulation of liver growth by drugs II. Biochemical analysis. Proc. Eur. Soc. Study Drug Tox., *7*:138-153, 1966.

Kunz, W., Schaude, G., Schmid, W., and Siess, M.: Stimulation of liver growth by drugs I. Morphological analysis. Proc. Eur. Soc. Study Drug Tox., *7*:113-137, 1966.

Lakshmanan, M. R., Phillips, W. E. J., and Brien, R. L.: Effect of p-chlorophenoxyisobutyrate (CPIB) fed to rats on hepatic biosynthesis and catabolism of ubiquinone. J. Lipid Res., *9*:353-356, 1968.

Langer, T., and Levy, R. I.: Acute muscular syndrome associated with administration of clofibrate. New Engl. J. Med., *279*:856-858, 1968.

Magee, P. N., and Barnes, J. M.: Carcinogenic nitroso compounds. Adv. Cancer Res., *10*:163-246, 1967.

Manktelow, B. W.: The loss of pulmonary surfactant in paraquat poisoning: a model for the study of the respiratory distress syndrome. Brit. J. Exp. Path., *48*:366-369, 1967.

Mattocks, A. R.: Toxicity of pyrrolizidine alkaloids. Nature, *217*:723-728, 1968.

Middleton, M. D., Roth, G. J., Smuckler, E. A., and Nyhus, L. M.: The effect of high concentration of halothane on the isolated perfused bovine liver. Surg. Gynec Obstet., *122*:817-825, 1966.

Miller, F., and Wieland, O.: Elektronenmikroskopische Untersuchungen der Leber von Maus und Ratte bei akuter Phalloidin-Vergiftung. Virchows Arch. path. Anat., *343*:83-99, 1967.

Moulé, Y., and Fraysinnet, C.: Effect of aflatoxin on transcription in liver cell. Nature, *218*:93-95, 1968.

Musa, B. U., Ogilvie, J. T., and Dowling, J. T.: Effects of ethyl chlorophenoxyisobutyrate on thyroxine distribution, transport and metabolism in man. Metabolism, *17*:909-915, 1968.

Mutschler, L. E., and Gordon, A. H.: Plasma protein synthesis by the isolated perfused regenerating rat liver. Biochim. Biophys. Acta, *130*:486-492, 1966.

Nievel, J. G., and Golberg, L.: Primary effects on liver microsomal protein synthesis of compounds producing hepatomegaly. Fourth Mtg. Fed. Europ. Biochem. Soc., Oslo. Abstr. No. 196: 49, 1967.

Nievel, J. G., and Golberg, L.: Effect of coumarin and other compounds on ribosomal protein synthesis in the rat liver. Nature, *219*:858-860, 1968.

Oppenheimer, J. H., Bernstein, G., and Surks, M. I.: Increased thyroxine turnover and thyroidal function after stimulation of hepatocellular binding of thyroxine by phenobarbital. J. Clin. Invest., *47*:1399-1406, 1968.

Osorio, C., Walton, K. W., Browne, C. H. W., West, D., and Whystock, P.: The effect of chlorophenoxyisobutyrate ('Atromid-S') on the biliary excretion and distribution of thyroxine in the rat. Biochem. Pharmacol., *14*:1479-1481, 1965.

Paget, G. E.: Experimental studies of the toxicity of Atromid with particular reference to fine structural changes in the livers of rodents. J. Atherosclerosis Res., *3*:729-736, 1963.

Paul, J. S., Reynolds, R. C., and Montgomery, P. O'B. Jr.: Inhibition of DNA-dependent RNA polymerase by 4-nitroquinoline-N-oxide in isolated nuclei. Nature, *215*:749-750, 1967.

Platt, D. S., and Cockrill, B. L.: Changes in the liver concentrations of the nicotinamide adenine dinucleotide coenzymes and in the activities of oxidoreductase enzymes following treatment of the rat with ethyl chlorophenosyisobutyrate (Atromid-S). Biochem. Pharmacol., *15*:927-935, 1966.

Platt, D. S., and Cockrill, B. L.: Liver enlargement and hepatotoxicity: an investigation into the effects of several agents on rat liver enzyme activities. Biochem. Pharmacol., *16*:2257-2270, 1967.

PLATT, D. S., and THORP, J. M.: Changes in the weight and composition of the liver in the rat, dog and monkey treated with ethyl chlorophenoxyisobutyrate. Biochem. Pharmacol., *15*:915-925, 1966.

PRIEST, J. H.: Human cell culture: an important tool for the diagnosis and understanding of disease. J. Pediat., *72*:415-423, 1968.

REES, K. R., and VARCOE, J. S.: The interaction of tritiated p-dimethylaminoazobenzene with rat liver nuclear proteins. Brit. J. Cancer, *21*:174-177, 1967.

REES, K. R., and ZUCKERMAN, A. J.: Lack of toxicity of halothane on differentiated liver cell cultures. Brit. J. Anaesth., *39*:857-860, 1967.

SESSA, G., and WEISSMANN, G.: Effects of four components of the polyene antibiotic, filipin, on phospholipid spherules (liposomes) and erythrocytes. J. Biol. Chem., *243*:4364-4371, 1968b.

SESSA, G., and WEISSMANN, G.: Phospholipid spherules (liposomes) as a model for biological membranes. J. Lipid Res., *9*:310-318, 1968a.

SCHIMASSEK, H., KUNZ, W., and GALLWITZ, D.: Differentiation of liver metabolism on the molecular level during chronic application of halothane. Biochem. Pharmacol., *15*:1957-1964, 1966.

SCHLICHT, I., KORANSKY, W., MAGOUR, S., and SCHULTE-HERMANN, R.: Grösse und DNS-Synthese der Leber unter dem Einfluss körperfremder Stoffe. Arch. Pharmak, exp. Path., *261*:26-41, 1968.

SCHULTE-HERMANN, R., THOM, R., SCHLICHT, I., and KORANSKY, W.: Zahl und Ploidiegrad der Zellkerne der Leber unter dem Einfluss körperfremder Stoffe. Arch. Pharmak. exp. Path., *261*:42-58, 1968.

SMUCKLER, E. A., and BENDITT, E. P.: Carbon tetrachloride poisoning in rats: alteration in the ribosomes of the liver. Science, *140*:308-310, 1963.

SMUCKLER, E. A., and BENDITT, E. P.: Studies in carbon tetrachloride intoxication. III. A subcellular defect in protein synthesis. Biochemistry, *4*:671-679, 1965.

SMUCKLER, E. A., BOMBECK, C. T., and NYHUS, L. M.: Structural and functional changes in the isolated perfused liver associated with halothane and chloroform. *In, Toxicity of Anesthetics,* Ed. B. R. Fink. The Williams & Wilkins Co., Baltimore, 1968, pp. 176-185.

SMUCKLER, E. A., PARTHIER, B., and HULTIN, T.: The effects of polyuridylic acid on phenylalanine incorporation by subcellular fractions from carbon tetrachloride-poisoned rat liver. Biochem. J., *107*:151-163, 1968.

SMYTH, H. F. JR., WEIL, C. S., ADAMS, E. M., and HOLLINGSWORTH, R. L.: Efficiency of criteria of stress in toxicological tests. Arch. Indust. Hyg. Occup. Med., *6*:32-36, 1952.

STIER, A.: The biotransformation of halothane. Anesthesiology, *29*:388-390, 1968.

STITZEL, R. E., TEPHLY, T. R., and MANNERING, G. J.: Inhibition of drug metabolism VI. Inhibition of hexobarbital metabolism in the isolated perfused liver of the rat. Molec. Pharmacol., *4*:15-19, 1968.

SUNDERMAN, F. W. JR.: Nickel carbonyl inhibition of phenobarbital induction of hepatic cytochrome P-450. Cancer Res., *28*:465-470, 1968.

SVOBODA, D. J., and AZARNOFF, D. L.: Response of hepatic microbodies to a hypolipidemic agent, ethyl chlorophenoxyisobutyrate (CPIB). J. Cell Biol., *30*:442-450, 1966.

SVOBODA, D., and HIGGINSON, J.: A comparison of ultrastructural changes in rat liver due to chemical carcinogens. Cancer Res., *28*:1703-1733, 1968.

SVOBODA, D., RACELA, A., and HIGGINSON, J.: Variations in ultrastructural changes in hepatocarcinogenesis. Biochem. Pharmacol., *16*:651-657, 1967.

THORP, J. M.: An experimental approach to the problem of disordered lipid metabolism. J. Atheroscler. Res., *3*:351-360, 1963a.

THORP, J. M.: Biochemical aspects of toxicology of Atromid. J. Atheroscler. Res., *3*:737-739, 1963b.

THORP, J. M.: Experimental evaluation of orally active combination of androsterone with ethyl chlorophenoxy*iso*butyrate. Lancet, *i*:1323-1326, 1962.

VAN DYKE, R. A., and CHENOWETH, M. B.: Metabolism of volatile anesthetics. Anesthesiology, *26*:348-357, 1965.

VILLA-TREVINO, S.: A possible mechanism of inhibition of protein synthesis by dimethylnitrosamine. Biochem. J., *105*:625-631, 1967.

VILLA-TREVINO, S., and LEAVER, D. D.: Effects of the hepatotoxic agents retrorsine and aflatoxin B_1 on hepatic protein synthesis in the rat. Biochem. J., *109*:87-91, 1968.

WEIL, C. S., and MCCOLLISTER, D. D.: Safety Evaluation of Chemicals. Relationship between short- and long-term feeding studies in designing an effective toxicity test. J. Agr. Food Chem., *11*:486-491, 1963.

WESTERFELD, W. W., RICHERT, D. A., and RUEGAMER, W. R.: The role of the thyroid hormone in the effect of p-chlorophenosyisobutyrate in rats. Biochem. Pharmacol., *17*:1003-1016, 1968.

WITSCHI, H.: Inhibition of deoxyribonucleic acid synthesis in regenerating rat liver by beryllium. Lab. Invest., *19*:67-70, 1968.

ZEIDENBERG, P., ORRENIUS, S., and ERNSTER, L.: Increase in levels of glucuronylating enzymes and associated rise in activities of mitochondrial oxidative enzymes upon phenobarbital administration in the rat. J. Cell Biol., *32*:528-531, 1967.

Chapter 2A

Selective Toxicity-Genetic Implications

M. S. LEGATOR, Ph.D., and F. SPERLING, Ph.D.

INTRODUCTION

Numerous definitions of toxicity are available, each developed from specific points of view. This is particularly true in the Federal statutes regulating consumer-oriented products where each definition has been prepared to handle a specific type of commodity.[8, 9, 10]

The companion terms "adverse effect" and "side effect" are frequently used in self-contradictory ways with vague and elastic meanings. Consequently, it is important that a reasonable but rigorous definition be established in order to discuss the various aspects of the problem.

Toxicity is an undesirable pharmacological action. This definition has many implications, for pharmacological actions are considered to vary with dose. It implies that the response to a single molecule would be expected to differ from the response to a million molecules; that, therefore, there would be a continuum of effects from zero to maximum; that the beneficial compound of today may become the harmful compound of tomorrow; that the evaluation of effect be on a single system; and that the pharmacological effect on each system be independently evaluated. By this definition, "selectivity toxicity" is a redundancy, for the definition implies selective effect, involving selective action on specific targets. The action may be specific within an individual, within a population or within a species.

The pharmacological action of any substance may be considered to represent an interference with some homeostatic mechanism and when such interference is undesirable, the action is toxic. Inhibition of coagulation by the dicoumarols and the indandiones or central nervous system depression by the barbiturates results from an interference of some metabolic mechanism. In each instance, a predetermined degree of effect is a therapeutic goal; effects of greater degree are considered toxic. The rodenticidal action of the dicoumarols and the indandiones differs from their therapeutic action only in degree. The target is the same.

The effect on the specific target may be considered to represent selective action. Atropine administered to quiet the gut may also cause cycloplegia and dry mouth. The latter two effects represent the same target as that of the gut, i.e., blockage of cholinergic activity, even though these "side effects" are not intended. However, blood dyscrasias induced by the antiepileptic hydantoins involve target systems other than the one intended and the toxicity of the hydantoins differs *qualitatively* from that of atropine, barbiturates, or anticoagulants. Toxic action — undesirable action — may thus involve degree of effect on a specific target, multiple responses of a diffuse target, or multiple responses of multiple targets.

The ideal drug, according to Goldstein, has a perfectly selective biological action; it has no side effect and no toxicity. There is no such drug.[13] To cite examples of the attempts to develop the ideal "selective drug," by 1964 over 10,000 sulfonamides, 25,000 anti-malarials, 30,000 antitubercular compounds, and over 125,000 anti-neoplastic agents had been evaluated.[2] Similar figures could no doubt be cited in other areas, such as in the development of selective weed killers, fungicides, and pesticides. No drug was found which had only the single selective effect. The contrasting themes of unity and diversity in biological systems are the opposing factors in our attempt to develop a greater degree of selectivity. To achieve a greater degree of selectrivity, we frequently capitalize on the diversity of biological phenomena and minimize the similarities.

It is almost a certainty that among our various drugs, food additives, pesticides, and herbicides, there are compounds with toxic properties which have not yet been identified. The type of toxicity that is most difficult to measure, that does not have a readily apparent cause and effect relationship in man, is in the areas of teratogenicity, carcinogenicity, and mutagenicity. It is in this sphere of genetic effects that we should look for unsuspected toxicity in compounds presently regarded as safe and in current use. After a brief examination of some of the more common mechanisms of selective toxic agents, a few examples will be presented of commercial compounds whose potential genetic effects may have been overlooked.

Mechanism of Action

The mechanisms that can be exploited to develop certain selectivity among various agents are numerous and well defined. The following is a list of some of the obvious ones:

1. *Rate of absorption or penetration.* Waxy insect cuticle and waxy coat of *Mycobacterium tuberculosis* permit penetration of drugs with lipophilic properties.
2. *Distribution.* Carbon tetrachloride localizes to a great extent in the liver.
3. *Qualitative differences in metabolic processes.* Penicillin blocks cross-linking polymerization that yields complete cell wall mucopolypeptide in sensitive bacteria. Sulfonamides are not acetylated by dogs as they are in humans.
4. *Excretion.* The elimination rate of phenobarbital varies among the species.

Phylogenetic differences with respect to drug metabolism are numerous. Fish have no oxidative drug-metabolizing enzymes, nor can they form glucuronides or sulfuric acid esters. Amphibia are also unable to oxidize foreign compounds but can form glucuronides and sulfuric acid esters. Reptiles, birds, and mammals have oxidative drug-metabolizing enzymes and can form glucuronides and sulfates; they also have the necessary enzymatic mechanisms for increasing the polarity of lipoid-soluble compounds and thus can rapidly excrete them. Insects can also increase the polarity of lipoid-soluble compounds, but the enzymes are different in many ways from those of the vertebrates.[24] The number of qualitative metabolic differences that have been exploited in our attempt to eliminate an uneconomic species from among economic species are comparatively few, although many opportunities exist.

Selected Examples in Chemotherapy

One of the oldest divisions of selective toxicity, and probably the most productive in terms of benefit to mankind, is the field of chemotherapy. The following are representative examples:

1. The development of the sulfonamides is a classic example of the utilization of a metabolite analog to selectively act on one organism in the presence of another. The selectivity of the antibacterial sulfonamides depends on the essential requirements of many microorganisms for p-aminobenzoic acid which is needed for the synthesis of folic acid. The substitution of sulfonamide prevents this necessary synthesis. Mammals and resistant organisms do not synthesize folic acid but absorb it from the diet. Therefore, the action is selective.[1]
2. An elegant but still not fully understood mechanism of selective toxicity is illustrated by streptomycin. Evidence has now been accumulated to show that ribosomes from streptomycin-sensitive cells bind to the drug in such a manner that the specific codon-anticodon interaction is distorted. Thus the wrong tRNA is permitted at a fairly high frequency with resulting faulty protein synthesis. The new protein is not compatible with the survival of the cell. The 30S ribosome subunit seems to carry the resistance or sensitivity to streptomycin.[12]
3. The inhibition of leukemia in man by L-asparaginase is an example of the use of selective toxicity in the field of cancer chemotherapy. The cells of tumors that respond to L-asparaginase all require L-asparagine. Insensitive tumors and normal cells are independent of an external source of this amino acid. L-asparaginase thus has a unique property as a chemotherapeutic agent; its effect depends on a specific metabolic defect of certain malignant cells.[17]

Genetic Damage

The examples of selectively toxic agents capitalizing on biological diversities are numerous. In the vast majority of cases the proposed mechanism of selectivity was advanced after the agent had been discovered by empirical testing and had been on the market for several years. In evaluating the safety of these agents, there has been difficulty in developing meaningful tests for measuring their potential for genetic damage. It is also precisely in this area that the greatest amount of unity exists in biological systems. The level of replication, transcription and translation represents the common denominator of all living matter. The term genetic damage is used here in its broadest sense and involves any modification or alteration of DNA. The consequence of genetic damage includes the following:

Target
Immature, embryonic cell
Mature cells
Germinal cells

Effect
Teratogenic
Neoplasm induction (somatic mutation)
Mutagenic (succeeding generation)

Our assessment of substances for their carcinogenic potential is time-consuming and because of little feed-back from human experience, difficult to evaluate. Screening for teratogenic effects is dependent on four events occurring in a testing protocol: administration of (1) a specific substance, (2) at a particular dose, (3) to a genetically susceptible animal, and (4) when embryos are in a susceptible stage of development.[18] Screening for teratogenic effects depends so critically upon giving the correct dose to the right type of animal at the right stage of pregnancy that all negative results must be viewed with caution. In the third area, that of characterizing mutagenic agents by the genetic damage produced, no really extensive approach has yet been made. The area of mutation research is important not only to our contemporary generation, but also to the generations yet to come. Although the magnitude of the problem in terms of incidence of effective mutagens in the total environment is unknown, the consequences of incorrect decisions are so far-reaching that high priority must be given to the development of methods and the use of current methods for identifying those compounds which might cause mutation in man.

Examples of Overlooked Genetic Toxicity

Can any examples of agents be cited which are currently on the market that were considered highly selective agents at the time of their initial introduction, but whose selective action must be questioned in the light of new knowledge? A single investigator has provided us with two possible examples. Epstein has determined the carcinogenic properties of the herbicide, maleic hydrazide, and of a commonly used fungicide, griseofulvin.[5, 6]

Maleic hydrazide (1,2-dihydro-3,6-pyridazinedione) was introduced in 1949, and its growth-inhibiting properties on plants and its delaying action on blossoming were described.[3] Its commercial uses now include inhibition of sprouting in vegetables and stored root crops, prevention of sucker production in tobacco plants, and growth control of grasses and foliage.[20] Maleic hydrazide is claimed to be selectively toxic to plants, but not to bacteria, fungi, rodents, or dogs.[6] Its selective toxicity was attributed to a difference in permeability. It has been shown to be mutagenic in drosophila and bacteria, and to produce cytotoxicity, mitotic inhibition, and unbalanced growth in cultured mammalian cells.[6] Shortly after its introduction, the finding that maleic hydrazide induced breakage of chromosomes in *Vicia faba* prompted this warning: "Since nearly all chromosome-breaking agents have so far proved to be cancer-producing as well, we must hope that the agricultural use of this new agent will not be encouraged before suitable tests are made."[4]

In a recent investigation, this compound was found to produce a high incidence of remote tumors and hepatomas after subcutaneous injection in infant mice. An incidence of 73% hepatomas as compared to 8% in controls was reported.[6]

Griseofulvin (7-chloro-2′,4,6-trimethoxy-6′-methylspiro [benzofuran-2(3H)-1′-[2]cyclohexene]-3,4′-dione) is a potent antibiotic that is commonly used by prolonged oral administration to treat a variety of dermatomycosis. It has also been suggested for use as an insecticide. The selective action of this fungicide was attributed to its complexing to nucleic acid and protein of sensitive fungi. In insects, this fungicide inhibits cuticle formation and morphogenesis. In cultured mammalian cells, this compound produces metaphase delay. Epsein reported that after subcutaneous injection into infant mice a high incidence of hepatomas occurred (44% in male mice at 49 weeks as compared to 8% in controls) .[5]

Captan (N-trichloromethylthio-4-cyclohexene-1,2-dicarboximide) is one of the most widely used agricultural fungicides both in this country and abroad. It has been on the market for well over ten years and is supposedly one of the "safest" known agricultural products. The oral LD_{50} of this compound is 9-15 g/kg in laboratory animals. Its chronic effects are not competely understood. There is some evidence that it breaks down to thiophosgene which in turn reacts with cysteine in sensitive fungi.[16] Recent studies with this fungicide indicate that it prevents mitosis, breaks chromosomes in cultured mammalian cells, is mutagenic in bacteria, increases breaks in both miotic and germinal cells in rats, and is highly teratogenic to the chick embryo.[15,19] Further studies are required to resolve the implications of these recent findings.

Thalidomide is a prime example of a drug that was claimed, because of superficial investigation, to be among the safest compounds to be marketed. The detrimental effect of the drug on the fetus during early pregnancy was not even considered when the drug was introduced overseas after clinical trials. The teratogenic effect of this agent might never have been discovered if it caused a common form of congenital malformation rather than phocomelia. This compound, which was so free of major toxic effects that a lethal oral dose could not be approached, has altered our entire screening protocol.

Conclusion

The factors of absorption, distribution, metabolic transformation, and excretion apply to genetic toxicity as well as to nongenetic toxicity. There are striking differences, however, between genetic and nongenetic damage. The long latent period in carcinogenic and mutagenic response is one outstanding difference. In order for a compound to manifest its mutagenic activity, several generations will have to be followed. In terms of carcinogenicity, several decades is not an unreasonable figure. This long latent period does not diminish the importance of this type of damage, but merely underlines our inability to define a direct cause and effect relationship. Thus, the mere fact that a compound has been used for years with apparent impunity cannot be taken as evidence of its freedom from genetic effects.

Additional method development in this area is obviously required. The nature of response to genetic damage means that we may be forced to extrapolate to a greater extent, at least initially, from simple test and animal data than in most other areas of toxicity studies. Fortunately, newer techniques such as cytogenetic evaluation, dominant lethal studies,[7] and the host-mediated assays[11] offer promise of characterizing even the most difficult area of genetic damage, mutagenic effects. The development of new methods and our recognition of the importance of this area should provide us with chemicals in the future that have been adequately tested and that have minimal genetic toxicity. The concern for commonly used compounds that are already on the market will constitute a serious problem in terms of identification.

It is important to realize that toxicity consists only of those manifestations which are capable of being recognized today. A new era is probably being approached where all forms of genetic damage will be taken into account before concluding that an agent is "selectively" toxic.

REFERENCES

1. Albert, A.: *Selective Toxicity.* John Wiley & Sons, New York, 1965, pp. 147-152.
2. Burger, A.: Approaches to drug discovery. New Eng. J. Med., *270*:1098-1101, 1964.
3. Crafts, A. S.: *The Chemistry and Mode of Action of Herbicides.* Interscience, New York, 1961, pp. 188-192.
4. Darlington, C. D., and McLeish, J.: Action of maleic hydrazide on the cell. Nature, *167*:407-408, 1951.
5. Epstein, S. S., Andrea, J., Joshi, S., and Mantel, N.: Hepatocarcinogenicity of griseofulvin following parenteral administration to infant mice. Cancer Res., *27*:1900-1906, 1967.
6. Epstein, S. S., and Mantel, N.: Hepatocarcinogenicity of the herbicide maleic hydrazide following parenteral administration to infant Swiss mice. Intern. J. Cancer, *3*:325-335, 1968.
7. Epstein, S. S., and Shafner, H.: Chemical mutagens in the human environment. Nature, *219:* 385-387, 1968.
8. Federal Insecticide, Fungicide and Rodenticide Act as amended 1959.
9. Federal Hazardous Substances Act, 1967.
10. Federal Food, Drug, and Cosmetic Act as amended 1968.
11. Gabridge, M. G., and Legator, M.: A host-mediated microbial assay for the detection of mutagenic activity. Proc. Soc. Exptl. Biol. Med., *130:* 831-834 (1969).
12. Goldstein, A., Arokow, L., and Kalman, S. M.: *Principles of Drug Action.* Harper & Row, New York, 1968, p. 738.
13. Goldstein, A., *et al.*: *Ibid.*, 1968, 266.
14. Goldstein, A., *et al.*: *Ibid.*, 1968, 549-552.
15. Legator, M. S., Kelly, F. J., Green, S., and Oswald, E. J.: *Mutagenic Effects of Captan.* Presented at New York Academy of Science Symposium on Pesticides, May 1967.
16. Lukens, R. J., and Sisler, H. D.: Chemical reactions involved in the fungitoxicity of captan. Phytopathol., *48*:235-244, 1958.
17. Oettgen, H. F., Old, L. O., Boyse, E. A., Campbell, H. A., Philips, F. S., Clarkson, B. D., Taccal, L., Leeper, R. D., Schwarz, M. K., and Nokin, J.: Inhibition of leukemias in man by L-Asparaginase. Cancer Res., *27*:2619-2631, 1967.
18. Runner, M. N.: Comparative pharmacology in relation to teratogenesis. *Proc. of an International Symposium of Comparative Pharmacology, 26:*1131-1136, 1967.
19. Verrett, M. J., Mutchler, M. K., Scott, W. F., Reynaldo, E. F., and McLaughlin, J.: *Teratogenic Effects of Captan and Related Compounds in the Developing Chicken Embryo.* Presented at the New York Academy of Science Symposium on Pesticides, May 1967.
20. Zurel, J. W.: *A Literature Summary of Maleic Hydrazide.* U. S. Rubber Co., Naugatuck, Conn., 1963.

Chapter 2B

Detection of Cytogenetic Effects of Toxic Agents in Mammalian Systems

MARVIN S. LEGATOR, PH.D., and CECIL B. JACOBSON, M.D.

INTRODUCTION

Satisfactory techniques for the detailed examination of mammalian chromosomes is a little over ten years old, but the impact of these new techniques has had a profound effect on all branches of biology. A bond has been forged by workers in this field between medicine, agriculture, and the physical sciences. In clinical medicine, chromosome abnormalities have been identified in cases of mental retardation, congenital anomalies, infertility and in about 28% of all cases of spontaneous abortions.[6] Cytogenetic analysis has added a new dimension to genetic counseling, and its use in medical diagnosis, prognosis, and possible prevention of certain specific syndromes are just being realized. Of equal importance to the immediate medical significance of cytogenetic studies is the potential usefulness of this type of analysis in detecting and identifying specific agents in our environment that may have detrimental genetic effects, i.e., radiation, chemicals, and viruses.[9] The long-range genetic effect of chemicals that can be simply identified by chromosome analysis may be one of the most practical means of curtailing the genetic wasteage in our human population. We would like to discuss a few fundamental facts concerning chromosomes and chromosome analysis, refer to a few specific examples of chemical effects on chromosomes, and finally present some of the advanced automated technique in this field.

Chromosome Organization

In the biological organization of hereditary material, three levels of complexity can be identified.

1. At the first level, characterized by viruses, single or double stranded nucleic acid can be identified which is associated at some stage of the life cycle with proteins that aid in their dissemination.

2. At the second level of organization, the hereditary material is contained in long fibrillar DNA-rich elements about 140A in length and 30A in diameter. There is no typical nuclear membrane and the fibrillar elements are contained in intracytoplasmic regions. Most bacteria are typical of this level of organization.

3. In the third level of organization,

which is typical of higher organisms, the cells have a nucleus which is clearly differentiated from the cytoplasm.

Practically all of the DNA resides in the nuclei where it is organized into chromosome structures. The average chemical composition of a mammalian chromosome (HeLa cell) shows 16% DNA, 12% RNA, and 72% protein.[11] In terms of chromosome structure, present evidence bearing on this question indicates that the nucleic acid is continuous from one end of the chromosome to the other. The HCl soluble, non-tryptophan containing proteins (histones) made during the DNA synthesis period of the cell and intimately connected with DNA are believed to play a regulatory role. The non-histone proteins are probably important in maintenance of chromosome morphology.

During most of the life cycle of a cell, the chromosomes appear as long, fine filaments. However, during metaphase, the chromosomes appear as long, fine short and thick. Almost all cytogenetic evaluations are carried out during the metaphase stage where the highly condensed chromosome can be most easily observed.

Methodology

There is a great deal of similarity in the techniques employed in the study of chromosomes, whether cultured mammalian cells, animals, or man are being evaluated. The methods used are usually a modification of the one reported by Moorhead *et al.*[12] The basic prerequisites enumerated by Bartalos and Baramki[1] include the following points:

1. Availability of cells in active division (either natural cell division as in cultured cells, or by use of mitogenic stimulating agent such as phytohemagglutinin in leukocyte culture).
2. Accumulation of sufficient metaphase plates usually through the use of a mitotic arresting agent (colcemide*).
3. Hypotonic swelling to further disperse the chromosomes within the cell.
4. Preparation of a cellular suspension and its fixation.
5. Slide preparation with rupture of the swollen cells to spread the chromosomes in one optical plane.
6. Photomicroscopy to obtain proper plates for analysis.

Types of Aberrations

Two major types of chromosomal aberrations can be identified, numerical changes and structural changes. The numerical changes represent a departure from the normal diploid number. If the deviation from the normal diploid number is an exact multiple, it is referred to as euploidy. Polyploidy is an exact multiple greater than the diploid state. A second type of numerical abnormality, where an irregular number of chromosomes are present, is referred to as aneuploidy.

Structural abnormalities including gaps, breaks, deletions, fragments, and various exchange figures can be visualized as occurring by a primary breaking of the linear structure of the chromo-

*CIBA

some followed by a typical union of broken ends with or without subsequent divisions. If breaks occur during resting stage or interphase, the broken ends are referred to as "sticky" and they will usually join again (restitution). If the breaks occur when the chromosome is condensed (at mitosis or in spermatozoa), restitution does not occur, and structural aberrations result. If a break occurs in only a single chromatid, it is referred to as a chromatid break, gap, etc.; if both chromatids are altered, it is called a chromosome (isolocus, or isochromosome) effect. Figures 1, 2, and 3 illustrate typical structural abnormalities.

In cytogenetic analysis, four levels of significance or importance can be determined.

1. *Greatest significance* is attributed to persistent clonal aneusomy, second generation translocation figures (exchanges), structural markers (dicentrics, rings) and endoreduplication.

2. *Moderate significance* is awarded to non-clonal hyperdiploidy, persistent polyploidy, fragmentation, and chromosomal (isochromatid) breaks at non secondary constriction sites, also to inconsistent karyotypic anomalies suggesting deletion or translocation.

3. *Mild significance* is attributed to chromatid breaks, telomere blebs, chromatid fragments, and non-clonal hypodiploidy.

4. *No significance* has been attributed of chromosome gaps and sporatic hemologue asymmetry.

A minimum of 20 randomly selected metaphase spreads are analyzed from each tissue (approximate total 100 per specimen). Coded 8 x 11 photographic enlargements are independently scored by two investigators.

Chemical Effects

Human chromosomes have been shown to be susceptible to breakage and rearrangement following cellular damage by a number of agents including viruses, chemicals, and radiation. The effect of drugs on animal and plant chromosomes were known before techniques for satisfactory metaphase preparations were available.[3] Alkylating agents, nucleotide analogs, and compounds that inhibit nucleotide synthesis are the major classes of compounds that are known to break human chromosomes either *in vivo* or *in vitro*. One of the earliest studies on chromosome effects in humans was reported by Conen and Lansky[2] after therapeutic use of nitrogen mustards in a patient with bronchogenic carinoma. Just as radiation is known to be carcinogenic, teratogenic, and mutagenic in mammalian systems, the manifestations of many of the chemicals that cause chromosome aberrations are also known to produce the same types of genetic damage. Although one frequently cannot differentiate the end product of genetic damage caused by either radiation of chemicals, nor would one be able to determine if any individual chromatid aberration is chemically or radiation induced, there are cytogenic differences between the two agents. Chemicals have a delayed effect, while radiation has an immediate effect; radiation effects are usually randomly distributed among the chromosomes, while chemical effects are usually localized; and chemical effects are indifferent to

CHROMATID ABERRATION

Structural variation either in a single chromatid or at different loci on sister chromatids.

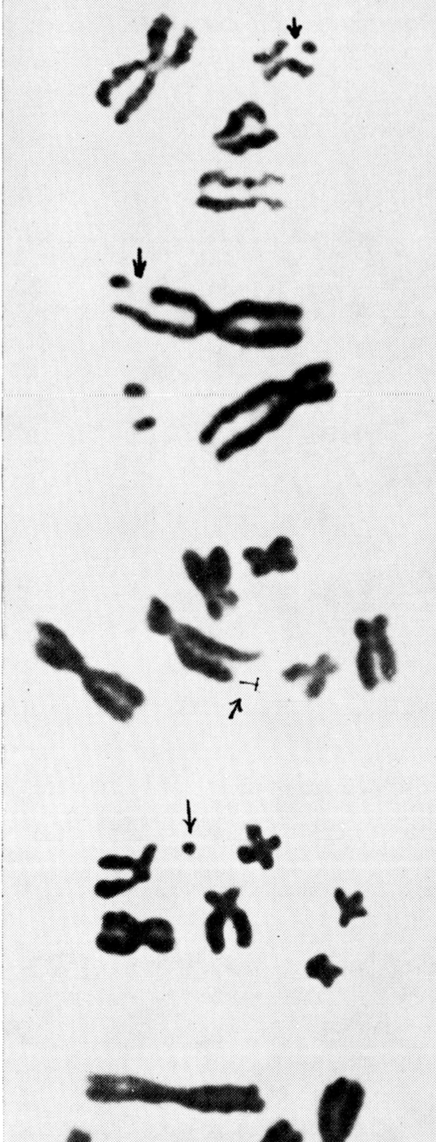

GAP (g)

- Chromatid interstitial deletion (less than 1 chromatid width)
- No linear displacement involved
- Thought to be an incomplete break

BREAK (b)

- Chromatid interstitial deletion (greater than 1 chromatid width)
- Often accompanied by slight axial displacement (less than 30°)
- No chromatid connection (bridge)

DELETION (d)

- Interstitial or terminal chromatid loss (in excess of 3 chromatid widths) as compared with sister chromatid
- Not identifiable as an associated fragment

FRAGMENT (f)

- A free chromatid piece displaced either more than 30° from chromosome axis, or more than three chromatid widths from parent chromosome

TERMINAL BLEBS (tb)

- Single chromatid telomere fragmentation
- Circular shape (1 chromatid width diameter)
- Terminal position within one chromatid width

Figure 1.

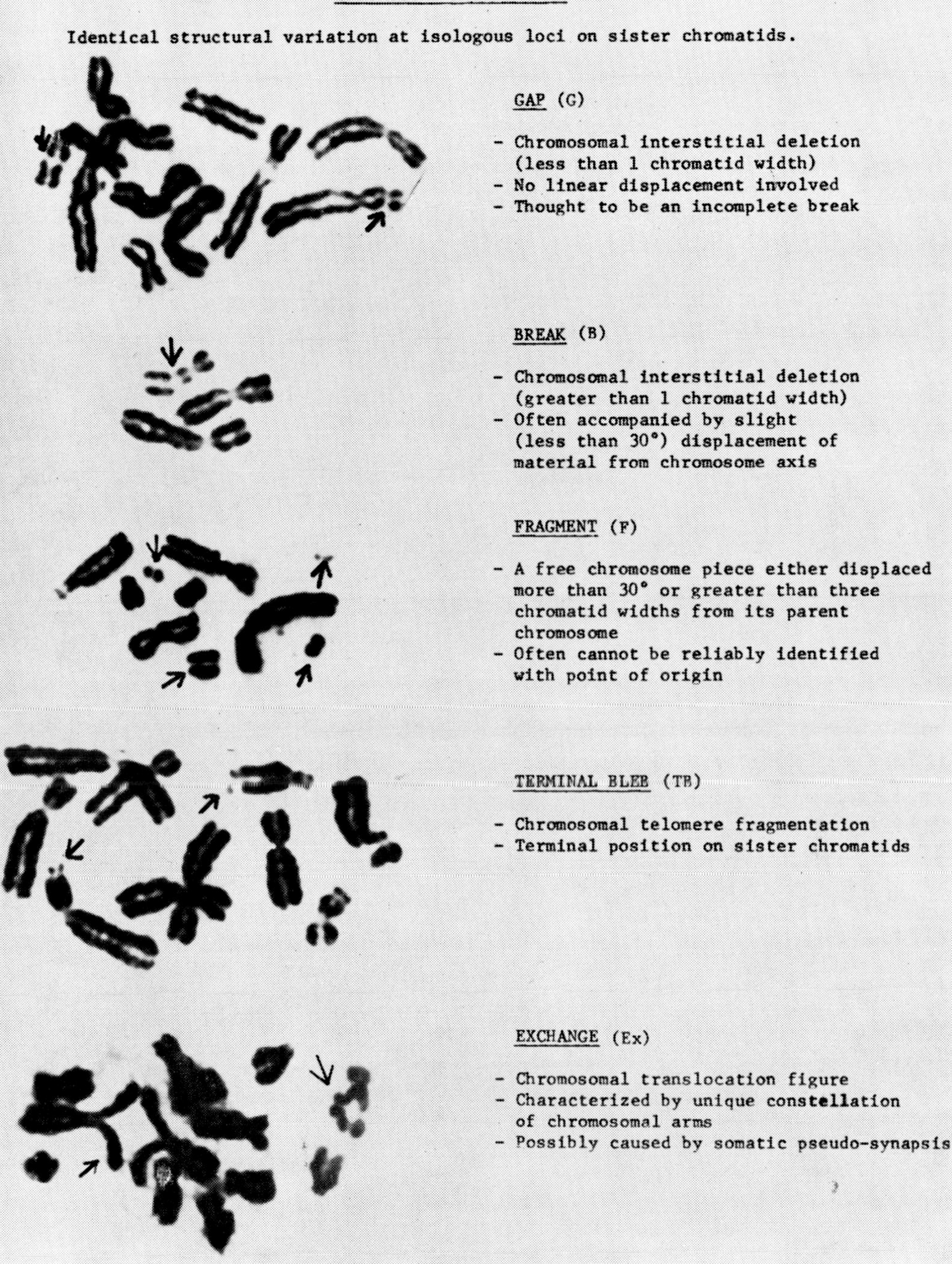
CHROMOSOME ABERRATIONS
Identical structural variation at isologous loci on sister chromatids.
GAP (G)
- Chromosomal interstitial deletion (less than 1 chromatid width)
- No linear displacement involved
- Thought to be an incomplete break
BREAK (B)
- Chromosomal interstitial deletion (greater than 1 chromatid width)
- Often accompanied by slight (less than 30°) displacement of material from chromosome axis
FRAGMENT (F)
- A free chromosome piece either displaced more than 30° or greater than three chromatid widths from its parent chromosome
- Often cannot be reliably identified with point of origin
TERMINAL BLEB (TB)
- Chromosomal telomere fragmentation
- Terminal position on sister chromatids
EXCHANGE (Ex)
- Chromosomal translocation figure
- Characterized by unique constellation of chromosomal arms
- Possibly caused by somatic pseudo-synapsis

Figure 2.

MARKER CHROMOSOMES

Unique structural alteration reflective of translocation, deletion or centromere rearrangements which allows consistent chromosomal identification.

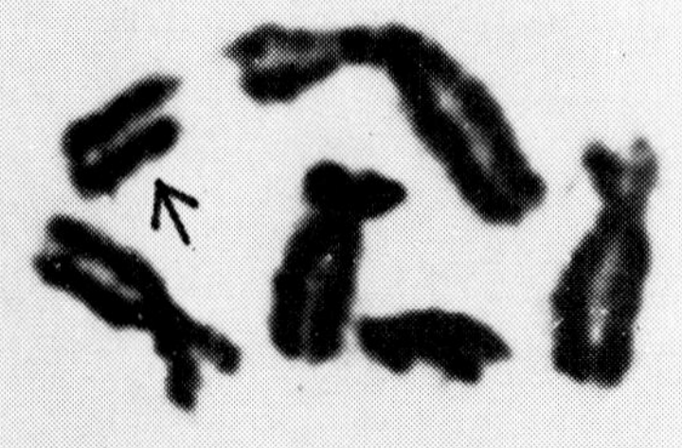

ACENTRIC (A)

- Chromosomal fragment larger than Group G
- No identifiable centromere region

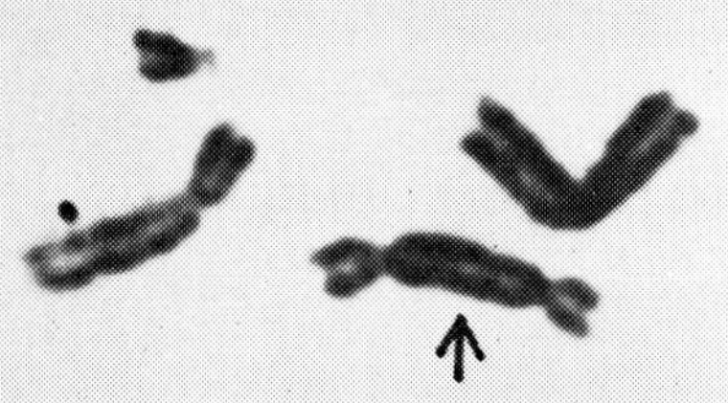

DICENTRIC (D)

- Chromosome with two centromeres
- May also include multi-centrics

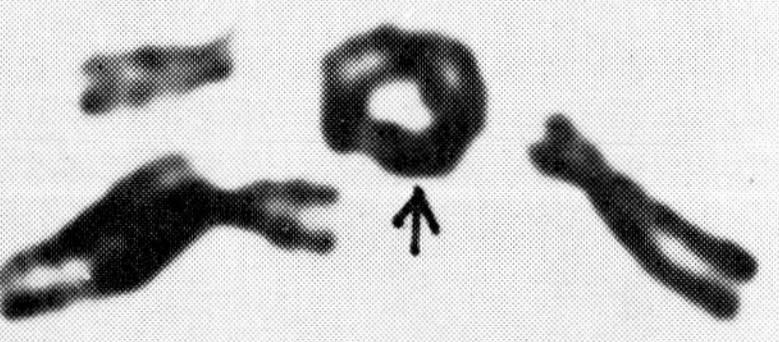

RING (R)

- Chromosome with appearance of a ring
- Either acentric or multi-centric
- Either inter-lapping or overlapping

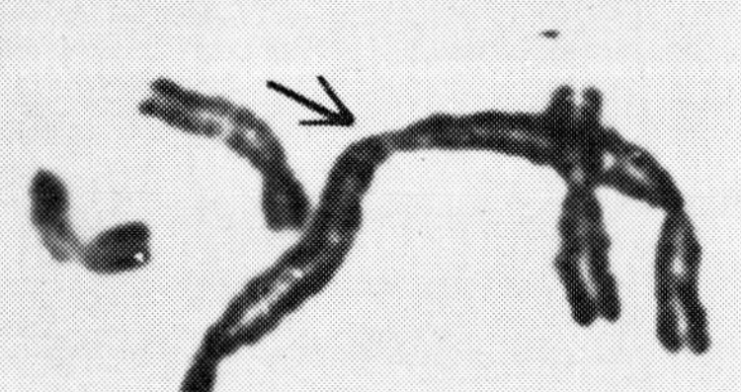

MARKER (M)

- Unique chromosomal structure which can be consistently identified
- Excludes centromere aberrations and exchanges
- Produced by non-reciprocal translocations, deletions or pericentric inversions

Figure 3.

the presence or absence of oxygen changes during treatment in contrast to radiation; and the proportion of intra to interchanges is always considerably higher with chemicals (alkylating agents) than with x-rays. The following table lists some of the representative classes of chromosome breaking compounds:

TABLE I. CHROMOSOME BREAKING CHEMICALS*

I. Inhibitors of DNA Synthesis
   Deoxyadenosine
   Cytosine Arabinoside
   S-flurodeoxy Uridine
II. Chemicals that denature or degrade DNA
   Actinomycin
   Streptonigrin
III. Compound that react with resting DNA Alkylating agents including:
   Mustards
   Epoxides
   Lactones
   Mitomycin
IV. Abnormal precursors producing labile DNA
   S-Bromodeoxyuridine
   Maleic hydrazide

*Modified from Kihlman.[7]

The number of compounds that have been evaluated for cytogenetic effects is increasing at a rapid rate. Examples of compounds that cannot be classified as yet in terms of known chromosome breaking agents can now be found in the literature. Recently, the cytogenetic effect of a naturally occurring toxin produced by a mold *A. flavus* has been reported.[4] Figure 4 illustrates the effect of this compound on human leukocyte cultures. Captan, a widely used fungicide, has been found to break chromosomes in cultured embryonic lung cells.[10]

One can anticipate exciting results in this field as additional compounds are evaluated in cultured cells, animals, and man. The technique involved in germinal cell analysis is essentially no more difficult to perform than somatic cell analysis, and there is a definite need for evaluation of compounds on germinal cells.

Automation of Chromosome Analysis

In addition to routine morphological analysis of chromosomes, there have been several methods employed to improve cytogenetic studies. Electron microscopy, fluorescent staining, quantitative estimation of DNA in individual chromosomes, measures to exaggerate secondary constriction or to produce decontraction, and computer analysis are a few of the techniques used to improve chromosome analysis.[5]

Considerable progress has been made in the use of pattern recognition instrumentation coupled with computer analysis for extending and improving current analysis, in classifying chromosomes and establishing relationships between chromosome abnormalities and pathological conditions in animal and man. In terms of man hours, approximately one hour of total time (including culturing, fixing, etc.), is spent in analyzing a single metaphase plate. Approximately 50 to 200 plates should be analyzed for each clinical condition, chemical treatment, etc., before reaching a conclusion. An automated analysis should greatly reduce the manual labor involved in chromosome analysis, but even more important, the data generated should be more complete and less subject to human error. There are several systems currently under development for scanning chromosome spreads either from slide preparations or from a photographic image. In one such system, a series of photomicrographs on a roll of film are read directly into the unit of a computer by a scanning device called FIDAC (film imput to digital automatic computer).[8] The computer is programmed to recognize and classify the objects under consideration. Total number of chromosomes, centromere location, area, length of the various segments can be recognized and classified by this system. The automation or partial automation of chromosome analysis should greatly advance the utility of this technique.

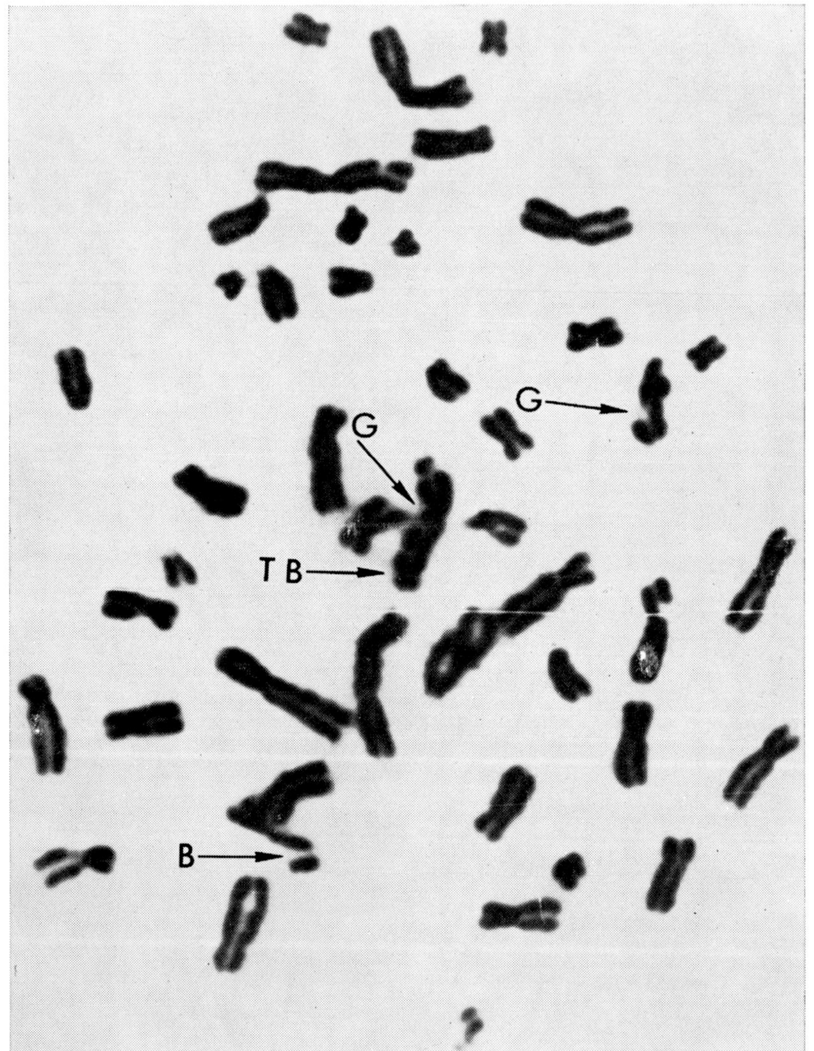

Figure 4.

Conclusion

Impressive advances have been made within the last eight years in the field of cytogenetics. In addition to clinical syndromes that have been described, human chromosomes have been shown to be susceptible to damage by agents such as radiation, viruses, and drugs. Cytogenetic analysis is a routine procedure in several clinical and research laboratories throughout the country. The advent of automated procedures should further simplify chromosome analysis. From the examples available of chromosome breaking agents, acting either *in vivo* or *in vitro* in either somatic or germinal cells, one would have to conclude that this is a powerful tool in characterizing genetically active agents. In the hands of a competent investigator where practical concentrations are used and where proper standards are used, this is a highly selective technique. It may well be that cytogenetic analysis will prove to be one of the most practical tools available for characterizing teratogenic, mutagenic, and carcinogenic agents.

REFERENCES

1. Bartalos, M., and Baramki, T. A.: *Medical Cytogenetics.* Baltimore, Williams and Wilkins Co., 1967.
2. Conen, P. E., and Lansky, G. S.: Chromosome damage during nitrogen mustard therapy. A case report. Brit. Med. J., *1055*:1961.
3. Darlington, C. D., and Koller, P. C.: The chemical breakage of chromosomes. Heredity, *1*:187-221, 1947.
4. Dolimpio, D., Jacobson, C., and Legator, M.: Effect of aflatoxin on human leukocytes. Proc. Soc. Exptl. Biol. Med., *127*:559-562, 1968.
5. German, J.: Autoradiographic studies of human chromosomes. Proc. Third Int. Cong. of Human Genetics, 123-136, 1966.
6. Jacobson, C. B.: Reproductive cytogenetics. Clin. Obstet. and Gynec. New York, Hoeber, 1969 (in preparation).
7. Kihlman, B. A.: *Actions of Chemicals on Dividing Cells.* Englewood Cliffs, N. J., Prentice-Hall, Inc., 1966.
8. Ledley, R. S.: High speed analysis of biomedical pictures. Science, *146*:216-233, 1964.
9. Legator, M., and Jacobson, C.: Chemical mutagens as a genetic hazard. Clin. Proc. Children's Hosp., *14*:184-189, 1968.
10. Legator, M., Kelly, F. J., Green, S., and Oswald, E. J.: Mutagenic effects of Captan. Symp. on Pesticides, N.Y. Acad. of Sci., 1967.
11. Maio, J. J., and Schildkraut, C. L.: Isolated mammalian metaphase chromosomes. 1. General characteristics of nucleic acids and proteins. J. Mol. Biology, *24*:29-40, 1967.
12. Moorhead, P. S., Nowell, R. C., Mellman, W. J., Battips, D. M., and Hungerford, D. A.: Chromosome preparations of leukocytes cultured from peripheral blood. Expl. Cell Res., *20*:613, 1960.

Chapter 3

Metabolism and Excretion of Toxic Agents[1]

E. W. MAYNERT, M.D., PH.D.

In the metabolism and excretion of foreign compounds, the human body makes few, if any, distinctions between toxic agents and clinically useful drugs. Thus, this chapter is concerned with generalizations derived from pharmacological as well as toxicological research. Most organic compounds are subjected to chemical changes in the body and are eliminated as metabolites rather than the substance administered. Therefore, the few drugs and poisons excreted completely unchanged are of some interest in revealing that their biological activity does not depend upon direct involvement in a chemical reaction, i.e., the formation or cleavage of a covalent bond. The diversity of structure in organic compounds might suggest that a brief review of patterns of biotransformation would not only be inadequate, but fruitless. Fortunately, this is not so. Every organic chemical can be regarded as composed of a rather limited number of component parts (alkyl chains, carbocyclic or aromatic rings and various groups such as hydroxyl, amino, carboxyl, etc.), and the fate of these separate parts is now well enough known to permit meaningful qualitative predictions about the routes of metabolism of drugs and poisons. However, quantitative predictions are not feasible. The end-products of drug metabolism are usually somewhat complex in that several of the theoretically possible routes are exploited to some extent. Moreover, many of the reactions discussed below do not proceed to completion.

Patterns of Metabolism

The great majority, if not all, of the reactions involved in the metabolism of toxic agents can be classified as oxidation, reduction, hydrolysis or synthesis. Oxidation is undoubtedly the most common reaction.

Oxidation. If a poison containing only carbon, hydrogen and oxygen were completely metabolized, the products would, of course, be carbon dioxide and water. However, very few drugs are completely degraded in the body. Ethyl alcohol,

[1] Some of the research described in this paper was supported by U.S.P.H.S. Research Grant NB-06288.

which is usually metabolized to the extent of 90% or more, is one of the rare exceptions. The sequence of reactions involved in its degradation will serve to bring out some other generalizations about the fate of toxic agents. Primary

$$CH_3CH_2OH \rightleftarrows CH_3CHO \rightarrow CH_3COOH \rightarrow CO_2 + H_2O$$

alcohols are extensively oxidized to aldehydes, and aldehydes to carboxylic acids. Primary alcohols and aldehydes are rarely end-products of metabolism, but carboxylic acids are common.

The following two reactions illustrate that alkyl chains are also subject to oxidation *in vivo*. The mechanism is direct hydroxylation (1). This process prob-

$$RCH_2CH_3 \rightarrow RCH_2CH_2OH \rightleftarrows RCH_2CHO \rightarrow RCH_2COOH$$

$$\rightarrow RCHOHCH_3 \rightleftarrows RCOCH_3$$

ably occurs to some extent at all carbon atoms in the chain, but overwhelming preference is given to the terminal (ω) and penultimate (ω-1) atoms (9). Secondary alcohols derived from penultimate oxidation are more resistant to metabolism than primary alcohols but are often excreted in part as ketones. These reactions are responsible for the detoxification of the commonly used dialkylbarbiturates and many other drugs and poisons. The various saturated ring systems, including the steroid nucleus, behave like alkyl chains in that they are also metabolized by hydroxylation.

Aliphatic olefins are often excreted in part as glycols, but a few toxic agents such as the insecticides heptachlor and Aldrin yield epoxides as final products. Recent research (16) has demonstrated that

$$RCH = CH_2 \rightarrow (RCH - CH_2)\ O \rightarrow RCHOHCH_2OH$$

epoxides are obligatory intermediates in the biological formation of glycols. The relatively rare occurrence of epoxides as end-products can be attributed to a microsomal enzyme which readily accomplishes hydrolysis to the *trans* form of the glycol (7, 15). In man secobarbital is converted in large part to a glycolic metabolite (13, 14).

Most aromatic compounds are hydroxylated to phenolic products. This widely-studied process is still poorly understood, but the available evidence indicates several possible pathways, the relative importance of which may depend upon substituents in the ring and animal species (10, 11). In some aromatic compounds the mechanism may be similar to that in saturated aliphatic compounds. However, alkyl chains and saturated rings are more readily hydroxylated than aromatic systems (3). The metabolism of certain aromatic compounds (e.g., naphthalene) has been

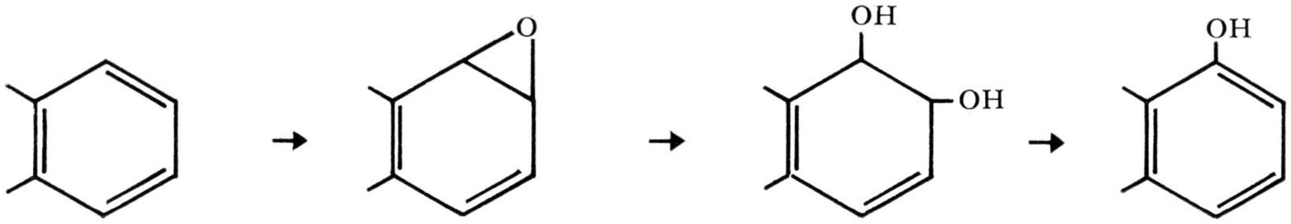

O

OH

OH

OH

shown quite clearly to involve epoxide intermediates (2, 5). The phenol could arise by rearrangement of the epoxide or by the process illustrated above, i.e., hydrolysis followed by dehydration. Epoxide intermediates provide a facile explanation for the formation of catechol metabolites as well as mercapturic acids (*vide infra*).

Many toxic agents are metabolized by the removal of methyl groups attached to nitrogen, oxygen or sulfur. These reactions are usually classified as dealkylations (e.g., N-dealkylation, O-dealkylation), but they have been shown quite clearly to involve oxidation to hydroxymethyl compounds, which decompose spontaneously to yield formaldehyde. Dealkylation is not restricted to the methyl group but is usually of minor significance when the chain contains more than two carbon atoms. The nature of the R group is not crucial in N- or S-dealkylation, but O-dealkylation is largely confined to arylalkyl ethers.

$$R_2NCH_3 \rightarrow R_2NCH_2OH \rightarrow R_2NH + HCHO$$
$$ROCH_3 \rightarrow ROCH_2OH \rightarrow ROH + HCHO$$
$$RSCH_3 \rightarrow RSCH_2OH \rightarrow RSH + HCHO$$

Certain foreign amines such as amphetamine are deaminated in the rabbit by a process which appears to involve primary hydroxylation rather than the formation of an ketimine ($R_2C = NH$) intermediate. However, the microsomal enzyme responsible for this reaction has not been clearly demonstrated in other species. Desulfuration may be considered as analogous to deamination. Although the intermediates are unknown, the process is clearly oxidative. Desulfuration is of crucial importance in connection with the toxicity of phosphorothionate insecticides and occurs to some extent in the metabolism of thiobarbiturates. The liberation of sulfide ion in this reaction has been thought to be of some significance in the toxicity of the rodenticide α-naphthylthiourea.

$$C_6H_5CH_2CH(NH_2)CH_3 \rightarrow [C_6H_5CH_2C(OH)(NH_2)CH_3] \rightarrow C_6H_5CH_2COCH_3 + NH_3$$

$$R_2C = S \rightarrow R_2C = O$$

The nitrogen in primary and secondary aromatic amines and urethane may be hydroxylated to yield hydroxylamino compounds. These are usually only minor products, but they may be responsible for the carcinogenic activity of 2-acetamidofluorene and certain other poisons (2). The rearrangement of hydroxylamines can result in *ortho*-hydroxylation. Oxidation of tertiary amines yields amine oxides. Certain compounds of this kind containing methyl groups may rearrange spontaneously to liberate formaldehyde and the corresponding secondary amine. The formation of amine oxides is analogous to the formation of sulfoxides and sulfones from thioethers. These reactions are important in the metabolism of phenothiazine tranquilizing agents and the industrial solvent dimethyl sulfoxide.

$$RNH_2 \rightarrow RNHOH$$

$$R_3N \rightarrow R_3NO$$

$$R_2S \rightarrow R_2SO \rightarrow R_2SO_2$$

Reduction. In the metabolism of toxic agents reduction is a much less common process than oxidation. However, this reaction is known to involve aldehydes and ketones, certain carbon-carbon double bonds (particularly in terpenes), azo, hydrazo, and nitro groups, amine oxides, sulfoxides, disulfides and halogen compounds. The conversion of chloral hydrate, an aldehyde, to trichloroethanol is of special interest in that it appears to account for the depressant activity of this

$$CCl_3CH(OH)_2 \rightarrow CCl_3CH_2OH$$

widely used hypnotic. The reductive cleavage of the prontosils to yield sulfanilamide likewise provided an explanation for the antibacterial action of these

$$NH_2SO_2C_6H_5N = NR \rightarrow NH_2SO_2C_6H_5NHNHR \rightarrow NH_2SO_2C_6H_5NH_2 + H_2NR$$

azo compounds. The reduction of nitro compounds to amines has been shown to involve nitroso and hydroxylamino intermediates. Amine oxides and sulfoxides merely lose their oxygen atoms. The conversion of tetrathylthiuram disulfide (disulfiram) to diethyldithiocarbamic acid may account for its pharmacological activity in the treatment of alcoholism. The chlorine and bromine atoms in certain

$$(C_2H_5)_2NCSS\text{-}SSCN(C_2H_5)_2 \rightarrow (C_2H_5)_2NCSSH$$

alifatic compounds are also subject to reduction. For example, CCl_4 is metabolized in part to $CHCl_3$, and halothane ($CF_3CHBrCl$) to 1,1,1-trifluoroethane (CF_3CH_3).

Hydrolysis. From the point of view of patterns of metabolism hydrolysis is easy to discuss, because it is largely restricted to esters and amides. However, the enzymology of this process is rather complex, for the body contains a variety of hydrolytic ferments which differ in their substrate specificities from tissue to tissue. In general, esters are metabolized more readily than amides. Thus, the ester procaine is hydrolyzed faster than procaine amide (pronestyl). The hydrolysis of esters often proceeds to completion, but amides, only if other pathways of metabolism are not available.

Aromatic nitriles are hydrolyzed to the corresponding carboxylic acid and ammonia. In contrast, aliphatic nitriles are largely metabolized to cyanide. These different pathways probably explain the greater toxicity characteristic of aliphatic nitriles.

Hydrolysis also appears to be involved in the biotransformation of certain natural products of toxicological importance. These include not only a variety of polypeptides and polysaccharides but some of the common cardiac glycosides. For example, the metabolism of digitoxin involves the stepwise cleavage of digitoxose moieties.

Synthesis (Conjugation). Many toxic agents and their metabolites combine with natural constituents of the body and are excreted as conjugates. The endogenous chemicals most commonly involved in these synthetic reactions are glucuronate, sulfate, acetate (or their precursors), certain amino acids and the methyl group. Although many foreign compounds offer the possibility of multiple conjugation, only rarely is a molecule conjugated in more than one place.

In all mammals except the cat, conjugation with glucuronic acid is the most important synthetic reaction of drugs and poisons. The products are formulated and named as follows:

$$\overset{\frown O \frown}{\mathrm{ROCH(CHOH)_3CHCOOH}}$$
ether glucuronide

$$\overset{\frown O \frown}{\mathrm{RCOOCH(CHOH)_3CHCOOH}}$$
ester glucuronide

$$\overset{\frown O \frown}{\mathrm{RNHCH(CHOH)_3CHCOOH}}$$
N-glucuronide

$$\overset{\frown O \frown}{\mathrm{RSCH(CHOH)_3CHCOOH}}$$
S-glucuronide

Almost any hydroxyl group, whether alcoholic or phenolic, can participate in the formation of ether glucuronides. In contrast, ester glucuronides are largely restricted to aromatic carboxylic acids. The ethers are stable in alkaline solution, but the esters are readily hydrolyzed. N-Glucuronides can be derived from aromatic amines, sulfonamides, carbamates and heterocyclic nitrogen compounds. The amine conjugates are labile in acid solution, but the amide derivatives are rather stable. S-Glucuronides have not been encountered very widely. However, thiophenol and the diethyldithiocarbamate derived from the metabolism of disulfiram have been shown to yield products of this kind.

Conjugation with sulfate yields products which are often called ethereal sulfates. For many years this reaction was thought to be confined to phenols and sterols. However, it is now recognized

$$C_6H_5OH \rightarrow C_6H_5OSO_3H$$

that aliphatic alcohols, including ethanol, utilize this metabolic pathway to some extent. Moreover, aromatic amines are conjugated to form sulfamates. Phenolic metabolites are usually excreted

$$C_6H_5NH_2 \rightarrow C_6H_5NHSO_3H$$

partly as the glucuronide and partly as the ethereal sulfate. However, the ability of the body to form sulfate conjugates is rather limited. Thus, when large quantities of phenols are administered or formed metabolically, the ratio of ethereal sulfate to glucuronide in the urine diminishes. Several authors have expressed curiosity about the rarity of conjugation of foreign compounds with phosphate, which is much more abundant than sulfate in mammalian tissues. One example of this reaction is the formation of *bis* (2-amino-1-naphthyl) phosphate from 2-naphthylamine in dogs.

Many drugs and poisons containing primary amino or amido groups are metabolized to a large extent by acetylation. However, this reaction does not embrace aliphatic amines.

$$NH_2C_6H_5SO_2NH_2 \begin{array}{l} \nearrow CH_3CONHC_6H_5SO_2NH_2 \searrow \\ \searrow NH_2C_6H_5SO_2NHCOCH_3 \nearrow \end{array} CH_3CONHC_6H_5SO_2NHCOCH_3$$

A good example of acetylation is provided by sulfanilamide, which is subjected to conjugation at both ends of the molecule. Isoniazid is metabolized primarily by acetylation of the hydrazid moiety.

$$RCONHNH_2 \rightarrow RCONHNHCOCH_3$$

Glycine is involved in the conjugation of a variety of aromatic and heterocyclic carboxylic acids. The products are generally called hippuric acids, although this name is properly applied only to benzoylglycine. Occasionally, other amino acids are incorporated into similar

$$C_6H_5COOH \rightarrow C_6H_5CONHCH_2COOH$$

end-products of drug metabolism. For

example, in man 3,4-dihydroxy-5-methoxyphenacetyl glutamine has been detected as a metabolite of mescaline.

The formation of mercapturic acids by conjugation with glutathione has received careful study, although the importance of this reaction in man is still obscure. Benzene, naphthalene and a number of other aromatic substances appear to react with tissue glutathione by means of epoxide intermediates *(vide supra)*. However, benzyl chloride and certain other compounds containing labile halogen atoms may alkylate the tripeptide directly. The products of these reactions are subjected *in vivo* to enzymatic removal of the glutamine and glycine moieties of glutathione followed by acetylation. Urinary metabolites derived from epoxides are called premercapturic acids. Treatment with mineral acid to effect the removal of water yields

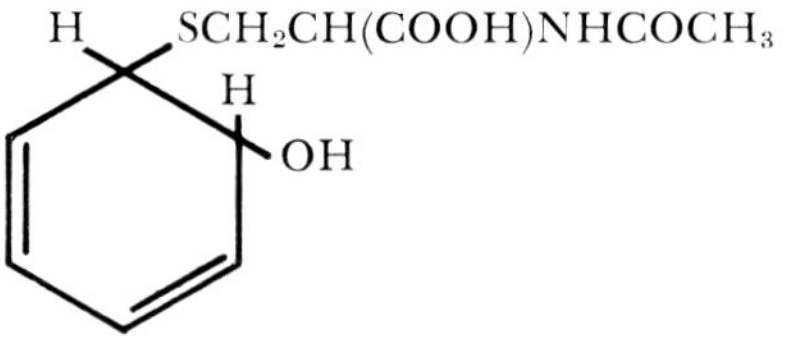

H $SCH_2CH(COOH)NHCOCH_3$ H OH

premercapturic acid

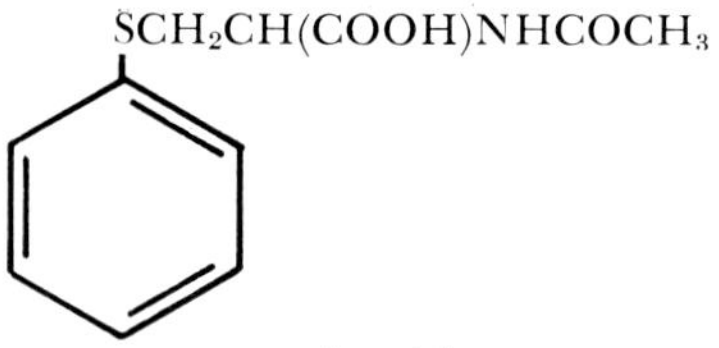

$SCH_2CH(COOH)NHCOCH_3$

mercapturic acid

a mercapturic acid. The excretory products of the halogen compounds are mercapturic acids rather than premercapturic acids.

The methyl group in S-adenosyl metheionine may be transferred to a variety of amines, phenols and thiols. The scope and limitations of N-methylation are not yet clear. However, selected primary, secondary and tertiary amines have been shown to participate in this reaction. O-methylation is of great quantitative significance in the metabolism of catechols, catecholamines and catechol acids. In these compounds usually only one hydroxyl group is conjugated. The location

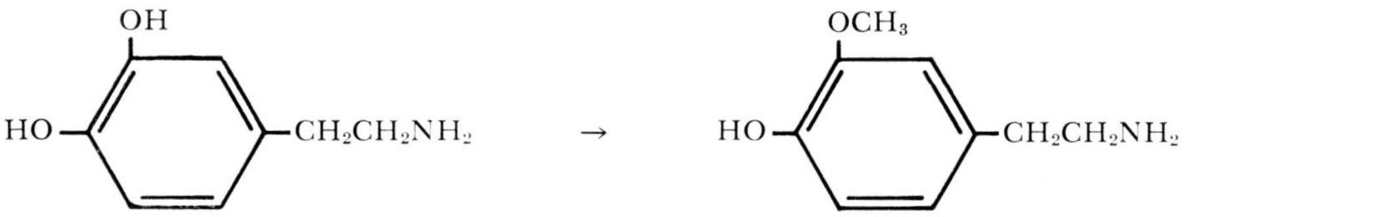

OH HO $CH_2CH_2NH_2$ → OCH_3 HO $CH_2CH_2NH_2$

of the methylation depends upon the nature and position of other substituents in the molecule. The best known examples of S-methylation involve aliphatic thiols and thiouracil.

No discussion of conjugation reactions would be complete without some mention of the conversion of cyanide to thiocyanate. This reaction is catalyzed by the enzyme rhodanese. No cofactor is needed. The source of the sulfur is probably thiosulfate.

$$CN^- \rightarrow CNS^-$$

Relation to Detoxification. Several of the reactions discussed above increase rather than decrease the pharmacological activity of foreign compounds. The conversion of parathion to paraoxon is a classical example of an oxidative reaction leading to a toxic metabolite. However, other oxidative products such as aldehydes, epoxides and hydroxylamines may also be more inimical than their precursors. Increased toxicity resulting from biochemical reduction is illustrated by the transformation of nitro compounds to hydroxylamines, azo compounds to amines, and chloral hydrate to trichloroethanol. The hydroxylation of aliphatic molecules usually produces a marked decrease in pharmacological activity, but the products of aromatic hydroxylation and dealkylation often differ only slightly from the parent compounds. Conjugation with glucuronic acid or sulfuric acid usually results in such a marked decrease in biological activity than these processes may be regarded as true detoxification. The most important feature of detoxification appears to be the production of molecules of sufficient polarity to resist reabsorption in the renal tubules or in the intestine after excretion in the bile.

Enzymatic Mechanisms

All of the reactions discussed above occur predominantly in the liver. Many of them cannot be detected in other tissues even when abundantly supplied with cofactors. The hydroxylation of toxic agents is rather tightly restricted to the liver. However, the enzymes responsible for hydrolysis, glucuronidation, sulfation, acetylation, methylation and the oxidation of alcohols and aldehydes seem to be more widely distributed.

The reactions presented above as involving hydroxylation appear to take place almost exclusively in the endoplasmic reticulum of hepatic cells. The minimum *in vitro* requirements are smooth microsomes, NADPH and gaseous oxygen. Despite an impressive volume of research, the exact mechanism of hydroxylation is not yet clear. The electron transport system has been formulated as follows:

NADPH / NADP ⇄ Ox. Flavoprotein / Flavoprotein Red. ⇄ Fe^{++} Protein / Fe^{+++} Protein ⇄ Ox. P-450 / P-450 Red. ⇄ RH → ROH / O_2 → H_2O

Cytochrome P-450 is believed to function as the oxygen-activating component of a variety, but still undefined number, of drug metabolizing hydroxylases. An authoritative review of this problem is now available (4).

The enzymes responsible for desulfuration and the oxidation of olefins, thioethers and amines are also located in microsomes and resemble very closely those involved in hydroxylation. In contrast, the conversion of alcohols to aldehydes or ketones is catalyzed by dehydrogenases present in the cell sap. These enzymes require either NAD or NADP as a cofactor. The oxidation of aldehydes to carboxylic acids involves to a varying extent aldehyde oxidase, xanthine oxidase and a NAD-specific aldehyde dehydrogenase. These enzymes are also found in the soluble fraction of liver homogenates.

The reduction of the azo and nitro groups is carried out in the endoplasmic reticulum of the liver. The responsible enzymes appear to be flavoproteins. Reductive dehalogenation also occurs in microsomes, but the hydrogenation of olefins, disulfides, sulfoxides and amine oxides does not. The location and nature of the enzymes involved in many of these processes are still unknown.

Hepatic microsomes catalyze the hydrolysis of foreign esters and amides. In view of the wide distribution of esterases in tissues it is interesting to note that microsomes can cleave certain esters not acted upon by the plasma enzymes. A distinctive feature of the hydrolytic enzymes is that they do not require a cofactor.

The necessary reactant in the formation of all kinds of glucuronide conjugates is uridine diphosphate α-D-glucosiduronic acid, abbreviated UDPGA. Enzymes called UDP transglucuronylases exchange UDP with the drug. These enzymes are deficient in the newborn and in certain patients with congenital nonhemolytic jaundice.

The formation of ethereal sulfates also involves a nucleotide and a group of transferases. The nucleotide, often called "active sulfate," is 3′-phosphoadenosine-5′-phosphosulfate, abbreviated PAPS. The enzymes which transfer sulfate to the drug are found in the soluble fraction of tissue homogenates and are designated as sulfotransferases or sulfokinases.

$$\text{PAPS} + \text{ROH} \rightarrow \text{ROSO}_3\text{H} + \text{ADP}$$

The methylation of drugs and poisons resembles glucuronidation and sulfation in involving a nucleotide cofactor, *viz.*, S-adenosylmethionine. Magnesium or other divalent ions are required in the transfer of the methyl group to oxygen, nitrogen or sulfur. Three different N-methyl- and at least two O-methyltransferases are soluble enzymes. However, S-methyltransferase and one O-methyl enzyme are found in hepatic microsomes.

The acetylation of amines and the conjugation of aromatic acids with glycine involve coenzyme A. In the first of these processes, acetyl coenzyme A, which occurs naturally in tissues, is the necessary reactant. The formation of hippuric acids involves conversion of the foreign acid to aroyl conenzyme A which then reacts with glycine. The enzymes which catalyze all these reactions are called acylases. They are found primarily in the mitochondria of liver and kidney.

$$\text{CH}_3\text{CO-S-CoA} + \text{RNH}_2 \rightarrow \text{CH}_3\text{CONHR} + \text{CoA-SH}$$

$$\text{RCOOH} + \text{CoA-SH} \rightarrow \text{RCO-S-CoA} + \text{H}_2\text{O}$$

$$\text{RCO-S-CoA} + \text{NH}_2\text{CH}_2\text{COOH} \rightarrow \text{RCONHCH}_2\text{COOH} + \text{CoA-SH}$$

The enzymes responsible for the first step in mercapturic acid formation are called glutathione S-aryl or S-alkyl transferases. Both are found in the soluble fraction of liver homogenates.

Excretion

Toxic agents may be eliminated in the urine, feces, breath, sweat or milk. The latter two routes will be ignored here, for they are rarely quantitatively significant; the interested reader is referred to a recent review (12). Excretion in the breath is of major clinical significance in connection with volatile anesthetics and poisons such as methanol. The process is well-understood and has been reviewed in depth (6). Volatile foreign compounds usually behave like the normal respiratory gases in that during passage through the pulmonary capillaries they are readily equilibrated with alveolar air. Thus, the elimination of such agents depends upon two physiological factors (ventilation and pulmonary blood flow) and one physicochemical factor (the blood/air solubility coefficient). Differences in solubility in blood explain the major differences in rates of excretion. For example, under conditions of normal circulation and ventilation the elimination of the insoluble gas ethylene (Ostwald coefficient, 0.14) is 90% complete is less than 10 minutes, whereas the removal of the soluble drug ether (Ostwald coefficient, 12) requires many hours. The mechanism of the excretion of carbon monoxide and other poisons which bind to tissue proteins is more complex (8).

Urinary Route. Urinary excretion is the process by which most drugs and poisons ultimately leave the body. Entry into the urine is achieved by glomerular filtration and proximal tubular secretion. Filtration is a passive process. The quantity of drug entering the lumen depends entirely upon the volume of plasma water filtered. Drugs bound to plasma proteins are excluded. Tubular secretion involves the transport of ions from the blood to the urine. This process embraces bound as well as free constituents of the blood. The renal tubules contain at least two active transport systems directed toward the lumen. One of these handles a wide variety of organic acids including sulfonic, carboxylic and uric acids and sulfonamides. The other is concerned with quaternary ammonium compounds and amine salts.

After entering the tubular lumen, foreign compounds are concentrated by the extensive reabsorption of water. They may then diffuse back into the blood stream according to the concentration gradient. The cells of the tubular epithelium have the properties of a lipid barrier. Thus, the laws of nonionic diffusion govern the passive reabsorption of drugs. Unionized compounds with high oil/water partition coefficients are readily reabsorbed. Polar metabolites and ions are poorly reabsorbed. It seems probable that some drugs and metabolites may also be actively reabsorbed in the renal tubules. However, this process has not yet been clearly demonstrated.

By means of the systemic administration of bicarbonate or other alkalinizing ions, the pH of the urine may be raised as high as 8. This alteration can markedly enhance the excretion of weak acids reabsorbed by nonionic diffusion. The practical usefulness of this procedure in the treatment of poisoning from salicylates and phenobarbital is now well-recognized. Acidification of the urine may likewise facilitate the excretion of amines. However, inasmuch as the urine in normally acidic, this maneuver is generally less effective than is alkalinization for the removal of acids. The excretion of acids and bases as well as neutral metabolites may be strikingly increased by an increased urine flow. The quantitative aspects of these methods are detailed in a superlative review (17).

Hepatic metabolism and urinary excretion may be regarded as acting in concert toward detoxification. Most of the reactions of drug metabolism lead to compounds of increasing polarity. Thus, reabsorption in the renal tubules is diminished. Moreover, many of the products (e.g., glucuronides, ethereal sulfates, hippurates, mercapturates, etc.) are acids. Thus, tubular secretion, the most facile mechanism of renal elimination, may be utilized.

Fecal Route. Toxic agents found in the feces are derived from three sources: (1) drug which has merely resisted intestinal absorption; (2) drug secreted into the intestinal tract (e.g., an amine concentrated in gastric juice as a result of nonionic diffusion), and (3) drug excreted in the bile. Biliary excretion involves both active and passive processes. The parenchymal cells of the liver contain active transport systems for the secretion of both acids and bases. However, the role of chemical structure, dissociation constants and lipid solubility have not yet been clearly defined. Glucuronides, which are moderately strong acids, seem particularly likely to be secreted in the bile. Inasmuch as drugs are not readily reabsorbed from the gall bladder, and the emptying of this viscus is periodic, the discharge of drug into the intestine may be greatly delayed. After entering the gut, the drug may be reabsorbed. The combined processes of biliary secretion and intestinal reabsorption are sometimes referred to as the enterohepatic circulation.

The enterohepatic circulation may play an important role in the ability of 4-aminobiphenyl and 4-amino-3,2′-dimethylbiphenyl to produce intestinal tumors in rats. These substances are metabolized in the liver to ortho-hydroxyamines and excreted in the bile as the corresponding glucuronides. The conjugates are then hydrolyzed in the intestine to the free ortho-hydroxyamines, which are carcinogenic (18).

REFERENCES

1. Brodie, B. B., Gillette, J. R., and LaDu, B. N.: Enzymatic metabolism of drugs and other foreign compounds. Ann. Rev. Biochem., *27:* 427-454, 1958.
2. Boyland, E., and Booth, J.: The metabolic fate and excretion of drugs. Ann. Rev. Pharmacol., *2:*129-142, 1962.
3. Elliott, T. H., Hanam, J., Parke, D. V., and Williams, R. T.: The metabolism of I-(^{14}C) tetralin in rabbits. Biochem. J., *92:*52P-53P, 1964.
4. Gillette, J. R: Biochemistry of drug oxidation and reduction by enzymes in hepatic endoplasmic reticulum. Advances in Pharmacol., *4:* 219-261, 1966.
5. Holtzman, J. L., Milne, Q. W. A., and Gillette, J. R.: The incorporation of ^{18}O into naphthalene in the formation of 1,2-dihydronapthalene 1,2-diol and 1-naphthol. Pharmacologist, *8:*190, 1967.
6. Kety, S. S.: The theory and applications of the exchange of inert gas at the lungs and tissues. Pharmacol. Rev., *3:*1-41, 1951.
7. Leibman, K. C., and Ortiz, E.: Microsomal hydration of epoxides. Fed. Proc., *27:*302, 1968.
8. Lilienthal, J. L.: Carbon monoxide. Pharmac. Rev., *2:*324-354, 1950.
9. Maynert, E. W.. On the specificity of penultimate oxidation. The fate of 5-ethl 5-*n*-hexylbarbituric acid. J. Pharmac. Exper. Therap., *150:*476-483, 1965.
10. Parke, D. V.: *The Biochemistry of Foreign Compounds.* Pergamon Press, 1968.
11. Sloan, N. H.: Hydroxymethylation of the benzene ring. 1. Microsomal formation of phenol via prior hydroxymethylation of benzene. Biochem. Biophys. Acta, *107:*599-602, 1965.
12. Stowe, C. M., and Plaa, G. L.: Extrarenal excretion of drugs and chemicals. Ann. Rev. Pharmacol., *8:*337-356, 1968.
13. Toki, S., and Maynert, E. W.: Species differences in dihydroxysecobarbital excretion. Fed. Proc., *25:*531, 1966.
14. Waddell, W. J.: The metabolic fate of 5-allyl-5-(1-methylbutyl) barbituric acid (secobarbital). J. Pharmacol. Exper. Therap., *149:*23-28, 1965.
15. Watabe, T., and Maynert, E. W.: Evidence for a microsomal epoxide hydroxylase. Fed. Proc., *27:*302, 1968.
16. Watabe, T., and Maynert, E. W.: Role of epoxides in the metabolism of olefins. Pharmacologist, *10:*276, 1968.

17. Weiner, I. M., and Mudge, G. H.: Renal tubular mechanisms for excretion of organic acids and bases. Am. J. Med., *36:*743-762, 1964.
18. Williams, R. T., Millburn, P., and Smith, R. L.: The influence of enterohepatic circulation on toxicity of drugs. Annals. N.Y. Acad. Sci., *123:* 110-122, 1965.

Chapter 4

Predictive Value of Human Toxicity from Animal Data

HARRY W. HAYS, PH.D.

Among all the laboratory animals used in research, there is still no established animal that simulates man. The introduction of new species in toxicity tests has provided more information on interspecies differences than it has in predicting effects in man. The introduction of a new drug is usually marked by enthusiastic acclaim for its great therapeutic benefits, but is soon followed by condemnation because of limited use and adverse reactions.

The predictive value of animal data is not limited to drugs, but includes all chemicals to which man may be exposed and which have been tested as rigorously as drugs. The physician must be constantly aware of the reactions that may occur from exposure to food, cosmetics, industrial chemicals, pesticides, and air pollutants. Indeed, when one considers the total environment of man and the well-controlled environment of the laboratory test animal, it would not be surprising that some adverse reactions may occur that could never be predicted from laboratory tests.

There is no standard procedure for pharmacological or toxicological studies that is universally acceptable, or which would necessarily be applicable, for every chemical. The nature of the test is dictated by the intended use, the physical-chemical properties, the chemical structure, absorption, distribution, excretion, metabolism, and what may already be known from experimental and clinical reports. The laboratory tests for evaluating drug toxicity include acute, subacute, chronic, reproduction, and teratogenicity studies on at least two species of animals, one of which should be a nonrodent. Of particular importance is the clinical chemistry, hematology, organ function tests, and histopathology, as well as pharmacological studies involving the neuromuscular and cardiovascular systems, These should be done in considerable depth for it is important to establish as early as possible, the site or sites of action.

There are many factors that may influence the outcome of toxicity tests not only making it difficult to predict the effect in man, but also to interpret the significance of the data within the test species. The type of response depends in part upon the route of administration. Magnesium sulfate produces a cathartic effect when given by mouth, but given intravenously produces CNS depression. A chemical may be distributed throughout the body or may concentrate in certain organs. The site of maximum concentration may or may not be in tissues upon which it exerts its characteristic effect. The cardiac glycoside, digitoxin, acts on cardiac muscle but is found in highest concentration in the liver. The principal routes of excretion are the lungs, kidney, bile, and large intestine. If considerable reabsorption occurs by the kidney, accumulation and undesirable effects may result.

Impaired nutrition may influence the outcome of toxicological tests by causing a variety of tissue changes unrelated to the chemical being tested. Female rats are usually more sensitive than males, and young animals are usually more responsive than adults, so that testing various age groups becomes a matter of practical importance. One observes quite frequently increased toxicity with increased temperature. Spontaneous diseases, such as infection in the middle ear and lungs of rats may be severe enough to invalidate a long-term study. Genetic factors may determine the response to a particular compound and may not be representative of most strains of the same species. Amphetamine is much more toxic in aggregated mice than in isolated animals. However, in the BDF strain, amphetamine does not produce excitation, but instead the animals exhibit depression. A deficiency in the red cells of glucose-6-phosphate is recognized as rendering the cells susceptible to destruction by a number of chemicals and drugs, such as 8-aminoquinolines, sulfonamides, sulfones, nitrofurans, acetanilid, and aminopyrene.

Perhaps the most important factor to be considered is the species variation in the biotransformation of chemicals entering the circulation. A chemical may be esterified in the rat, conjugated in the dog, and acetylated in man. The differences in response may be qualitative as in the case of morphine, which is depressant in the dog and man, but a stimulant in the mouse and cat. In the case of butylated hydroxyanisole, the difference is only quantitative. Of equal importance is the rate of metabolism, for this determines to a great extent the biological effects. The rate may be expressed in two ways: the percent metabolized per hour, or the biologic half-life, i.e., the time taken for the plasma level to fall to 50% of its original value. For example, a single dose of meperidine in man lasts 3 to 4 hours, but in the dog produces only a transient effect. The difference lies in the rate of metabolism which is 20% in man and 90% in the dog. Chemicals are metabolized by such reactions as oxidation, reduction, hydrolysis, demethylation, acetylation, and conjugation. Compounds may not only be inactivated but may give rise to metabolites as shown with phenylbutazone, which upon hydroxylation yields a metabolite with antirheumatic effects and a metabolite with urocosuric effects. It would, therefore, seem highly desirable to select a species that metabolizes the chemical in the same way as man before embarking on extensive toxicological studies.

It has been said that the conventional procedures for carrying out chronic toxicity studies in the laboratory are empirical and have little scientific basis and that the extrapolation of the animal data to man is a matter of guesswork. While there may be an element of truth in this statement, everyone will agree that such studies provide valuable information in taking that first step toward clinical trials.

Litchfield made a retrospective study of six drugs that had been tested on rats, dogs, and man, and his analysis showed that most of the effects observed in man were also observed in the dog. It must be emphasized that what is observed in animals are signs and not symptoms, and what is very often reported as adverse reactions in man, such as tinnitus and visual disturbances, cannot be measured in any laboratory animal. There are some clinical reactions, such as contact dermatitis, eczematous sensitivity, and photo sensitivity, that cannot be predicted from animal studies.

While it is recognized that the predictive value of human toxicity from animal data is open to serious question, nevertheless there is need for this valuable laboratory data. More thought should be given to planning, selecting the appropriate species, measuring those things which are pertinent, and observing the animal as if it were a patient. The evolution of animal experimentation and predictability of toxicity in man lends some justification for the pessimism of the value of animal studies. It was customary in the beginning to use a few mice, an odd rabbit, and a rat or two. It soon became clear that toxicity in man could not be predicted in this way, so the number of rats increased. Dogs came in. Rabbits went out. Cats became scarce. Predictions improved, but soon more species were added. Tests became longer — ten days, two months, two years. One stopped counting the dead and began weighing everything that could be removed, and slicing everything that could be sliced.

Well, the methods haven't changed much. One still weighs everything that can be removed, slices everything that can be sliced, feeds everything that can be fed for the life span of the animal. Unless the current approach to toxicology changes significantly, the predictive value of human toxicity from animal data will become even more obscure.

REFERENCES

1. Brodie, B. B.: Difficulties in extrapolating data on metabolism of drugs from animal to man. Clin. Pharm. Therap., *3*:274-278, 1962.
2. Edson, E. F.: Pesticides. Chapter 13 *in, Toxicity Testing*. Pergamon Press, To be published.
3. Hays, H. W.: Pharmacological aspects of toxicology. Pages 143-153 *in A Symposium on Toxicity in the Closed Ecological System*. Palo Alto, Calif., 1963.
4. Hays, H. W.: Problems in the interpretation and extrapolation of animal data to man. Pages 166-173 *in Proceedings of the Conference on Atmospheric Contamination in Confined Spaces*. Dayton, Ohio, 1965. AMRL-TR-65-230.
5. Litchfield, J. T., Jr.: Forecasting drug effects in man from studies in laboratory animals. J.A.M.A., *177*:104-107, 1961.
6. Litchfield, J. T., Jr.: Predictability of conventional animal toxicity tests. Ann. N.Y. Acad. Sci., *123*:268-272, 1965.
7. Zbinden, G.: Experimental and clinical aspects of drug toxicity. Advances in Pharm., *2*:1-111, 1963.

Chapter 5

Approaches to Fetal Pharmacology and Toxicology

HERBERT S. POSNER, PH.D.

I. Introduction

The developing fetus has been studied from many different orientations: embryologic, genetic, immunologic, developmental biochemistry, pathology, diagnosis, therapy, etc. Although the intended orientation of this report is pharmacologic and toxicologic, research in related fields is included so that appropriate associations can be made. The approaches chosen include: the ability of chemical or physical agents to produce immediate or delayed defects; the potential roles of the placenta, fetal immaturity, and mechanical pressure in bringing about the defects; the concept of overcoming genetic defects; and newer techniques of diagnosis and drug administration.

When considering the effects that chemical or physical agents might have on the developing organism, one should be aware of the parameters of reactability. For example, the agent might act: acutely or chronically, or singly or in combination with other agents. If it acts in combination, inhibitory, additive, or potentiating effects might be produced. It might also act prenatally, perinatally, or postnatally. The organism might be resistant, sensitive, or develop hypersensitivity. The exposure might be accidental or deliberate. The effects might be: immediate or delayed, transient or permanent, non-cumulative or cumulative, detrimental or beneficial. Finally, the effects may be at the molecular level only, at the level of cells and tissues, or manifest at higher levels of structure or function.

The problem is difficult. Shirkey (182) feels, that with respect to drugs, we are producing a class of "therapeutic orphans," infants and children who are perhaps not getting the drugs that they need because insufficient testing has been done on this age group. Testing must be done but under appropriate conditions. Very hard decisions have to be made on the basis of the knowledge at hand, the knowledge that can be developed, the need for the drug, alternate possibilities, and the risk involved. With respect to exposure of pregnant women to potentially deleterious environmental agents, one must continue to seek those agents that are deleterious, and those that might alter the response to drugs. What we don't know may hurt us.

More deleterious, and in some cases permanent effects, either manifest quickly or delayed, are discussed first.

II. Ability of Chemical or Physical Agents to Produce Immediate or Delayed Defects

CONGENITAL MALFORMATIONS AND ANOMALIES

Many reviews and symposium volumes have been written since 1959 on the subject of teratogenesis—the production of overt congenital malformations or of other forms of anomalies. Just a few of the more extensive reviews, from a variety of orientations, are referenced (2, 20, 29, 64, 97, 108, 109, 110, 154, 159, 178, 184). It is not that this is a newly recognized problem. Rather, the hormone and cancer chemotherapeutic drug malformations of the fifties and the thalidomide malformations of the sixties brought the problem into focus for pharmacologists and toxicologists. Embryologists and geneticists had been concerned with the problem for many years. Obstetricians and pediatricians took more cognizance of it later.

To assess the extent of the burden in humans, and without distinguishing between genetic, environmental, or a combination of causes, Apgar and Stickle (14) recently reviewed the incidences of a number of conditions: 1) loss of fetuses associated with the presence of malformation (30% or higher; Nishimura (158) has studied the malformations, and Inhorn (102) the chromosomal abnormalities, associated with spontaneous human abortions); 2) the incidence of defects found at birth or shortly thereafter (7%, with less than half of these evident at birth); 3) the number of yearly deaths from congenital conditions identifiable from the International Classification of Diseases, U. S., 1965 (62,000, with about one-half of these associated with diabetes mellitus, one-third with congenital malformations, and the remainder distributed between seventeen other categories); and 4) the prevelance of birth defects in the population ("at least 15 million persons in the United States have one or more congenital defects that affect their daily lives"). They also presented a graph of eighteen late-appearing birth defects with age of onset varying from one year to 40-60 years of age, some of which can be influenced, at least postnatally, by environmental factors.

Kennedy (113) also reviewed the epidemiological aspects of congenital malformations, from 238 reports covering about 20 million births. Incidences as low as 0.15% were found when birth certificates and official records were used, a mean of 1.26% when data was derived from hospital records, and a mean of 4.50% when data was obtained after special examination. It is interesting to note with respect to the latter, that in Britain, Europe (excluding Germany), Germany, and in "other countries", the incidences varied from 2.20% to 2.96%, while in the United States the incidence was 8.76% as a result of the inclusion of "a wide range of minor anomalies." Without the minor anomalies and allowing for under-reporting, Kennedy feels that the real incidence must be at least 2%, detectable at birth or shortly thereafter.

In recognition of the increased cognizance given to birth defects, the Eighth Revision of the *International Classification of Diseases* (ICD) and the same, adapted for use in the United States (ICDA) (62), have increased the number of gross structural malformations categorized from ten in the Seventh Revision of 1965, to twenty-three in 1968. The ICDA contains, in addition, many subdivisions of the twenty-three in order to provide greater specificity for epidemiological analysis.

Etiological factors for the production of congenital malformations are known to be multiple: genetic, mechanical, ionizing radiation, imbalances of vitamins, minerals, and hormones, viruses, drugs, environmental chemicals, and combinations of these. At present, we are thinking mainly in terms of omission of the offending environmental agents. This is a good approach when practical. With further knowledge, additional euphenic and eugenic* means of control over development should also become possible. In sections III-V, some experimental approaches to the control of development are discussed.

Briefly, malformations were first produced experimentally during the last century by puncturing avian embryos (see 29). Many experiments involving physical manipulation of the fetus followed. Then x-rays were used in the early part of this century to produce malformations. Dekaban (48) has recently compared abnormalities seen in children and in rats. Both groups were prenatally exposed to x-ray at different times of gestation. A recent review of the effects of ionizing radiations on mammalian development is that of Hicks and D'Amato (97).

That vitamin imbalances could lead to the production of malformations was first reported for *hypo*vitaminosis A by Hale (90, 91). Since then, *hypo*vitaminnoses of folic acid, pantothenic acid, riboflavin, or Vitamin E have been shown to produce malformations, as have the *hyper*vitaminoses of A or D. Imbalances in the mineral content of the diet, as for example deficiencies of zinc, copper, or manganese produce malformations. Symposia on many of the nutritional aspects of prenatal and postnatal development have recently been held (100, 180a). Excesses of some of the elements also produce malformations, as for example in the case of mercury (145), lead (65), and cadmium (66).

By means of estrone administration, intersexuality was produced in the chick, in 1935 (207). Since then much work has been done on the effects of hormones on development (131, 179, 213).

In 1941, Gregg (83) established a relationship between the production of birth defects and maternal infection with rubella virus. Several other viral groups have now been implicated in the production of birth defects (92, 200).

In the 1950's and 1960's, some cancer chemotherapeutic agents and antibiotics were found to be capable of producing malformations.

In 1963, it was reported that sheep grazing on the plant Veratrum californicum produced some young with cyclopia (24). The active principles have recently been isolated and identified (111).

It was only after malformations were reported in human infants in cases where the mother had received thalidomide, a relatively non-toxic drug (130, 139), that more investigators became interested in the problems of maldevelopment. Although the drugs used as cancer chemotherapeutic agents or as antibi-

*In Section IV, the meanings and implications of the terms euphenics and eugenics are discussed.

otics were shown previously to produce malformations, this was not as surprising since they were known to affect growth processes. Thus, after an incubation period, experimental teratology came of age.

Whether or not an agent will be teratogenic is dependent upon a number of factors. First, it has to be active at a dose that does not kill the embryo or fetus. The slope of the dose-response curve varies considerably, being quite steep in some cases. Second, it has to be either: present at a time when a target tissue is at a sensitive stage, persist unchanged or as an active metabolite (s) until that time, produce an initiating effect earlier, which then acts in a secondary manner, or it has to damage the tissue after the tissue has undergone development. In some cases, teratogenesis can follow a single dose, and in other cases, administration of multiple doses are necessary. Long-term administration, or co-administration of compounds that stimulate the production of the metabolizing enzymes can also sometimes either reduce or increase the degree of teratogenicity by altering the relative concentrations of the parent compound and its metabolites. Sex, species, age, maternal weight, route of administration, etc. can all play their part. Sometimes the developing fetus is more sensitive to the agent than the mother, and sometimes less sensitive.

The difficulty in finding both a proper animal model and a set of conditions for teratogenesis testing, the varied potential end-points of the test (gross structure, internal organs, enzyme activity, behavior, hypertension, etc.) and the large number of compounds that have been shown to be teratogenic in animals, introduced a degree of chaos. Luckily, and as would be expected, many fewer compounds have been demonstrated to be teratogenic in man (29, 110, 184), although it is mainly the more visible malformations that have been sought.

INTRAUTERINE GROWTH RETARDATION (IUGR) vs. PREMATURITY

Brent and Jensh (27) stress in their review what is recognized now, the importance of distinguishing between *intrauterine growth retardation* (IUGR) and *prematurity*. The fomer term, *low birth weight,* should be used only to describe small infants for whom the gestational age is unknown, or generically, for a large heterogenous group of infants that include both IUGR and prematurity. IUGR should be used to describe small infants that have failed to maintain their expected growth potential at any of the stages of gestation. *Prematurity* should be used to describe infants of small size due to shortened gestation, i.e., usually below 37 weeks.

The effects of IUGR and prematurity can be manifest differently as differences in mortality, morbidity, congenital anomaly rates, and growth potential. Now that accurate growth data for the development of human fetuses has been obtained (85, 133, 134), it is possible to look for correlative effects of low, normal, or high birth weights; early, normal, or late parturition; twinning; disease states; genetic factors; drug administration; and the effects of other types of environmental agents (21, 86, 87, 153, 180, 198).

Brent and Jensh (27) reviewed the many etiological factors potentially responsible for either IUGR or prematurity. IUGR is primarily associated with the following conditions: a) nutritional deprivation, b) genetic and cytogenetic pathology, c) irradiation, d) clinical syndromes of unknown etiology, e) some drugs, or f) hypoxia and/or high altitude. Prematurity, on the other hand, may be associated with the following etiological categories: a) placenta praevia, b) abruptio placentae, c) placental separation, d) attempted abortion, e) acute uterine trauma, f) uterine tumors, g) uterine malformations, h) incompetent cervix, cervical prolapse, or other cervical pathology, or i) maternal haemorrhagic disease. In infants where there appears to be a combination of IUGR and prematurity, etiological factors may be among the following: a) placental dysfunction — both subacute and chronic, b) toxemia of pregnancy, c) maternal hypertensive disease, d) multiple births, e) smoking, f) certain drugs, or g) rubella, syphillis, toxoplasmosis, or cytomegalic inclusion disease.

With respect to prognosis, infants suffering primarily from IUGR demonstrate a quite variable prognosis. Nutritional deprivation, if not too extreme, is a least partially overcome by later growth. Other conditions causing IUGR can result in permanent retardation of growth or development.

Infants that are primarily of the premature type have higher mortality and morbidity rates and lag somewhat behind their full-term counterparts. Their growth potential is reasonably good. Thus, neurologic sequelae, associated with premature morbidity, is a much greater problem for these infants than is their postpartum physical growth lag.

Infants that show a combination of IUGR and prematurity are a heterogenous group from the standpoint of prognosis. For example, the infant from a toxemic pregnancy may show normal development while the infant exposed to rubella can be permanently affected.

Brent and Jensh sought to compare the ability of drugs to produce teratogenesis and/or growth retardation in animals. Few drugs fit neatly into the specified categories and it would be erroneous to list them here, out of context with their discussion. However, they categorized four groups: Group 1 — those for which teratogenic and growth retarding effects are essentially inseparable, Group 2 — those that produce a relatively specific teratogenic effect in the fetus or a recognizable syndrome, but for which there is a less predictable effect on fetal growth, Group 3 — drugs that are teratogenic but do not produce IUGR, and Group 4 — the largest group, those for which the therapeutic dose is neither teratogenic nor growth-retarding.

Several other primarily clinical reviews or books are recommended (1, 19, 93, 135).

CARCINOGENESIS

The problem of cancer in childhood raises a question of etiology. Is it possible that initiation could have occurred during the gestational or early postnatal period; and could an environmental agent have been involved?

Teratomas, for example, have been of long interest to both biologists and pathologists (165, 190). Teratomas can be considered to be congenital malformations that are also neoplasms, either benign or highly malignant. They can be of a relatively simple type or may be composed of many types of tissues. In some instances they produce structures that resemble embryonic stages of the host species (embryoid bodies). The teratocarcinogenic process resembles carcinogenesis in that it results in tumor formation, and parthenogenesis in that it results in the activation of development of the germ cells. Although teratomas can be found at other sites in the body, they are much more common in the gonads. Commonly used synonyms or subgroups of teratoma include: embryonal carinoma, embryoma, teratocarcinoma, disembryoma, dermoid cyst, and teratoid tumor.

Either sex can show a predilection for teratomas and the predilection varies between species. In humans, ovarian teratomas or dermoid cysts are common and are usually benign. In contrast, the homologous tumor in males is rare but is usually highly malignant.

The highly malignant choriocarcinoma, composed of cytotrophoblast and syncytial trophoblast is one of the teratomas. Friedman (75) considers that no clear dividing line can be drawn between the morphologically classic choriocarcinoma and many embryonic carcinomas. It is generally agreed that embryonic carcinoma is the precsursor of both the trophoblastic and the teratoid tumors.

Experimentally, teratomas can be produced in fowl by the administration of zinc or copper salts or by zinc salts plus gonadotropic hormone. In adult mice, teratomas can be produced by the administration again, of zinc or copper salts, or by copper salts plus testosterone. They can also be produced in fetal genital ridges by transplanting of the ridges to the testis of adults. Several reports (77, 103, 132, 164) have also indicated that the cryptorchid testis is more likely to undergo malignant transformation than the normal scrotal testis, in man.

Miller (147) reviewed data with respect to neoplasms in children that show mortality or morbidity peaks either below or above the age of five. For example, there is a peak of leukemia mortality at four years of age in United States white children, although not in the non-white population, which is attributable entirely to the acute lymphocytic rather than to the myelogenous form (38). There are also peaks in mortality, at about four with respect to Wilms' tumor (61) and neuroblastoma (148), cancers whose intrauterine origins are indicated not only by their early occurrence, but also by the frequency with which they are found *in situ,* at autopsy before three months of age but not thereafter (22). A similar age distribution is seen for primary liver cancer (71), and at least with respect to age at diagnosis, for adrenocortical neoplasia (70).

Neoplasms with peak morbidity below the age of five included retinoblastoma, rhabdomyosarcoma and teratoma, and several brain tumors: ependymoma, medulloblastoma, and basal cell nevis syndrome.

Neoplasms with mortality peaks above five years include gonadal tumors, lymphoma, and bone neoplasia.

Miller (147) now reports, in his epidemiological investigation, that some of the neoplasms above are accompanied by congenital defects. Thus, leukemia is associated with chromosomal abnormalities; medulloblastoma with certain phakomatoses (tuberous sclerosis and multiple neurofibromatosis); Wilms' tumor, primary liver cancer, and adrenocortical neoplasia with congenital hemihypertrophy, the hemihypertrophy in turn being associated with two other forms of growth excess, hamartomas and congenital visceral cytomegaly. Wilms' tumor was also associated with aniridia, independent of the hemihypertrophy. On the contrary, neuroblastoma, despite both epidemiologic and pathologic characteristics similar to the neoplasms that are found with hemihypertrophy, does not occur excessively with congenital defects. Finally, there was an increased incidence of lymphoma among persons with dysgenetic gonads.

Prenatal administration of a number of chemicals to animals can lead to the production of cancers up to one and one-half years after birth. In 1940, Law reported (127) that when he injected dibenz [a, h] anthracene into the amniotic fluid of fetal mice, he obtained 19 of 23 young that showed primary lung tumors at ages up to five months. A fibrocarcinoma in the skull area was also noted in one female, and a carcinoma of the liver, in addition to the carcinoma of the lung, was seen in a male. Control animals yielded only one carcinoma of the lung.

Larsen (126), Klein (119), and DiPaolo (52) obtained lung tumors following the prenatal administration of urethan. The incidence of tumor production increased both when administration was nearer to the time of delivery (52, 119, 126) and when the animals were maintained under hypoxic or hyperoxic conditions from the time of injection until birth (52).

More recently, Spatz and Laqueur (187) reported the production of tumors in the offspring of Sprague-Dawley rats fed a diet containing an extract from the Cycad plant, either during the first, second, or third week of gestation, or for the full three weeks of pregnancy. They obtained neoplasms on all schedules, with an overall incidence of 18.5% affected. Induction time for tumor formation was 6 to 16 months, similar to the length of time found earlier when Cycad meal was fed to young adult rats. The neoplasms were frequently found in the brain and jejunum, organs infrequently found to be involved in studies on older animals. The offending component is believed to be the glucoside of methylazoxymethanol, cycasin. This compound can be hydrolyzed by a microbial glucosidase present in the maternal intestine (124, 189) and the glucoside is not carcinogenic in germ-free animals (124, 125, 189). The glucoside can be hydrolyzed, however, in the skin of the embryo or young animal, but not in the skin of an older animal (188). Methylazoxymethanol is believed to be the more proximate carcinogen.

Ethyl nitrosourea (57), when administered to pregnant BD rats after the twelfth day of gestation, produced tumors of the brain, spinal cord, or peripheral nerves in progeny at postnatal ages of 150-300 days. Even a single dose as low as 5 mg/kg, corresponding to 2% of the LD_{50}, was effective (59). In subsequent work (58), tumors of the brain and peripheral nerves were obtained by single-day administration of 1,2-diethylhydrazine or azoxyethane (50 mg/kg, i.v., on day 15) or by azoethane inhalation (300 or 600 mg/kg for 1 hour). The overall incidence of tumors in the young was 94% (107 of 114) and the histological types of tumors were the same in all groups. The tumors were isomorphic (oligodendrogliomas, ependymomas, or astrocytomas) or polymorphic gliomas and gliosarcomas. Tumors were found in the brain, the spinal cord, the trigeminus vagus, or in the peripheral nerves (plexus brachialis and lumbosacralis). In contrast to the high yield of tumors in the young, only one brain tumor, four carcinomas of the ovaries and two nephroblastomas were found in the 32 treated mothers indicating, as had been found earlier with ethyl nitrosourea, the higher susceptibility of the prenatal nervous system. In contrast, following prenatal administration of hydrazo- and azoxymethane, no tumors were found in the young up to 525 days of age. These compounds, however, are potent carcinogens when administered to adult rats.

Prenatal (138) or postnatal (196) x-ray exposure of children can lead to the production of tumors.

The problem, therefore, of prenatal carcinogenic induction, as well as its possible relationship to congenital malformations is important. In humans, although the overall incidence is quite low, cancer is the second most common cause of death of childhood in Britain and in the United States (144). An editorial in *Lancet* (30) outlined the dimensions of the problem and called for increased centralization of activities in order to attack the problem in a more meaningful manner. It is stressed that, at present there is no general agreement on the entities that should be included as childhood cancer, and that if the natural history of childhood cancer is to be understood, some benign tumors will also have to be included and studied. They, and Miller (147), call for improved classification in this area, and for improvement of the histological basis of diagnosis.

DiPaolo and Kotin (53) reviewed possible relationships between teratogenesis and carcinogenesis.

GENETIC EFFECTS

Genetic effects from x-ray exposure of the germ cell line of Drosophila, in earlier experiments, and in mice (177) more recently, are unquestioned. In mice, the ability to obtain clear-cut results was made possible by the technique of breeding irradiated wild-type mice with mice homozygous for seven autosomal, recessive, visible traits. If a mutation occurred at one or more of the genetic loci under study, the offspring would appear abnormal. In humans, positive data are more difficult to obtain. Neel (157) surveyed the results obtained in the studies following the atomic bomb explosions and concluded, that of the various possible indicators of genetic damage employed, only with respect to one, the sex ratio, is there an effect which "taken in conjunction with the results of the other studies on the offspring of radiated individuals, appears to be of possible significance." The other studies included the demonstrated effects of radiation on somatic cells, such as chromosome damage both *in vivo* and *in vitro,* and the induction of leukemia. Follow-up reports continue on cytogenetic investigations of the *in utero* exposed of Hiroshima and Nagasaki (25). A more recent review of the effects of radiation on mammalian populations is that of Green (82).

Crow (54) presented the position for the study of chemicals as a potential source of mutagenesis in man. He argued, as does Neel for radiation, from the standpoint of the known effects on lower organisms and the common nature of DNA as the genetic material. He proposes tests for mutations and for cytogenetic effects, such as chromosome breakage, chromosome loss, non-disjunction, translocation, and deletion, either in infra-human species or in human tissue cultures. He also proposes a monitoring system for the human population in order to detect evidence of mutagenesis or chromosome damage. Rules for the standardization of human cytogenetics have been agreed upon (32). Soukop *et al.* (186) reported chromosome changes in animal embryos exposed to various teratogens.

There have been many theories of carcinogenesis, one of which is that carcinogenesis is associated with somatic mutation. Though inherently attractive, the concept has been difficult to test. It has been found, for example, that although some alkylating agents are both mutagenic and carcinogenic, no consistent correlation could be found for the majority of compounds studied (see 142). Some of the reasons for this may be: that many carcinogens have to be metabolized to active forms which may not be present under the conditions of the mutagenicity tests; the half-lives of some mutagens are so short that they may not survive long enough to get to their targets; and permeability barriers may prevent absorption of the compound in a mutagenicity or carcinogenicity test.

Maher *et al.* (142), in an *in vitro* system, demonstrated that the higher reactivities and mutagenicities of three derivatives of two carcinogenic amines toward a bacterial transformaing DNA, correlated well with the carcinogenicity of the compounds. They also found that the half-lives of two of the compounds at pH 7.5 and at room temperature, were indeed, very short, i.e., less than a minute and twelve minutes. Although they state that the mutational hypothesis is supported but not proven by this type of experiment, they suggest that mutagenicity assays in non-metabolizing systems appear to be, at least, useful tools for the determination of the active forms of chemicals.

Price *et al.* (172) recently determined the ability of a monofunctional nitrogen mustard to react at individual sites on nucleic acid bases. And Kihlman (114) wrote on the effects of chemicals on dividing cells.

In rats Alexander *et al.* (5) reported inherited abnormalities in three generations of offspring treated with LSD. The abnormalities included stillborns, deaths shortly after birth, and stunted young. The cause of the effect is unknown, and the data on effects of LSD have been highly contradictory. The report of Jacobson, in this volume, should be referred to for additional comments on LSD.

In addition to the possibility of mutation, chromosomal damage, or effects on the mitotic process, some compounds can damage the germ cell line and produce sterility. Thus, busulfan has been reported to produce sterility in rats (26) and marked hypoplasia of the ovaries and thyroid of an infant that was also hypotrophic (50); cyclophosphamide produced loss of the germ cell line in apparently normal rabbit embryos (76); and cadmium ion is destructive of testicular tissue, and its effect can be counteracted by zinc ion (33, 66, 163).

DNA repair, for some types of damage, is a process known in microorganisms (99). The extent to which this is operable in humans is unknown. The reviews in this volume by Legator and by Jacobson should be referred to.

BEHAVIORAL EFFECTS

Behavioral effects are, perhaps, among the most difficult indicators of toxicology to assess for relevance; the morphological correlates can be considerably less visible, and it is difficult, in many cases, to compare animal reactions and learning with the human situation. Effects can be of two types: retardation of learning ability, and emotionality. A few examples will be given.

The effects of androgens or estrogens administered at the end of gestation or in the first few days after birth in animals are now well known (131 179, 213). A single administration at the appropriate time can permanently alter the animals sex behavior. Recently, it was reported (13) that the progestational combination of norethynodrel plus mestranol, administered to mice as a single dose on either days 7, 10, 12, 15, or 17 of gestation, demonstrated two "critical periods." When administered on day 10, the male progeny isolated after weaning in order to induce aggressiveness, were less aggressive than controls in the test; when the drugs were given on day 17, however, the mice were more aggressive than were the controls.

Ordy *et al.* (160) reported behavioral effects of chlorpromazine administered prenatally, in addition to reporting many other effects on rat progeny (such as effects on birth weight, survival time, and activities of liver enzymes). The young, in these experiments, were cross-fostered in order to eliminate the possibility of postnatal transfer of drug via the milk.

Xintaras *et al.* (210, 211) studied the effects of ozone, carbon monoxide, and phenobarbital: 1) on the evoked electrophysiological response to a light flash, in unanethetized, unrestrained animals having steriotaxically implanted electrodes, and 2) on behavior, as measured by lever pressing for food reward. They found that the effect of ozone on the evoked EEG response was different from that of either carbon monoxide or phenobarbital. The latter two produced similar responses which were similar, again, to that obtained during the normal transition from wakefulness to spontaneous sleep. The lever pressing response was not affected with the concentrations of carbon monoxide used. Mention was not made of the effect, or lack of effect, of the other two agents on lever pressing.

OTHER DELAYED EFFECTS

Friedler and Cochin (72) found differences in the postnatal growth rates of young rats when the maternal rat received morphine sulfate for a six day period, terminating five days before mating, and the effect was unchanged even though the young were cross-fostered (73). More recently it has been found (74) that there is a reduced reaction of the young in hot-plate response, at 7 weeks of age, to a challenging dose of morphine sulfate.

Another delayed effect is that of the production of hypertension. Grollman and Grollman (84) demonstrated that increased blood pressure could be produced in rats, one year after birth, when maternal rats were administered either a high-sodium diet, low potassium diet, choline-free diet, aldosterone, cortisone, deoxycorticosterone, progesterone, or chlorthiazide. For a review of postnatal experimental work in rats and also the clinical and epidemiological investigations in infants and adults, on the question of a possible relationship between hypertension and increased intake of dietary sodium chloride the report of Guthrie (88) and the guest editorial of Dahl (43) should be referred to.

III. Some Potential Mediating Influences

THE PALACENTA

As evidenced, in part, by the four Rochester Trophoblast Conferences (137), a considerable amount of work has been done in recent years on the normal and abnormal development, pathology, and functional aspects of the placenta. Several good reviews of normal development and comparative morphology are those of Wynn (209), Wilkin (206), and Mossman (151). Normal and abnormal placental ultrastructure, as determined by electron microscopy, was reviewed by Wynn (208). Dawes (44) considered the placenta more from the physiological standpoint.

Pathology

Benirschke (23) reviewed placental abnormalities due to many causes and considered: twin placentas, the umbilical cord, tumors, abnormalities of the amnion and chorion, abnormalities of gross structure, abnormalities of the villous tissue, and inflammation of the placenta, membranes or umbilical cord. The villous tissue is the "exchange organ proper," and was discussed at length, although according to Benirschke, it was reported upon least. Aladjem (3) performed phase contrast microscopic examination of 900 normal and abnormal human placentas, from age six weeks to term. The samples included 25% from normal term pregnancies, 28% from prematurities (reported in greater detail subsequently (4), 13% from cases of preeclamptic toxemia, and the remainder were from ten other categories. Aladjem found that hypoplasia and edema were associated primarily with spontaneous abortion, abruptio placentae, prematurity and stillbirths, while the avascular villus and hyperplasia of the syncytium were associated primarily with diabetes, preeclampsia or prolonged pregnancy. An 11% incidence of perinatal mortality occurred when placental pathology was present, while only an 0.9% incidence was found when placental pathology was absent. Normal term pregnancies yielded a 15% incidence of "pathology" by the method used, while the other categories yielded similar or higher incidences, up to an 80% incidence. As stressed by Aladjem, the type of pathology was more important than the presence of indiscriminate pathology.

Transfer Function

Some reviews of transfer function in the placenta are those of Page (161), Moya and Thorndike (152) and Assali *et al.* (17). Page dealt with the range of small molecules to proteins and whole cells, Moya and Thorndike with drugs of major interest to the areas of obstetrics and anaesthesiology, and Assali *et al.* reviewed isotopic studies with anions, cations, the alkaline earth elements, carbohydrates, lipids, and proteins, as well as non-isotopic studies on the passage of respiratory gases, water, and electrolytes. Several mechanisms are available for transport, as outlined in the three reports.

Moya and Thorndike (152) concluded that, as in the case of the blood brain barrier, drugs cross the placenta as though the placenta had the characteristics of a lipoid barrier. Thus, the rate of transfer is primarily governed by the lipid solubility of the non-ionized form of the compound. Other factors such as concentration gradient and molecular weight appear to be of secondary import. They pointed out, however, that for multiple reasons, the majority of the studies reviewed were done under considerably less than optimal experimental conditions, a sentiment echoed by Assali *et al*· (17). Some of the difficulties, and the ways of circumventing them are outlined (17, 152, 166).

Important questions remain: under what conditions might transfer be altered, and when might this be detrimental or beneficial?

Flexner *et al.* (67) reported that ^{24}Na transport was half that of normal in a case of preeclamptic toxemia. Cox and Chalmers (39), following up this report, found two groups of toxemic patients, one in which no deviation occurred (14 cases), and another in which sodium transport was from a third to half that in uncomplicated pregnancies (7 cases). McGaughey *et al.* (140) studied transport of both antipyrine and sodium and concluded that the transport of antipyrine varied in both directions from the norm, and that transport of sodium followed that found with antipyrine, a result at some variance with those above. And Clemetson and Churchman (36), reported reduced transport of amino acids in mild toxemia and a greater reduction in severe toxemia.

In a study designed to attempt the alteration of transport of antigenic determinants Nathan *et al.* (156) studied the responsiveness of rabbit progeny to maternal skin transplants following treatment of the pregnant rabbit. They found that skin transplants were retained longer in progeny of rabbits that received a single low dose of hyaluronidase in addition to the maternal antigen, when compared to antigen treatment alone. Najarian and Dixon (155) subsequently found that repeated high doses of hyaluronidase or histamine, but not chymotrypsin, from days 11 to term, allowed the transplants to survive longer. A few of the progeny even showed tolerance to a second transplant. In a few cases, reverse transplants (i.e., from progeny to mother) survived, indicating a reciprocal transfer of antigen. Reciprocal transfer, however, was demonstrable for about half of the cases. More recently, Tai and Halasz (191) found some tolerance when non-maternal rather than maternal antigens were administered along with the high doses of hyaluronidase. Like Najarian and Dixon, they found evidence for reciprocal transfer, that is, both maternal-fetal and fetal-maternal transfer. Uteroplacental trauma, at mid-gestation, was tried, but with modest success (149).

Assali *et al.* (17), in reviewing the transfer of oxygen across the sheep placenta, as studied by his group (118, 136) and by that of Dawes (45), concluded that transfer and consumption of oxygen remain relatively stable, due largely to reciprocal changes between blood flow and arteriovenous oxygen difference. Only when one of these parameters changes drastically does transfer and consumption change. Conditions that were able to alter transfer or consumption of oxygen were circulatory shock, hyperbaric oxygenation, and the breathing of 6% oxygen.

Finally, Hensleigh and Krantz (95)

perfused human placentas *in vitro,* and found that either oxytocin or papaverine, when added to the perfusion medium, reduced the rate of transport of added ascorbic acid. Meperidine and a mixture of synthetic progestins, however, did not show the effect. The authors rightly point out that these are very important findings. "If the amount of oxytocin in labor, natural or employed, achieves this effect with ascorbic acid, what does it do to other necessary compounds? . . . In addition, apparently innocuous compounds may play a significant role in maternal: fetal transfer. This would require us to re-examine many of our accepted therapeutic agents as well as methods of evaluation."

Blood Flow

Blood flow via the placenta is a process dependent upon several regional blood flows: flow to the uterus, flow in the uterine tissue, flow in the placenta itself, flow in the umbilical vessels, and flow in the fetus (16, 46, 47, 201). Some of these flows are subject to neural regulation while others are not.

Flow has been measured by several techniques and on several types of preparations. It has been measured by passage or dilution of marker compounds such as nitrous oxide, 4-aminoantipyrene, ^{22}Na or ^{24}Na, by the use of electromagnetic flow meters attached directly to blood vessels, or by the volume of fluid collected in perfusion experiments. It has been measured *in vivo* in the gravid uterus, or *in vitro* on isolated placentas or on the umbilical cord.

The degree of flow will regulate both the amount of oxygen and other nutrient that is supplied to the fetus, and the rate at which waste can be removed. It is also a factor in the proper maintenance of fluid balance in the various fluid compartments (e.g., amniotic fluid and fetus).

Panigel (162) reviewed placental perfusion experiments that were carried out prior to 1962, both preliminary to the study of placental anatomy and for the study of vasomotor responsiveness. He reviewed initial studies that had been performed on the responses of the umbilical cord arteries, the umbilical cord vein, on isolated perfused placental cotyledons and on the whole placenta. Gautieri and his co-workers (34, 35, 202, 203) and Klinge *et al.* (120) studied the effects of many contrictor and dilator substances and their antagonists on flow through isolated, perfused human placentas. Marley *et al.* (143) investigated the embryotoxic action of 5-hydroxytryptamine *in vivo,* in rats, using ^{22}Na. They found that transport of the ^{22}Na was inhibited following the 5-hydroxytryptamine. And Assali and Dilts (16) presented both their data and a critique of the various methods for determination of blood flow.

Enzymatic and Hormonal Capabilities

The placenta contains many enzymes (89, 199). Hagerman (89) concludes that the placenta is an organ of very generalized metabolic capabilities, containing many of the capabilities of liver, kidneys, and lungs, combined. Not only does the placenta contain enzymes related to the normal cellular reactions of anabolism and catabolism and those related to steroid metabolism, but also, at least one enzyme which is inducible by an environmental agent. Thus, while benzpyrene hydroxylating activity was below detectable levels when placental homogenates from non-smoking women were incubated *in vitro,* the placentas from women who smoked 10-30 cigarettes daily metabolized benzpyrene quite well (205). There was, however, not a dose-response relationship for possible reasons listed. When, however, a single dose of benzpyrene was administered to rats on day 19 of gestation, benzpyrene hydroxylating activity increased within a 24 hour period according to a normal dose-response relationship. The role of interactions of this type in the general well-being of the mother and fetus are interesting to contemplate. An excellent review of the nature and implications of microsomal enzyme induction, in general, has appeared (37).

The human placenta can synthesize the two protein hormones, human chorionic gonadotropin and human placental lactogen. In addition, it can synthesize gestagens including progesterone, and estrogens such as estriol, 17β-estradiol, and estrone. The interrelationships of biosynthesis and degradation in the "fetoplacental unit" and in the mother are highly complex. The comprehensive reviews of Diczfalusy (51) Simmer (183) and Solomon and Friesen (185) should be sought for details of biosynthesis, metabolism, and the roles of the hormones.

THE IMMATURE STATUS OF THE FETUS

The organs of the fetus develop at different rates, and thus the fetus manifests varying degrees of immaturity of structure or of function at different stages of its development. The immaturity of the fetus can be considered with respect to enzymes, hormones, metabolic processes, cell types and organs, or on the basis of pharmacologic responses.

The development of enzymes and metabolic pathways was reviewed by Herrmann and Tootle (96) and by Sereni and Principi (181), as was the biochemical basis of immaturity by Kretchmer *et al.* (122). Some enzymes are present early in gestation and develop over a period of time to the adult levels. Still others are seen at an early time but wane as development proceeds. Others cannot be detected until the last days before parturition or do not become manifest until the first days or weeks after birth. Thus, microsomal drug metabolizing enzymes develop at the end of gestation and soon after birth (60, 68, 69, 104) while the skin of the fetal golden hamster contains a glucosidase activity that wanes in the early postnatal period (188).

Enzyme induction has been studied for many years for both the microsomal and non-microsomal enzymes. It is also known that many drugs and chemicals can induce the microsomal enzymes (37, 121). Is it possible that enzyme induction in the fetus, placenta or mother, in response to drugs or other chemicals, might present a hazard; might it be beneficial or might induction be used therapeutically? Induction would present a hazard if innocuous compounds were metabolized to active metabolites. Although inactivation is more common, there are many examples of activation by metabolism (168). If hazardous compounds were converted to compounds of lesser hazard, the effect would potentially be beneficial. An example of the latter was given in the last section. Induction of a placental enzyme converted a more carcinogenic compound to less carcinogenic metabolites (205).

Therapeutically, an attempt has been made to induce the activity of the conjugating enzyme that combines glucuronic acid with bilirubin. Following the first reports that phenobarbital administration reduced bilirubin levels in two children under the age of one (40, 212), and other reports that indicated a more variable response, which was possibly dependent upon the nature of the genetic defect (41, 49, 176), Trolle (197) reported reduced serum bilirubin levels following phenobarbital administration in the first week of life, and Maurer *et al.* (146) found similar results when administration was in the last two weeks before delivery. In four adult patients with obstructive jaundice, Thompson and Williams (194) found up to a 50% reduction of serum bilirubin.

Hormones develop in the fetal organs according to varying time schedules. Jost published much on the potential role of hormones produced by the fetus (105, 106, 107). The fetus participates as part of an active feto-placental unit for synthesis and degradation of the steroids.

At the level of the organs, some organs develop quite early, while others complete their development later in gestation or even long after birth. The kidney, for example, continues to develop in childhood, and the reproductive organs renew their development after a lag of many years. Also, while mylenization of some nerves had already been known to extend into the postnatal period, it has now been demonstrated that some neurons (7, 11) and glial cells (6) continue their development postnatally, even in the guinea pig which is fairly mature at birth (12). The newer cells, as studied in the rat (9, 10) and kitten (8), are also more sensitive to irradiation.

Pharmacologic responses to drugs and environmental chemicals are dependent upon the above levels of maturity. Done (55, 56) reviewed the degree of sensitivity to drugs during the latter stages of gestation (from 27 weeks in the human) and in the perinatal period. It should be well recognized by now that for many drugs and other chemicals, the fetus and infant cannot be considered as a smaller version of the adult.

MECHANICAL PRESSURES

Browne (28) recently summarized all of his work. He attempted to demonstrate how intrauterine postures or pressures might lead to the production of a variety of malformations. He discussed four classes of conditions: malposition, increased spatial pressure, increased hydrostatic pressure, and membranous perforation. The third, increased hydrostatic pressure, will be considered here because of a more direct, potential association with pharmacology and toxicology.

Grabowski and his co-workers, in their studies on the mechanism of teratogenic action of hypoxia (78), and more recently on that of epinephrine and vasopressin (31), demonstrated what they call the "edema syndrome." Short term hypoxia with 6% oxygen, yielded a transient edema in chicks, followed by the formation of clear subcutaneous blisters and hematomas (78). The sites of malformations correlated with the sites of production of hematomas. Subsequently, (79) Grabowski found that mild hypoxia caused a reduction of the differences that are normally present in the concentrations of serum and extraembryonic fluid anions, cations, and carbon dioxide. Time-lapse photography (80) further clarified the picture and demonstrated, in addition, general swelling of the fetus, transient swelling of the neural tube and flexion of the fetus. Measurement of embryonic blood pressure (81) showed that the peak of increase coincided with the time of maximum occurrence of hemmorhage of blood vessels. Grabowski (78) reviewed other reports that indicate a possible edema syndrome in chicks, amphibia and mammals, both resulting from environmental manipulation or from genetic factors.

Chernoff (31) demonstrated that vasopressin or epinephrine, administered to rats on day 17 of gestation, produced limb abnormalities after 15 hours. He demonstrated, further, that both the heart beat and blood pressure of the fetus decreased in proportion to the dose, and that necrotic loci (opacities) and hemmorhages occurred prior to the restoration of normal circulation. The virtually complete cessation of circulation observed, was opposite to the effect produced in adult animals.

Meclizine produces a biphasic effect on the volume of amniotic fluid of rats (112). This compound and several other benzhydrylpiperazine drugs, produce cleft palate, micrognathia, fusion of the tongue to the palate, and shortened limbs and edema at higher doses in the fetus, when administered to pregnant rats or mice (115, 116, 117). Posner and Darr (169, 170) found that an increased water content of the fetus could be demonstrated at doses of drug that were on the dose-response curve for cleft palate formation. Edema occurred partly in the thorax and caused an approximately 25% increase in thoracic cross-sectional area, at a dose of drug that produced a 50% incidence of cleft palate. The thoracic edema was found on days 17 and 18 of gestation. In addition, there was a 1-2 day delay in closure of the 50% of the palates that succeeded in closing (167). It was hypothesized that some of the facial malformations might result secondary to production of the edema (170).

The earlier work of Holtfreter, on the effects of chemical and mechanical factors in development, can be entered via one of his reports (98).

IV. Overcoming Genetic Defects

Reference has been made, primarily, to the ability of chemicals to interfere with normal development so as to produce aberrations. Part of man's ills, however, are the result of defective genetic information, such that development is aberrant despite the presence of a normal environment. McKusick (141) catalogued an annotated bibliography of almost 1500 dominant, recessive and X-linked human conditions. Many collections are available for the lower animals. If one wished to think broadly, the concept of "toxicity of genes", could be stated. The next step would then be to think in terms of diagnosis and treatment, in the same way that one would for an environmental toxicant. Eugenics was discussed for many years. Now euphenics is also being discussed.

Euphenics is a concept and area of endeavor, that aims at the optimalization of biologic development rather than at modification of genes, themselves. Control of development, as Lederberg states (128, 129), changes both the means and the ends of eugenics, and opens the way for a more comprehensive eugenics partly through the systematization of the knowledge of gene action. Euphenics has been alternately referred to as "the engineering of human development."

Tatum (193) reviewed the differences between eugenics, genetic engineering, and euphenic engineering.

For example, postnatally, either treatment of children with Human Growth Hormone to compensate for hypopituitarism (94), or lowering the amount of phenylalanine or galactose in the diets of either phenylketonuric or galactosemic children, respectively, are types of euphenic modulation. The treatment permits a more normal development in the face of a genetic defect although it does not correct the gene, itself. Likewise, treatment of a strain of mice that genetically develops ataxia, by feeding pregnant mice a diet very high in manganese, normalizes development of the inner ear and prevents production of the ataxia (63, 101). This, too, is euphenic modulation. The latter can be obtained in phenocopy, by feeding genetically normal pregnant mice a low-manganese diet (63). Thus, the extension drawn to "genetic toxicities" is not unreasonable, at the very least with respect to the study of the mechanisms of pathologic development.

V. Newer Techniques of Diagnosis and Drug Administration

Kumar (123) outlined methods of diagnosis that are available for assessing the status of the developing fetus and placenta. Some are commonly used and others are not because of the excessive hazard or because the techniques are still in an experimental stage.

In addition to important clinical examinations that are outlined, he discusses: hormone assays on maternal urine or serum and the examination of vaginal cells for known hormonal effects; gross examination of the amniotic fluid as well as for respiratory gases, bilirubin, steroids or for the chromosomal status of fetal cells that slough into the fluid; placental function by blood flow, atropine transfer or by placental biopsy; direct examination of the fetus by ultrasound, EEG, ECG, phonocardiography, cardiotacography, or by fetal scalp blood analyses; and maternal serum protein and enzyme analyses. In addition, scanning the placenta after administration of radionuclide (42, 195) and thermoplacentography (175) have also been applied. Three methods for amniotic fluid analysis for erythroblastosis faetalis (bilirubin analyses) have been compared (174) and the applicability and acceptability of the fetal scalp blood method has been considered (192).

Queenan (173) prepared a monograph on the modern management of the Rh problem. In it he discusses intrauterine exchange transfusion, contrast radiography, amniotic fluid analysis, and amniocentesis.

Direct fetal surgery and transfusion is being practiced in primates but it is still a very highly experimental technique in the human (15).

Of the types of intrauterine treatment possible, Kumar (123) mentions intrauterine transfusion as the one practiced most. It is reviewed in the book by Queenan (173) and also in a chapter by Montague (150). Blood is injected into the peritonium of the fetus. When this is done, the erythrocytes are absorbed from the peritoneal cavity into the fetal blood stream. It should also be possible to administer other substances this way.

Since the fetus swallows amniotic fluid, drugs could also be administered into the amniotic fluid. Drug would then be absorbed via the fetal, oral route. Intramuscular injection of the fetus is also a possibility.

In all of these instances, the ability of the therapeutic agent to pass the placenta in an active form should be balanced against the safety and effectiveness of the intrauterine route.

Examinaiton of the newborn is discussed by Avery et al. (18) .

Summary

Some aspects of pharmacology and toxicology associated with prenatal growth and development have been considered. Although drugs and other chemicals were primarily discussed, some of the considerations could also apply to physical and microbiological agents. In all, an attempt has been made to concentrate on approaches to a fairly wide number of problems, considering some of these in depth.

REFERENCES

1. Abramowicz, M., and Kass, E. H.: Pathogenesis and prognosis of prematurity. New Engl. J. Med., *275*:878-85, 935-43, 1001-7, 1053-59, 1966.
2. Adamsons, Jr., K., and Joellson, I.: The effects of pharmacologic agents upon the fetus and newborn. Am. J. Obstet. Gynec., *96*:437-60, 1966.
3. Aladjem, S.: Phase contrast microscopic observations of the human placenta from six weeks to term. Obstet. Gynec., *32*:28-39, 1968.
4. Aladjem, S.: Placenta of the premature infant. Am. J. Obstet. Gynec., *102*:311-12, 1968.
5. Alexander, G. J., Machiz, S., and Alexander, R. B.: Inherited abnormalities in three generations of offspring of LSD-treated rats. Federation Proc., *27*:No. 2, 220, 1968.
6. Altman, J.: Proliferation and migration of undifferentiated precursor cells in the rat during postnatal gliogenesis. Exptl. Neurol., *16*:263-78, 1966.
7. Altman, J.: Autoradiographic and histological studies of postnatal neurogenesis. II. J. Comp. Neurol., *128*:431-74, 1966.
8. Altman, J., Anderson, W. J., and Wright, K. A.: Selective destruction of precursors of microneurons of the cerebellar cortex with fractionated low-dose x-rays. Exptl. Neurol., *17*:481-97, 1967.
9. Altman, J., Anderson, W. J., and Wright, K. A.: Gross morphological consequences of irradiation of the cerebellum in infant rats with repeated doses of low-level x-ray. Exptl. Neurol., *21*:69-91, 1968.
10. Altman, J., Anderson, W. J., and Wright, K. A.: Differential radio-sensitivity of stationary and migratory primitive cells in the brains of infant rats. Exptl. Neurol., *22*:52-74, 1968.
11. Altman, J., and Das, G.D.: Autoradiographic and histological studies of postnatal neurogenesis I. A longitudinal investigation of the kinetics, migration and transformation of cells incorporating tritiated thymidine in neonate rats, with special reference to postnatal neurogenesis in some brain regions. J. Comp. Neurol., *126*:337-90, 1966.
12. Altman, J., and Das, G. D.: Postnatal neurogenesis in the guinea pig. Nature, *214*:1098-1101, 1967.
13. Antonita, Sr. M., Scudder, C., and Karczmar, A.: The effect of norethynodrel with mestranol treatment of female mice on the isolation induced agression of their male offspring. The Pharmacologist, *10*:No. 2, 168, 1968.
14. Apgar, V., and Stickle, G.: Birth defects: their significance as a public health problem. J.A.M.A,. *204*:371-74, 1968.
15. Asensio, S. H., Figuero-Longo, J. G., and Pelegrina, I. A.: Intrauterine exchange transfusion. Obstet. Gynec., *32*:350-55, 1968.
16. Assali, N. S., and Dilts, Jr. P. V.: Uteroplacental circulation. in *Biology of Gestation*, Vol. 1. Assali, N. S. (Ed.) , Academic Press, N. Y., 1968, 186-203.
17. Assali, N. S., Kirschbaum, T., and Gross, S.: Placental transfer—transport systems and transfer of specific substances. in *Biology of Gestation*, Vol 1. Assali, N. S. (Ed.) . Academic Press, N. Y., 1968, 250-73.

18. Avery, G. B., Kraybill, E. N., and Mullick, U. C.: Examination of the newborn infant. G. P., *37*:78-94, 1968.
19. Babson, S. G., and Benson, R. C.: *Primer on Prematurity and High-risk Pregnancy*. C. V. Mosby Co., St. Louis, 1966.
20. Baker, J. B. E.: The effects of drugs on the foetus. Pharmacol. Rev., *12*:37-90, 1960.
21. Battaglia, F. C., Frazier, T. M., and Hellegers, A. E.: Birth weight, gestational age, and pregnancy outcome, with special reference to high birth weight — low gestational age infant. Pediatrics, *37*:417-22, 1966.
22. Beckwith, J. B., and Perrin, E. V.: *In situ* neuroblastomas: a contribution to the natural history of neural crest tumors. Amer. J. Path., *43*:1089-1104, 1963.
23. Benirschke, K.: A review of the pathologic anatomy of the human placenta. Am. J. Obstet. Gynec., *84*:1595-1622, 1962.
24. Binns, W., James, L. F., Shupe, J. L., and Everett, G.: A congenital cyclopian-type malformation in lambs induced by maternal ingestion of a range plant, Veratrum californicum. Am. J. Vet. Res., *24*:1164-75, 1963.
25. Bloom, A. D., Neriishi, S., and Archer, P. G.: Cytogenetics of the *in-utero* exposed of Hiroshima and Nagasaki. Lancet, *2:* No. 7558, 10-12, 1968.
26. Bollag, W.: Der einfluss von Myleran auf die keimdrüsen von ratten. Experientia, *9*:268, 1953.
27. Brent, R. L., and Jensh, R. P.: Intrauterine growth retardation. Adv. Teratology, *2*:139-227, 1967.
28. Browne, D.: A mechanistic interpretation of certain malformations. Adv. Teratology, *2*:11-36, 1967.
29. Cahen, R. L.: Experimental and clinical chemoteratogenesis. Adv. Pharmacol., *4*:263-349, 1966.
30. Cancer in children. Lancet, *2:* No. 7558, 32-3, 1968.
31. Chernoff, N.: Effects of vasopressin and adrenalin on fetal blood pressure. Teratology, *2*:212-13, 1968.
32. Chicago conference: standardization in human cytogenetics. Birth Defects Original Article Series *2:* No. 2, 1-21, 1966.
33. Chiquoine, A. D.: Effect of cadmium chloride on the pregnant albino mouse. J. Reprod. Fertil., *10*:263-65, 1965.
34. Ciuchta, H. P., and Gautieri, R. F.: Effects of certain drugs on perfused human placentas II. Vasodilators. J. Pharm. Sci., *52*:974-78, 1963.
35. Ciuchta, H. P., and Gautieri, R. F.: Effects of certain drugs on perfused human placentas III. Sympathomimetics, acetylcholine and histamine. J. Pharm. Sci., *53*:184-88, 1964.
36. Clemetson, C. A. B., and Churchman, J.: The placental transfer of amino acids in normal and toxaemic pregnancy. J. Obstet. Gynaec. Brit. Emp., *61*:364-71, 1954.
37. Conney, A. H.: Pharmacologic implications of microsomal enzyme induction. Pharmacol. Rev., *19*:317-66, 1967.
38. Court Brown, W. M., and Doll, R.: Leukaemia in childhood and young adult life. Trends in mortality in relation to aetiology. Brit. Med. J., *1*:981-88, 1961.
39. Cox, L. W., and Chalmers, T. A.: The effect of pre-eclamptic toxaemia on the exchange of sodium in the body and the transfer of sodium across the placenta, measured by ^{24}Na tracer methods. J. Obstet. Gynec. Brit. Emp., *60*:214-21, 1953.
40. Crigler, Jr., J. F., and Gold, N. I.: Sodium phenobarbital-induced decrease in serum bilirubin in an infant with congenital nonhemolytic jaundice and kernicterus. J. Clin. Invest., *45*:998-99, 1966.
41. Crigler, Jr., J. F., and Gold, N. I.: Effect of sodium phenobarbital on the metabolism of bilirubin-^{3}H and ^{14}C in an infant with congenital nonhemolytic jaundice and kernicterus. J. Clin. Invest., *46*:1047, 1967.
42. Curry, G. C., and Bonte, F. J.: Radionuclide scanning of the placenta in abdominal pregnancy. J.A.M.A., *203*:225-7, 1968.
43. Dahl, L. K.: Salt in processed baby foods. Am. J. Clin. Nutrition, *21*:787-92, 1968.
44. Dawes, G. S.: *Foetal and Neonatal Physiology*. Yearbook Medical Publishers, Inc., Chicago, 1968, pp. 18-78.
45. Dawes, G. S.: *Ibid.*, Chap. 3.
46. Dawes, G. S.: *Ibid.*, Chap. 5.
47. Dawes, G. S.: *Ibid.*, Chap. 6.
48. Dekaban, A. S.: Abnormalities in children exposed to X-radiation during various stages of gestation: tentative timetable of radiation injury to the human fetus, Part 1. J. Nucl. Med., *9*:471-77, 1968.
49. DeLeon, A., Gartner, L., and Arias, I. M.: The effect of phenobarbital on hyperbilirubinemia in glucuronyl transferase deficient rats. J. Lab. Clin. Med., *70*:273-78, 1967.
50. Diamond, I., Anderson, M. M., and McCreadie, S. R.: Transplacental transmission of busulfan (Myleran) in a mother with leukemia. Pediatrics, *25*:85-90, 1960.
51. Diczfalusy, E.: Endocrine functions of the human fetoplacental unit. Federation Proc, *23:* 791-98, 1964.
52. DiPaolo, J. A.: Effects of oxygen concentration on carcinogenesis induced by transplacental exposure to urethan. Cancer Res., *22*:299-304, 1962.

53. DiPaolo, J. A., and Kotin, P.: Teratogenesis-oncogenesis: a study in possible relationships. Arch. Pathology, *81*:3-23, 1966.

54. Do chemicals sow seeds of genetic change? Med. World News, 21-23, April 28, 1968.

55. Done, A. K.: Developmental pharmacology. Clin. Pharmacol. Therap., *5*:423-79, 1964.

56. Done, A. K.: Perinatal pharmacology. Ann. Rev. Pharmacol., *6*:189-208, 1966.

57. Druckrey, H., Ivankovic, S., and Preussmann, R.: Teratogenic and carcinogenic effects in the offspring after single injection of ethylnitrosourea to pregnant rats. Nature, *210*:1378-79, 1966.

58. Druckrey, H., Ivankovic, S., Preussmann, R., Landschütz, C., Stekar, J., Brunner, U., and Schagen, B.: Transplacental induction of neurogenic malignomas by 1,2-diethylhydrazine, azo-, and azoxyethane in rats. Experientia, *24:* 561-2, 1968.

59. Druckrey, H., Preussmann, R., Ivankovic, S., and Schmähl, D.: Organotropic carcinogenic effects of 65 different n-nitroso-compounds on BD-rats. Z. Krebsforschung, *69*:103-201, 1967

60. Dutton, G. J., Langelaan, D. E., and Ross. P. E.: High glucuronide synthesis in newborn liver: choice of species and substrate. Biochem. J., *93*:4P, 1964.

61. Ederer, F., Miller, R. W., and Scotto, J.: U. S. childhood cancer mortality patterns, 1950-1959: etiological implications. J.A.M.A., *192*:593-96, 1965.

62. Eighth Revision *International Classification of Diseases:* Adapted for Use in the United States (ICDA). Vol. 1, Public Health Service Publ. No. 1693, U. S. Govt. Printing Office, 1968.

63. Erway, L., Hurley, L. S., and Fraser, A.: Neurological defect: manganese in phenocopy and prevention of a genetic abnormality of inner ear. Science, *152*:1766-68, 1966.

64. Fave, A.: Les embryopathies provoquées chez les mammiferes. Thérapie, *1*:1-122, 1964.

65. Ferm, V. H., and Carpenter, S. J.: Developmental malformations resulting from the administration of lead salts. Exptl. Molec. Path., *7*:208-13, 1967.

66. Ferm, V. H., and Carpenter, S. J.: The relationship of cadmium and zinc in experimental mammalian teratogenesis. Lab. Investig., *18:* 429-32, 1968.

67. Flexner, L. B., Cowie, D. B., Hellman, L. M., Wilde, W. S., and Vosburgh, G. J.: The permeability of the human placenta to sodium in normal and abnormal pregnancies and the supply of sodium to the human fetus as determined with radioactive sodium. Am. J. Obstet. Gynec., *55*:469-80, 1948.

68. Fouts, J. R, and Adamson, R. H.: Drug metabolism in the newborn rabbit. Science, *129:* 897-98, 1959.

69. Fouts, J. R., and Hart, L. G.: Hepatic drug metabolism during the perinatal period. Ann. N. Y. Acad. Sci., *123*:245-51, 1965.

70. Fraumeni, Jr., J. F., and Miller, R. W.: Adrenocortical neoplasms with hemihypertrophy, brain tumors, and other disorders. J. Pediat., *70*:129-38, 1967.

71. Fraumeni, Jr., J. F., Miller, R. W., and Hill, J. A.: Primary carcinoma of the liver in childhood: an epidemiological study. J. Nat. Cancer Inst., *40*:1087-99, 1968.

72. Friedler, G., and Cochin, J.: Altered post-natal growth pattern of offspring of female rats chronically treated with morphine prior to mating. The Pharmacologist, *9:* No. 2, 230, 1967.

73. Friedler, G., and Cochin, J.: The effect of cross-fostering on growth patterns in offspring of morphinized and withdrawn female rats. Federation Proc., *27:* No. 2, 754, 1968.

74. Friedler, G., and Cochin, J.: Sensitivity and tolerance to morphine sulfate (MS) in the rat as affected by neonatal thymectomy or MS-pretreatment of the mother. The Pharmacologist, *10:* No. 2, 188, 1968.

75. Friedman, N. B.: Choriocarcinoma of the testis and extragenital choriocarcinoma in men. Ann. N. Y. Acad. Sci., *80*:161-77, 1959.

76. Gerlinger, P., and Clavert, J.: Action des cyclophosphamide injecté à des lapines gestantes sur les gonades embryonnairres. Compt. Rend., *258*:2899-2901, 1964.

77. Gilbert, J. B., and Hamilton, J. B.: Studies in malignant testis tumors III. Incidence and nature of tumors in ectopic testes. Surg. Gynecol. Obstet., *71*:731-43, 1940.

78. Grabowski, C. T.: The etiology of hypoxia-induced malformations in the chick embryo. J. Exptl. Zool., *157*:307-26, 1964.

79. Grabowski, C. T.: Physiological changes in the bloodstream of chick embryos exposed to teratogenic doses of hypoxia. Developmental Biol., *13*:199-213, 1966.

80. Grabowski, C. T., and Schroeder, R. E.: A time-lapse photographic study of chick embryos exposed to teratogenic doses of hypoxia. J. Embryol. Exp. Morph., *19*:347-62, 1968.

81. Grabowski, C. T., and Tsai, E. N. C.: The effects of teratogenic doses of hypoxia on the blood pressure of 3-day chick embryos. Teratology, *1*:215, 1968.

82. Green E. L.: Genetic effects of radiation on mammalian populations. Ann. Rev. Genetics, *2*:87-120, 1968.

83. Gregg, N. M.: Congenital cataract following

German Measles in the mother. Trans. Ophthalmol. Soc. Australia, *3*:35-46, 1941.

84. Grollman, A., and Grollman, E. F.: The teratogenic induction of hypertension. J. Clin. Investig., *41*:710-14, 1962.
85. Gruenwald, P.: Growth of the human fetus I. Normal growth and its variation. Am. J. Obstet. Gynec., *94*:1112-19, 1966.
86. Gruenwald, P.: Growth of the human fetus II. Abnormal growth in twins and infants of mothers with diabetes, hypertension, or isoimmunization. Am. J. Obstet. Gynec., *94*:1120-32, 1966.
87. Gruenwald, P., Funakawa, H., Mitani, S., Nishimura, T., and Takeuchi, S.: Influence of environmental factors on foetal growth in man. Lancet, *1*:1026-29, 1967.
88. Guthrie, H. A.: Infant feeding practices — a predisposing factor in hypertension? Am. J. Clin. Nutrition, *21*:863-67, 1968.
89. Hagerman, D. D.: Enzymatic capabilities of the placenta. Federation Proc., *23*:785-90, 1964.
90. Hale, F.: The relation of vitamin A to anophthalmos in pigs. Am. J. Ophth., *18*:1087-93, 1935.
91. Hale, F.: Relation of maternal vitamin A deficiency to microphthalmia in pigs. Texas State J. Med., *33*:228-32, 1937.
92. Hardy, J. B.: Viruses and the fetus. Postgraduate Med., 156-65, 1968.
93. Harper, P. A., and Wiener, G.: Sequelae of low birth weight. Ann. Rev. Med., *16*:405-20, 1965.
94. Henneman, P. H.: The effect of human growth hormone on growth of patients with hypopituitarism: a combined study. J.A.M.A., *205*:828-36, 1968.
95. Hensleigh, P. A., and Krantz, K E.: Extracorporeal perfusion of the human placenta I. Placental transfer of ascorbic acid. Am. J. Obstet. Gynec., *96*:5-13, 1966.
96. Herrmann, H., and Tootle, M. L.: Specific and general aspects of the development of enzymes and metabolic pathways. Physiol. Rev., *44*: 289-371, 1964.
97. Hicks, S. P., and D'Amato, C. J.: Effects of ionizing radiations on mammalian development. Adv. Teratol., *1*:195-250, 1966.
98. Holtfreter, J.: Differential inhibition of growth and differentiation by mechanical and chemical means. Anat. Rec., *93*:59-74, 1945.
99. Howard-Flanders, P.: DNA repair. Ann. Rev. Biochem., *37*:175-200, 1968.
100. Hurley, L. S. (Ed.) : Nutrition and prenatal development. Federation Proc., *27:* No. 1, 162-204, 1968.
101. Hurley, L. S.: Approaches to the study of nutrition in mammalian development. Federation Proc., *27:* No. 1, 193-98, 1968.
102. Inhorn, S. L.: Chromosomal studies of spontaneous human abortions. Adv. Teratology, *2:* 37-99, 1967.
103. Johnson, D. E., Woodhead, D. M., Pohl, D. R., and Robison, J. R.: Cryptorchism and testicular tumorigenesis Surgery, *63*:919-22, 1968.
104. Jondorf, W. R., Maickel, R. P., and Brodie, B. B.: Inability of newborn mice and guinea pigs to metabolize drugs. Biochem. Pharmacol., *1:* 352-54, 1959.
105. Jost, A.: Anterior pituitary function in foetal life, in The Pituitary Gland, Harris, G. W., and Donovan, B. T. (Eds.) Univ. California Press, Berkeley, Vol. 2, 299-323, 1966.
106. Jost, A.: Problems of fetal endocrinology: the adrenal glands. Recent progr. Hormone Res., *22*:541-74, 1966.
107. Jost, A.: Full or partial maturation of fetal endocrine systems under pituitary control. Perspectives in Biol. and Med., 371-4, Spring 1968.
108. Kalter, H.: *Teratology of the Central Nervous System*. Univ. Chicago Press, Chicago, 1968.
109. Kalter, H., and Warkany, J.: Experimental production of congenital malformations in mammals by metabolic procedure. Physiol. Rev., *39*:69-115, 1959.
110. Karnofsky, D. A.: Drugs as teratogens in animal and man. Ann. Rev. Pharmacol., *5*:447-72, 1965.
111. Keeler, R. F., and Binns, W.: Teratogenic compounds of Veratrum californicum (Durand) V. Comparison of cyclopian effects of steroidal alkaloids from the plant and structurally related compounds from other sources. Teratology, *1*:5-10, 1968.
112. Kendrick, F. J., and Weaver, S. A.: Alteration in amniotic fluid volume and other findings in meclizine hydrochloride induced anomalies. Proc. Soc. exp. Biol. Med., *114*:747-50, 1963.
113. Kennedy, W. P.: Epidemiological aspects of the problem of congenital malformations. Birth Defects Original Article Series *3*, No. 2, 1967.
114. Kihlman, B. A.: *Actions of Chemicals on Dividing Cells*. Prentice Hall, Englewood Cliffs, N. J,. 1966.
115. King, C. T. G.: Teratogenic effects of meclizine hydrochloride on the rat. Science, *141*:353-55, 1963.
116. King, C. T. G., and Howell, J.: Teratogenic effect of buclizine and hydroxyzine in the rat and chlorcyclizine in the mouse. Am. J. Obstet. Gynec., *95*:109-11, 1966.
117. King, C. T. G., Weaver, S. A., and Narrod, S. A.: Antihistamines and teratogenicity in the rat. J. Pharmac. exp. Therap., *147*:391-98, 1965.
118. Kirschbaum, T. H., Lucus, W. E., DeHaven, J. C., and Assali, N. S.: The dynamics of placental oxygen transfer I. Effects of maternal

hyperoxia in pregnant ewes and fetal lambs. Am. J. Obstet. Gynec., *98*:429-43, 1967.

119. Klein, M.: The transplacental effect of urethan on lung tumorigenesis in mice. J. Nat. Cancer Inst., *12*:1003-10, 1952.

120. Klinge, E, Matilla, M. J., Penttilä, O., and Jukarainen, E.: Influence of drugs on vasoactive peptides and amines in perfused human placenta. Ann. Med. exp. Fenn., *44*:369-75, 1966.

121. Koransky, W., Magour, S., Merker, H. J., Schlickt, I., and Schulte-Hermann, R.: Influence of inducing substances on growth of liver and microsomal electron transport systems. *Third International Pharmacological Meeting*, Rašková, H. (Ed.) . Pergamon Press, N. Y., *4*: 55-63, 1968.

122. Kretchmer, N., Greenberg, R. E., and Serini, F.: Biochemical basis of immaturity. Ann. Rev. Med., *14*:407-26, 1963.

123. Kumar, D.: Intrauterine diagnosis, indices of fetal jeopardy and intrauterine therapy. In, *Intrauterine Development*, Barnes, A. C. (Ed.) . Lea and Febiger, Philadelphia, 1968, Chap. 26, 477-97.

124. Laqueur, G. L.: Carcinogenic effects of cycad meal and cycasin, methylazoxymethanol glycoside, in rats and effects of cycasin in germfree rats. in Third Conference on Toxicity of Cycads. Federation Proc., *23*:1386-7, 1964.

125. Laqueur, G. L., McDaniel, E. G., and Matsumoto, H.: Tumor induction in germfree rats with methylazoxymethanol (MAM) and synthetic MAM acetate. J. Nat. Cancer Inst., *39*: 355-71, 1967.

126. Larsen, C. D.: Pulmonary tumor induction by transplacental exposure to urethane. J. Nat. Cancer Inst., *8*:63-70, 1947.

127. Law, L. W.: The production of tumors by injection of a carcinogen into the amniotic fluid of mice. Science, *91*:96-7, 1940.

128. Lederberg, J.: Molecular biology, eugenics and euphenics. Nature, *198*:428-29, 1963.

129. Lederberg, J.: Biological future of man. In *Man and His Future*, Wolstenholme, G. (Ed.) . Little Brown and Co., Boston, 1963, 263-73.

130. Lenz, W.: Thalidomide and congenital abnormalities. Lancet, *I*:45, 1962.

131. Levine, S., and Mullins, Jr., R. F.: Hormonal influences on brain organization in infant rats. Science, *152*:1585-92, 1966.

132. Lewis, L. G.: Testis tumors. Adv. Surg., *2*:419-94, 1949.

133. Lubchenco, L O., Hansman, C., and Boyd, E.: Intrauterine growth in length and head circumference as estimated from live births at gestational ages from 26 to 42 weeks. Pediatrics, *37*:403-8, 1966.

134. Lubchenco, L. O., Hansman, C., Dressler, M., and Boyd, E.: Intrauterine growth as estimated from liveborn birth weight data at 24 to 42 weks of gestation. Pediatrics, *32*:793-800, 1963.

135 Lubchenco, L. O., Horner, F. A., Reed, L. H., Hix, Jr., J. E., Metcalf, D., Cohig, R., Elliott, H. C., and Bourg, M.: Sequelae of premature birth. Evaluation of premature infants of low birth weights at ten years of age. Am. J. Dis. Child., *106*:135-49, 1963.

136. Lucas, W. E., Kirschbaum, T. H., and Assali, N. S.: Effects of autonomic blockade with spinal anaesthesia on uterine and fetal hemodynamics and oxygen consumption in the sheep. Biol. Neonat., *10*:166-69, 1966.

137. Lund, C. J., and Thiede, H. A. (Eds.) : Transcripts of the 1st, 2nd, 3rd and 4th Rochester Trophoblast Conferences, 1961, 1963, 1965, 1967.

138. MacMahon, B.: Prenatal x-ray exposure and childhood cancer. J. Nat. Cancer Inst., *28*:1173-91, 1962.

139. McBride, W. G.: Thalidomide and congenital abnormalities. Lancet, *II*:1358, 1961.

140. McGaughey, Jr., H. S., Jones, H. C., Talbert, L., and Anslow, Jr., W. P.: Placental transfer in normal and toxic gestation. Am. J. Obstet. Gynec., *75*:482-95, 1958.

141. McKusick, V. A.: *Mendelian Inheritance in Man: Catalogues of Autosomal Dominant, Autosomal Recessive, and X-linked Phenotypes.* The Johns Hopkins Press, Baltimore, 1966.

142. Maher, V. M., Miller, E C., Miller, J. A., and Szybalski, W.: Mutations and decreases in density of transforming DNA produced by derivatives of the carcinogens 2-acetylaminofluorene and n-methyl-4-aminoazobenzene. Mol. Pharmacol., *4*:411-26, 1968.

143. Marley, P. B., Robson, J. M., and Sullivan, F. M.: Embryotoxic and teratogenic action of 5-hydroxytryptamine: mechanism of action in the rat. Br. J. Pharmac. Chemother., *31*:494-505, 1967.

144. Marsden, H. B., and Steward, J. K.: Tumours in children. In *Recent Results in Cancer Research*, Vol. 13. Springer-Verlag New York, Inc., 1968.

145. Matsumoto, H., Koya, G., and Takeuchi, T.: Fetal Minamata disease. A neuropathological study of two cases of intrauterine intoxication by a methyl mercury compound. J. Neuropath. Exp. Neurol., *24*:562-74, 1965.

146. Maurer, H. M., Wolff, J. A., Finster, M., Poppers, P. J., Pantuck, E., Kuntzman, R., and Conney, A. H.: Reduction in concentration of total serum-bilirubin in offspring of women treated with phenobarbitone during pregnancy. Lancet, *2*:122-24, 1968.

147. Miller, R. W.: Relation between cancer and congenital defects: an epidemiological evaluation. J. Nat. Cancer. Inst., *40*:1079-85, 1968.
148. Miller, R. W., Fraumeni, Jr., J. F., and Hill, J. A.: Neuroblastoma: epidemiological approach to its origin. Amer. J. Dis. Child., *115*: 253-61, 1968.
149. Monroe, C. W., Andresen, R. H., Hass, G. M., Madden, D. A., and Schwartzbaugh, S.: Uteroplacental trauma as a method of conditioning the maternal host to adult homografts. Ann. N. Y. Acad. Sci., *99*:733-42, 1962.
150. Montague, A. C. W.: Hemolytic disease of the fetus. In *Intrauterine Development,* Barnes, A. C. (Ed.). Lea and Febiger, Philadelphia, 1968, Chap. 24, 443-66.
151. Mossman, H. W.: The principle interchange vessels of the chorioallantoic placenta of mammals. In, *Organogenesis,* DeHaan, R. L., and Ursprung, H. (Ed.). Holt, Rinehart and Winston, N. Y., 1965, 771-86.
152. Moya, F., and Thorndike, V.: Passage of drugs across the placenta. Am. J. Obstet Gynec., *84*: 1778-98, 1962.
153. Naeye, R. L, Benirschke, K., Hagstrom, J. W. C., and Marcus, C. C.: Intrauterine growth of twins as estimated from liveborn birth-weight data. Pediatrics, *37*:409-16, 1966.
154. Nair, V., and DuBois, K. P.: Prenatal and early postnatal exposure to environmental toxicants. Chicago Med. Sch. Quart., *27*:75-89, 1968.
155. Najarian, J. S., and Dixon, F. J.: Induction of tolerance to skin homografts in rabbits by alterations of placental permeability. Proc. Soc. exp. Biol. Med., *112*:136-38, 1963.
156. Nathan, P., Gonzales, E., and Miller, B. F.: Tolerance to maternal skin grafts in rabbits induced by hyaluronidase. Nature, *188*:77-78, 1960.
157. Neel, J. V.: *Changing Perspectives on the Genetic Effects of Radiation.* The Beaumont Lecture, Thomas, 1962.
158. Nishimura, H., Takano, K., Tanimura, T., Yasuda, M., and Uchida, T.: High incidence of several malformations in the early human embryos as compared with infants. Biol. Neonat., *10*:93-107, 1966.
159. Nyhan, W. L.: Toxicity of drugs in the neonatal period. J. Pediat., *59*:1-20, 1961.
160. Ordy, J. M., Samorajski, T., Collins, R. L., and Rolsten, C.: Prenatal chlorpromazine effects on liver, survival and behavior of mice offspring. J. Pharmacol. exp. Therap., *151*:110-25, 1966.
161. Page, E. W.: Transfer of materials across the human placenta. Am. J. Obstet. Gynec., *74*: 705-18, 1957.
162. Panigel, M.: Placental perfusion experiments. Am. J. Obstet. Gynec., *84*:1664-83, 1962.
163. Pařízek, J.: The destructive effect of cadmium ion on testicular tissue and its prevention by zinc. J. Endocrinol., *15*:56-63, 1957.
164. Patton, J. F., Seitzman, D. N., and Zone, R. A.: Diagnosis and treatment of testicular tumors. Am. J. Surg., *99*:525-32, 1960.
165. Pierce, G. B.: Teratocarcinoma: model for a developmental concept of cancer. In *Current Topics in Developmental Biology,* Moscona, A. A., and Monroy, A. (Eds.). Academic Press, N. Y. 1967, 223-46.
166. Plentl, A. V.: Placental transfer — the use of tracer methods for the study of placental transmission. In, *Biology of Gestation,* Vol. 1. Assali, N. S. (Ed.). Academic Press, N. Y., 1968, 203-49.
167. Posner, H. S. and Darr, A.: Fetal effects of benzhydrylpiperazines: 1. Fetal edema as a possible cause of the oral-facial malformation in rats. Toxicol. Appl. Pharm. (in press).
168. Posner, H. S.: Modification of structure and activity of drugs by the liver. In *Laboratory Diagnosis of Liver Disease,* Sunderman, F. W., and Sunderman, Jr., F. W., (Eds.). Warren H. Green, Inc., St. Louis, 1968, 337-48.
169. Posner, H. S., and Darr, A.: Chlorcyclizine effects in rat fetuses: organ weights and water content. Federation Proc., *26*:539, 1967.
170. Posner, H. S., and Darr, A.: Fetal edema and oral-facial malformations. The Pharmacologist, *9* (2), 206, Fall 1967.
171. Posner, H. S., Graves, A., King, C. T. G., and Wilk, A.: Experimental alteration of the metabolism of chlorcyclizine and the incidence of cleft palate in rats. J. Pharmac exp. Therap., *155*:494-505, 1967.
172. Price, C. C., Gaucher, G. M., Koneru, P., Shibakawa, R., Sowa, J. R., and Yamaguchi, M.: Relative reactivities for monofunctional nitrogen mustard alkylation of nucleic acid components. Biochem. Biophys. Acta, *166*:327-59, 1968.
173. Queenan, J. T.: *Modern Management of the Rh Problem.* Hoeber, N. Y., 1967.
174. Queenan, J. T., and Goetschel, E.: Amniotic fluid analysis for erythroblastosis fetalis. Obstet. Gynec., *32*:120-33, 1968.
175. Reynolds, W. A., Ayers, M. A., and Parker, G. M.: Thermoplacentography: a report of 83 cases. Radiology, *89*:825-7, 1967.
176. Robinson, S. H., Lester, R., Crigler, Jr., J. F., and Tsong, M.: Early-labeled peak of bile pigment in man: studies with glycine-^{14}C and delta-aminolevulinic acid-^{3}H. New Engl. J. Med., *277*:1323-29, 1967.
177. Russell, W. L., Russell, L. B., and Oakberg, E. F.: Radiation genetics of mammals. In *Radiation Biology and Medicine,* W. D. Claus

(Ed.), Addison-Wesley Publishing Co., Reading, Mass. 1958, 189-205.

178. Salzgeber, G., and Wolff, E.: Experimental production of malformations of the limbs by means of chemical substances. Intl. Rev. Exptl. Pathol., *3*:329-63, 1964.

179. Saunders, F. J.: Effects of sex steroids and related compounds on pregnancy and on development of the young. Physiol. Rev., *48*:601-43, 1968.

180. Schutt, W.: Foetal factors in intrauterine growth retardation. Clin. in Develop. Med., *19*: 1-9, 1965.

180a. Scrimshaw, N. S., and Gordon, J. E. (Eds.): *Malnutriton, Learning and Behavior*. Massachusetts Institute of Technology Press, Cambridge, Mass., 1968.

181. Serini, F., and Principi, N.: The development of enzyme systems. Pediat. Clin. N. Amer., *12*: 515-34, 1965.

182. Shirkey, H. C.: Editorial comment: therapeutic orphans. J. Pediat., *72*:119-20, 1968.

183. Simmer, H. H.: Placental hormones. In *Biology of Gestation,* Vol. 1. Assali, N. S. (Ed.). Academic Press, N. Y., 1968, 290-354.

184. Smithells, R. W.: Drugs and human malformations. Adv. Teratology, *1*:251-78, 1966.

185. Solomon, S., and Friesen, H. G.: Endocrine relations between mother and fetus. Ann. Rev. Med., *19*:399-430, 1968.

186. Soukup, S., Takacs, E., and Warkany, J.: Chromosome changes in embryos treated with various teratogens. J. Embryol. exp. Morphol, *18*:215-26, 1967.

187. Spatz, M., and Laqueur, G. L.: Transplacental induction of tumors in Sprague-Dawley rats with crude cycad material. J. Nat. Cancer Inst., *38*:233-39, 1967.

188. Spatz, M., Laqueur, G. L., and Hirono, I.: Hydrolysis of cycasin by β-D-glucosidase in subcutis of newborns. Federation Proc., *27*: No. 2, 722, 1968.

189. Spatz, M., Smith, D. W. E., McDaniel, E. G., and Laqueur, G. L.: Role of intestinal microorganisms in determining cycasin toxicity. Proc. Soc. Exp. Biol. Med., *124*:691-97, 1967.

190. Stevens, L. C.: The biology of teratomas. Adv. Morphogenesis, *6*:1-31, 1967.

191. Tai, C., and Halasz, N. A.: Histocompatability antigen transfer *in utero:* tolerance in progeny and sensitization in mother. Science, *158*:127-28, 1967.

192. Tatelbaum, R. C.: Applicability and acceptability of fetal scalp blood sampling technic. Obstet. Gynec., *32*:290-91, 1968.

193. Tatum, E. L.: Perspectives from physiological genetics. In *The Control of Human Heredity and Evolution*. Sonnenborn, T. M. (Ed.). Macmillan Co., N. Y. 1965, 20-47.

194. Thompson, R. P. H., and Williams, R.: Treatment of chronic intrahepatic cholestasis with phenobarbitone. Lancet, *2*:646-48, 1967.

195. Thompson, W., Bell, T. K., and Pinkerton, J. H. M.: Location of placenta by means of a colour antoscan technique. Brit. Med. J., *4*: 390-1, 1967.

196. Toyooka, E. T., Pifer, J. W., Crump, S. L., Dutton, A. M., and Hempelmann, L. H.: Neoplasms in children treated with x-rays for thymic enlargement II. Tumor incidence as a function of radiation factors. J. Nat. Cancer Inst., *31*:1357-77, 1963.

197. Trolle, D.: Decrease of total serum-bilirubin concentration in newborn infants after phenobarbitone treatment. Lancet, *2*:705-8, 1968.

198. Van den Berg, B. J., and Yerushalmy, J.: The relationship of the rate of intrauterine growth of infants of low birth weight to mortality, morbidity and congenital anomalies. J. Pediatrics, *69*:531-45, 1966.

199. Villee, C. A.: Biochemical aspects of the mammalian placenta. In *Biochemistry of Animal Development,* Vol. 2. Weber, R. (Ed.). Academic Press, N. Y., 1967, 390-95, 407-8.

200. *Viral Etiology of Congenital Malformations.* May 19-20, 1967. U. S. Govt. Printing Office, 1968.

201. Ward, C. O.: Role of the placenta in teratogenesis. New Engl. J. Med., *279*:720-1, 1968.

202. Ward, C. O., and Gautieri, R. F.: Effects of certain drugs on perfused human placenta VI. Serotonin antagonists. J. Pharm. Sci., *55*:474-78, 1966.

203. Ward, C. O., and Gautieri, R. F.: Effect of certain drugs on perfused human placenta VIII. Angiotensin-II antagonists. J. Pharm. Sci., *57*:287-92, 1968.

204. Warkany, J., and Takacs, E.: Changes of endocrine glands produced by teratogenic methods: the pituitary gland. Arch. Path., *85*:101-13, 1968.

205. Welch, R. M., Harrison, Y. E., Conney, A. H., Poppers, P. J., and Finster, M.: Cigarette smoking: stimulatory effect on metabolism of 3,4-benzpyrene by enzymes in human placenta. Science, *160*:541-2, 1968.

206. Wilkin, P. G.: Organogenesis of the human placenta. In *Organogenesis,* DeHaan, R. L., and Ursprung, H. (Eds.). Holt, Rinehart and Winston, N. Y., 1965, 743-69.

207. Wolff, E., and Ginglinger, A.: Sur la transformation des poulets mâles en intersexués par injection d'hormone femelle (folliculine) aux

embryons. Arch. Anat. Histol. Embryol., *20:* 219-78, 1935.

208. Wynn, R. W.: The interpretation of placental ultrastructure. In, *Advances in Obstetrics and Gynecology,* Vol. 1, Marcus, S. L., and Marcus, C. C. (Eds.). Williams and Wilkins, Baltimore, 1967, 21-37.
209. Wynn, R. W.: Morphology of the placenta. In, *Biology of Gestation,* Vol. 1, Assali, N. S. (Ed.). Academic Press, N. Y., 1968, 93-184.
210. Xintaras, C., Johnson, B. L., Ulrich, C. E., Terrill, R. E., and Sobecki, M. F.: Application of the evoked response technique in air pollution toxicology. Toxicol. Appl. Pharmacol., *8:* 77-87, 1966.
211. Xintaras, C., Ulrich, C. E., Sobecki, M. F., and Terrill, R. E.: Brain potentials studied by computer analysis. Arch. Environ. Health, *13:* 223-32, 1966.
212. Yaffee, S. J., Levy, G., Matzauzawa, T., and Baliah, T.: Enhancement of glucuronide-conjugating capacity in a hyperbilirubinemic infant due to apparent enzyme induction by phenobarbital. New Engl. J. Med., *275:*1461-65, 1966.
213. Young, R. D.: Drug administration to neonatal rats: effects on later emotionality and learning. Science, *143:*1055-57, 1964.

Chapter 6

Modifications in Toxicity from the Interactions of Drugs and Chemicals

ABRAHAM STOLMAN, PH.D.

The combined action of two or more drugs present together in the body may cause a variety of effects. The nature of the combined actions is not clearly understood.

The use and presence of several drugs simultaneously in the body produces pharmacological effects which are obviously of considerable importance clinically and also may lead to a form of toxicity that would not occur if single drugs are used or administered alone. It is possible, therefore, that the administration of doses of two or more drugs, not sufficient to produce hypnosis or toxic effects when administered alone, will produce very definite responses when they are present in combination. Understandably, toxic effects appear to be more frequent when the drugs are used in combination.

The hazards associated with the administration of drug combinations cannot be evaluated from the toxicity of the individual drugs or compounds.

It has become increasingly evident that many factors or independent variables besides the dose of drug can markedly influence the duration of action of the drugs and contribute to the toxicity of drug or drug combination. Toxicities of drug combinations involve not merely the enhancement of the potency of one drug with another but also an interaction between the drugs and the subject.

Marked individual differences exist in the metabolism of many drugs. Some individuals metabolize a drug so rapidly that therapeutically effective blood and tissue levels are not achieved while others may metabolize the same drug so slowly as to result in accumulation of the drug which will then produce toxic effects.

It is well established that prolonged administration of drugs can speed up their own metabolism. In one case, evidence for this was found in a patient who was treated with 75 mg dicumarol per day for seven months. When the subject was given 1 grain of phenobarbital daily for 4 weeks there was a substantial lowering of the plasma dicoumarol level and a decrease in the anticoagulant activity as measured by the prothrombin time. Upon discontinuing the barbiturate, the plasma dicoumarol level and prothrombin time returned to their original level.

Interest in the combined effects of drugs, in the toxicological field was originally aroused by the observations of the suddenness of death in some known instances or where the available evidence suggested that death may have supervened after several drugs in small quantities were ingested. Workers have observed that in persons who had taken both alcohol and barbiturates, death was more rapid and the clinical picture different from that produced by either one acting alone. They were impressed with the relative suddenness at which the onset of death occurred.

Ethanol and barbiturates, because of their widespread use, are the drugs most frequently encountered in deaths by poisoning and are of considerable practical interest. Experience has shown that the severity of the symptoms of the ethanol and barbiturate combinations were greater if the ethanol concerned had been taken as hard liquor (whiskey, gin) rather than beer or in other dilute forms though the total quantity of ethanol so consumed was no more. A much more severe coma in the drinkers of hard liquors was found than in the drinkers of beer and wines. The explanation was given that hard liquors irritated the gastric and duodenal mucosa and thus promoted the absorption of those drugs that were subsequently swallowed.

Some data presented from eleven pairs of matching patients suffering from acute barbiturate poisoning of moderate severity indicated that the severity of symptoms was greater in alcoholics than in non-alcoholics, and in drinkers of hard liquors than in drinkers of beer and ale. The ratio expressing the degree of coma was 8:1 in favor of the individuals drinking hard liquor.

It is apparent that from presently available data, alcohol and barbiturates can make a most dangerous combination. Even if the actions are simply additive, the effect may easily reach alarming proportions. The volume and concentration of the alcohol is an important factor as a speedier attainment of the peak level of blood alcohol would allow an earlier and fuller development of the barbiturate-alcohol synergism.

When ethanol was present in the tissues of the victims of fatal barbiturate intoxication, the barbiturate levels were lower than in cases where ethanol was absent. Only about 2/3 of the "normal" lethal concentrations were found in cases where ethanol was also present. The blood concentrations of fast acting barbiturates (amobarbital, pentobarbital) in cases of death due exclusively to barbiturates were about 2.7 mg/100 ml compared with about 1.7 mg/100 ml in those cases where barbiturates were found in combination with alcohol (0.05%).

Clinical signs of intoxication were observed in a patient who was treated with diphenylhydantoin (Dilantin) and dicoumarol. Investigation revealed an increase in the serum diphenylhydantoin level and a very considerable increase in the half-life of the blood diphenlyhydantoin. Before dicoumarol therapy, the diphenylhydantoin half-life in blood was 9 hours. After one week of dicoumarol therapy, the half-life was strikingly prolonged to 36 hours. The substance accumulating in the blood was found to be diphenylhydantoin and not a metabolite.

Serious hypoglycemic reactions were seen in a number of tolbutamide-treated diabetics who had previously been in good balance and the obvious cause of these attacks seemed to be sulphaphenazole. One diabetic individual who was receiving 0.5 gm tolbutamide per day had blood glucose levels ranging from 120-150 mg per 100 ml. The individual was treated for urinary infection with 2 gm sulphaphenazole daily for 3 days and 1 gm daily for the next 16 days. Five days later at a time when tolbutamide and sulphaphenazole had been given concurrently for 2 days the blood glucose levels dropped to between 63 and 76 mg/100 ml. After the tolbutamide was stopped, the blood glucose levels were in the range of 110 – 160 mg/100 ml. Some 13 days later the patient was again given 0.5 gm tolbutamide daily while still taking sulphaphenazole. This caused a lowering of the blood glucose values to 62-78 mg/100 ml. Sulphaphenazole when given to well balanced non-tolbutamide-treated diabetics showed no decrease in their blood glucose values.

The half-life of a 1 gm dose of tolbutamide intravenously in non-diabetics before and after the administration of sulphaphenazole was found to increase from 4½ to 18½ hours.

Hypoglycemic attacks rarely occur during treatment with chlorpropamide in therapeutic doses. However, during the past few years there have been a number of reports of such attacks. Three diabetic patients who had been receiving treatment with 250 mg chlorpropamide daily for at least 2 weeks were given dicoumarol in such doses as to produce prothrombin-proconvertin values of 40%. There was a clear increase in the plasma chlorpropamide concentration from an average of 7.6 mg/100 ml before treatment to 13.3 mg/100 ml after dicoumarol treatment. The chlorpropamide concentration did not return to "predicoumarol levels" until 17 days after the withdrawal of dicoumarol. Chromatography of the serum revealed that these samples contained only chlorpropamide and no metabolites.

Illicit narcotic pushers have learned of and taken advantage of the synergistic or additive effect of drug combinations. Previously it was common practice to cut heroin with milk sugar. Today it is more usual to find the heroin cut with quinine.

Experiments with rats, given 100 mg quinine/kg orally 30 minutes before 1 to 8 mg morphine/kg subcutaneously, showed that quinine increased the potency of morphine 2.7 times. About 17 mg quinine/kg was required to double the total analgesic effect of 2 mg morphine/kg. Potentiation could be obtained only when the quinine was given with or prior to the injection of the narcotic, never when administered after the analgesic agent. This was true no matter what the route of administration of quinine.

REFERENCES

1. Bonnichsen, R., Maehly, A. C., and Frank, A.: J. Forensic Sci., *6*:411, 1961.
2. Burn, J. J., Cucinelli, S. A., Koster, R., and Conney, A. H.: Ann. N.Y. Acad. Sci., *123*:273, 1965.
3. Christensen, L. K., Hansen, J. M., and Kristensen, M.: Lancet, *II*:1298, 1963.
4. Graham, J. D. P.: Toxicol. Appl. Pharmacol., *2*: 14, 1960.
5. Hansen, J. M., Kristensen, M., Skovsted, L., and Christensen, L. K.: Lancet, *II*:265, 1966.
6. Kristensen, M., and Hansen, J. M.: Acta Med. Scand., *183*:83, 1968.
7. Orahovats, P. D., Lehman, E. G., and Chapin, E. W.: Arch. Int. Pharmacodyn. Ther., *90*:245, 1957.
8. Stolman, A.: *Progress in Chemical Toxicology*, Vol. 3, A. Stolman (Ed.). Academic Press, N. Y., 1967, p. 305.

Chapter 7

Toxicity of Food Additives and Cosmetics

LEON GOLBERG, D.Sc., D.Phil., M.B.

Is there a Hazard?

Toxic effects of food additives in man are manifested so rarely that consideration of potential harmfulness usually centers on the possibility, albeit remote, of unexpected and perhaps unrecognized long-term effects, or on the likelihood that some chance combination of chemicals in the diet, among them perhaps natural food ingredients, may have an adverse action that could not have been anticipated. The present system of safety evaluation relies heavily on studies of individual compounds carried out in animals. The relatively small number of investigations in man, with single compounds, have mostly been of short duration; they cannot be expected to resolve the doubts voiced above.

Where cosmetics and toiletries are concerned, any immediate effect is usually readily noted and may be correctly attributed to its cause, but the possibility of some more subtle long-term harmful action remains, though it is rarely demonstrable in practice. Despite the shortcomings of existing tests of safety of food additives and cosmetics, they have a remarkable record of success in protecting the consumer or user from harm. It is instructive, therefore, to review some of the main considerations that underlie safety evaluation of these classes of products and to take note of some of the problems that have arisen.

Defining the Responsible Agent

Not infrequently, it is difficult to be sure which product ought to be tested. Doubt may arise, for instance, over the nature and amount of impurities present, even in food grade chemicals. Because commercial products must be used, specification and quality control are all-important. Some additives are inherently ill-defined in composition, either because of their natural origin (as in flavorings) or process of manufacture (as with "caramel," a term that covers over 100 distinct technical products). Irradiated foods probably constitute the most complex current problem of this sort.

A number of additives break down during processing of food: azodicarbonamide gives rise to biurea and diethyl pyrocarbonate to carbon dioxide, ethanol and carbethoxy derivatives of constituents of beverages. The transformation products formed from additives by reaction with ingredients of food are of greater importance. Some of these have been tabulated by Golberg (1967a). The formation of the neurotoxin methionine sulfoximine from "agene" (nitrogen trichloride) probably represents the closest that man has come to disaster from the use of modern food additives (Campbell and Morrison, 1966).

Even more varied are the transformation products of food additives formed through the action of intestinal flora. Most azo coloring undergo reductive cleavage of the azo link (Radomski and Mellinger, 1962; Scheline and Longberg, 1965) and the resulting amino compounds are largely absorbed into the body. In the case of the coloring Brown FK, which comprises at least six component dyes (Fore and Walker, 1967) not only does reductive cleavage of azo links occur but the polyamine moeities so formed condense to yield 1, 4, 7-triaminophenazine and possibly other phenazines (Fore, Walker and Golberg, 1967). The effects of Brown FK in rats and mice are decidedly unusual (Grasso, Gaunt, Hall, Golberg and Batstone, 1968; Grasso, Muir, Golberg and Batstone, 1968) and are largely, if not entirely, attributable to the intestinal transformation products. Similarly, the antioxidant nordihydroguaiaretic acid is converted to an *o*-quinone in the lower third of the ileum and cecum of the rat, and it is probably this product that induces cystic reticuloendotheliosis of the paracecal lymph nodes and vacuolation of renal tubular epithelium (Grice, Becking and Goodman, 1968).

Changes Brought About by the Body

Metabolic and pharmacokinetic studies in several animal species, as well as in man, are now generally required for new drugs. Such information is available for very few food additives. Yet, its importance is undeniable, as shown recently by the case of the antioxidant butylated hydroxytoluene whose metabolism in man proved to be radically different from the pathways in rat and dog, thus accounting for species differences in excretion (Daniel, Gage, Jones and Stevens, 1967; Daniel, Gage and Jones, 1968).

Orthodoxy demands a "margin of safety" (ratio of highest no-effect level in animals to the level of intended use in man) of at least 100. To achieve this margin sometimes involves levels of exposure so high as to produce artefacts, such as overflow pathways of metabolism when the capacity of the main pathway is exceeded, or derangements in the balance of microbial population in the intestine and consequently in their degradative reactions.

When a food additive is composed of, or gives rise to, common physiological body constituents, what level of such compounds is acceptable in the diet? We know that even essential amino acids such as methionine are highly toxic to rats when added to the diet at a level of 2% (Klavins, Kinney and Kaufman, 1963). An interesting problem involves the increasingly widespread use of monosodium glutamate, which currently stands accused as the cause of the so-called "post-sino-cibal syndrome" (Kwok, 1968; Editorial, 1968a) more euphoniously known as "Kwok's Quease" (Leading article, 1968). How such ubiquitous ions as sodium and glutamate can bring about the reported disturbances, or if indeed they do, remains a mystery. That glutamate in high doses is toxic to the eye is well recognized (Potts, Modrell and Kingsbury, 1960; Cohen, 1967).

In passing, it is worth drawing attention to the increasing number of environmental chemicals of all kinds capable of exercising deleterious effects on the eye (Marzulli, 1968). No one has sought to explore the possibilities of pejorative combinations of such chemicals acting on the sensitive metabolism of lens, retina and other ocular structures.

The metabolism of food additives is usually studied in animals that have not been exposed to stimulators of microsomal processing (drug-metabolising) enzymes. Man, on the other hand, can hardly avoid being in a state of enhanced activity of these enzymes, not only through the use of drugs but by consumption of alcohol, coffee, by smoking, exposure to pesticides and other means. The transformations undergone by a test compound may be very different, qualitatively and quantitatively, if processing enzymes have been stimulated in the liver, kidney, small intestine and placenta. Thus, the metabolic capacity of the rat liver for butylated hydroxytoluene rises from an initial value of 42 mg/kg/day to 330 mg/kg/day after five large daily doses (Gilbert and Golberg, 1967).

Finally, consider the question of those food additives which are said not to undergo metabolism in the body. Modern techniques have revealed that cyclamate often gives rise to cyclohexylamine in man; occasionally a substantial proportion of the ingested material is converted to this product, and possibly other compounds (Wills, Jameson, Stoewsand and Coulston, 1968). Other additives for which "no metabolism" has been claimed include saccharin and tartaric acid.

Extent of Exposure

In the field under discussion, the key phrase in assessment of hazard refers to "conditions of intended use." These conditions are not as readily defined or limited as in the case of drugs. When it comes to food or toiletries, what provision should be made for extremes: the food faddist or the compulsive user of deodorants? According to British recommendations, food containing the additive should be considered to furnish "as much as one half of the daily calorie requirements of man for the greater part of his life" (Ministry of Agriculture, Fisheries and Food, 1965). An unexpected instance of this problem arose recently over the addition of cobalt to beer at levels up to 1.2 ppm. Beer drinkers consuming many liters daily for many years develop a characteristic cardiomyopathy (Rona, 1968) apparently attributable to the action of ionic cobalt, probably in association with alcohol (Morin and Daniel, 1967).

Consideration of the extent of use of a food additive entails the obligation to continue monitoring the total intake of any one food additive from all possible sources. The whole nature of safety evaluation alters when an additive formerly used in trace amounts attains appreciable proportions in the total diet, as has happened with phosphates, glutamate and cyclamate. The case of caffeine is typical, an additive that enjoys GRAS (generally recognized as safe) status and is, of course, present in several natural materials. A cup of perculator coffee provides about 150 mg of caffeine, of instant coffee 80-90 mg and of decaffeinated coffee 15-25 mg (Wolman, 1955). Caffeine is also present in tea, cocoa and in the naturally-derived flavorings kola nut extract, guarana and guarana gum. Caffeine and/or kola nut extract are added to cola drinks and root beer at levels up to 200 ppm (average maximum of 120 ppm) and kola nut extract to beverages, ice cream, ices, candy and baked goods at average maximum levels of 120-220 ppm, rising in some instances to 400 ppm or more (Food Protection Committee, 1965). While it is difficult to calculate an accurate total average intake of caffeine from all these sources, 20 mg/kg daily may not be unattainable.

This figure lends interest to the host of experimental findings on the biochemical, physiologic, pharmacologic and pathologic effects of caffeine (Bellet, Kershbaum and Finck, 1968; Cheraskin and Ringsdorf, 1968). The most unusual of these is the syndrome of psychotic-like self-mutilation that develops when rats are on a restricted diet (20% of the usual intake) containing caffeine at a daily intake of 18 mg/kg (Hofnagel, 1968; Nyhan, 1968; Peters, 1966; Peters and Boyd, 1966). This effect is also brought about by theophylline, but not by theobromine. The mutagenicity of caffeine has also been studied extensively (see below).

Numerous other instances beside caffeine, cyclamates and glutamate can be adduced to emphasize the need for periodic reexamination of GRAS status and, indeed, of all safety evaluations to bring them into line with fresh knowledge and new conditions of use.

Effects on the Body

The destruction of essential nutrients, such as thiamin by sulfites or of vitamin E by flour improvers (Golberg, 1967a) is well recognized. More subtle dangers lie in the convergence of effects of several compounds on a common pathway; as in the case of thyroxine biosynthesis, where a variety of naturally-occurring goitrogens elicit a synergistic effect (Langer, 1966). Interaction with environmental chemicals such as drugs, as in the "cheese syndrome" involving monoamine oxidase inhibitors (Sjögvist 1968) or deviation of metabolism from oxidative to reductive pathways, as induced by ingestion of alcohol (Davis, Brown, Huff and Cashaw, 1967) may have as yet unrecognized implications.

The issue of reversibility of observed effects, and its relationship to reserves of function, must never be lost sight of. Methemoglobinemia is a familiar example. Similarly, the safety of 2-chloroethanol absorbed from the intestine, as opposed to the hazard of inhaling this compound, is dependent on rapid transport to, and detoxication by the liver (Johnson, 1967). The capacity of this "hoovering" mechanism in man has never been studied; hence the safety of the compound in the rat, dog and monkey given 2-chloroethanol in the diet for 90 days scarcely justifies a confident extrapolation to man.

Studies carried out directly in man with food additives or cosmetics have so far not taken account of pharmacogenetic aspects, even though these are well known in drug studies. A case in point is individual susceptibility to excessive intake of iodide. While most subjects respond to prolonged iodide load by decreasing thyroid uptake, a few fail to compensate in this way and develop iodide goiter (Murray and Stewart, 1967). Such a failure of normal adaptation could be significant where iodide is derived from deiodination of erythrosine (FD&C Red No. 3), lipstick colorings, iodised throat lozenges and various other sources.

Carcinogenesis, Teratogenesis and Mutagenesis

For at least half a century, public fear of cancer following unexpectedly upon the chronic use of "chemicals" in food or cosmetics has never been dispelled. In recent years, numerous food additives, both of natural and synthetic origin, have been banned on grounds of carcinogenicity, particularly to the liver of rats and mice. The aminotriazole "cranberry incident" and the early detection of carcinogenicity of acetylaminofluorene represent victories for the protection of the public. On the other hand, there is the sad history of polyoxyethylene-8-stearate and of ethylene glycol, in regard to the production of bladder papillomas and carcinomas in the rat. The work of Weil, Carpenter and Smyth (1965) established that such tumors in the rat are secondary effects of the presence of bladder stones, produced by the long-term administration of excessively high doses of compound. Nevertheless, it is unlikely that the use of these compounds as food additives will be permitted. Similarly, many countries have taken action to delete colorings and other additives from permitted lists if they elicit local sarcomas on repeated subcutaneous injection in the rat. Despite the fact that such neoplasia has now been demonstrated to be associated with purely physical properties, such as surface activity, of the test materials and to have no relevance to their use in food, it remains to be seen whether their status as food additives will ever be restored. (Grasso and Golberg, 1966; Gangolli, Grasso and Golberg, 1967).

Barnes (1966) has provided an objective assessment of carcinogenic hazard from pesticide residues in food. He refers to the case against DDT, dieldrin and aldrin, as well as maleic hydrazide — all of which illustrate the difficulty and danger of extrapolating from results in animals directly to man.

Druckrey and others have elicited neoplasms of various types in the offspring of animals treated during the later stages of pregnancy with nitrosamines and related compounds, often given in a single dose (Druckrey, Schmähl, Preussmann and Ivankovic, 1964; Ivankovic, Druckrey and Preussmann, 1966; Wrba, Pielsticker and Mohr, 1967; Thomas and Bollmann, 1968). It is too early to say whether this approach, using exceptionally potent carcinogens, has any practical implications. It does, however, underline the need for careful study of all situations in which the use of nitrite or other chemical may introduce even traces of such powerful carcinogens into food or on to skin or mucous membranes (Editorial, 1868b; Hedler and Marquardt, 1968).

Embryotoxic and embryopathic effects have been induced with salicylates, including methyl salicylate (Takacs and

Warkany, 1968) caffeine and theophylline (Georges and Denef, 1968) lead salts (Ferm and Carpenter, 1967) and a variety of pesticides, including methylparathion (Tanimura, Katsuya and Nishimura, 1967) parathion and diazinon (Khera and Bedok, 1967) and carbaryl (Robens, 1968). The relevance to man of such effects, brought about by relatively large doses, in chick and duck embryos, rats, mice, hamsters, rabbits and dogs is difficult to assess. Strenuous efforts are in progress to study teratogenicity in the primate; when success is achieved the question of dosage employed, as well as other circumstances of exposure, will then arise.

In the area of mutagenesis, many "natural" food components, such as caffeine and coumarin, ethanol and adenine, are active chromosome breakers or have other effects. Heavy metal chelators, by complexing the DNA-bound metals, induce chromosomal aberrations and enhance chromosome breakage induced by x-rays (Kihlman, 1966). Since formaldehyde is such a powerful agent in this respect, the use of hexamethylene tetramine (which breaks down to formaldehyde) as a fish preservative has caused some concern, probably wholly unjustifiably. Among agricultural chemicals, maleic hydrazide is notoriously active in inducing chromosome breaks and other aberrations (Kihlman, 1966). A detailed study has been carried out of the mutagenic effect of xanthene dyes on *E. coli*. Some of those used in food and cosmetics showed distinct activity (Lück, Wallnöffer and Bach, 1963). Induction of mutation in yeast has been reported by Nagai (1959) using basic triphenylmethane dyes and xanthenes.

It is appropriate to conclude this section by referring to the baffling enigma of irradiated foods (Epstein, S.S., 1968). Whether or not some of them constitute a carcinogenic, teratogenic or mutagenic hazard only time will tell.

Allergic Sensitisation

Food allergy is commonplace. The capacity of the sensitised individual to respond to the minutest traces of a chemical is well recognized in the case of penicillin but may come as a surprise when it manifests itself as beet sensitivity to what is ostensibly 100% pure sucrose derived from beet and monosodium glutamate produced from beet molasses (Randolph and Rollins, 1950). Thus, while manifestations of hypersensitivity to food additives would be anticipated, they are surprisingly rare in practice. Feingold (1968) has stressed the difficulty of attributing such sensitivity to its correct cause. Food, drug and cosmetics colors are a source of allergic reactions. So are some flavorings, particularly when used in relatively high concentrations, or when they supplement naturally-occurring compounds such as salicylates, which are important in view of the frequency of aspirin sensitivity. Allergy to perfumes in toilet soaps and detergents was found in 4% of Danish patients with dermatitis; 75% of these reactions were associated with sensitivity to benzyl salicylate (Rothenborg and Hjorth, 1968).

Contact dermatitis from pesticides is rare (Wilkinson, 1968) and is often due to impurities or other ingredients of technical formulations. Pesticide residues in foodstuffs do not constitute a problem, probably because the minute amounts involved in the total daily exposure of the mass population are far below the critical threshold for sensitisation. Hayes (1967) has pointed out that in this sphere of hypersensitivity too, the relationship to dosage usually applies.

Turning to cosmetics and toiletries, the possibility of sensitisation is of paramount importance both to user and manufacturer. Extreme care is taken to avoid any such risk. Accounts of contact dermatitis arising from the use of cosmetics stress the relative frequency of lipstick and nail varnish sensitisation (Cronin, 1967; Calnan, 1967; Golberg, 1967b). The traditional source of hazard, the "para" group of hair dyes has been very considerably reduced but the possibilities of cross-reaction remain with any one of a host of drugs and other structurally-related chemicals. An interesting group here are the parabens, valuable preservatives for cosmetics and pharmaceuticals, and used also in some countries in food and beverages. In recent years, reports have accumulated of insidious and unrecognized paraben contact dermatitis, probably stemming from the use of the preservatives in high concentrations in topically-applied medicaments (Epstein, S., 1968). Parabens sensitize guinea pigs (Klaschka, 1966). This example illustrates how slowly awareness of a hazard is disseminated; yet only when this has happened does the offending agent stand much chance of being identified. The index of suspicion of specific materials is very low.

No account of this increasingly important form of toxicity would be complete without reference to what Calnan (1964) has called the 'climate of contact dermatitis' — the endogenous and exogenous factors that predispose to hypersensitivity. The fact is that the majority of skin diseases, not only those atopic in origin, increase susceptibility to the common sensitizing chemicals (Sipos, 1967).

Photosensitivity

Much of what was said above about hypersensitivity applies equally to photosensitivity in response to chemicals. The rapidly-extending list of photosensitising compounds has created increasing problems in recent years — not only the large number of drugs but the widely-used antibacterial agents in toilet soap, shampoos, rinses and antiseptic creams. In addition to the halogenated salicylanilides and carbanilides, other halogen compounds such as bithionol, hexachlorophene and fentichlor have been implicated. Apart from the undoubted photosensitising potency of 3,3′,4′,5-tetrachlorosalicylanilide, the responsibility of some of the other compounds, for example 3,4′,5-tribromosalicylanilide, for photosensitisation is a matter of dispute and the subject of a rising tide of publications (Ison and Tucker, 1968; Osmundsen, 1968; Harber, Targovnik and Baer, 1967).

Among food additives, reports of photosensitisation are rare, and often poorly documented. Both common nonnutritive sweeteners have given rise to photosensitivity (cyclamate: Lamberg, 1967; saccharin: Kennedy, O'Quinn, Perret, Tilley and Hennington, 1961; Kingsley, 1967) but in relation to the volume of use, the incidence of such reactions is negligible. In fact, some reported examples may represent cross-reaction to structurally related and much more powerful photosensitisers such as sulfonamides, thiazide diuretics or sulfones (Patiala and Raekallio, 1951).

Conclusion

Despite the exceptional record of safe use of food additives, constant vigilance is always necessary if toxicity is to be avoided. Such vigilance is not necessarily best expressed as demands for more and more and longer and longer routine animal tests on the part of government nor a servile readiness on the part of industry to satisfy these demands. The power of common sense, judgment and intellect achieves infinitely more for safety than the power of the dollar. Experience in man is the thing that counts, provided it is based on the right questions having been asked and answered correctly and competently. Finally, safety is an edifice that cannot be built all at once; nor can it be expected to last forever without periodic reconstruction.

BIBLIOGRAPHY

BARNES, J. M.: Carcinogenic hazards from pesticide residues. Residue Rev., *13*:69-82, 1966.

BELLET, S., KERSHBAUM, A., and FINCK, E. M.: Response of free fatty acids to coffee and caffeine. Metabolism, *17*:702-706, 1968.

CALNAN, C. D.: The climate of contact dermatitis. Acta derm. Venereol., *44*:33-43, 1964.

CALNAN, C. D.: Reactions to artificial colouring materials. J. Soc. Cosmetic Chemists, *18*:215-223, 1967.

CAMPBELL, J. A., and MORRISON, A. B.: Nutritional impact of modern food processing. Fed. Proc., *25*:130-136, 1966.

CHERASKIN, E., and RINGSDORF, W. M. JR.: Blood-glucose levels after caffeine. Lancet, *ii*:689, 1968.

COHEN, A. I.: An electron microscopic study of the modification by monosodium glutamate of the retinas of normal and "rodless" mice. Amer. J. Anat., *120*:319-356, 1967.

CRONIN, E.: Contact dermatitis from cosmetics. J. Soc. Cosmetic Chemists, *18*:681-691, 1967.

DANIEL, J. W., GAGE, J. C., and JONES, D. I.: The metabolism of 3,5-di-tert-butyl-4-hydroxytoluene in the rat and in man. Biochem. J., *106*:783-790, 1968.

DANIEL, J. W., GAGE, J. C., JONES, D. I., and STEVENS, M. A.: Excretion of butylated hydroxytoluene (BHT) and butylated hydroxyanisole (BHA) in man. Food Cosmet. Toxicol., *5*:475-479, 1967.

DAVIS, V. E., BROWN, H., HUFF, J. A., and CASHAW, J. L.: The alteration of serotonin metabolism to 5-hydroxytryptophol by ethanol ingestion in man. J. Lab. Clin Med., *69*:132-140, 1967.

DRUCKREY, H., SCHMÄHL, D., PREUSSMANN, R., and IVANKOVIC, S.: Krebserzeugung durch einmalige Dosis von Methylnitrosoharnstoff und verschiedenen Dialkyl-nitrosaminen. Naturwiss., *50*:735, 1964.

Editorial: Post-sino-cibal syndrome. New Engl. J. Med., *278*:1122, 1968a.

Editorial: Nitrites, nitrosamines and cancer. Lancet, *i*:1071-1072, 1968b.

EPSTEIN, S.: Paraben sensitivity: subtle trouble. Ann. Allergy, *26*:185-189, 1968.

EPSTEIN, S. S.: Irradiated foods warning. Science, *161*:741, 1968.

FEINGOLD, B. F.: Recognition of food additives as a cause of symptoms of allergy. Ann. Allergy, *26*: 309-313, 1968.

FERM, V. H., and CARPENTER, S. J.: Developmental malformations resulting from the administration of lead salts. Exp. Molec. Pathol., *7*.208-213, 1967.

Food Protection Committee: *Chemicals Used in Food Processing*. Publ. 1274, 1965. National Academy of Sciences-National Research Council, Washington, D.C.

FORE, H., and WALKER, R.: Studies of Brown FK. I. Composition and synthesis of components. Food Cosmet. Toxicol., *5*:1-9, 1967.

FORE, H., WALKER, R., and GOLBERG, L.: Studies on Brown FK. II. Degradative changes undergone in vitro and in vivo. Food Cosmet. Toxicol., *5*: 459-473, 1967.

GANGOLLI, S. D., GRASSO, P., and GOLBERG, L.: Physical factors determining the early local tissue reactions produced by food colourings and other compounds injected subcutaneously. Food Cosmet. Toxicol., *5*:601-621, 1967.

GEORGES, A., and DENEF, J.: Les anomalies digitales: manifestations teratogéniques des dérivés xanthiques chez le rat. Arch. Int. Pharmacodyn., *172*:219-222, 1968.

GILBERT, D., and GOLBERG, L.: BHT oxidase. A liver-microsomal enzyme induced by the treatment of rats with butylated hydroxytoluene. Food Cosmet. Toxicol., *5*:481-490, 1967.

GOLBERG, L.: The amelioration of food. The Milroy Lectures. J. Roy. Coll. Phycns. Lond., *1*:385-426, 1967a.

GOLBERG, L.: The toxicology of artificial colouring materials. J. Soc. Cosmetic Chemists, *18*:421-432, 1967b.

GRASSO, P., and GOLBERG, L.: Subcutaneous sarcoma as an index of carcinogenic potency. Food Cosmet. Toxicol., *4*:297-320, 1966.

GRASSO, P., GAUNT, I. F., HALL, D. E., GOLBERG, L., and BATSTONE, E.: Studies on Brown FK. III. Administration of high doses to rats and mice. Food Cosmet. Toxicol., *6*:1-11, 1968.

GRASSO, P., MUIR, A., GOLBERG, L., and BATSTONE, E.: Studies on Brown FK. IV. Cytopathic effects of Brown FK on cardiac and skeletal muscle in the rat. Food Cosmet. Toxicol., *6*:13-24, 1968.

GRICE, H. C., BECKING, G., and GOODMAN, T.: Toxic properties of nordihydroguaiaretic acid. Food Cosmet. Toxicol., *6*:155-161, 1968.

HARBER, L. C., TARGOVNIK, S. E., and BAER, R. L.: Contact photosensitivity patterns to halogenated salicylanilides in man and guinea pigs. Arch. Derm., *96*:646-656, 1967.

HAYES, W. J., JR.: Toxicity of pesticides to man: risks from present levels. Proc. Roy. Soc. B., *167*: 101-127, 1967.

HEDLER, L., and MARQUARDT, P.: Uber das Vorkommen von Nitrosaminen in Nahrungs-und Futtermitteln. Arch. fur Pharmakol., *259*:176-177, 1968.

HOFNAGEL, D.: Clinical features of the Lesch-Nyhan Syndrome. Pathology and pathologic physiology. Summary. Fed. Proc., *27*:1042-1046, 1968.

ISON, A. E., and TUCKER, J. B.: Photosensitive dermatitis from soaps. New Engl. J. Med., *278*:81-84, 1968.

IVANKOVIC, S., DRUCKREY, H., and PREUSSMANN, R.: Erzeugung neurogener Tumoren nach einmaliger Injektion von Äthylnitrosoharnstoff an schwangere Ratten. Naturwiss, *16*:410, 1966.

JOHNSON, M. K.: Detoxication of ethylene chlorohydrin. Food Cosmet. Toxicol., *5*:449, 1967.

KENNEDY, B., O'QUINN, S., PERRET, W. J., TILLEY, J. C., and HENINGTON, V. M.: Phototoxic and photoallergic skin reactions resulting from modern drug therapy. J. Louisiana State Med. Soc., *113*: 365-371, 1961.

KHERA, K S., and BEDOK, S.: Effects of thiol phosphates on notochordal and vertebral morphogenesis in chick and duck embryos. Food Cosmet. Toxicol., *5*:359-365, 1967.

KIHLMAN, B. A.: *Actions of Chemicals on Dividing Cells*. Prentice-Hall, Inc., Englewood Cliffs, New Jersey, 1966.

KINGSLEY, H. J.: Action of saccharin. Brit. Med. J., *i*:427, 1967.

KLASCHKA, F.: Tierexperimentelle Studien zum Kontaktekzem. III. Sensibilisierung von Meerschweinchen mit p-Hydroxybenzoesaureestern. Epicutantestung mit einem p-Hydroxybenzoesaureester-Stoffwechselproduk bei paragruppen-Kontaktekzematikern. Archiv. fur klin exper. Dermatol., *225*:384-397, 1966.

KLAVINS, J. V., KINNEY, T. D., and KAUFMAN, N.: Histopathologic changes in methionine excess. Arch. Path., *75*:661-673, 1963.

KWOK, R. H. M.: Chinese-restaurant syndrome. New Engl. J. Med., *278*:796, 1968.

LAMBERG, S. I.: A new photosensitizer. The artificial sweetener cyclamate. J.A.M.A., *201*:121-124, 1967.

LANGER, P.: Antithyroid action in rats of small doses of some naturally occurring compounds. Endocrinol., *79*:1117-1122, 1966.

Leading Article: Kwok's Quease. Brit. Med. J., *ii*: 447, 1968.

LÜCK, H., WALLNÖFER, P., and BACH, H.: Lebensmittelzusatzstoffe und mutagene Wirkung. VII. Mitteilung. Prüfung einiger Xanthen-Farbstoffe auf Wirkung an Escherichia coli. Path. Microbiol., Basel, *26*:206-224, 1963.

MARZULLI, F. N.: Ocular side effects of drugs. Fd Cosmet. Toxicol., *6*:221-234, 1968.

Ministry of Agriculture, Fisheries and Food: *Memorandum on Procedure for Submissions on Food Additives and on Methods of Toxicity Testing*. Her Majesty's Stationery Office, London, 1965.

MORIN, Y. L., and DANIEL, P.: Quebec Beer-Drinkers' Cardiomyopathy: Etiological Considerations. Canad. Med. Ass. J., *97*:926-928, 1967.

MURRAY, I. P. C., and STEWART, R. D. H.: Iodide goitre. Lancet, *i*:922-926, 1967.

NAGAI, S.: Induction of the respiration deficient mutation in yeast by various synthetic dyes. Science, *130*:1188-1189, 1959.

NYHAN, W. L.: Discussion. Fed. Proc., *27*:1044, 1968.

OSMUNDSEN, P. E.: Contact photodermatitis due to tribromsalicylanilide. Brit. J. Dermatol., *80*:228-234, 1968.

PATIALA, R., and RAEKALLIO, T.: Saccharin as an allergic agent. Report of a case of simultaneous cross sensitization against various sulfonamide drugs and saccharin. Ann. Med. Exper. Biol. Fenniae (Helsinki), *29*:191-196, 1951.

PETERS, J. M.: Caffeine toxicity in starved rats. Toxicol. Appl. Pharmacol., *9*:390-397, 1966.

PETERS, J. M., and BOYD, E. M.: Diet and caffeine toxicity in rats. Toxicol. Appl. Pharmacol., *8*: 350-351, 1966.

POTTS, A. M., MODRELL, R. W., and KINGSBURY, C.: Permanent fractionation of the electroretinogram by sodium glutamate. Amer. J. Ophthalmol., *50*:900-905, 1960.

RADOMSKI, J. L., and MELLINGER, T. J.: The absorption, fate and excretion in rats of the water-soluble azo dyes, FD&C Red No. 2, FD&C Red No. 4, and FD&C Yellow No. 6. J. Pharm. Exp. Ther., *136*:259-266, 1962.

Randolph, T. O., and Rollins, J. P.: Beet sensitivity: allergic reactions from the ingestion of beet sugar (sucrose) and monosodium glutamate of beet origin. J. Lab. Clin. Med., *36*:407-415, 1950.

Robens, J. F.: Teratogenic effects of carbaryl and other pesticides in the hamster, the rabbit, and the guinea pig. Toxicol. Appl. Pharmacol., *12:* 294, 1968.

Rona, G.: Endemic cardiomyopathy of beer consumers. Acta Morphologica Acad. Sci. Hung. *16:* 103-114, 1968.

Rothenborg, H. W., and Hjorth, N.: Allergy to perfumes from toilet soaps and detergents in patients with dermatitis. Arch. Derm., *97*:417-421, 1968.

Scheline, R. R., and Longberg, B.: The absorption, metabolism and excretion of the sulphonated azo dye. Acid Yellow, in rats. Acta Pharmacol. et Toxicol., *23*:1-14, 1965.

Sipos, K.: Chemical hypersensitivity and dermatological diseases. Dermatologica, *135*:421-432, 1967.

Sjöqvist, F.: Toxic interactions between monoamine oxidase inhibitors (MAOI) and other drugs. *Proc. 3rd Internat. Pharmacol. Meeting,* Ed. J. Cheymol and J. R. Boissier, *10*:61-74, 1968. Pergamon Press, Oxford.

Takacs, E., and Warkany, J.: Experimental production of congenital cardiovascular malformations in rats by salicylate poisoning. Teratology, *1*:109-111, 1968.

Tanimura, T., Katsuya, T., and Nishimura, H.: Embryotoxicity of acute exposure to methyl parathion in rats and mice. Arch. Environ. Health, *15*:609-613, 1967.

Thomas, C., and Bollmann, R.: Untersuchungen zur diaplacentaren krebserzeugenden Wirkung des Diäthylnitrosamins an Ratten. Ztschr. für Krebsforsch., *71*:129-134, 1968.

Weil, C. S., Carpenter, C. P., and Smyth, H. F.: Urinary bladder response to diethylene glycol. Arch. Env. Health, *11*:569-581, 1965.

Wilkinson, D. S.: Contact dermatitis II Sensitization to pesticides. Brit. J. Dermatol., *80*:272-274, 1968.

Wills, J. H., Jameson, E., Stoewsand, G., and Coulston, F.: A three-month study of daily intake of sodium cyclamate by man. Toxicol. Appl. Pharmacol., *12*:292, 1968.

Wolman, W.: Instant and decaffeinated coffee. J.A.M.A., *159*:250, 1955.

Wrba, H., Pielsticker, K., and Mohr, V.: Die diaplacentar carcinogene Wirkung von Diäthylnitrosamin bei Ratten. Naturwiss., *54*:47, 1967.

PART II

GENERAL METHODOLOGIC CONSIDERATIONS

Chapter 8

Isolation and Separation of Toxic Substances From Tissues

HENRY C. FREIMUTH, PH.D.

The scheme which is presented here is one which would be adequate for the so-called "general unknown" type of analysis. In those instances in which specific knowledge of a toxic substance involved in a case is available, consultation of the literature will usually provide specific qualitative and quantitative procedures for the suspected substance.

In general, toxic substances may be divided into five groups which are determined by the procedure used for isolation. These groups are:

1. *Gaseous poisons.* With the exception of carbon monoxide, it is difficult to detect gases in tissues and analytical procedures are usually confined to analysis of samples of air obtained at the scene of the poisoning.
2. *Steam volatile poisons.* Included in this group are organic and inorganic substances which may be isolated by steam distillation.
3. *Metallic poisons.* Metals which are non-volatile below 400°C are separated by dry ashing while those which are volatile at such temperatures are separated by wet ashing.
4. *Non-volatile organic poisons.* These are isolated by solvent extraction using ether or chloroform after appropriate adjustment of pH.
5. *Poisons not classifiable in the other groups.* Included in this group are most inorganic anions as well as water — and alcohol — insoluble organic compounds. Special procedures must usually be employed for the isolation of each substance in this group.

For analysis, large samples of tissue (100 to 500 gm) are preferred to smaller ones since the yield of the toxic substance would be greater and would thus make identification simpler. After qualitative tests have resulted in identification of a toxic agent, a separate smaller portion of tissue can then be used for quantitation.

Negative or questionable results obtained as a result of analysis of very small samples of tissue may be due to inadequacy of the sample. Hence, the pathologist bears the burden of collecting adequate samples of tissues so that proper analysis may be done.

The general scheme for isolation is shown in Figure 1. It will be noted that there is an indication for reservation of 1/3 of the tissue sample for future use. In medical-legal work, this is important

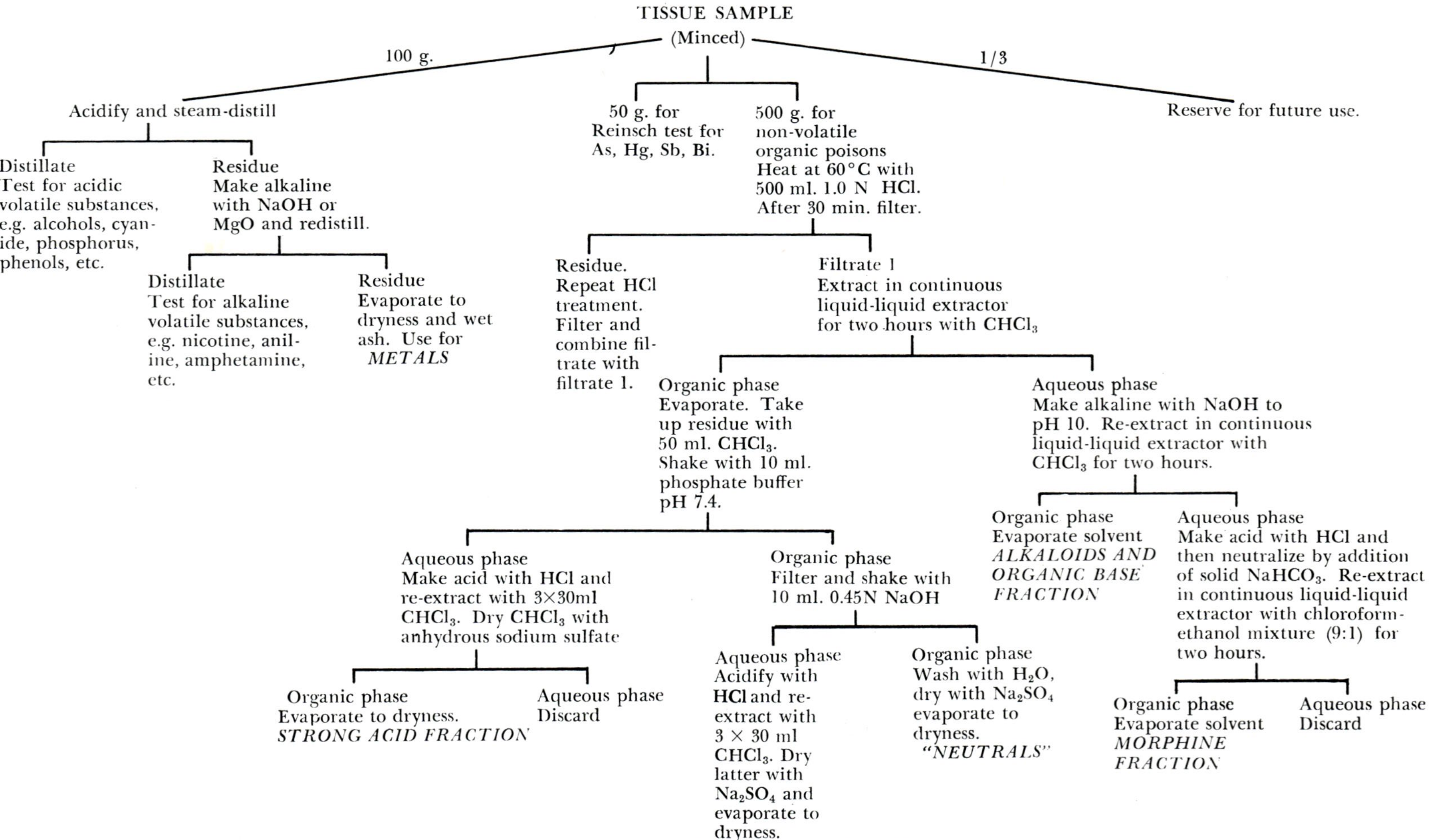

Figure 1. Schema for Isolation of Poisons

since a request might be made for tissue for independent analysis. The stipulation of 1/3 of the sample is the minimum for this purpose.

The various steps indicated in Figure 1 are self-explanatory but some elaboration on the procedure used for ashing for metals may be desirable. In dry ashing, which may be used for metals like lead, a weighed sample of minced tissue (50 to 100 gm) is dried at 110°C in a silica dish. The dried sample is then ashed in a muffle furnace which is gradually heated to 450°C and maintained at this temperature until a white or gray ash remains. This usually requires five to six hours of heating. In the initial stages of heating, the sample should be inspected and any crust which forms should be broken with a spatula to permit escape of gases. Failure to do this may result in the tissue swelling to the point of overflowing the container.

When the ashing has been completed, leaching with mineral acid will yield the metals in solution. The latter may then be tested by the usual chemical tests for the metal in question.

For wet ashing, a weighed sample of tissue is covered with twice its volume of concentrated nitric acid and after standing in a warm place for two to three hours is placed on a steam bath for five to six hours or overnight. Upon cooling, a layer of fat will separate on the surface. This is removed by quantitatively filtering the mixture through a funnel containing a glass wool plug in its apex. The filtrate is collected in a 500 ml Kjeldahl flask.

Five to 10 ml of concentrated sulfuric acid and a few glass beads are added to the flask and the mixture is heated to evaporate the nitric acid. This evaporation is carried out until the mixture just begins to show evidence of charring by darkening in color. At this point, a mixture containing two parts nitric acid and one part perchloric acid is added dropwise while heating is continued. This process is continued until an amber colored residue remains. After cooling, an equal volume of water is added and the mixture is boiled until sulfur trioxide fumes appear. This removes the last traces of nitric and perchloric acids and upon cooling the digest is diluted with water yielding a solution which can be used for metal analysis.

Reference to the literature citations which are appended will give more detail concerning various steps involved in the isolation scheme.

REFERENCES

1. Curry, A. S., and Phang, S. E.: J. Pharm. and Pharmacol., 1960.
2. Daubney, C. G., and Nickolls, L. C.: Analyst, *62:*851, 1937.
3. Daubney, C. G., and Nickolls, L. C.: Analyst, *63:* 560, 1938.
4. Feldstein, M., and Klendshoj, N. C.: Analyst, *78:*43, 1953.
5. Feldstein, M., and Klendshoj, N. C.: J. Forensic Sci., *2:*39, 1957.
6. Gettler, A. O., and Siegel, H.: A.M.A. Arch. Pathol., *19:*208, 1935.
7. Gonzales, T. A., Vance, B. M., Helpern, M., and Umberger, C. J.: *Legal Medicine, Pathology and Toxicology,* 2nd ed. Appleton-Century-Crofts, New York, 1954, p. 1064.
8. Lundsgaard, C., and Holboll, S. A.: J. Bio. Chem., *68:*439, 1926.
9. Pfeiffer, H., and Diller, H. A.: Anal. Chem., *149:* 264, 1956.
10. Plaa, G. L., Hall, F. B., and Hine, C. H.: J. Forensic Sci., *3:*201, 1958.
11. Stewart, C. P., and Stolman, A.: *Toxicology Mechanisms and Analytical Methods,* Vol. I, Chapters 7 and 8. Academic Press, New York, 1960.
12. Umberger, C. J., Stolman, A., and Schwartz, H.: Proc. Am. Acad. Forensic Sci., *1:*250, 1951.
13. Zsigmondy, R., and Heyer, R. Z.: Anorg. Chem., *68:*169, 1910.

Chapter 9

Thin Layer Chromatography in Toxicology

HENRY C. FREIMUTH, PH.D.

INTRODUCTION

Thin layer chromatography, or TLC, is a comparatively recently adopted technique which has found widespread use in analytical toxicology. The principle involved in this technique is the same as in all other chromatographic separation methods, i.e., a mobile phase moves over a stationary phase and, in so doing, carries different substances at different rates in the direction of flow of the mobile system. The mobile phase in TLC is usually a mixture of organic solvents and the stationary phase consists of a thin layer film of adsorbent applied to an inert support. If a mixture of substances, soluble in the mobile phase, is permitted to pass along the film, the components of the solute mixture will be separated because of their differences in adsorption characteristics with respect to the thin film.

Most of the components of a solute mixture would be colorless and therefore could not be located on the thin layer of adsorbent. Hence, a reagent which will react to produce colored products with the solutes is then applied, by spraying, in order to locate the different solute components. This is a very brief exposition of the general techniques in TLC. Space does not permit greater elaboration on theory and the reader is referred to the excellent discussion of these details in the book by Stahl cited in the bibliography.

In the following discussion, it is assumed that the major application of TLC in toxicological analysis is in the separation and identification of non-volatile organic compounds which may be present in tissues or drug products. Using common extraction techniques, the substances of interest are first isolated in an impure state as acidic, basic, or neutral groups of compounds. These residues are then examined by TLC techniques.

Equipment and Reagents

1. *TLC plate or sheets.* Polyester sheets coated with a layer of silica gel 100 microns in thickness are available as Chromagram sheets from Eastman Kodak Company. These sheets are quite satisfactory for many TLC procedures.

In preference to the polyester sheets, glass plates coated with silica gel are more commonly used. Such pre-coated plates are available commercially from Mallinckrodt Chemical Company and from Brinkmann Instruments Inc., Westbury, N.Y. However, many workers prefer to prepare their own plates.

If the latter course is followed, a special spreader or applicator, an application tray, and 20 x 20 cm (or 10 x 20 cm) glass plates must be available. The cleaned glass plates are aligned on the applicator tray and the spreader is placed in position on the first plate with its guide bar adjusted to a thickness of 250 microns. A slurry of Silica Gel G (E. Merck A.G., Darmstadt) is prepared by shaking 25 gm of adsorbent with 60 ml of distilled water for 30 seconds. This is poured into the spreader which is then drawn across the surface of the aligned plates in a smooth, continuous motion. The usual applicator tray will hold five 20 cm plates and the entire coating operation should take about 5 to 6 seconds. The plates are then allowed to remain on the tray until the water evaporates. This is shown by a change in the appearance of the coating from an initial shiny surface to an opaque white surface. The plates are then placed in a carrier rack which, with the plates in a vertical position, is put into a drying oven at 110°C. for 30 minutes. The rack, with the plates, is then stored in a desiccator from which the plates are removed as needed.

2. *Developing jars.* Rectangular glass jars measuring approximately 22 x 22 x 10 cm having ground edges are most satisfactory. The jars are lined on all sides to a height of 18 cm with filter paper (Whatman 3 MM). After placing the appropriate mobile phase in the jar, saturating the filter paper in the process, the jar is covered with a glass cover, sealing with a starch-glycerine paste. Preferably, a flat, heavy weight should be placed over the glass cover to ensure complete sealing.

3. *Application pipettes.* These may be either Drummond "Microcaps" or hand drawn capillary pipettes with a rubber squeeze bulb attached.

4. *Spotting template.* This is a transparent plastic bridge used as a guide for marking the plate and for placing sample spots on the plate. It serves also to prevent damage to the thin layer during sample application.

5. *Spray applicators.* These are used for spraying reagents over the plate after chromatographic development. They may be glass nebulizers operated with compressed air or commercially available sprayers which are operated by pressurized cans.

6. *Compressor,* attached to a drying tower, to provide a source of dry air used during the application of samples to the plate.

7. *Mobile phases.* These are used for chromatographic development of the plates. Many systems are described in the literature for such development and it would not be possible to include them in this discussion. A few representative systems only will be described.

All solvents and chemicals should be of reagent grade quality and the solvents preferably should be redistilled before use.

a. *Mobile phase for acid substances.*

Chloroform	— 210 ml
N-butanol	— 120 ml
ammonia	— 10 ml

The mixture is shaken in a separatory funnel and allowed to stand overnight until clear. The organic layer is allowed to drain into a developing jar, making certain that the paper liner is thoroughly saturated. The ammonia layer is placed in a small beaker which is, in turn, placed in the developing jar. This serves to prolong the life of the jar. The jar is covered and allowed to stand for 6 hours before use.

b. *Mobile phase for alkaloids and other basic substances.*

Benzene	— 150 ml
Dioxane	— 120 ml
Ethanol	— 15 ml
Ammonia	— 15 ml

This is prepared in the same manner as the above mixture and introduced into the jar in the same way. The ammonia layer is also placed in the jar in a small beaker, as above.

Re-distilled dioxane for the preparation of this mixture remains stable (free of peroxides) when stored under nitrogen in a refrigerator.

c. *Mobile phase for phenothiazines.*

Chloroform	— 150 ml
Cyclohexane	— 120 ml
Diethylamine	— 30 ml

The components of this system are completely miscible and the mixture is introduced into the jar immediately after mixing in the manner described above.

d. *Methanol*

As was mentioned previously, many other solvent systems are described in the literature. The choice of solvent is dependent on two factors, i.e., the polarity of the substances to be separated and the polarity of the solvent. In general, the more polar the substance, the greater should be the polarity of the solvent used for its separation.

8. *Spray reagents.* These are chemical compounds or mixtures which will react with the substances separated on the plate to produce a colored product thus locating the substance. Many such spray reagents are used in TLC and only a few will be mentioned here.

a. *Potassium iodoplatinate.* This reagent will produce purplish spots with most organic bases. It is prepared by dissolving 1 gm of $PtCl_4 \cdot 2\ HCl$ in 10 to 50 ml of H_2O, adding a solution of 10 gm KI in 250 ml of H_2O and diluting to 500 ml.

b. *Sulfuric acid – ethanol.* This produces colored spots with phenothiazines. It is made by mixing 4 parts of 50% sulfuric acid with 1 part ethanol and must be prepared freshly before use.

c. *Mercuric nitrate – diphenylcarbazone.* This reacts with barbiturates and many other substances. s-diphenylcarbazone is prepared as a 0.1 percent (w/v) solution in 95 percent alcohol. This is sprayed over the plate to a slight rose color and allowed to dry for five minutes. The plate is then sprayed with 0.33 percent mercuric nitrate in 0.04N nitric acid.

d. *Furfural – hydrochloric acid.* This reacts with carbamates. Redistilled furfural will remain stable for 1 month if stored in a dark bottle under refrigeration. This is first sprayed on the plate and, after drying, followed by a spray of concentrated HCl.

TLC Procedure

The chromatographic jars containing the various solvent systems should be maintained at as nearly constant temperature as possible. This helps to maintain stability of the jar atmospheres and permits greater reproducibility from run to run.

Although other methods are possible,

the usual and most easily carried out method is that of ascending development of the TLC plates which will be the only one discussed here.

When TLC plates are prepared, the spreader forms a thinner layer at the edges of the plate than that on the rest of the glass. This would cause uneven migration of the solvent and therefore the edges of the plate should be stripped to a distance of about 5 mm before use. This may be done using the thumb nail with the forefinger acting as a guide. Alternatively, a razor blade mounted in a holder may be used.

The plate is placed on a sheet of paper which is used to record the various samples applied and their points of application. The template is placed over the plate, positioning its edge 30 mm from the edge of the plate. The substances to be applied are then spotted on the plate at intervals of 15 to 20 mm. It is generally advisable to apply no more than ten samples to a 20 cm plate.

In the application of toxicological samples, the residues obtained as the result of tissue extraction are dissolved in 2 ml of 95% ethanol. Aliquots of this ethanol solution are then transferred immediately to each of two small test tubes. The usual aliquots are 1 ml and 0.2 ml, representing respectively, 50% and 10% of the original tissue sample. The solvent in each tube is evaporated by placing the tube in a beaker of warm water and applying a gentle flow of filtered, dry air from a compressor to the mouth of the tube. The residues in the tubes are then dissolved in two to three drops of 1:1 chloroform-methanol mixture and these solutions are applied quantitatively to the plate. The application of the spots to the plates involves intermittent application of minute drops (using a Drummond Microcap or self-drawn capillary) with subsequent drying by a gentle flow of filtered, dry air from a compressor between applications of the droplets. This is continued until all of the sample has been transferred to the plate. It is essential that the spot covers the smallest possible area. On each plate, there are also applied pilot spots of known compounds in the group being investigated. These known compounds can be made up as 500 mg% solutions in ethanol, so that the application of 10 microliters of such a solution will yield a spot containing 50 micrograms of the known substance.

In narcotic analysis, a good pilot spot to use is an ethanol solution containing 500 mg each of morphine, codeine, heroin and demerol per 100 ml. Ten microliters of this will represent 50 micrograms of each of the component substances. For barbiturates, a similar mixture of barbital, phenobarbital and pentobarbital may be used as a pilot spot.

After all samples have been applied, a line is scribed across the plate exactly 15 cm from the line of application of the spots. It is a good idea to mark the location of each spot by making a small dot in the silica gel by touching it with the tip of the applicator pipette after the last portion of sample has been applied.

The plate is now placed in the appropriate developing jar with the end containing the spots at the bottom of the jar. The jar is sealed and the solvent permitted to migrate until it reaches the prescribed 15 cm line. The progress of the solvent is easily noticed because the wet layer is darker than the unwetted surface. When the 15 cm line is reached, the plate is immediately removed from the jar (which is immediately re-covered for further use) and allowed to dry. This is best done at room temperature in a fume hood where the flow of air across the plate surface will facilitate drying.

The dried plate is then examined under ultra-violet light to locate any substances which fluoresce. This is particularly important in narcotics examinations since quinine, commonly used as an adulterant in illegal narcotic traffic, can be readily detected in this way.

Following the ultra-violet examination, the plate is sprayed with the appropriate spray reagent and allowed to dry again. Colored spots will locate the various substances on the plate. The distance from the starting line to the center of the spot is measured. This distance divided by the distance of solvent flow (15 cm) is the R_f value of the substance. Reference to a table of previously determined R_f values will indicate the nature of the unknown substance. However, absolute R_f values are frequently misleading since it is difficult to duplicate all experimental parameters each time. Hence, a better procedure is to use a relative R_f value which is the ratio of the R_f value of the substance to the R_f value of a standard substance. For example, codeine is frequently used as the standard substance in narcotics analysis. On a given plate, one determines the R_f value of the unknown and the R_f value of codeine, thus establishing the relative R_f value of the unknown. Reference is then made to a previously constructed table of relative R_f values based upon codeine as the standard.

After the sprayed plate has dried, a permanent record may be made by photocopying on an ordinary office copying machine such as a Verifax or Thermofax copier. This photocopy is usually more easily used for the measurement of R_f values than the original plate.

R_f values, of themselves, do not characterize a substance since many compounds in a group have identical or similar R_f values. A minimum difference of 0.05 in R_f value must be present in order to make a distinction between any two substances. For example, in the benzene-dioxane system, a difference of only 0.02 exists between morphine and dilaudid so that one could not distinguish between these two compounds by TLC in this system. Furthermore, if both were present in a sample, the resolution would be so poor as to lack usefulness. However, the spot on the plate could be eluted as described below and then re-applied to a sodium hydroxide impregnated silica gel G plate. The latter is made in the same way as an ordinary plate with the exception that 0.1N sodium hydroxide is used in place of water in preparing the slurry. The plate is then developed in methanol. In this system, the difference between the R_f values of morphine and dilaudid is 0.15 thus serving as a means of characterization and separation.

In general, TLC techniques serve as another analytical tool which, if used in conjunction with other techniques, will assist in characterizing a substance. It serves as a preliminary indication of identity and also serves to produce the substance in a pure state so that other identifying characteristics are not interfered with.

In the case of alkaloids and other basic compounds located on a plate with iodoplatinate spray, the spot on the plate is outlined by scribing a rectangular area well around the spot. The silica gel within the rectangle is carefully scraped off and transferred to a 60 ml separatory funnel. Five to ten ml of 0.1N hydrochloric acid plus a few crystals of sodium bisulfite are added. This mixture is shaken with two portions (15 to 20 ml) of ether, retaining the aqueous phase. The combined ether extracts are re-extracted with two portions (3 to 5 ml) of 0.1N hydrochloric acid and the latter extracts are added to the aqueous phase above. The ether is discarded.

The aqueous phase is made alkaline by addition of solid sodium bicarbonate until no further effervescence occurs. It is then extracted with three 20 ml portions of chloroform containing 10% ethanol. Each chloroform extract is passed through the same filter containing anhydrous sodium sulfate and collected in a dry 60 ml separatory funnel. The combined chloroform extract is then extracted with two 2 ml portions of 0.1N hydrochloric acid. The clear aqueous phases are combined and used for ultra-violet spectrophotometry. The sample is measured against a blank prepared by extracting 60 ml of chloroform containing 10% ethanol with two 2 ml portions of 0.1N hydrochloric acid. Characteristic absorption maxima may be used for quantitation.

Since many narcotics are poor absorbers in the ultra-violet region, the absence of spectra does not exclude their presence. Color reactions and precipitation reactions may be used for identification. The hydrochloric acid solution used above is made alkaline by addition of sodium bicarbonate as before and extracted with three 10 ml portions of chloroform containing 10% ethanol. The combined chloroform extracts, filtered through anhydrous sodium sulfate, are collected in a small beaker. This is evaporated to near dryness on a water bath, and the last few drops are allowed to evaporate at room temperature. The residue may then be used for color tests, precipitation reactions, infra-red spectra, and/or gas chromatography as described in the literature.

Similar confirming procedures may be applied to barbiturates and like compounds separated by TLC. The spot scraped off the plate is placed in a separatory funnel to which 10 ml of 0.1N hydrochloric acid is added. This is extracted with three 30 ml portions of chloroform. The combined, filtered chloroform is extracted with 5 ml of 0.45N sodium hydroxide. The clear sodium hydroxide is subjected to ultra-violet spectrophotometry for characterization.

Reference to the bibliography will give more specific information concerning many of the applications of this technique.

REFERENCES

1. Curry, A. S.: *Methods of Forensic Science,* Vol. III, 1964; Vol. IV, 1966. Interscience Publishers, New York.
2. Stewart, C. P., and Stolman, A.: *Toxicology, Mechanisms and Analytical Methods,* Vol. I, 1961; Vol. II, 1962. Academic Press, New York.
3. Stolman, A.: *Progress in Chemical Toxicology,* Vol. I, 1963; Vol. II, 1965; Vol. III, 1967. Academic Press, New York.
4. Stahl, E.: *Thin Layer Chromatography, A Laboratory Handbook.* Academic Press, New York. 1965.
5. Mule, S. J.: Determination of narcotic analgesics in human biological materials. Application of UV spectrophotometry, thin layer and gas liquid chromatography. Anal. Chem., *36:*1907, 1964.
6. Eberhardt, H., *et al.*: Thin layer chromatographic detection of habit forming analgesics as pure substances and after passing through the body. Arzneimittel-Forsch., *14* (12) :1354, 1964 (German) .
7. Davidow, B., *et al.*: A thin layer chromatographic screening test for the detection of users of morphine and heroin. Am. J. Clin. Path., *46:* 58, 1966.
8. Cochin, J., *et al.*: Rapid identification of analgesic drugs in urine with thin layer chromatography. Experientia, *18:*294, 1962.
9. Cochin, J., *et al.*: The use of thin layer chromatography for the analysis of drugs. Isolation and identification of barbiturates and non-barbiturate hypnotics from urine, blood and tissues. The Pharmacologist, *4:*171, 1962.

10. Sunshine, I.: Use of thin layer chromatography in the diagnosis of poisoning. Am. J. Clin. Path., *40*:576, 1963.
11. Sunshine, I.: Identification of therapeutically significant organic bases by TLC. J. Forensic Sci., *11*:428, 1966.
12. Schweda, P.: Thin layer chromatography of toxicologically significant substances on silica gel coated glass plates and polyester sheets. Anal. Chem., *39*:1019, 1967.

Chapter 10

Measurement of Toxic Agents by Gas Chromatography

JOHN SAVORY, PH.D.

Applications of gas chromatography to chemical toxicology are at the present time in an early developmental stage. Eventually, the chief uses of gas chromatography will involve the screening of specimens in the general unknown category. However, current uses are in special procedures designed for the identification of a single compound or class of compounds. Measurements by gas chromatography rely to a large extent on the volatility of compounds rather than depending on specific chemical properties. Thus, a large number of compounds possessing volatility, but having different chemical properties, can be identified by a single gas chromatographic analysis. The remarkable sensitivity of the technique is also attractive to the chemical toxicologist who frequently has only microgram quantities of material available for analysis.

Principles of Gas Chromatography

Most of the applications of gas chromatography in the biomedical field have involved gas-liquid chromatography. However, gas-solid chromatography has been developed and uses adsorptive materials on a solid support as a column packing. A schematic representation of the basic design of a gas chromatograph is shown in Figure 1. Gas-liquid chromatography is a variety of partition chromatography in which the stationary phase is a liquid film supported by a column of inert particles inside a long tube. The tube, or column, is housed in a thermostatically controlled oven and is maintained at a temperature high enough to ensure that all compounds to be detected are kept in the vapor state inside the column. The mobile phase involved in the chromatographic separation is an inert gas such as helium, which flows through the column over the surface of the liquid film. The sample is injected into one end of the gas chromatographic column where a flash heater causes vaporization of all volatile constituents of the mixture. These constituents become separated into zones as they travel along the column. The separated compounds finally emerge from the other end of the column in a sequence which is dependent upon their respective partition coefficients between the gas and liquid phases. The partition coefficients of com-

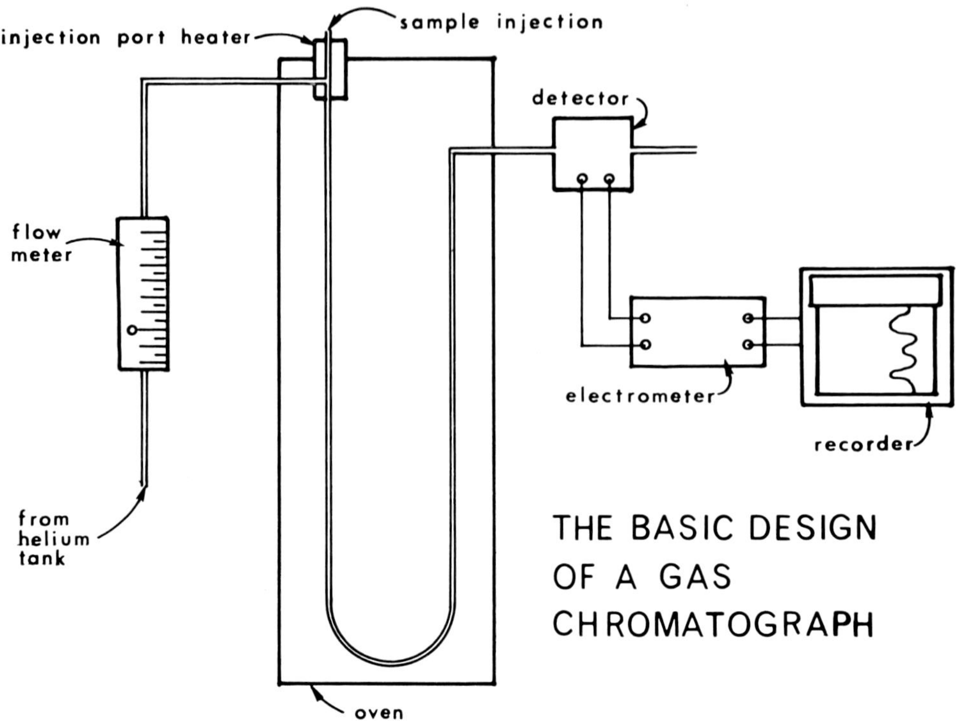

Figure 1. The basic design of a gas chromatograph.

pounds may be adjusted by changing the temperature of the chromatographic column. The emergence of a compound from the end of the column is usually detected by the alteration it produces in the ionization, thermal conductivity, or electron capture capabilities of the effluent gas. The detector response is amplified by an electrometer and is visualized graphically as a peak upon a continuous recording of the detector response. This graphic recording is known as a "gas chromatogram."

Qualitative identification of a compound by gas chromatography is based upon measurements of its "retention time" upon the column. The retention time of a compound is a parameter which is analogous to an R_f value in paper chromatography. Quantitative estimation of a compound is made by comparing the area or height of its peak on the gas chromatogram with corresponding measurements made with standard samples of the same compound. The capability of performing simultaneous qualitative and quantitative analyses is one of the principal advantages of gas chromatography. Additional advantages include: (1) great resolution for the separation of mixtures, with theoretical plate values ranging from 2,000 to 1,000,000; (2) high sensitivity, with limits of detection at the submicrogram level; (3) speed, with fractionations usually being completed within a few minutes; and (4) versatility, with a wide variety of possible analytical applications in chemical toxicology. Identification and determination of alcohols and drugs are among the most important applications of gas chromatography, and will be reviewed as examples of the contribution of this technique to chemical toxicology.

In addition, a review of procedures presently being developed for the gas chromatographic determination of metals will be presented to illustrate the immense potential of gas chromatograph as an analytical tool in the area of chemical toxicology.

Gas Chromatography of Alcohols

Among the first applications of gas chromatography to the detection of toxic compounds in biological materials was the determination of volatile organic poisons. Particular emphasis has been placed on ethanol because of the frequency of tests requested, but most methods described for ethanol can be extended to many more compounds, for example, methanol, n- and isopropyl alcohol, the butyl alcohols, acetone, diethyl ether, benzene, toluene, chloroform, carbon tetrachloride, etc.

A gas chromatographic method for the quantitative determination of ethanol in blood or serum was described by Fox[21] in 1958 and has been modified by numerous subsequent investigators.[8, 10, 14, 16, 17, 22, 23, 36, 37, 40, 42, 51, 55, 61, 69, 76, 82] These modifications differ primarily in the techniques for handling the samples of blood or serum prior to the injection onto the columns of gas chromatographs. Fox[21] separated ethanol from blood proteins by distillation and injected an aliquot of the distillate onto the column of the gas chromatography. McCord and Gasden[42] used a similar distillation technique and achieved a separation of acetone and the volatile aliphatic alcohols using a di-isodecylphthalate column. Cadman[8] and other workers[61] described the extraction of ethanol from blood and urine with n-propyl acetate followed by gas chromatographic determination of ethanol in the extract. Lyons and Bard[36] performed a similar extraction using a combination of n-butanol with anhydrous calcium sulfate. Goldbaum and associates[24] described a method in which vapor in equilibrium with a sample of blood was injected into the gas chromatograph. This method has limited accuracy due to variations in the gas-liquid partition ratio of alcohol caused by variations in the composition of the biological specimens. Wallace and Dahl[82] minimized variations in this gas-liquid partition ratio by adding greater than saturation amounts of sodium chloride to the samples. Protein precipitation prior to injection of the serum sample into the column has also been employed.[16, 40] Most other procedures,[10, 14, 22, 23, 37, 55, 76] however, involve the addition of a volatile internal standard to the blood samples and injection into the gas chromatographic column. Proteins and other nonvolatile constituents are retained on the column around the injection port and in some procedures a provision has been made to replace this part of the column at frequent intervals. In 1965, Natelson and Stellate[51] reported a novel technique whereby the serum sample was dehydrated by addition of anhydrous copper sulfate, and the liberated ethanol swept by a stream of carrier gas onto the gas chromatographic column. The Natelson-Stellate procedure has been employed in our laboratory during the past three years, and has undergone a number of modifications,[69] which have significantly improved the sensitivity, precision, and adaptability of the technique for routine use in clinical laboratories. In many respects, this modified procedure is similar to the gas chromatographic method for determination of lactic acid in blood which has been described by Savory and Kaplan.[66] Serum is injected into a gas-tight dehydration tube which contains an excess of anhydrous copper sulfate. Water is rapidly extracted from the serum by the formation of copper sulfate pentahydrate, an exothermic reaction which simultaneously liberates serum ethanol as a vapor. The ethanol vapor is swept onto the column of a gas chromatograph, where it is separated from the other volatile constituents of serum. Ethanol is detected and measured in the effluent gas from the chromatographic column by means of a hydrogen-flame ionization detector.

Thus, gas chromatographic procedures for the measurement of alcohols and similar compounds in biological materials have been developed to a stage where they are reliable and suitable for routine determinations. The over-all sensitivity, speed of analysis, and capability of identifying several compounds on a single chromatogram makes gas chromatography the method of choice for this type of analysis.

Gas Chromatography of Drugs

Gas chromatographic methods have been developed over the past few years for the separation and identification of a large number of drugs including barbiturates, analgesics, hypnotics, amphetamines, tranquilizers and antihistaminics.

Janak,[31] in 1960, employed pyrolysis of a sample at 800° prior to gas chromatography and was able to identify barbiturates. Nelson and Kirk[52] described a similar procedure and reported pyrolysis patterns for 27 barbiturates. These procedures were probably satisfactory for samples containing only one unknown compound, but their application to analysis of mixtures of unknown compounds in biological materials would give extremely complicated patterns. Cook and co-workers[12] achieved gas chromatographic separations of barbiturates using the dimethyl derivatives formed by reaction of the barbiturates with diazomethane. Stevenson[75] carried out a methylation reaction on the gas chromatographic column itself by injecting the barbiturate in a solution of tetramethylammonium hydroxide.

Parker and Kirk,[56] in 1961, attempted to apply gas chromatography to the separation of barbiturates as the free acids. Barbiturates were extracted from blood by conventional procedures using chloroform and 0.45 N sodium hydroxide. After a concentration step, an aliquot of the final chloroform extract was injected onto the column of the gas chromatograph and separation of several barbiturates was achieved. Several papers[5, 7, 11, 26, 43] have appeared since 1961 describing gas chromatographic conditions for the separation of barbituric acid derivatives and related compounds in non-biological systems. Various column packings, column temperatures and detectors have been employed to obtain these separations.

In 1963, Kazyak and Knoblock[33] described the application of gas chromatography to analytic toxicology. They obtained acid, neutral, and basic chloroform extracts of biological specimens and succeeded in detecting microquantities of barbiturates, tranquilizers, histamines, sympathomimetic amines and many of the alkaloids. To achieve adequate sensitivity, the chloroform extracts were concentrated prior to gas chromatographic measurements. Other workers have developed similar procedures for screening biological specimens to identify a wide variety of drugs.[24, 30, 44, 54, 79] In addition, several procedures have been described for the determination of specific drugs.[15, 20, 29, 35, 41, 60, 74, 77, 83] Many procedures for extracting drugs from blood and other biological materials have involved solvent extraction of the aqueous fluids and evaporation to dryness. After reconstitution the residue has been injected into the gas chromatograph.[20, 24, 30, 33, 35, 41, 44, 74, 77, 79] However, in certain instances adequate sensitivity has been achieved without the evaporation step. Anders[2] extracted barbiturates from blood by mixing one volume of blood with one volume of chloroform and injecting an aliquot of the extract. Winsten and Brody[83] similarly extracted glutethimide from one ml of serum by mixing with 0.4 ml of chloroform. Methods where the evaporation step is eliminated are more adaptable to emergency situations where simplified and rapid procedures are desirable.

Gas Chromatography of Chromium

Measurements of levels of chromium in biological materials are important from both a toxicological aspect, and from the functioning of chromium as a trace element essential to normal metabolic processes in man. Chromium (VI) has been considered a toxic metal for many years and toxicity studies of subjects exposed to industrial dichromates have been reported.[3, 6, 25, 38, 39, 49, 57] Chromium (III) is less toxic than chromium (VI) and evidence is accumulating that this trivalent ion has biological activity.[13, 45, 46, 70, 71, 72]

Gas chromatography is a specific and extremely sensitive method for the detection of metals as their β-diketone chelates. Extensive studies have been made of the basic problems involved in these measurements and much of this work has been reviewed.[50, 65] β-diketone chelates of chromium derived from acetylacetone,[28, 62] trifluoroacetylacetone,[1, 28, 62, 64, 78, 81] hexafluoroacetylacetone,[28, 32, 62, 63] and heptafluoro-dimethyloctanedione[73] have been detected by gas chromatography and exceptional sensitivity has been obtained from the fluoro-β-diketones using the electron capture detector.[1, 62, 63, 64, 73]

A method was developed in the authors' laboratory[67, 68] for the determination of chromium in serum and urine using the gas chromatographic properties of chromium trifluoroacetylacetonate [$Cr(TFA)_3$], and was the first reported procedure where gas chromatography has been used to determine metals in biological samples. This method was found to be more sensitive than previous chromium methods which have utilized the various techniques of spectrophotometry,[9, 47, 80] arc emission spectrography,[27, 34, 48, 53] spark source mass spectrography,[84] atomic absorption spectrometry,[19, 58] coulometry,[18] polarography,[57] and neutron activation analysis.[4, 59] The method involved a preliminary acid digestion step to destroy all organic material in the serum or urine sample. Conditions were adjusted to assure that all chromium present was in the trivalent ionic state and a reaction was carried out with trifluoroacetylacetone to produce chromium trifluoroacetylacetone. Gas chromatographic analysis of the resulting reaction mixture was used to determine the amount of chromium trifluoroacetylacetonate present.

Extension of this technique to the determination of other metals is feasible since stable volatile chelates can be prepared from many metals.

Summary

A resume has been presented of the basic principles of gas chromatography with applications in the area of measuring blood alcohols and drugs. The development of a method for the measurement of chromium indicates future applications of gas chromatography to chemical toxicology in the area of trace metal measurements.

REFERENCES

1. Albert, D. K.: Comparison of electron capture and hydrogen flame detectors for gas chromatographic determination of trace amounts of metal chelates. Anal. Chem., *36*:2034-2035, 1964.
2. Anders, M. W.: Rapid micromethod for gas chromatographic determination of blood barbiturates. Anal. Chem., *38*:1945-1947, 1966.
3. Baetjer, A. M., Damron, C., and Budacz, V.: The distribution and retention of chromium in men and animals. A.M.A. Arch. Indust. Health, *20*:136-150, 1959.
4. Bowen, H. J. M.: Determination of chromium in biological materials by radioactivation. Analyst, *89*:658-661, 1964.
5. Braddock, L. I., and Marec, N.: The gas chromatographic analysis of submicrogram quantities of barbiturates using a flame ionization detector. J. of Gas Chromatog., pp. 274-277, 1965.
6. Brieger, H.: Zur Klinik der akuten Chromatovergiftung. Ztschr. f. exper. Path. u. Therap., *21*:393-408, 1920.
7. Brochmann-Hanssen, E., and Svendsen, A. B.: Separation and identification of barbiturates and some related compounds by means of gas-liquid chromatography. J. Pharm. Sci., *51*:318-320, 1962.
8. Cadman, W. J., and Johns, T.: Application of the gas chromatograph in the laboratory of criminalistics. J. Forensic Sci., *5*:369-385, 1960.
9. Cahnmann, H. J., and Bisen, R.: Microdetermination of chromium in blood. Anal. Chem., *24*: 1341-1345, 1952.
10. Chundela, B., and Janak, J.: Quantitative determinations of ethanol besides other volatile substances in blood and other body liquids by gas chromatography. J. Forensic Med., *7*:153-161, 1960.
11. Cieplinski, E. W.: Prevention of peak tailing in the direct gas chromatographic analysis of barbiturates. Anal. Chem., *35*:256-257, 1963.
12. Cook, J. G. H., Riley, C., Nunn, R. F., and Budgen, D. E.: Gas Chromatography of methyl derivatives of some barbiturates. J. Chromatog., *6*:182-185, 1961.
13. Curran, G. L.: Effect of certain transition group elements on hepatic synthesis of cholesterol in the rat. J. Biol. Chem., *210*:765-770, 1954.
14. Curry, A. S., Walker, G. W., and Simpson, G. S.: Determination of ethanol in blood by gas chromatography. Analyst, *91*:742-743, 1966.
15. Curry, S. H.: Determination of nanogram quantities of chlorpromazine and some of its metabolites in plasma using gas-liquid chromatography with an electron capture detector. Anal. Chem., *40*:1251-1255, 1968.
16. Davis, R. A.: The determination of ethanol in blood or tissue by gas chromatography. J. Forensic Sci., *11*:205-213, 1966.
17. Drawert, F., and Kupfer, G.: Reaction gas chromatography V. Blood alcohol analysis. Hoppe Seyler Z. Physiol. Chem, *329*:90-96, 1962.
18. Feldman, F. J., Christian, G. D., and Purcy, W. C.: Coulometric determination of chromium in biologic materials. Am. J. Clin. Path., *49*: 826-833, 1968.
19. Feldman, F. J., Knoblock, E. C., and Purdy, W. C.: The determination of chromium in biological materials by atomic absorption spectroscopy. Anal. Chim. Acta., *38*:489-497, 1967.
20. Finkle, B. S.: The identification, quantitative determination, and distribution of meprobamate and glutethimide in biological material. J. Forensic Sci., *12*:509-528, 1967.
21. Fox, J. E.: Gas chromatographic analysis of alcohol and certain other volatiles in biological materials for forensic purposes. Proc. Soc. Exp. Biol. Med., *97*:236-237, 1958.
22. Freudiger, J. B., and Vignau, J. A.: Determination of alcohols in body fluids by gas-liquid chromatography. J. Forensic Sci., *10*:73-76, 1965.
23. Freund, G.: Exchangeable injection port cartridge for gas chromatographic determination of volatile substances in aqueous fluids. Anal. Chem., *39*:545-546, 1967.

24. Goldbaum, L. R., and Domanski, T. J.: Detection and identification of micrograms of neutral drugs in biological samples. J. Forensic Sci., *11:* 233-242, 1966.
25. Goldman, M., and Karotkin, R. H.: Acute potassium bichromatic poisoning. Am. J. M. Sci., *189:*400-403, 1935.
26. Gudzinowicz, B. J., and Clark, S. J.: The gas chromatographic analysis of low concentrations of barbiturates using an electron affinity detector. J. of Gas Chromatog., pp. 147-151, 1965.
27. Herring, W. B., Leavell, B. S., Paixao, Z. M., and Yoe, J. H.: Trace metals in human plasma and red blood cells. Am. J. Clin. Nutrition, *8:*846-854, 1960.
28. Hill, R. D., and Gesser, H.: An investigation into the quantitative gas chromatographic analysis of metal chelates using a hydrogen-flame ionization detector. J. Gas Chromatog., pp. 11-14, 1963.
29. Jain, N. C., Crim, D., Kaplan, H. L., Forney, R. B., and Hughes, F. W.: A rapid gas chromatographic method for the determination of chloral hydrate and trichloroethanol in blood and other biological materials. J. Forensic Sci. *12:*497-508, 1967.
30. Jain, N. C., and Kirk, P. L.: Systematic applications of gas-liquid chromatography in toxicology. 1. Extraction procedure and the alkaloids. Microchem. J., *12:*229-240, 1967.
31. Janak, J.: Identification of the structure of non-volatile organic substances by gas chromatography of pyrolytic products. Nature, *185:*684-686, 1960.
32. Juvet, R S., and Durbin, R. P.. Flame photometric detection of metal chelates separated by gas chromatography. J. Gas Chromatog., pp. 14-17, 1963.
33. Kazyak, L., and Knoblock, E. C.: Application of gas chromatography to analytical toxicology. Anal. Chem., *35:*1448-1452, 1963.
34. Koch, H. J., Jr., Smith, E. R., Shimp, N. F., and Conner, J.: Analysis of trace elements in human tissues. Cancer, *9:*499-511, 1956.
35. Korzun, B. P., Brody, S. M., Keegan, P. G., Lunders, R. C., and Rehm, C. R.: Rapid chromatographic method for the identification and estimation of glutethimide (Doriden) in blood. J. Lab. Clin. Med., *68:*333-338, 1966.
36. Lyons, H., and Bard, J.: Gas chromatographic determination of lower alcohols in biologic samples. Clin. Chem., *10:*429-432, 1964.
37. Machata, G.: Routine determination of blood alcohol concentration by gas chromatography. Mikrochim. Acta., *4:*691-700, 1962.
38. Major, R. H.: Case of chronic acid nephritis. Bull, John Hopkins Hosp., *33:*56-61, 1922.
39. Mancuso, T. F.: Occupational cancer and other health hazards in a chromate plant: A medical appraisal. II. Clinical and toxicological aspects. Industrial Med. and Surgery, *20:*393-407, 1951.
40. Maricq, L., and Molle, L.: Investigation on the determination of blood alcohol levels by gas chromatography. Bull. Acad. Med. Belg., Series 6, *24:*199-232, 1959.
41. Martin, H. F., and Driscoll, J. L.: Gas chromatographic identification and determination of barbiturates. Anal. Chem., *38:*345-346, 1966.
42. McCord, W. M., and Gadsden, R. H.: The identification and determination of alcohols in blood by gas chromatography. J. Gas Chromatog., pp. 38-39, 1964.
43 McMartin, C., and Street, H. V.: Gas-liquid chromatography of submicrogram amounts of drugs. 1. Preparation, scope and limitation of columns J. Chromatog., *22:*274-285, 1966.
44. McMartin, C. and Street, H. V.: Gas-liquid chromatography of submicrogram amounts of drugs. II. Analysis of barbiturates and related drugs in biological media. J. Chromatog., *23:* 232-241, 1966.
45. Mertz, W., Roginski, E. E., and Reba, R. C.: Biological activity and fate of trace quantities of intravenous chromium (III) in the rat. Am. J. Physiol., *209:*489-494, 1965.
46. Mertz, W., and Schwarz, K.: Chromium (III) and the glucose tolerance factor. in: "Measurements of exocrine and endocrine functions of the pancreas," J.B. Lippincott Co., Philadelphia, Pa., pp. 123-127.
47. Miller, D. O., and Yoe, J. H.: Spectrophotometric determination of chromium in human plasma and red cells Clin. Chim. Acta., *4:*378-383, 1959.
48. Monacelli, R., Tanaka, H., and Yoe, J. H.: Spectrochemical determination of magnesium, chromium, nickel, copper and zinc in human plasma. Clin. Chim. Acta., *1:*577-582, 1956.
49. Morris, G. E.: Chrome dermatitis. A.M.A. Arch. of Dermatology, *78:*612-618, 1958.
50. Moshier, R. W., and Sievers, R. E.: Gas chromatography of metal chelates. Pergamon Press, Oxford, 1965, and references cited therein.
51. Natelson, S., and Stellate, R. L.: Instrumentation for the concentration of trace components of a mixture for gas chromatography. Application to the determination of acetone, ethanol, methanol, and 2-propanol in blood. Microchem. J., *9:*245-256, 1965.
52. Nelson, D. F., and Kirk, P. L.: Identification of substituted barbituric acids by gas chromatography of their pyrolysis products. Anal. Chem., *34:*899-903, 1962.
53. Paixao, L. M., and Yoe, J. H.: Spectrochemical determination of magnesium, chromium, nickel, copper and zinc in human plasma and red cells. Clin. Chim. Acta., *4:*507-514, 1959.

54. Parker, K. D., Fontan, C. R., and Kirk, P. L.: Rapid gas chromatographic method for screening of toxicological extracts for alkaloids, barbiturates, sympathomimetic amines and tranquilizers. Anal. Chem., *35:*356-359, 1963.
55. Parker, K. D., Fontan, C. R., Yee, J. L., and Kirk, P. L.: Gas chromatographic determination of ethyl alcohol in blood for medicolegal purposes. Anal. Chem., *34:*1234-1236, 1962.
56. Parker, K. D., and Kirk, P. L.: Separation of identification of barbiturates by gas chromatography. Anal. Chem., *33:*1378-1381, 1961.
57. Pascale, L. R., Waldstein, S. S., Engbring, G., Dubin, A., and Szanto, P. B.: Chromium intoxication with special reference to hepatic injury. J.A.M.A., *149:*1385-1389, 1952.
58. Pierce, J. O, and Cholak, J.: Lead, chromium and moylbdenum by atomic absorption. Arch. Environ. Health, *13:*208-212, 1966.
59. Pijek, J., Gillis, J., and Hoste, J.: Preparative radiation chemistry. Intern. J. Appl. Radiation and Isotopes, *10:*149-157, 1961.
60. Resnick, G. L., Corbin, D., and Sandberg, D. H.: Determination of serum chloramphenicol utilizing gas-liquid chromatography and electron capture spectrometry. Anal. Chem., *38:*582-585, 1966.
61. Rockerbie, R. A.: The quantitative determination of ethanol in blood by gas chromatography. Canad. Phar. J., *96:*38-39, 1963.
62. Ross, W. D.: Detection of metal chelates in gas-liquid chromatography by electron capture. Anal. Chem., *35:*1596-1598, 1963.
63. Ross, W. D., and Wheeler, G.: Quantitative determination of chromium (III) hexafluoroacetylacetonate by gas chromatography. Anal. Chem., *36:*266-268, 1964.
64. Ross, W. D., and Sievers, R. E.: Quantitative ultra-trace analysis of mixtures of metal chelates by gas chromatography. Anal. Chem., *37:*598-600, 1965.
65. Ross, W. D., and Sievers, R. E.: Rapid ultratrace determination of beryllium by gas chromatography. Talanta, *15:*87-94, 1968.
66. Savory, J., and Kaplan, A.: A gas chromatographic method for the determination of lactic acid in blood. Clin. Chem., *12:*559-569, 1966.
67. Savory, J., Mushak, P., Roszel, N. O., and Sunderman, F. W., Jr.: Determination of chromium in serum by gas chromatography. Fed. Proc., *27:* 777, #3154, 1968.
68. Savory, J., Mushak, P., and Sunderman, F. W., Jr.: Gas chromatographic determination of chromium in serum. Advances in Chromatog., in press.
69. Savory, J., Sunderman, F. W., Jr., Roszel, N. O., and Mushak, P.: An improved procedure for the determination of serum ethanol by gas chromatography. Clin. Chem., *14:*132-144, 1968.
70. Schroeder, H. A.: Chromium deficiency in rats: a syndrome simulating diabetes mellitus with retarded growth. J. Nutr., *88:*439-445, 1966.
71. Schroeder, H. A., Balassa, J. J., and Tipton, I. H.: Abnormal trace metals in man-chromium. J. Chron. Dis., *15:*941-964, 1962.
72. Schwarz, K., and Mertz, W.: Chromium (III) and the glucose tolerance factor. Arch. Biochem. Biophys., *85:*292-295, 1959.
73. Sievers, R. E., Connolly, J. W., and Ross, W. D.: Metal analysis by gas chromatography of chelates of heptafluorodimethyloctanedione. J. Gas Chromatog., pp. 241-247, 1967.
74. Skinner, R. F.: The determination of meprobamate in blood, urine, and liver by gas chromatography. J. Forensic Sci., *12:*230-237, 1967.
75. Stevenson, G. W.: On-column methylation of barbituric acids. Anal. Chem., *38:*1948-1949, 1966.
76. Sturner, W. Q., and Coumbis, R. J.: The quantitation of ethyl alcohol in vitreous humor and blood by gas chromatography. Am. J. Clin. Path., *46:*349-351, 1966.
77. Sunshine, I., Maes, R., and Faracci, R.: Determination of glutethimide (Doriden) and its metabolites in biologic specimens. Clin. Chem., *14:*595-609, 1968.
78. Tanikawa, K., Hirano, K., and Arakawa, K.: Organometallic compounds. V. Gas chromatographic analysis of metal trifluoroacetylacetonates. Chem. Pharm. Bull., *15:*915-920, 1967.
79. Thompson, H. L., and Decker, W. J.: Analysis of blood. A simplified gas chromatographic approach for toxicological purposes. Am. J. Clin. Path., *49:*103-107, 1968.
80. Urone, P. F., and Anders, H. K.: Determination of small amounts of chromium in human blood, tissues, and urine. Anal. Chem., *22:*1317-1321, 1950.
81. Veening, H., and Huber, J. F. K.: Phenomena which influence the retention of metal fluoroacetylacetonates in gas-liquid chromatography. J. Gas Chromatog., pp. 326-330, 1968.
82. Wallace, J. E., and Dahl, E. V.: Rapid vapor phase method for determining ethanol in blood and urine by gas chromatography. Am. J. Clin. Path., *46:*152-154, 1966.
83. Winsten, S., and Brody, D.: Rapid determination of glutethimide (Doriden) by gas-liquid chromatography. Clin. Chem., *14:*589-594, 1967.
84. Wolstenholme, W. A.: Analysis of dried blood plasma by spark source mass spectrometry. Nature, *203:*1284-1285, 1964.

Chapter 11

Measurement of Toxic Metals by Atomic Absorption Spectrophotometry

M. LUBRAN, M.D.

Exposure to many metals or their salts, particularly over a long period of time, may result in toxic effects.[1] The amount of the metal in the tissues and body fluids is usually small, blood and urine concentrations often being lower than 1 $\mu g/ml$. Acute metal poisoning, either accidental or deliberate, frequently results in much higher concentrations. A major problem of industrial hygiene is the screening of urine or blood for unacceptable levels of toxic metals in exposed workers. Atomic absorption spectrophotometry (AAS) provides a suitable technique, combining sensitivity, specificity and convenience (Table 1).[2, 3, 4, 5] However in common with other techniques, it has its limitations; to obtain meaningful answers with AAS requires an understanding of the principles of the technique and the apparatus used.

In essence, AAS measures the amount of light of particular wavelengths (resonance energies) absorbed by neutral atoms in the ground state (i.e., unexcited and unionised). The basic apparatus for making this measurement consists of a source of the specific radiation, a device for producing atoms, a monochromator and slit system for selecting the specific radiation passing through the atoms, and a device for detecting and quantitating the transmitted radiation. Light of the correct wavelength is conveniently produced by a hollow-cathode lamp; atoms are in almost all cases produced by a flame into which a solution of the compound is introduced through a nebulizer. The monochromator need not have very high resolution: the width of the lines emitted by the hollow cathode lamp is very narrow. The detector is usually a photomultiplier tube with appropriate circuitry for amplification. Each part of the apparatus has its characteristics, which can affect the final answer, particularly when low concentrations of metal are being measured. The hollow-cathode lamp and the flame (with nebulizer) are responsible for most of the difficulties of AAS.

The hollow-cathode lamp produces many emission lines of the element concerned. Only a few of these lines are absorbed, and are therefore suitable for AAS; they are produced by transitions from the first excited level to the ground state. Usually, only one or two lines are

TABLE 1

Element	*Sources*	*Concentration* ($\mu g/ml$)	*Sensitivity* ($\mu g/ml$)	*Optimal Range* ($\mu g/ml$)
Antimony	Printing type, glazing, drugs	1-10(U)	0.5	10-100
Arsenic	Ores, insecticides	2(U) 0.3(B) (6μg/g hair)	5	20-200
Barium	$BaCO_3$	Very low	8	100-1000
Beryllium	Ores	0.01(U)	0.03	1-10
Bismuth	Drugs	0.5(U)	1	10-100
Cadmium	Boot, silver polish, EP	0.1(U) 0.05(B)	0.03	0.5-5
Chromium	Leather-glue, batteries	0.1(U)	0.05	2-20
Cobalt	Ores	0.1(U)	0.2	4-40
Copper	Ores, electrics	1-2(B) 0.1(U)	0.1	2-20
Gold	Drugs	0.5(U)	0.3	5-50
Iron	Drugs, $Fe(CO)_5$	5(B) 1(U)	0.1	2-20
Lead	Paint, batteries, tetraethyl Pb	0.7(B) 0.15(U)	0.3	6-60
Lithium	Drugs	7(B)	0.03	1-10
Manganese	Dry cells, alloys	0.07(B)	0.06	2-20
Mercury	Metal, amalgam, tanning, pesticides	0.01(B)	10	20-2000
Nickel	$Ni(CO)_4$	0.05(U)	0.13	2-25
Selenium	Glass, porcelain	5(U)	2	40-400
Tellurium	Glass, rubber	Very low	2	40-400
Thallium	Rodent poison	0.3(B) 0.1(U)	0.03	0.6-6
Vanadium	Alloys	0.02(U)	0.05	1-10
Zinc	Ores	7(B)	0.03	0.5-5

Notes: (i) B = Blood U = Urine
(ii) Sensitivity = 1% absorption
(iii) All measurements refer to aqueous solutions, without scale expansion. Sensitivities can be increased up to 100 times, in some cases, by solvent extraction and scale expansion.

sufficiently bright to be usable; these lines are, as a rule, widely separated from each other and can be easily isolated by the monochromator system and slit. Some metals, however, produce lines too close together for complete separation. If, as is almost always the case, these lines are absorbed to different degrees (some emission lines are not absorbed at all) a non-linear calibration curve results. The most sensitive absorption line for iron occurs at 2483.3 Å; another line with about half the sensitivity occurs at 2488.1 Å. A band of 2 Å or less is required to separate the most sensitive line; complete separation is difficult with most instruments. Nickel presents a more extreme example. The most sensitive line is at 2320.0 Å; there is a non-absorbing line at 2139.8 Å, and others at 2317.2 Å and 2321.4 Å. These cannot be separated by the usual monochromators used with AAS. (Table 2)

The most sensitive lines of some elements are very strongly absorbed by the flame (Table 2) ; arsenic, mercury and selenium are examples. In the case of mercury and selenium, other suitable lines can be used; however, there are no better lines for arsenic, making this element difficult to measure by AAS, unless its concentration is high. Copper used in the cathode of many lamps emits lines very close to the absorption lines of some elements, e.g. selenium and tellurium, creating non-linear calibration curves and

TABLE 2

Element	*Line*	*Interferences*
As	1937.0	Strong flame absorption
Ba	5535.6	Al, CaOH, PO_4 depress
Be	2348.6	Cu, H_2SO_4, HNO_3 enhance
Cd	2258.0	Si depresses
Cr	3578.7	Fe, MgOH depress; A lines at 3576.6 and 3582.3 (from lamp)
Co	2407.3	Co line at 2411.6
Cu	3247.5	OH in flame emits at 3247
Fe	2483.3	Fe line at 2488.1
Pb	2170.0	Some flame absorption; A line near 2170; Pb line at 2175.6
Li	6707.8	K, Na enhance, SrO depresses;
Mn	2794.8	Si, Mg depress; Mn line at 2798.3
Hg	1849.6	Strong flame absorption
	2536.5	Hg line at 2534.8
Ni	2320.0	Ni lines at 2319.8, 2317.2 and 2321.4
Se	1960.3	Strong flame absorption
	2039.9	Some flame absorption; Cu line at 2024.3
Te	2142.7	Te line at 2147.2; Cu line at 2143
V	3818.2	V line at 3817.8
Zn	2138.6	Some flame absorption; Si depresses

Interferences in AAS at the usual analytical lines
(Interferences have not been reported for toxic metals listed in the table)

loss of sensitivity. Argon, commonly used as a filler gas in hollow-cathode lamps, produces lines close to those of certain elements, such as chromium and lead. Hollow cathode lamps using different filler gases and different supporting metals are now available for the metals mentioned; this source of error should now be unimportant.

The major source of problems in AAS is the flame. The strong absorption of short wavelength light by the flame gases has been described. In addition, the flame contains many molecules and radicals which can absorb or emit light over a wide range of the spectrum, particularly at the higher wavelengths. Thus, OH in the flame interferes with copper determinations and CaOH with barium. Flame absorption or emission due to its constituents interferes to some degree with the measurement of almost every metal; its effect is of greatest importance with low concentrations of metals. Its magnitude can be estimated by measuring the absorption of a nearby non-absorbing line, if one exists. More conveniently, flame absorption can be measured by the use of a deuterium arc,[6] which provides an abundance of suitable lines.

If the flame contains a significant number of particles, scattering of light may occur, giving the false impression that specific absorption has taken place. Flame scattering occurs particularly when urine and other liquids with a high salt content are aspirated. It can be measured by the deuterium arc technique. Preferably, it can be avoided by the use of the solvent-extraction techniques described below.

Other interferences may occur in the flame. Some metals affect the absorption of others (Table 2). Thus, aluminum depresses the absorption of barium; copper enhances the absorption of beryllium; potassium and sodium enhance the absorption of lithium. These effects can be kept constant by the addition of a suitable amount of the interfering element to the solution under examination and the standard and blank solutions. Anions and radicals in the solution being aspirated into the flame may also affect the amount of light absorbed by particular metals. Thus, phosphate depresses the absorption of barium: sulphuric and nitric acids enhance the absorption of beryllium. These effects can be controlled by adding chemicals which combine preferentially with the interfering substance; lanthanum or strontium will remove the phosphate effect.

Flame temperature, which depends upon the nature and proportions of gases in the combustion mixture, seriously affects the sensitivity of the AAS methods. When the nebulized droplets of solution are introduced into the flame, the solvent is evaporated (or combusted, if organic) leaving a particle of solid in the flame. The solid is vaporized (usually through an intermediate molten state), producing molecules; these are broken up to yield atoms. Intermediate, unstable, compounds may be formed, of the nature of free radicals. Further, the atoms produced in the flame may be converted to excited atoms and then to ions. Only free atoms, unexcited and unionized, absorb the resonance energy light; therefore, conditions reducing the number of these atoms will diminish the sensitivity of the method, while conditions increasing the number of atoms will increase sensitivity.

The commonest combustion mixture used in AAS is acetylene and air, which can be used either in stoichiometric proportions, or with an excess of air (lean flame) or with an excess of acetylene (rich flame). The temperatures of these flames differ; further, the temperatures of different parts of the flames differ.[7] The correct type of flame for the measurement of each element has been determined experimentally; flame conditions are given in manuals on AAS. In practice, the best proportions of gas and air are determined empirically, to provide greatest sensitivity. Elements such as lead, mercury and zinc which have volatile salts are usually best measured in low temperature flames, e.g., propane and air flames or rich acetylene-air flames. Some elements, such as beryllium, produce very few atoms in an acetylene-air flame; acetylene-nitrous oxide is necessary.[8] Hot flames usually give rise to less interference than cooler flames; there are fewer radicals and interfering compounds in the hot flames; they also cause more dissociation of molecules. On the other hand, hot flames produce more excited atoms and ions than cooler flames, thus reducing atomic concentration. There is frequently an uneven distribution of atoms in the flame, making it essential for the optical axis of the system to be always the correct height above the burner top. The region of the flame yielding maximum sensitivity must also be determined empirically. It will not remain constant unless flame conditions remain constant. With many elements, the position of maximum sensitivity in the flame varies with the concentration of the element aspirated. It is sound practice always to use standard solutions of about the same concentration as the unknown solution, in order to avoid flame errors.

It would be convenient if it were possible to aspirate urine directly into the flame; fully automated techniques could then be easily devised. However, it is unwise to aspirate urine directly, if low concentrations of the element are present. The high salt content of urine affects the aspiration rate of the nebulizer, produces scattering of light in the flame, increases non-specific absorption in the flame, and, finally, clogs the burner. In addition, the concentration of many elements is too low to be measured directly.

Although burners exist, which are capable of handling liquids of high salt concentration, the small amounts of toxic metal present in most urines makes some form of concentration necessary.

Concentration is effected, in the case of metals, by adding a chelating agent and extracting the chelated metal complex into a suitable organic solvent. In routine work, it is convenient to use substituted dithiocarbamates; ammonium pyrrolidine dithiocarbamate combines with most of the toxic metals, including arsenic and selenium. The chelate is extracted into methylisobutyl ketone. In most cases, a concentration ratio of about 100 can be achieved. The limiting factors are the degree of chelate formation and the partition coefficient of the chelate between the aqueous and organic phases. Other chelating agents, such as disodium diethyldithiocarbamate have been used,[9] and other solvents.[10] Reagents used in the colorimetric determination of the metals may also be used in some cases; e.g., dithizone is suitable for lead.

Toxic metals are for the most part protein-bound in blood, either to plasma proteins or to the red cell envelope. The distribution of metal between red cell and plasma varies with the metal; lead is found mainly in the red cell, copper and iron (excluding hemoglobin) mainly in the serum. For chelation to be possible, it is necessary to detach the metal from protein combination. Although this can be achieved by digestion of the blood or serum with strong acids, in most cases the metal can be detached and the proteins precipitated at the same time, by addition of trichloroacetic acid. This technique is simple and rapid, but requires attention to detail and much experience. If the metal is in high enough concentration in the serum, as in patients treated with lithium or children suffering from acute iron poisoning, it is best to dilute the serum twenty or more times and aspirate the diluted serum directly into the flame. Variation in aspiration rate due to protein is small at these dilutions; it can be allowed for by the use of diluted serum standards.

In addition to providing more concentrated solutions, solvent extraction procedures have other merits. In most cases, the solvent enhances the sensitivity of the method. Thus, the sensitivity for lead is increased about three times by the use of methylisobutyl ketone. The non-specific nature of chelation and solvent extraction, although a serious limiting factor in colorimetric methods, is of little consequence in AAS, unless the other metals are present in such high concentrations that they interfere with the extraction of the metal under examination or produce spectral interferences. This situation is rare in biological materials, although it may occur in the analysis of alloys, ores and similar mineral material. Of more importance is the fact that metals such as sodium and potassium are not chelated and extracted into the organic solvent. These elements in aqueous solution are responsible for a great deal of interference in the flame. It is possible to make standard and blank solutions having essentially the same matrix as the unknowns, thereby removing the effect of chemical interferences. The solvent alters the flame conditions, which are different from those suitable for aqueous solutions. Once again, the best conditions must be determined empirically.

AAS can be used to measure the amounts of toxic metals in tissues, such as liver and kidney. The major problem is not that of AAS, but that of obtaining a solution of the metal suitable for aspiration. In conventional toxicological procedures, it is necessary to digest the tissues completely, either by dry ashing in a muffle furnace, or by wet ashing with a mixture of strong acids. This is unnecessary when AAS is used, provided that chelation and solvent-extraction are employed. Dry ashing should be avoided. Many metals are lost by volatilisation in considerable quantities, particularly if they are present in low concentration.[11, 12, 13] Arsenic, lead, mercury, zinc, antimony and silver are examples. Wet ashing causes little loss, but it is necessary to be meticulous about blanks and standards because even the purest acids may contain significant quantities of trace metals. Many tissues, e.g. liver, kidney and brain, can be adequately digested with 50% nitric acid, provided the tissues are first thoroughly homogenized. If the tissue does not go completely into solution, the centrifuged residue can be re-extracted into boiling hydrochloric acid. By adding water and boiling almost to dryness, most of the nitric acid can be removed. After adjusting the pH of the solution, a chelating agent can be added and the complex extracted into an organic solvent. This procedure avoids the use of perchloric acid, which, in unskilled hands, can prove dangerous.

Alternative methods of digestion of tissue exist, which are widely used by organic chemists in their analytical work, but which have been largely ignored by toxicologists. Examples are the peroxide bomb, and the oxygen bomb. The material is digested in a closed system, either with sodium peroxide or with gaseous oxygen. After combustion, the residue can be dissolved in a suitable hot acid, and analysed by AAS. In a recent method, the sample is placed in a tantalum boat, which is then introduced into the flame.[14] Other methods avoid the use of the flame; instead special means are employed to obtain an atomic vapor. In one method, which is useful for measuring very low concentrations of mercury in urine, the mercury is isolated by means of a copper strip, which it coats (as in the Reinsch test). The strip is introduced into an evacuated tube. The mercury is displaced from the copper by heating with an electric current and mercury vapor fills the tube. The absorption of mercury atoms in the tube can then be measured.[15] This technique seems suitable for any metal which can be deposited onto copper and removed from it by heat.

AAS is a new technique, although now widely used. Improvements of the apparatus are being made frequently. It appears, however, that unless some novel device is invented, improvements in the lamps, burners, nebulizers and detectors will improve the sensitivity of AAS by a factor of only two or three. We are still a long way away from an instrument of sufficient sensitivity and freedom from interferences to permit direct measurements of the low concentrations of toxic metals in urines of unexposed subjects, by convenient and preferably automated methods. Perhaps the sister technique of atomic fluorescence flame spectrometry,[16] now in its developmental stage, will mature as rapidly as AAS, and provide the basis for an automated system for the screening of urine for toxic metals.

REFERENCES

1. Moeschlin, S.: Poisoning. Grune and Stratton, New York, 1965.
2. Elwell, W. T., and Gidley, J A. F.: Atomic-absorption Spectrophotometry, 2nd Edition. Pergamon Press, New York, 1966.

3. Willis, J. B.: The analysis of biological materials by atomic-absorption spectroscopy. *In* Methods of Biochemical Analysis. Edited by D. Glick. Interscience Publishers, *11:*1-67, 1963.
4. Kahn, H. L.: Principles and practice of atomic absorption. Trace inorganics in water. Adv. Chem. Ser., *73:*183-229, 1968.
5. Koirtyohann, S. R.: Recent developments in atomic absorption and flame emission spectroscopy. Atomic Absorption Newsletter,* *6:*77-84, 1967.
6. Kahn, H. L.: A background compensation system for atomic absorption. Atomic Absorption Newsletter,* *7:*40-43, 1968.
7. Mavrodineanu, R., and Boiteux, H.: Flame Spectroscopy. J. Wiley & Sons, Inc., New York, 1965.
8. Manning, D. C.: The determination of boron, beryllium, germanium and niobium using the nitrous oxide-acetylene flame. Atomic Absorption Newsletter,* *6:*35-37, 1967.
9. Bode, H., and Neumann, F.: Disubstituted dithiocarbamates. VIII Extraction with solutions of diethylammonium diethyldithiocarbamate in organic solvents. Z. Anal. Chem., *172:*1-21, 1960.
10. Allan, J. E.: Use of organic solvents in atomic absorption spectrophotometry. Spectrochim. Acta, *17:*467-73, 1961.
11. Hamilton, E. I., Minski, M. J., and Cleary, J. J.: The loss of elements during the decomposition of biological materials with special reference to arsenic, sodium, strontium and zinc. Analyst, *92:* 257-259, 1967.
12. Gorsuch, T. T.: Radiochemical investigation on the recovery for analysis of trace elements in organic and biological materials. Analyst, *84:* 135-73, 1959.
13. Pijck, J. O., Gillis, J., and Hoste, J.: The determination of Cu, Cr, Zn and Co in the serum by radioactivation. Intern. J. Appl. Radiation and Isotopes, *10:*149-57, 1961.
14. Kahn, H. L., Peterson, G. E., and Schallis, J. E.: Atomic absorption microsampling with the "sampling boat" technique. Atomic Absorption Newsletter,* *7:*35-39, 1968.
15. Brandenberger, H., and Bader, H.: The determination of nanogram levels of mercury in solution by a flameless atomic absorption technique. Atomic Absorption Newsletter,* *6:*101-103, 1967.
16. Winefordner, J. D., and Mansfield, J. M.: Atomic fluorescence flame spectrometry, *In* Fluorescence. Edited by G. G. Guilbault. Marcel Dekker, Inc., New York, 565-625, 1967.

*The Perkin-Elmer Corporation, Norwalk, Connecticut.

Chapter 12

Application of Polarography to Toxicological Determinations

WILLIAM C. PURDY, PH.D.

Although it has long been known that polarography is an important analytical tool for the determination of metal ions, this technique has remained virtually unexplored by the biochemist and toxicologist in this country. To be sure, the biochemist does perform amperometric titrations and other voltammetric measurements such as oxygen electrode studies. However, the great body of polarogaphy has been practically neglected. Brezina and Zuman[1] have written a monograph dealing with the field of polarography in biochemistry and medicine. In this monograph are compiled a vast number of methods for the determination of reducible and oxidizable substances in body fluids, tissue, etc.

Many ions of toxicological interest undergo redox reactions in solutions of electrolytes. In most cases, these reactions occur at an electrical potential within the range normally associated with aqueous polarography 0 to -2.0 V. *vs.* SCE (saturated calomel electrode). If this is the case, the material can be identified and quantitated in a single operation. The location of the midpoint of the polarographic wave, the half-wave potential ($E_{\frac{1}{2}}$), serves to qualitatively identify the substance, and the height of the wave, the diffusion current (i_d), gives quantitative measure. The principles of polarography have been discussed by Purdy.[2] At the present time, it is sufficient to state that quantitation is achieved through use of the Ilkovic equation:

$$i_d = 607\ D^{\frac{1}{2}} n C m^{2/3} t^{1/6}$$

where i_d is the diffusion current in microamperes, D is the diffusion coefficient in cm^2 per second, n is the number of electrons involved in the reversible redox reaction, C is the concentration of the electroactive substance in millimoles per liter, m is the flowing mass of mercury to the dropping mercury electrode (DME) in mg per second, and t is the drop time in seconds. Although this equation looks complicated, for a particular reaction all quantities can be held constant with the exception of the current and the concentration. This reduces the Ilkovic equation simply to

$$i_d = kC$$

Knowing k and reading the current from the polarogram, it is a simple matter to determine the concentration. Or, more usually, the concentration is obtained from a calibration curve.

One of the elements that the toxicologist is frequently asked to determine is lead. A generally accepted method for the determination of this substance involves the formation of the lead-dithizone complex, which complex forms a deep purple color in chloroform solution. The intensity of this purple color can be determined spectrophotometrically.[3] Unfortunately, certain other elements, including copper cadmium, cobalt, and zinc, are extracted into chloroform under the same conditions as lead. These other elements form purple dithizonates and serve, therefore, as interferences in the lead determination.

The dithizone and the polarographic methods for lead have been compared on identical blood and urine samples.[4] In all cases, the polarographic method was found to be more specific for lead. Polarography has been employed to follow the efficacy of EDTA clearance therapy in removing lead, zinc, cadmium, and copper from the system. The use of polarography can prevent a wrong diagnosis or aid in discovering the source of intoxication. Two examples will serve to illustrate these points. A sample of tissue was obtained from a deceased serviceman. Toxicology, employing the dithizone method, determined that death was caused by high levels of lead. The polarographic method indicated that the level of lead in the tissue was normal, but that the sample contained high concentrations of cadmium.

A different sample was obtained from a serviceman suffering from lead intoxication. The source of the lead was unknown. Polarography indicated that there were high levels of lead involved, but that these were accompanied by high levels of zinc and tin. The source of the lead intoxication was subsequently traced to solder.

Owing to the specificity and sensitivity of the method for metal ions, polarography offers great potential both for the qualitative and quantitative determination of toxic substances.

REFERENCES

1. Brezina, M., and Zuman, P.: Polarography in Medicine, Biochemistry, and Pharmacy, Revised Eng. Ed. Interscience Publishers, Inc., New York, 1958.
2. Purdy, W. C.: Electroanalytical Methods in Biochemistry. McGraw-Hill Book Company, Inc., New York, 1965, pp. 87-190.
3. Cholak, J., Hubbard, D. M., and Burkey, R. E.: Determination of lead in freshly voided urine. J. Ind. Hyg. Toxicol., *30*:59-62, 1948.
4. Colony, J. A., Knoblock, E. C., and Purdy, W. C.: A comparative study of the dithizone and polarographic determinations for lead. Amer. J. Clin. Path., *39*:652-655, 1963.

Chapter 13

Identification of Chemicals by Infrared Spectroscopy

JOHN H. JONES, M.S.

The major purpose of this chapter is to point out how the analytical chemist can use infrared spectroscopy to identify unknown chemicals encountered in his work. The examples will be primarily from the field of cosmetic analysis; however, the general approach outlined should be applicable to other fields such as drugs, foods, etc.

Discussion of infrared theory, instrumentation, sampling techniques, and quantitative analysis, are not included. These important phases of infrared analysis are covered in many excellent books and manuals on the subject. The discussion will be limited to the wavelengths in 2-16 μ range because this is the most widely used region of the infrared spectrum.

The term "chemical," as used in this chapter, means a commercially available natural or synthetic product of reasonably fixed composition. If the "chemical" is a mixture of compounds, the mixture is one produced by more or less standard methods of isolation and/or synthesis. The term includes, therefore, pure chemicals, practical grade chemicals, technical grade chemicals and complex mixtures such as polymers, copolymers, natural products, etc.

Some may wonder why a chemist whose primary interest is in cosmetic analysis should be interested in the identification of chemicals. The reasons are very simple: The Food, Drug, and Cosmetic Act does not require that the ingredients of a cosmetic be declared on the label or that cosmetic formulas be pre-cleared with the Food and Drug Administration prior to marketing. In addition, there are only a few cosmetics whose formulations are more or less standardized. The FDA, therefore, has little or no knowledge of the composition of many samples which are submitted for analysis. Obviously, a valid and useful analysis of a cosmetic requires identification of the compounds present.

Estimates of the number of individual components used in cosmetics range from a few thousand to thirteen thousand. The components vary from the simple compounds used as propellants in aerosols to high molecular weight polymers. They cover a wide range of organic and inorganic compounds of both natural and synthetic origin. Because nearly all these materials give infrared spectra, infrared analysis is by far the most useful single technique available for their identification.

Except for a few simple compounds, the infrared spectrum of a compound can not be derived from theoretical considerations. As a practical matter, therefore, the only way to identify a spectrum as that of a particular chemical is to compare it with the spectrum of an authentic sample of the chemical. (This statement does not mean that useful and valid assumptions about a chemical cannot be obtained from its spectrum alone.) Fortunately, the analytical chemist has available a tremendous number of spectra to compare with the spectrum of his unknown. Numerous compilations and sets of spectra are commercially available or are published in books, pamphlets, and scientific journals; individual or small groups of spectra are often published as part of a scientific article. The number of available spectra is probably near 100,000 and is growing rapidly. The problem for the analytical chemist is: How can he utilize this tremendous volume of information to identify a single chemical?

One of the most useful features of infrared spectra is that there is a high degree of correlation between the structural groups present in the compound and its spectrum. That is, in general, all compounds containing the functional group A will also have an absorption band at or near wavelength X. This correlation between chemical structure and absorption bands in the infrared region has received much study by chemists and spectroscopists. Many useful empirical correlations are reported in the literature.

One of the most popular and useful methods presenting structure-band correlation data is by charts such as that shown in Figure 1. This is a simplified structure-band chart showing a few of the correlations found to be most useful and reliable. These are only a very few of the many correlations that have been proposed in the literature. Obviously, if one can obtain enough clues to the structure of the unknown from its spectrum to limit the number of possible structures to a few compounds, direct comparison of the unknown spectrum with the spectra of these compounds should identify the compound.

The structure-band correlation approach to the identification of compounds is a very useful technique but it does have several limitations. It is obvious from the very limited data shown in Figure 1 that a band at a particular wavelength may be assigned to several different chemical structures. Usually, it is impossible to say with certainty that a peak at a particular wavelength indicates that a particular structure is present. Consideration of other bands in the spectrum of an unknown may or may not resolve this problem. On the other hand, the absence of a band in a particular wavelength region is strong but not conclusive evidence that the compound does not contain any of the structures that give rise to bands in that region.

A major difficulty with the band-structure correlation chart is that the intensities of bands owing to the same structure may vary widely from compound to compound, depending on the other groups present. Another difficulty is that many of the most useful bands are weak bands and may not be identifiable in weak spectra and/or may be confused with bands due to impurities in the sample.

Many correlations giving precise location of the band for certain structures have been proposed, for example, the various carbonyl frequencies for acids, esters, amides, etc. These group frequency shifts are of considerable value in choosing between two different structures for a compound whose overall structure is reasonably well established. Caution should be used in applying these correlations to compounds that are not closely related to the group of compounds on which the original correlations were based. For this reason, the group frequency shifts are of limited value for general use in identifying "unknowns."

Another method of using the data mentioned is to develop a scheme to allow one to locate the infrared curve, or curves, which has peaks at certain wavelengths. For example, if the spectra of an unknown has peaks of 2.8, 3.4, 7.7, 8.1, 8.6, 11.6, 12.9 and 13 μ, the analyst obviously would be interested in comparing this curve with all other curves available to him which have peaks at the same wavelengths. There are at least three methods in use for locating spectra that have peaks corresponding to those of an unknown.

1. A printed list of spectra arranged by wavelength which can be examined by the analyst to locate spectra having the same peaks as the unknown compound. Usually, the list is based on the wavelength of the strongest peak in the spectrum and is subdivided by listing the other peaks in the spectrum. This system is quite satisfactory for small collections of spectra but becomes more and more cumbersome as the number of spectra

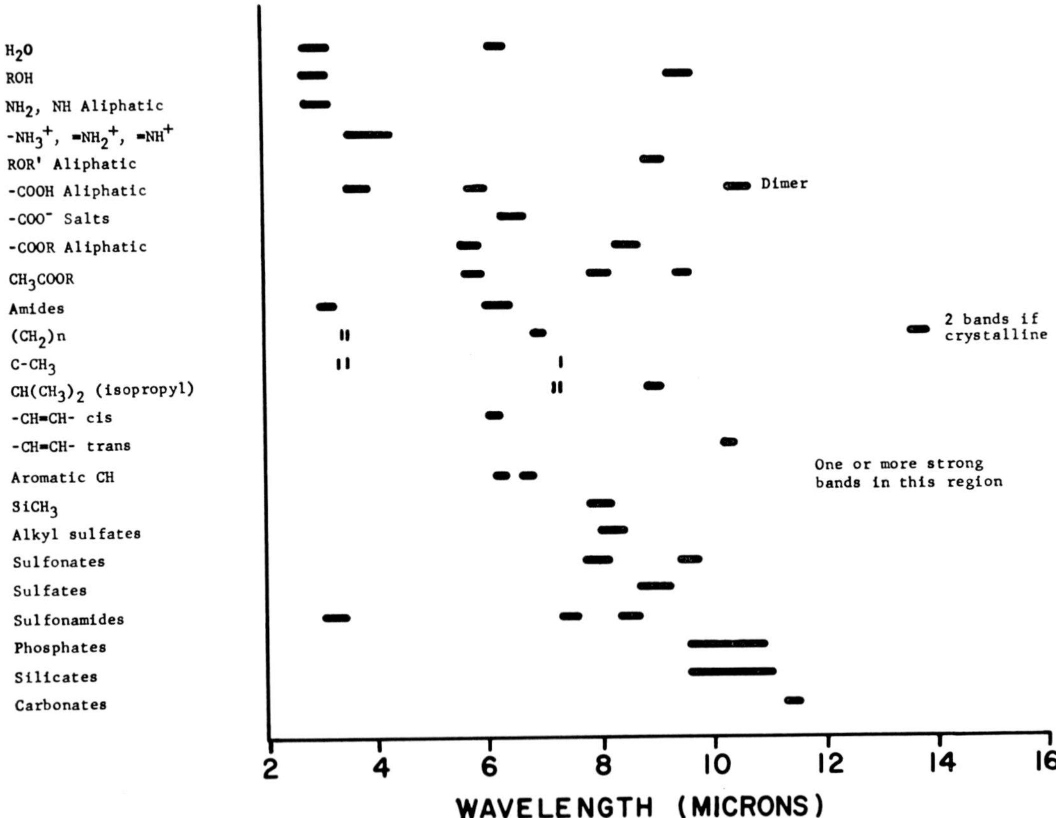

Figure. 1. Structure-band correlation chart.

to be considered increases. This type of listing is available for the largest collection of spectra (Sadtler Spec Finder, Sadtler Research Laboratories) and can be a useful tool in locating spectra in that collection.

2. Large collection of spectra can be sorted by entering the data on punch cards and sorting the cards on a mechanical sorter. The American Society for Testing Materials has been very active in making punched cards of this type available. More than 70,000 infrared cards are available at present. In addition to the spectral data, these cards may contain data on chemical structure, empirical formula, melting and boiling points, etc.

3. As the number of available spectra becomes larger and larger, the use of computers to store and retrieve spectral data becomes more attractive; in fact, it can be argued that computers are the only reasonable solution to the problem. The use of computers in spectral searches has received considerable attention and several systems have been developed. At least one firm (Sadtler Research Laboratories) offers computer searching on a fee basis.

It should be noted that none of the three methods of searching spectral data provides an identification of an unknown. They are simply methods for locating a spectrum (or preferably a number of spectra) which is similar to the spectrum of the unknown. The actual identification must be made by an overall comparison of the spectrum of the unknown with the spectrum of a known compound (s).

In Figure 2-7 are shown a few examples of the use of infrared to aid in the identification of chemicals isolated from cosmetics. All of the spectra shown were obtained with a Perkin-Elmer 137B spectrophotometer.

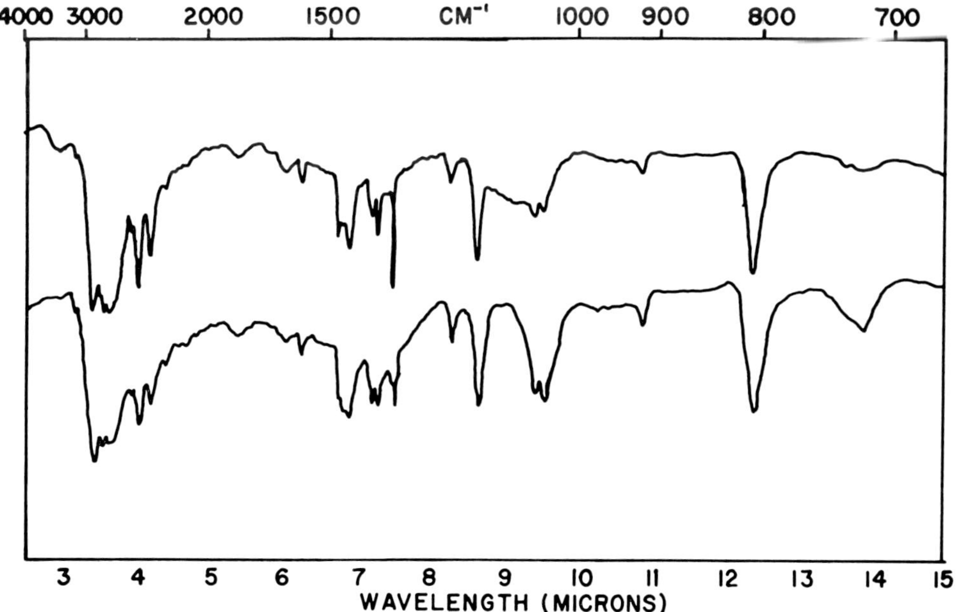

Figure 2. Identification of amine isolated from a cosmetic. Upper spectrum — Amine hydrochloride isolated from product. Lower spectrum — Diethylamine hydrochloride. Halocarbon® mull, 2.5-7.5 μ; mineral oil mull, 7-5-15.0 μ.

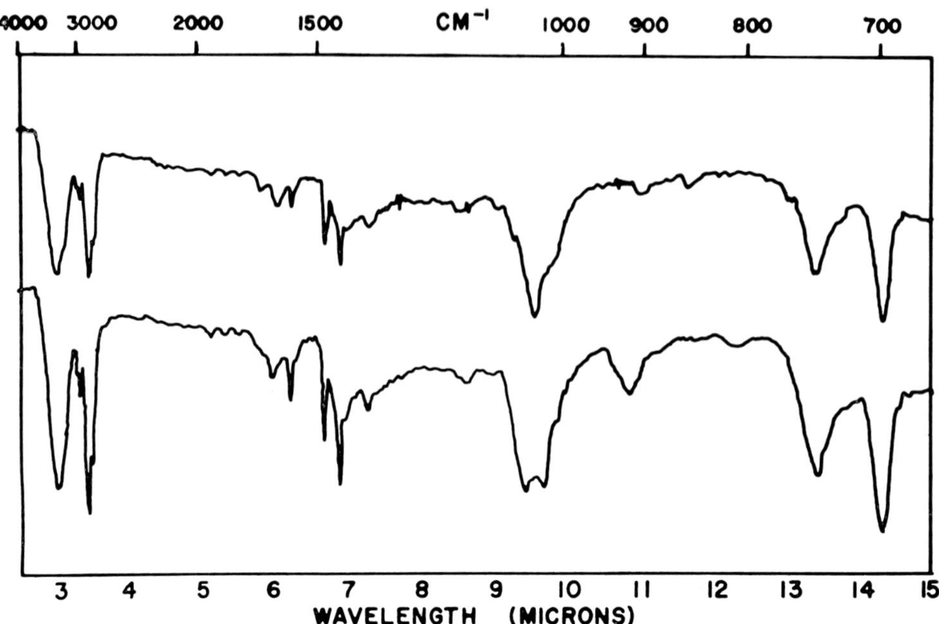

Figure 3. Spectra of compounds isolated from a perfume. Upper spectrum — identified as phenylethyl alcohol. Lower spectrum — identifed as 3-phenyl-propanol-1. Liquids between salt plates.

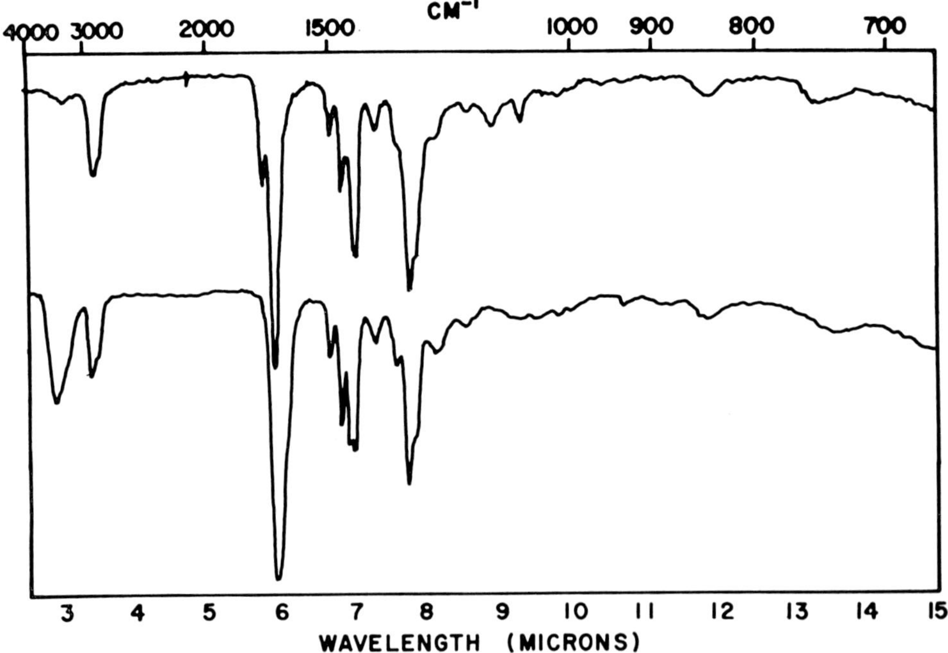

Figure 4. Identification of polymer by infrared. Upper spectrum — film from aerosol hair spray. Lower spectrum — film, from alcohol, of polyvinylpyrrolidone.

Preliminary examination of a sample submitted to our laboratory indicated that it contained a volatile amine. When the amine was extracted into ether and converted to its hydrochloride the upper spectrum shown in Figure 2 was obtained. The peaks around 4.0 μ are characteristic of amine hydrochlorides and confirm that the sample contained an amine. The spectrum of the unknown was compared, therefore, with the spectra of the hydrochlorides of a number of the lower aliphatic amines. As the lower curve indicates, the spectrum of diethylamine hydrochloride is a good match for the unknown spectrum. The melting point, the NMR spectrum, and the C, H, and N content of the isolated material agreed with that of diethylamine hydrochloride.

In Figure 3 are shown the spectra of two fractions isolated from a perfume by gas chromatography. The peaks at 3.0 and 9.5 μ indicate that the compounds contain an aliphatic hydroxyl group. The peaks at 6.2 and 6.7 μ indicate that the compound is aromatic. The peaks at 13.4 and 14.3 μ are typical of a monosubstituted benzene. With this information available it is easy to establish that the upper curve is that of B-phenylethyl alcohol and the lower curve that of 3-phenylpropanol-1. The differences between the two spectra are minor but appear to be real.

The spectrum shown in Figure 4 was obtained by spraying an aerosol hair spray on a salt plate and drying for a few minutes at 100° C. Comparison with the lower spectrum indicates that the nonvolatile material is chiefly polyvinylpyrrolidone. The minor peaks at 5.8, 8.9, and 9.3 μ are present in the phthalate plasticizers frequently used in such products; subsequently dibutyl phthalate was isolated from the sample and identified by its infrared spectrum.

The unknown sample giving the up-

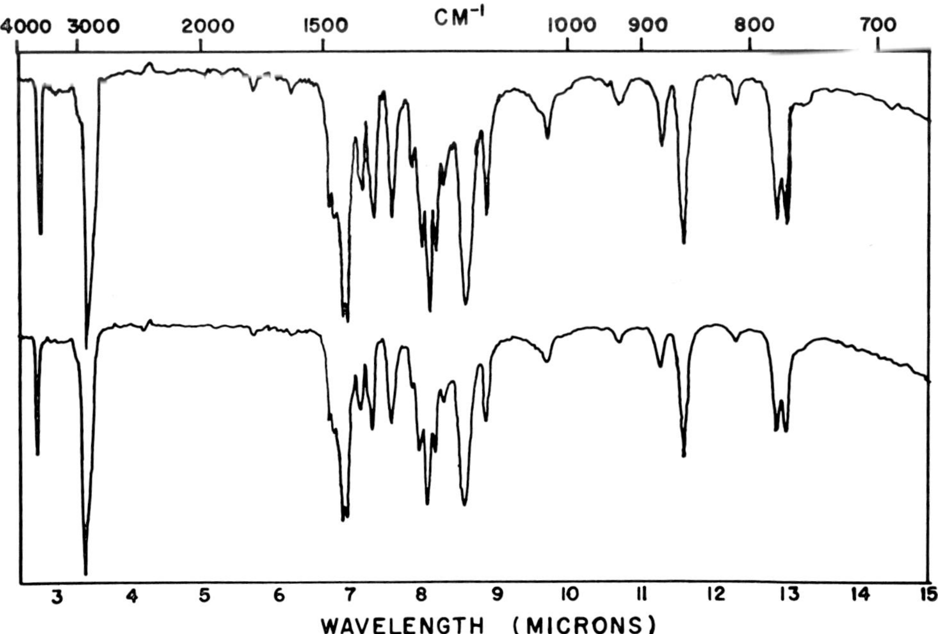

Figure 5. Identification of unknown by infrared. Upper spectrum — unknown. Lower spectrum — 2,6-di-tertiarybutyl-p-cresol. Liquids between salt plates.

per spectrum in Figure 5 consisted of a few milligrams of liquid material isolated by gas chromatography. No data other than the spectrum were available. It was possible to locate a matching spectrum in a few minutes by using an index of spectra arranged by wavelength. The two spectra are practically identical and there is little doubt that the unknown is 2,6-di-tertiary butyl-p-cresol, also known as BHT.

The spectrum of the next unknown (Fig. 6) contains only three bands, all of which are typical of aliphatic hydrocarbons. The interesting feature of the spectrum is the relative strength of the CH and CH_3 bands at 6.8 and 7.3. The ratio between these two peaks indicates the presence of a high proportion of CH_3 groups. This was confirmed by the NMR data on the sample which indicated a ratio of about 3 CH_3 hydrogens to 2 CH_2 and/or CH hydrogens. There are commercially available "isomerized" hyrocarbons whose spectra closely resemble the unknown spectra. It seems reasonable to assume that the unknown is such a material.

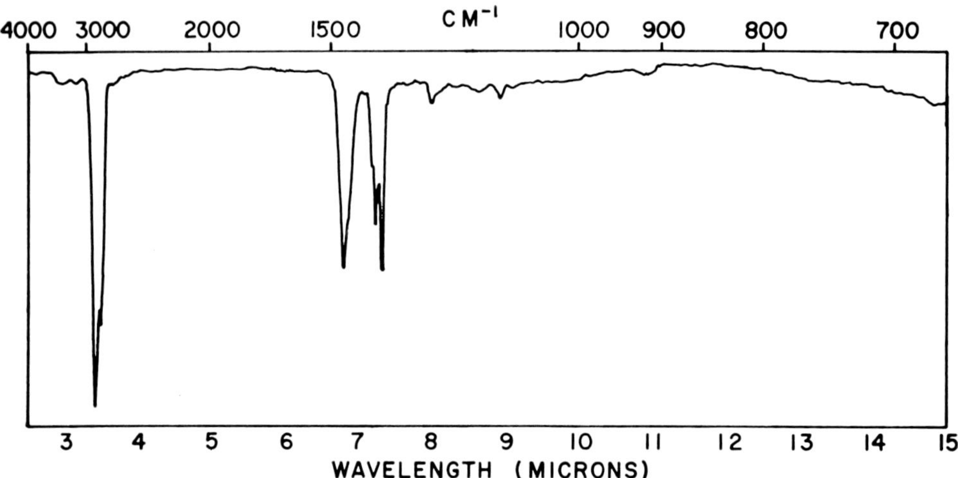

Figure 6. Spectrum of unknown isolated from cosmetic. Liquid between salt plates.

The next spectrum (Fig. 7) is shown primarily to illustrate the fact that infrared analysis will not always provide an identification for a chemical. This material was isolated from an essential oil by gas chromatography. It has not been possible to find a spectrum which matches the spectrum of the unknown. It appears likely that the unknown is a sesquiterpene alcohol; unfortunately few spectra of sesquiterpene alcohols are available and obtaining authentic samples of such compounds is difficult, if not impossible, at present.

In spite of the usefulness and overall simplicity of infrared identification of chemicals, there are a number of problems in the use of the technique.

One disadvantage of infrared spectroscopy is that, compared to some techniques, a fairly large sample is required. On most instruments, about 1 mg of sample is required to give reasonably strong spectrum. By using special techniques and instrumentation, such as beam condensing systems, the amount of sample can be drastically reduced; this naturally increases the cost of the equip-

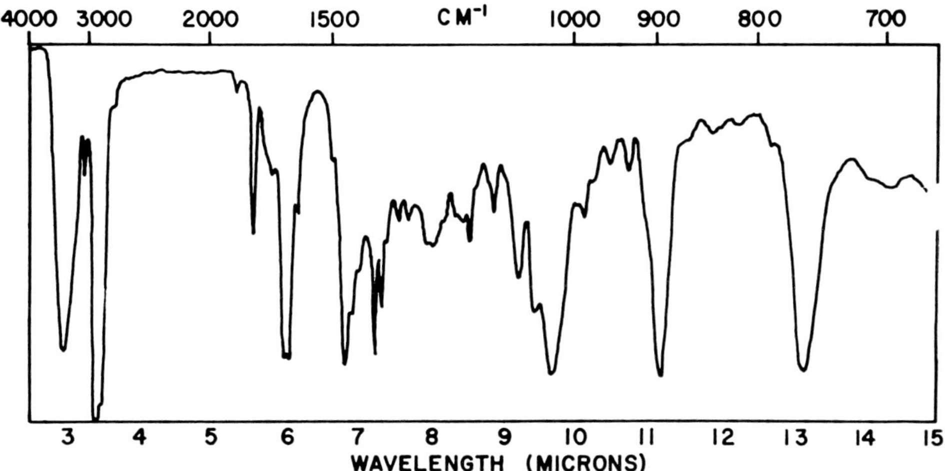

Figure 7. Spectrum of unknown isolated by gas chromatography from Oil of Vetiver. Liquid between salt plates.

ment and the experience required of the operator.

Another disadvantage of infrared identification is that usually the chemical to be identified must be separated from all other components of the sample. The infrared spectrum of a mixture is, of course, the sum of the spectra of the components. In Figure 8 are shown the spectra obtained at two different stages

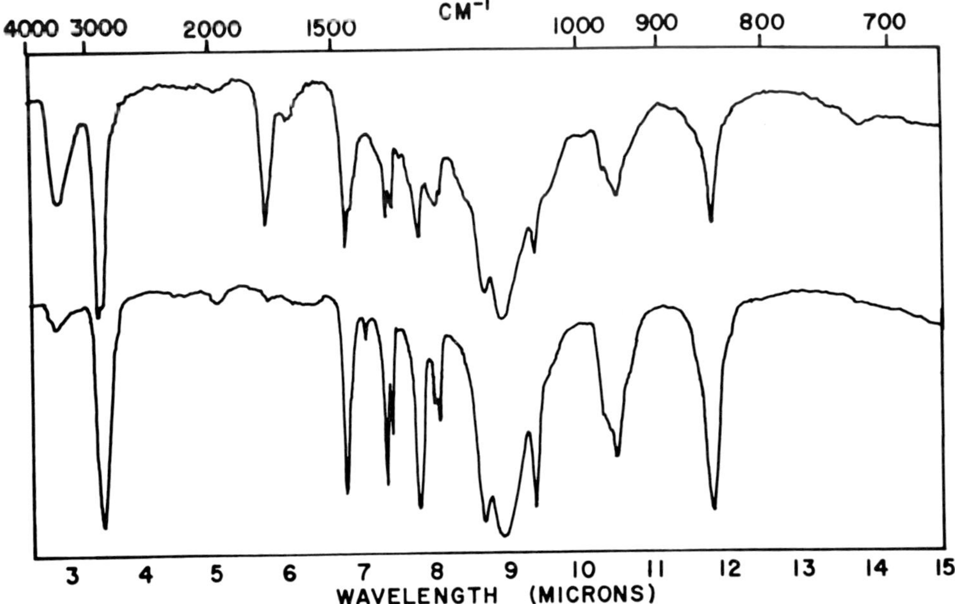

Figure 8. Spectra obtained during isolation of components of a cosmetic. Upper spectrum — fraction isolated from sample by solvent extraction. Lower spectrum — one component separated from solvent extract by partition chromatography — identified as a high molecular weight polyethylene glycol. Solidified melts.

in the isolation of a chemical from a cosmetic. The upper spectrum could have been logically identified as that of a fatty acid ester of a polyethylene glycol. Actually, this spectrum is that of a mixture. The lower spectrum shows that one of the components is a polyethylene glycol. The other component was identified as glycerol monostearate.

Another factor that must be considered in comparing infrared spectra is the physical state of the sample. The spectra of a compound as a gas, a liquid, in solution, or as a solid, usually are quite different. In addition, the spectrum of a compound in the solid state depends on whether it is amorphous or crystalline. The spectrum of a compound which crystallizes in more than one form will depend on the crystalline form examined. The spectra shown in Figure 9 were obtained from the same sample. Initially, the sample was melted between salt plates. The upper spectrum was obtained after the melt had apparently solidified; the lower, after the sample had staid at room temperature for about an hour. Presumably, the upper spectrum is that of the amorphous material and the lower spectrum that of the crystalline material. Numerous examples of the effect of the crystalline forms of a compound on its infrared spectra have appeared in the literature. Usually, spectral differences due to the effect of the crystalline form can be eliminated by dissolving both the unknown and authentic samples in a suitable solvent and evaporating both solutions under the same conditions.

One might gain the impression from reading the literature that the infrared spectrum of a compound is unique and that any compound can be identified by its infrared spectrum alone if enough authentic infrared spectra are available for comparison. From the practical standpoint this is not true, particularly

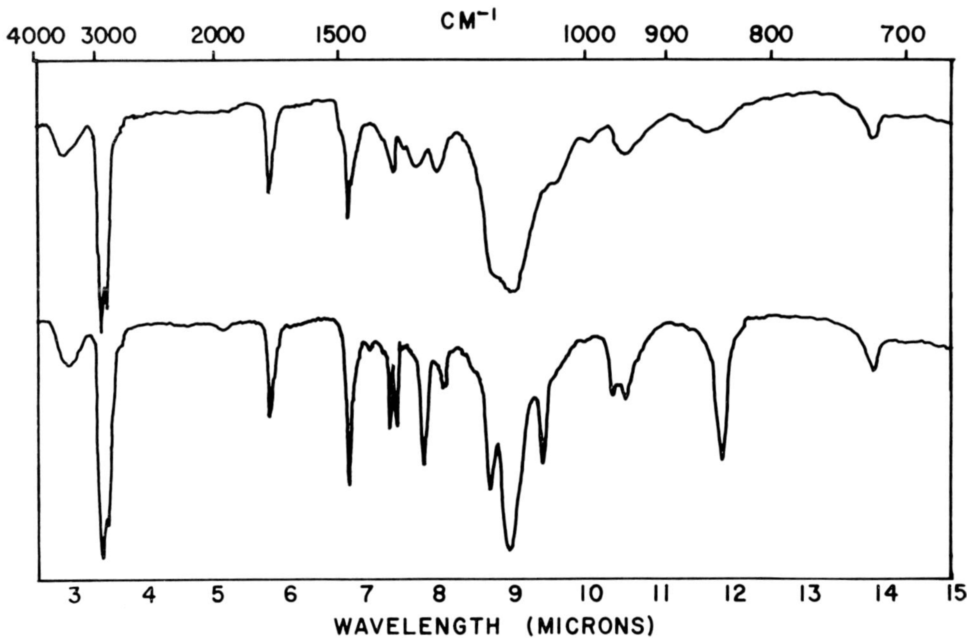

Figure 9. Effect of crystallinity on spectrum. Upper spectrum — solidified melt. Lower spectrum — same sample after aging for one hour at room temperature.

if one is identifying chemicals as originally defined. There are many pairs, or even groups, of chemicals whose infrared spectra are very similar. For example, in many homologous series, such as the higher fatty acids, alcohols, esters etc., the difference in the infrared spectra of consecutive members of the series is very small. These compounds are easily classified by their infrared spectra but it is very difficult to specify the exact chain length of the hydrocarbon portion of such compounds by infrared analysis alone. Certainly, in most cases, there are better means for determining the chain length of members of a homologous series.

Two compounds do not have to be members of a homologous series to give similar infrared spectra. One such case encountered in our work is shown in Figure 10. There are minor differences in these two spectra; however, the differences are not pronounced. It would be difficult to identify positively an unknown isolated from a mixture as one or the other of these chemicals. Fortunately, in actual practice, it is easy to differentiate between these two compounds. The infrared spectra of the acetates of these compounds differ more than the spectra of the compounds, and the acetates can be separated by gas chromatography.

The difficulty in exactly identifying a chemical naturally increases as the size and complexity of the molecule increases. It is not surprising, therefore, that the infrared spectra of synthetic or natural polymers give at best only an indication of the degree of polymerization.

Identification of a chemical by infrared spectroscopy depends upon the comparison of the spectrum of the unknown with the spectrum of an authentic sample of the chemical it is believed to be. The

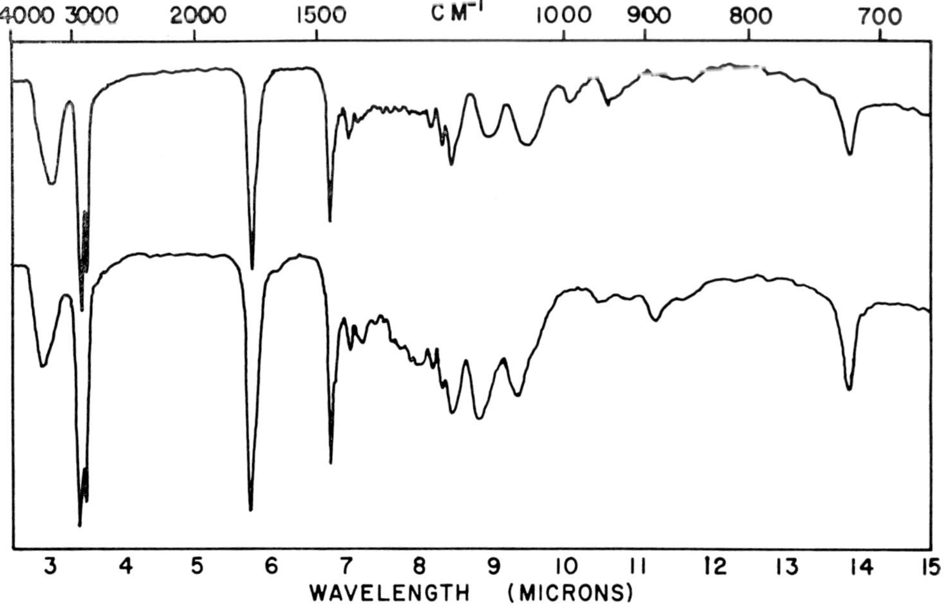

Figure 10. Spectra of two emulsifiers used in cosmetics. Upper spectrum — glyceryl monostearate. Lower spectrum — diethylene glycol monostearate. Solidified melts.

best way to be sure that the spectra are comparable is to run both the unknown and an authentic sample on the same instrument at nearly the same time. This serves to eliminate errors due to such factors as instrument calibration, effective resolution, etc. It also serves as a check on such errors as incorrect identification of spectra in collections, use of impure or non-representative samples in preparing the spectra in the collection, etc. It has been our experience that most of the published data are reliable both from the standpoint of quality of the spectrum (considering the instrument used) and the identity of the sample. Mistakes do occur, however, and the analyst should be on guard to detect them when they occur.

There is a tendency among chemists to equate "authentic" with "pure" when thinking about chemicals. It should be remembered that many commercial chemicals are mixtures. For example, commercial glycerol monostearate is a mixture of the distearate, the monostearate, glycerol, and stearic acid. In addition, the commercial stearic acid used in its preparation is a mixture of stearic and palmitic acids. Obviously it would be a mistake to expect the infrared spectrum of the commercial material to match that of pure glycerol monostearate.

On the other hand, the method used by the analyst to isolate a chemical from a mixture may give an unknown which is purer than any available sample of the chemical. For example, unknowns isolated by gas chromatography may be much purer than the best commercially available material. In such cases, to establish definitely the identity of the unknown, the analyst may need to subject the authentic chemical to the same separation procedure used to isolate the unknown.

In the examples given in this chapter, an attempt has been made to point out how supplemental data has been used to confirm the identification made by infrared. The importance of obtaining as much data as possible to supplement the infrared data cannot be over-emphasized. Obviously, if an unknown chemical has been correctly identified, all of its properties will agree with those of the authentic sample.

SELECTED REFERENCES

General

Manual on Recommended Practices in Spectrophotometry. Sponsored by ASTM Committee E-13. American Society for Testing and Materials, 1916 Race Street, Philadelphia, Pa. 19103 (1966).

Structural-Band Correlations

The Infra-red Spectra of Complex Molecules, Second Edition. By L. J. Bellamy. John Wiley and Sons, Inc., New York (1958).

Chemical Applications of Spectroscopy, W. Westy (Ed.), Chapter IV, The application of infrared and ramen structure to the elucidation of molecular structure. By R. Norman Jones and Camille Sandorfy. Interscience Publishers, New York, 1956.

Collections of Spectra

Sadtler Collections of Spectra. Sadtler Research Laboratories, 3316 Spring Garden Street, Philadelphia, Pa. 19104 (Various collections of Standard and Commercial Spectra, Indices, Spec-Finder, etc.).

Identification and Analysis of Surface Active Agents — Spectra Volume. By Dieter Hummel, translation by E. A. Wulkow. Interscience Publishers, New York, 1962. (Contains 466 spectra and several correlation charts useful for this class of compounds.)

Infrared, Ultraviolet, and Visible Absorption Spectra of Some USP and NF Reference Standards and Their Derivatives. J. Assoc. Offic. Anal. Chemists, *45*, No. 4, 797-900 (1962) by Alma L. Hayden, Oscar R. Sammul, George B. Selzer, and Jonas Carol (ca 200 spectra).

Infrared Spectra of Some Compounds of Pharmaceutical Interest. J. Assoc. Offic. Anal. Chemists, *47*, No. 5, 918-991, 1964. By Oscar R. Sammul,

Wilson L. Brannon, and Alma L. Hayden (ca 500 spectra).

Part II: Infrared Spectra of Some Compounds of Pharmaceutical Interest. J. Assoc. Offic. Anal. Chemists, *49,* No. 6, 1109-1153, 1966. By Alma L. Hayden, Wilson L. Brannon, and Charlotte A. Yaciw (ca 200 spectra).

Infrared Spectroscopy — Its Use as an Analytical Tool in the Field of Paints and Coatings. By Infrared Spectroscopy Committee of the Chicago Society For Paint Technology, 1350 South Kostner Avenue, Chicago 23, Illinois, 1961. (Contains ca 200 spectra and a brief, but useful, discussion of qualitative analysis by infrared spectroscopy.)

Infrared Spectra of Plastics and Resins, 1954; Infrared Spectra of Plastics and Resins, Part 2, Materials Developed Since 1954, 1966. U. S. Naval Research Laboratory, Washington, D. C. Copies available from Clearinghouse for Federal Scientific and Technical Information (CFSTI) Sills Building, 5285 Port Royal Road, Springfield, Virginia 22151.

Identification and Analysis of Plastics. By J. Haslam and H. A. Willis. D. Van Nostrand Company, Inc., Princeton, N. J., 1965. (ca 300 spectra of plastics and related products.)

The Infrared Spectra of Monoterpenes and Related Compounds. By B. M. Mitzner, E. T. Theimer, and S. K. Freeman. Applied Spectroscopy, *19:* 169 (1965).

Infrared Spectra of Monoterpenes and Related Compounds. II. Terpene Alcohols. By B. M. Mitzner, V. J. Mancini, S. Lemberg, and E. T. Theimer. Applied Spectroscopy, *22:*34, 1968. (These articles give the spectra of over 200 compounds of interest to workers in the fields of essential oils, perfumes, etc. Most of the compounds were purified by gas chromatography.)

Infrared Spectra and Characteristic Frequencies of Inorganic Ions. By F. A. Miller and C. H. Wilkens. Anal. Chem., *24:*1253, 1952. (Spectra of 160 compounds.)

These are only a few of the many collections of spectra available. Other collections can be found by searching the chemical literature in the usual manner. The *Annual Reviews* volumes of *Analytical Chemistry* are an excellent starting point for such a search.

Computer Searching

Fast Searching System for ASTM Infrared Data File. By Duncan S. Erley. Anal. Chem., *40:*894, 1968. (This article gives references to other reports on this topic.)

Sadtler Research Laboratories, 1517 Vine St., Philadelphia, Pa., offers computer searching on a fee basis.

Chapter 14

Electron Microprobe Analysis

(Study of Asbestos Fibers and Bodies from Lung Tissue)

ARTHUR M. LANGER, PH.D.

INTRODUCTION

The electron microprobe analyzer is an instrument which makes possible the chemical analysis of solid material by means of x-ray spectroscopy. The instrument incorporates two major components in a single unit. One is that of a scanning electron microscope capable of resolving surface morphologic details on a sample on the order of about 0.1 microns in size. Specimen image may be observed by means of raster sweep displays on a cathode ray tube. The scanning system, and its associated detection devices, permits detection and special display of sample current, secondary electrons, back-scattered electrons and x-ray emission. These differing display modes show sample morphology and give information as to the chemical nature of the substance. The second component instrument is an x-ray analyzer, equipped with x-ray spectrometers (analyzing crystals, detectors, and amplification and recording devices). Equipped with a light element attachment, the instrument is able to detect elements down to and including atomic number 5, Boron, and may achieve a sensitivity, depending on the specimen, instrumental conditions and geometry and elemental species examined, to about 10^{-15} grams (absolute) concentration. Analyses may be qualitative, semiquantitative, and in cases where proper instrumental controls and sample preparation are observed, quantitative in nature. The instrument is described fully in Birks (1963) and Andersen (1967). The electron probe used in the author's laboratory is the Applied Research Laboratories EMX model.

Current Study

A series of clinical, epidemiological and pathological studies by Selikoff *et al.* (1964; 1965; 1967; 1968) has shown that almost 50% of individuals working in the insulation trades die of lung cancer, pleural and peritoneal mesothelioma, and carcinoma of the gastrointestinal tract. These workmen are heavily exposed to asbestos and asbestos-containing materials. Histological examination of lung tissue taken from these individuals shows the presence of great numbers of asbestos fibers and bodies.

The analysis of these particles has met with limited success, details of which are presented in Beger, 1933; Sundius and Bygden, 1938; Beattie and Knox, 1961; Nagelschmidt, 1965; Berkley *et al.*, 1968a. These papers, with the exception of the most recent one, have dealt with the analysis of materials extracted as a bulk dust. Berkley *et al.* attempted analysis on single particles utilizing electron microscopy, electron diffraction and electron microprobe analysis. Some success at particle identification was achieved (Berkley *et al.*, 1968a/b). The necessity for single particle analysis has been emphasized by recent studies showing the occurrence of what appeared to be asbestos bodies in the lung tissue of half the individuals from the general population who come to autopsy in New York City (Baden and Schwartz, 1968). Because of the direct relationship between increased neoplastic diseases in individuals and exposure to asbestos, it remains to be determined epidemiologically if such an increased neoplastic risk occurs in individuals not occupationally exposed to asbestos. Positive identification of asbestos in the cores of the asbestos bodies in the general population is critical to this study.

Asbestos Materials

Asbestos is a generic term which includes six fibrous, hydrated, silicate minerals which may be subdivided readily into generally flexible fibers. These opened fibers possess a range of physical and chemical properties so that the insulation usage is now but one of literally thousands of applications of these materials. The mineralogy of the asbestos mineral group has been described fully in a number of review papers including those of Hendry (1965), Gaze (1965), and Speil and Leineweber (1969). Asbestos bulk chemistry is applicable to the current study in that fibers may be readily distinguished from each other on this basis. The commercial grade fibers possess narrow ranges of five major oxides, as follows:

TABLE 1: BULK CHEMISTRY RANGE OF THE ASBESTOS MINERALS

Major Oxide	*Crocidolite*	*Amosite*	*Anthophyllite*	*Actinolite-Tremolite*	*Chrysotile*
SiO_2	49.0-53.0	49.0-53.0	56.0-58.0	51.0-60.0	38.0-44.0
MgO	0.0- 3.0	1.0- 7.0	28.0-34.0	15.0-26.0	40.0-42.0
Total Fe Oxide	30.0-40.0	34.0-44.0	3.0-12.0	0.0-15.0	0.1- 4.0
CaO	0.3- 2.7	0.0	0.0	10.0-13.0	0.0- 1.0
Na_2O	4.0- 8.5	0.0	0.0	0.5- 1.5	0.0- Tr

Instrument Calibration

The microprobe spectrometers were calibrated with metal standards. The ratios of elemental emission for the chemical components in the asbestos types were determined on asbestos mineral specimens (Berkley *et al.*, 1968b). The elemental emission ratios of iron, silicon and magnesium (K alpha) x-rays are shown in Figure 1. This ternary diagram represents several thousand analyses taken on all the asbestos mineral types. It appears that the asbestos fibers may be made to produce characteristic x-ray emission which are discernible and unique. Each of the mineral type emission ratios was obtained on a number of samples; all from different geological localities. Therefore, even though asbestos types may originate from different localities, the fibers still possess similar chemical characteristics (Fig. 2). Individual asbestos types produced emission analyses which may be marked off as separate fields (Fig. 3). Although there is a characteristically wide range of emission values, the asbestos types form field maxima. Some of the specimens appear to have similar emission ratios in the system iron-silicon-magnesium. As shown in Table 1, those fields which lie in close proximity may still be differentiated on the basis of other components in their chemical make up. The fields of amosite and crocidolite, which lie juxtaposed on the iron-silicon join, may be differentiated from each other by measuring the sodium content of the fiber under observation. Sodium emission is almost nil in amosite and significant in crocidolite. In a similar manner, differences between chrysotile and tremolite may be found on the basis of calcium emission (Table 1). The anthophyllite fibers studied to date have shown a generally greater amount of iron emission than is observed in either chrysotile or tremolite.

To check the values of the emission ratios, the average chemical analysis for the asbestos types has been recalculated and plotted on the ternary diagram (Fig.

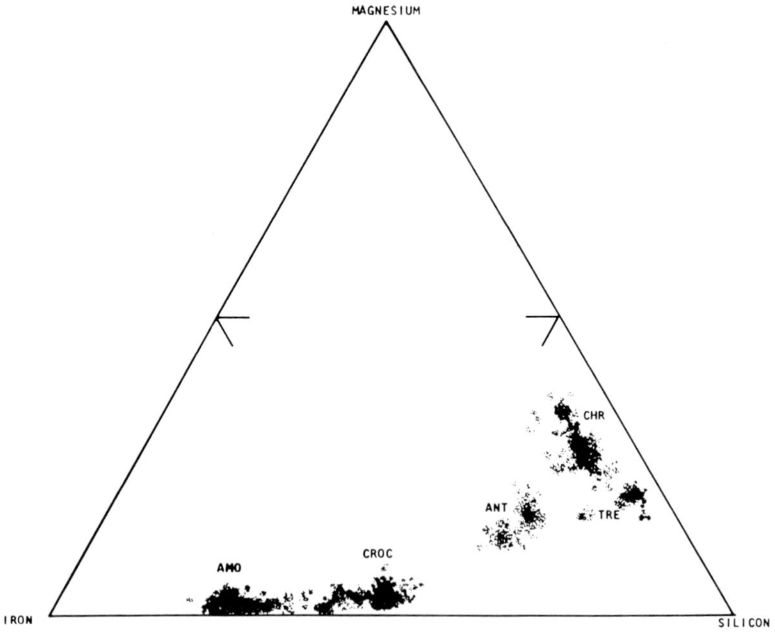

Figure 1. Emission ratios of iron-silicon-magnesium Ka* for the major asbestos mineral types. Each "dot" represents a single analysis: **AMO** = amosite; **CROC** = crocidolite; **ANT** = anthophyllite; **TRE** = tremolite; **CHR** = chrysotile. Actinolite member of the actinolite-tremolite series is not included.

*Ka = Kα (Greek "alpha")

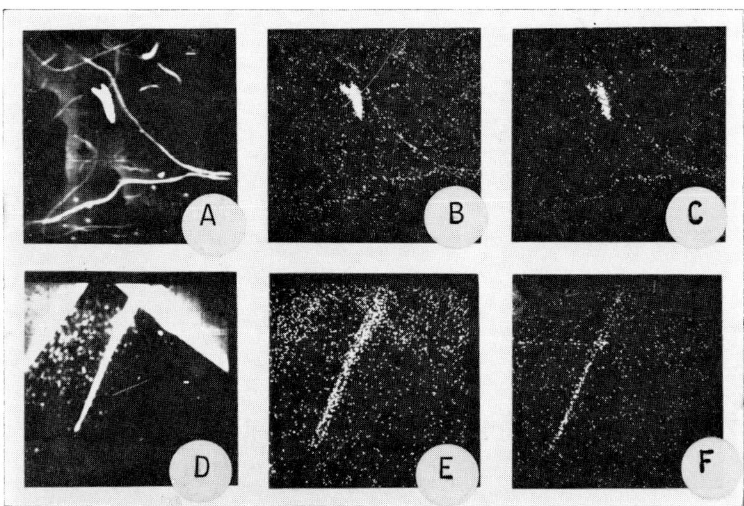

Figure 2. Analysis of "soft" (ABC) and "harsh" (DEF) chrysotile asbestos: **A** and **D** are sample current displays; **B**, **E** are 2000 counts of silicon Ka; **C**, **F** are 2000 counts of Mg Ka. Magnifications are indicated by grid markings on **A**, **D**; about 8 microns/division **A**, **B**, **C**; about 10 microns/division **D**, **E**, **F**. Although the "soft" fiber is from Canada and the "harsh" fiber is from Arizona, the analyses were identical.

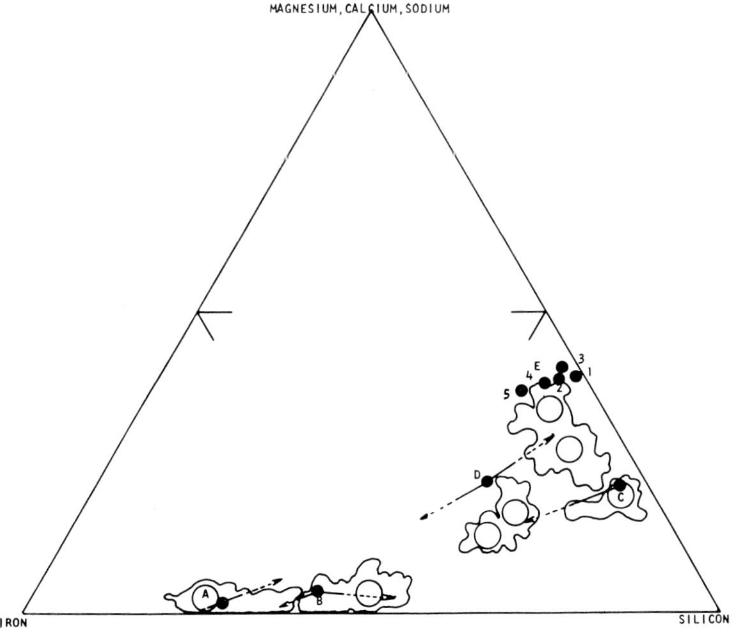

Figure 3. Asbestos fiber fields and emission characteristics. Dark circles indicate the areas where the average chemical composition of commercial fibers would yield emission values. Arrows indicate the direction and extent the fibers would produce corresponding changes in emission characteristics if the chemistry of the fibers changed within the points defined for "commercial grade" fibers.

3). The dark spots represent the average analysis for the various asbestos types. The E series of points 1 - 5 for the chrysotile asbestos was obtained for fibers from many commercially worked localities. All oxide values shown are also from localities from which fibers are mined commercially. The method of recalculation of bulk oxides into cation weight percents, and then into emission values, is outlined in Berkley *et al.* (1968b). This recalculation merely follows the "first order approximation" cited in Andersen (1967, p. 185), in which the emission of an element from a sample is approximately proportional to the elemental weight percent present in the sample.

Preparation of Materials for Probe Analysis

Much of the preliminary work on sample preparation was done on tissue specimens obtained from the lung of an asbestos worker. The reason for this is the fact that the greatest number of particles per volume of tissue occur in these individuals. Tissue sections were mounted on plastic substrates to avoid "background" fluorescence. The tissue was observed to "char" and "burst" under the beam making particles difficult to observe (Fig. 4). Also, the beam of the probe caused destruction of the tissue which caused the particles to dislodge and "fly off." Furthermore, particles were also observed to dislodge when carbon coated, and when placed in the vacuum system of the electron microprobe, and when they remained under the beam of the probe for a prolonged period of time. Where analyses could be made, however, good results were obtained. Sample current and x-ray emission pictures could be obtained from these materials (Fig. 5), as well as quantitative emission data for identification. The use of unashed tissue in particle analysis was considered a poor technique, especially for use on general population samples. The reason for this is obvious, in that the lungs from an individual in the general population have fewer bodies and fibers per unit volume of tissue. Therefore, the techniques which may have been acceptable for asbestos workers were not acceptable in a study of lung tissue from individuals in the general population.

A procedure was worked out whereby an ashed tissue section (the method worked out by Berkley *et al.*, 1965) from an individual exposed to asbestos was placed on a Leitz micromanipulator, and with the manipulator's finely drawn capillary needles, single fibers or groups of asbestos fibers and bodies were manipulated onto an Epoxy substrate on an EM grid. A review of these procedures, techniques and substrates, are given in Schwartz and Langer (1968) and Berkley *et al.* (1968b). The main problem connected with the manipulation of single particles is the development of a substrate which would permit the retention of the particles regardless of carbon coating methods, high vacuum systems of the coating device and the probe and attain stability under the electron beam. The procedure of manipulation is shown in Figure 6. Analysis of such a manipulated particle is shown in Figure 7. Morphological details of the fiber, including the segmentation, are clearly shown. Also, the analysis for silicon and iron clear-

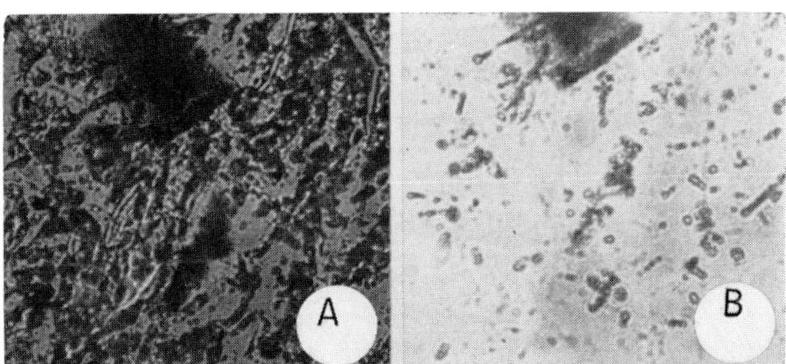

Figure 4. Beam sweeps of the probe produced "charred raster marks" on tissue sections. **A** shows the darkened tissue after exposure to the raster sweep of the beam; **B** is the same section after immersion in oil, showing the position of the fibers and bodies in the section.

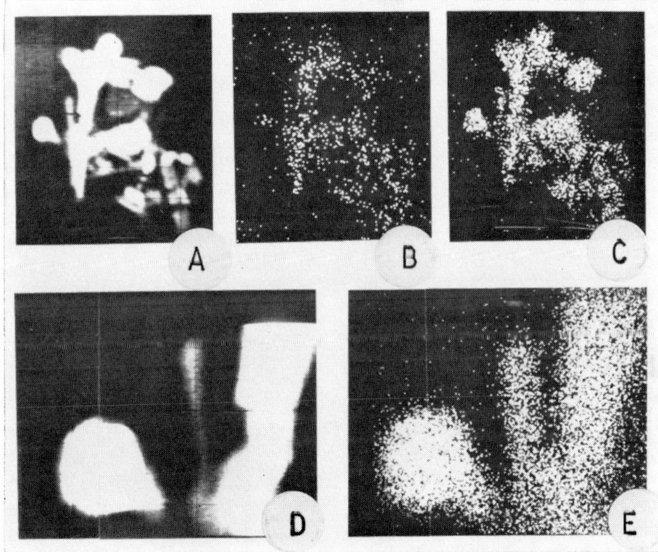

Figure 5. Group of asbestos bodies observed in the ashed lung tissue from an asbestos worker. The sample current display (A) SiK_a (B) FeK_a (C) at a magnification of about 13 microns/division. **D** and **E** are the sample current and Fe emission at a magnification of about 1 micron/division. Note that the resolution of the x-rays are about equal to that of the sample current resolution. Analyses indicate the bodies to be nucleated on amosite asbestos.

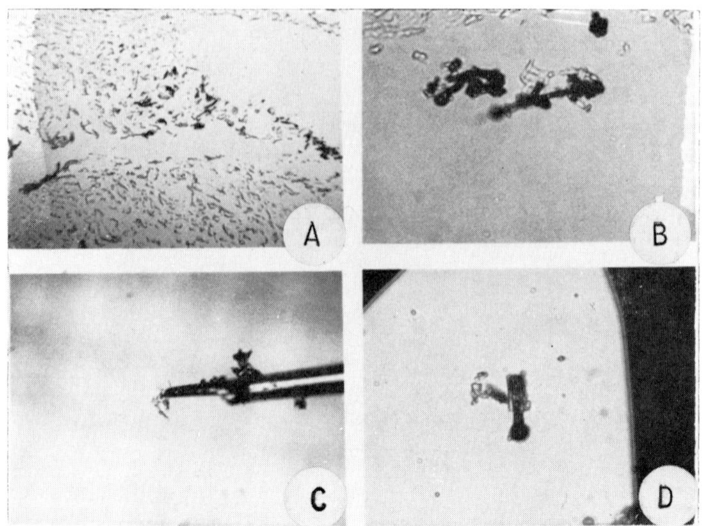

Figure 6. Manipulation of particles from an ashed tissue section: (A) ashed tissue section showing cellular outlines and a group of asbestos bodies (area of central photograph); (B) asbestos bodies as they appear in ashed tissue (compare with bodies in Figure 4A); (C) a cluster of asbestos bodies as they appear on the micromanipulator needle after manipulation; (D) the final stage of manipulation, the asbestos body after placement onto an EM grid.

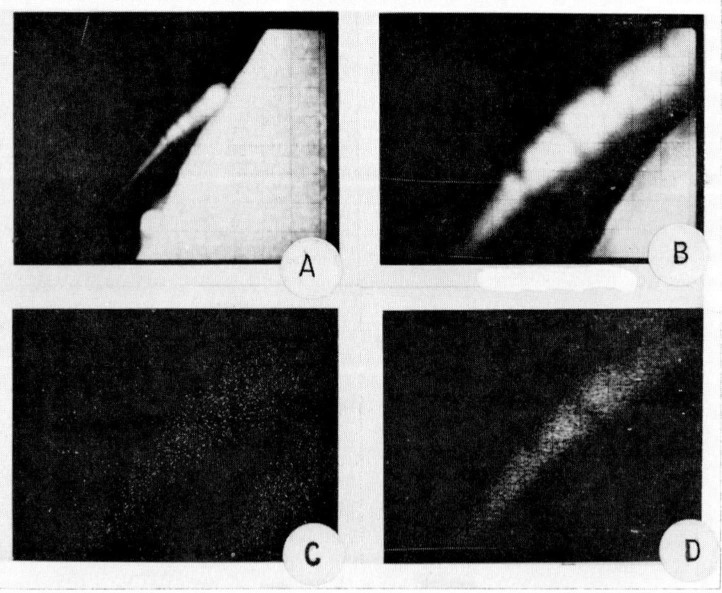

Figure 7. Analysis of a manipulated asbestos body: (A) and (B) are sample current pictures of the body at magnifications of 5 microns and 1 micron/division; (C) and (D) are Si and Fe Ka emission respectively. Chemical analysis of the fiber was possible at the ends of the body and in some of the segment areas.

ly shows the presence of both elements. This particle was analyzed as amosite in composition.

One of the unusual features of utilizing micromanipulation is that it occasionally picks up particles which are at the limits of, and are beyond, the resolution of light optical systems (Fig. 8). The body shown in Figure 8 was inadvertently manipulated onto an electron microscope grid along with larger fibers and bodies. It escaped detection until viewed under high resolution electron microscopy. This small body was analyzed on the electron microprobe and was found to be amosite asbestos.

Analyses have also been made on "pseudoasbestos bodies," which are differentiated from "classical" asbestos bodies on the basis of their morphology. The results of one such analysis is shown in Figure 9. This body was manipulated from ashed lung tissue onto an Epon coated electron microscope grid. The analysis showed quantities of iron, calcium and silicon present in the body. The elemental emission ratios of these elements did not indicate this core material to be asbestos in composition (Figure 10D).

Lung tissue was analyzed from a person who had worked in an asbestos factory in which only amosite asbestos was used. A sample of the fiber used within that factory was also analyzed. The analysis of the material used is shown in Figure 10A (marked as "Asbestos Fibers UNARCO"). The analyzed amosite fibers fell not only in the amosite field, but within and around the amosite maximum. Many analyses were made of fibers and bodies extracted from the workman's lung tissue. The analyses of thick asbestos bodies yield such a high proportion of iron emission from the iron rich coating material that it is not possible to evaluate the nature of the core material (Figure 10B). These are the analyses that lie near or at the iron apex. However, analyses of thin asbestos bodies, or those asbestos bodies in which little coating material is observed, fall near or at the amosite field maximum. What is remarkable about these analyses is the fact that this individual had not been employed in this factory for a peri-

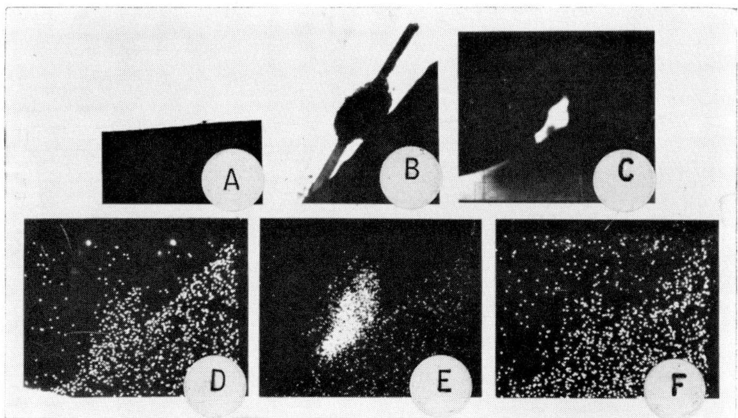

Figure 8. Analysis of a 2 micron long asbestos body. This body was inadvertently manipulated onto the EM grid during manipulation of much larger particles. (A) and (B) were taken with an electron microscope; (C) — (F) are sample current, Si, Fe Mg Ka emission. The particles analyzed as amosite.

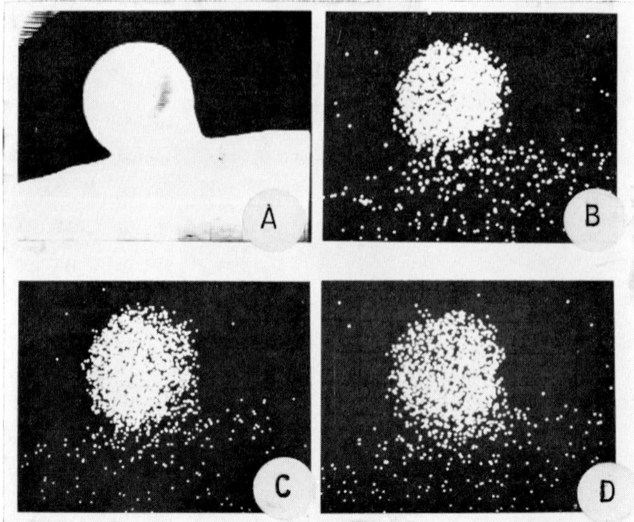

Figure 9. Analysis of a pseudoasbestos body manipulated from ashed lung tissue. The particle is about 5 microns in diameter as is shown by sample current (A) and Si, Fe, Ca Ka emission (B — D). The bulk chemistry is not related to any of the asbestos types (Fig. 10D).

od of ten years before his death. Therefore, the bulk chemistry of amosite had not altered appreciably during this period of biological residence. Amosite asbestos has been observed to be relatively easy to analyze; there is little doubt that chrysotile fibers are more difficult to analyze after biological residence. The rea-

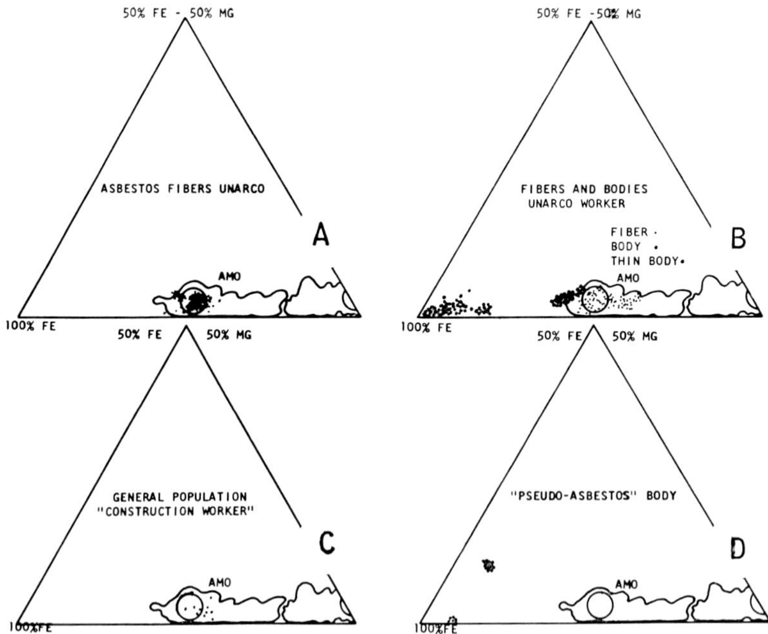

Figure 10. Analyses plotted on the emission ternary diagram (note that the entire diagram is not shown).

son for this lies in the physical and chemical nature of the fiber; chrysotile is easily broken down both chemically and physically.

Fibers and bodies from tissues of the general population have also been studied. It is of interest to note that a person from the general population had amosite asbestos present in his lung tissue (Figure 10C) and was found to have been employed as a construction worker.

Conclusion

The elemental emission ratios of the various asbestos types occur within fairly well-defined and characteristic fields thereby making it easy to differentiate the types. In cases where the fields appear to overlap, the fiber types may be differentiated on the basis of their calcium or sodium contents. Analyses thus obtained indicate that the first order approximation of chemical composition in relation to elemental emission has been obtained for the asbestos mineral types.

Analyses have been made on particles in ashed tissue residues and fibers and bodies which have been micromanipulated from tissue onto appropriate substrates. Success has been obtained in the analysis and identification of fibers which had been used in a specific factory environment. A comparison of the materials used in that factory with the fibers extracted from the lungs of an individual who had worked in that factory indicates they had the same bulk chemistry. The bulk chemistry of this fiber type had remained unaltered after at least 10 years of biological residence.

Preliminary results indicate that the electron microprobe may be used to identify and characterize particles observed in human lung tissue. It is possible to analyze material in the area of large particles thereby gaining information as to possible biological interaction. Particles beyond the resolution of light optical systems have been analyzed, extending and widening interpretations of histochemical techniques. Preliminary results utilizing the electron microprobe indicate it is a new and powerful tool in histochemistry.

ACKNOWLEDGMENTS

The author is presenting data which have accumulated through the joint effort of members of the probe group in the Environmental Sciences Laboratory: C. Berkley; A. Sastre; A. Arneson, and, J. Schwartz. He wishes to thank his colleagues for their permission to present the material.

REFERENCES

1. Andersen, C. A.: An introduction to the electron probe microanalyzer and its application to biochemistry. *In* Methods of Biochemical Analysis, Vol. 15, in SERIES, D. Glick (Ed.). Interscience Publishers, New York, 1967, 147-270.
2. Baden, V., and Schwartz, J.: Demonstration of asbestos bodies; comparison of available techniques. *In* Sec. Intl. Conf. Biol. Effects of Asbestos, Dresden Meeting. 1968. Anspach (Ed.). In press.
3. Beattie, J., and Knox, J. F.: Studies of mineral content and particle size distribution in the lungs of asbestos textile workers. *In* Inhaled Particles and Vapours. C. N. Davies (Ed.). Pergamon Press, New York, 1961, 419-433.
4. Beger, P. J.: Weiteres uber die asbestosiskorperchen. Virchows Arch., *290:*530-539, 1933.
5. Berkley, C., Churg, J., Selikoff, I. J., and Smith, W. E.: The detection and localization of mineral fibers in tissue. Ann. N.Y. Acad. Sci., *132:* 48-63, 1965.

6. Berkley, C., Langer, A. M., and Baden, V.: Instrumental analysis of inspired pulmonary fibrous particulates. Trans. N.Y. Acad. Sci., *30:* 331-350, 1968 (a) .
7. Berkley, C., Langer, A. M., Sastre, A., and Arneson, A.: Electron microprobe analysis of asbestos fibers and bodies. *In* Sec. Intl. Conf. Biol. Effects of Asbestos, Dresden Meeting. 1968. Anspach (Ed.) . In press, (b) .
8. Birks, L. S.: Electron probe microanalysis. *In* Monographs of Analytical Chemistry and its Applications. Interscience Publishers, New York, *17:*1-253, 1963.
9. Gaze, R.: The physical and molecular structure of asbestos. Ann. N.Y. Acad. Sci., *132:*23-30, 1965.
10. Hendry, N. W.: The geology, occurrences, and major uses of asbestos. Ann. N.Y. Acad. Sci., *132:*12-22, 1965.
11. Nagelschmidt, G.: Some observations of the dust content and composition in lungs with asbestosis, made during work on coal miners pneumoconiosis. Ann. N.Y. Acad. Sci., *132:*64-76, 1965.
12. Schwartz, J., and Langer, A. M.: Extraction techniques and instrumental analysis of asbestos bodies removed from human lung tissue. *In* Sec. Intl. Conf. Biol. Effects of Asbestos, Dresden Meeting. 1968. Anspach (Ed.) . In press.
13. Selikoff, I. J., Churg, J., and Hammond, C.: Asbestos exposure and neoplasia. J.A.M.A., *188:* 22-26, 1964.
14. Selikoff, I. J., Churg, J., and Hammond, E. C.: Relation between exposure to asbestos and mesothelioma. New Eng. J. Med., *272:*560-565, 1965.
15. Selikoff, I. J., Bader, R. A., Bader, M. E., Churg, J., and Hammond, E. C.: Asbestosis and neoplasia. Amer. J. Med., *42:*487-496, 1967.
16. Selikoff, I. J., Hammond, E. C., and Churg, J.: Asbestos exposure, smoking and neoplasia. J.A.M.A., *204:*106-112, 1968.
17. Speil, S., and Leineweber, J.: Asbestos minerals in modern technology. Environ. Res., *2:*166-208, 1969.
18. Sundius, N., and Bygden, A.: Der staubinhalt einer asbestosislunge und die beschaffenheit der sogenannten asbestosiskorperchen. Arch. Gewerbepath. Gewerbehyg., *8:*26-70, 1938.

Chapter 15

The Detection of Toxic Agents by the Mass Spectrometer

CHARLES J. UMBERGER, PH.D. and PARITOSH K. DE, PH.D.

Mass spectrometry is now included in the list of indispensible techniques for the elucidation of structure. Like the other techniques, mass spectrometry has definite applications for which there are no alternative procedures, and in common with various instrumental approaches, it has limitations that are difficult to circumvent by practical means.

In this chapter are discussed the limitations of mass spectroscopy in the detection of toxic organic compounds isolated from tissue and body fluids for routine toxicological analysis. Theoretical aspects and the mechanics of the instrumentation which have been adequately described,[1, 2, 3] are not included. The presentation is taken from the point of view of someone who must use the findings without needing to justify the mechanics by which it is obtained. Perhaps the title might better be named, "Practical Mass Spectroscopy in Forensic Applications."

Analytical toxicology is concerned with the separation, purification, qualitative detection and quantitative estimation of drugs and toxic substances from tissue and body fluids. Organic poisons can be isolated from tissue only by extraction with appropriate solvents, and during the isolation process there are always varying amounts of normal solvent soluble tissue components recovered with the toxic agents. The physical state of the tissue is a major factor in determining the amount of tissue impurities. Extracts from normal healthy tissue differ from the same organs in disease, and with putrefaction, potential tissue interference increases with the extent and nature of the putrefaction process. Purification procedures, which remove tissue components, are essential steps in toxicological analyses following the isolation process. In all purification methods, removal of solvent extractable tissue is accompanied by loss of compounds, and the more extensive the purification process the less the quantity of sample available for analysis. Since the sample contained in the tissue is limited, the tissue impurities vary in both quantity and composition, and once the tissue is processed, there is no other sample source, the question of where to stop in the preparation of the final sample for chemical examination requires more intuition than scientific judgment. To compound the problems further, the body invariably makes minor alterations in the chemical structure of the drug through

Contributed from: Laboratory of the Office of Chief Medical Examiner. Most of the views expressed here are those of the senior author.

detoxification and the degradation process, and these metabolites possess physical properties very similar to the present drug. Once the isolation and purification processes are completed, the toxicological analyses become a conventional chemical process with the restriction that the sample is rarely in a state of purity acceptable for the usual qualitative organic examination. This variable purity with variable composition in the nature of the impurities is the factor in toxicological analyses that limits and separates applications of mass spectrometry from other chemical applications. Because purity is a major mass requirement the toxicological application is limited to an empirical basis, which leaves few theoretical possibilities.

Despite such a shortcoming, the mass spectrometer has its place in the growing instrumental methology for forensic applications. The ideal mass situation would be a recording in which the molecular weight was the major peak (molecular mass) and fragmentation peaks were consistent with known structural relationships in the molecule. Unfortunately, this is not always attained. With some drugs, the molecular mass is an intense peak but seldom is it the strongest. With other compounds no $\frac{m}{e}$ corresponding to the molecular mass appears, yet fragment peaks are strong. In tissue extracts strong peaks due to impurities can appear at positions which are greater $\frac{m}{e}$ than the molecular mass. Nevertheless, the curves are reproducible under standardized conditions, varying in a constant manner with change in electron energy. Because of constancy and reproducibility in the curves, they may be used for identification by employing the empirical technique of spectroscopy in which the photographic recording of the metal spectrum is evaluated in order to differentiate spectral lines produced by a toxic metal from those of the metals that are normal components of tissue.

Texts on mass spectrometry[1, 2, 3] are informative for toxicological analyses but few of the principles are applicable, particularly the recommendations for recording data. Although the entire mass curve is generally not applicable to toxicological samples, the mass spectra from a tissue extract can be roughly divided into two fairly distinct regions; one for $\frac{m}{e}$ values below 100 and the other for $\frac{m}{e}$ values above 100. Tissue extractables undergo far more extensive fragmentation than drugs and most of the tissue peaks are below $\frac{m}{e}$ 100. The mass tissue spectrum is so complex in the lower molecular weight region that mass spectra is of questionable value for any compounds with molecular weights less than 100. Other complications from nitrogen, oxygen, carbon dioxide, carbon and their isotopes overlap peaks from tissue fragmentation and since purity is variable the contribution to the mass spectra of traces of tissue contaminants makes this an impractical area to resolve.

There is a relatively sharp cut off at $\frac{m}{e}$ 100 for tissue impurities. Most all drugs have molecular weights considerably greater than $\frac{m}{e}$ 100. Above $\frac{m}{e}$ 100 interference from contamination is minimal

[1]Introduction to Mass Spectrometry and Its Applications (Kiser). Prentice Hall, 1965.

[2]Applications to Mass Spectrometry to Organic Chemistry (Reed). Academic Press, 1966.

[3]Mass Spectrometry Organic Chemical Applications (Bremann). McGraw Hill, 1962.

to moderate depending on the volitalization temperature.

By controlling the volatilization temperature at the low vacuum of the instrument a partial separation between drug and tissue contaminants is possible. The situation is analogous to fractional vacuum sublimation[4] where the temperature at low vacuum is slowly raised through a temperature gradient in order to favor a preferential volatilization of the lower vapor pressure components. Variations due to mixed melting point phenomena produce the same type of variations on mass spectrometry as occur in sublimation. The toxicological operating procedure for mass spectrometry employing direct inlet techniques is to vary from room temperature up to around 160°C recording the different spectral responses and selecting that curve showing the best major peaks not associated with known tissue products.

Following this preliminary scanning to obtain optimum conditions for the unknown spectra and finding that it cannot be readily resolved in the $\frac{m}{e}$ area above 100, a second procedure is incorporated involving treatment of the sample by a purification process followed by another mass spectrum. This process has been successfully used in the infrared analysis of impure tissue samples.[5] This partial purification further separates tissue impurities from the drugs in the sample. Consequently, mass peaks due to tissue will be depressed while those from drugs will be enhanced. Comparison of the change in the ratios of the intensities in the spectra will differentiate those peaks in the $\frac{m}{e}$ region above 100 that are potential interferences in the pure mass spectra of the drug.

Purification procedures such as thin layer, paper, column and gas chromatography, vacuum sublimation and solvent extraction are all applicable. Solvent extraction is best carried out with a solid to organic solvent rather than immiscible liquid extraction in order to avoid variables due to the partition coefficient. Also, water vapor decreases the sensitivity and in excess is a pronounced interference. Difficulties in evaluating the spectra arise through the growing tendency toward the use of mixtures of drugs. With more complex mixtures, one involved purification such as counter current and elution column chromatography are indicated.

One major advantage of mass spectrometry is the extreme sensitivity of the method. It allows considerable loss of sample in purification and readily detects the small portions of sample subjected to thin layer and paper chromatography. It is equally applicable to those drugs for which good chemical indicating tests are lacking, particularly the neutral class of drugs and the acids.[6]

A prerequisite for the use of this method is that the suspected drug be first studied in the mass spectrometer and its spectrum compared with the normal tissue residues. This provides for the utilization of the most important feature of the method, namely the remarkable reproducibility of the spectra independent of the nature of the contaminants. It is an indispensable tool most valuable in

[4]Legal Medicine, Pathology and Toxicology (Gonzales, Vance, Helpern and Umberger). Appleton, Century and Croft, page 1157.

[5]Division of Absorption Spectrometry, Laboratory of Chief Medical Examiner, New York City.

[6]Legal Medicine, Pathology and Toxicology (Gonzales, Vance, Helpern and Umberger). Chapter 47, pages 1138-1142.

the final stage in a qualitative chemical process where confirmation is needed to confirm or exclude other physicochemical findings.

In the author's laboratory the isolation of acidic and neutral drugs from tissue and body fluids is carried out by the conventional procedures for toxicological processing,[7] and for mass spectrometry a Bendix Time-of-Flight Spectrometer (model 12 with 12-107 ion source and 30-12 analogs) is used. The mass spectra are recorded with a Honeywell 1508 Visicorder.[8] A heated crucible inlet system is used to introduce the sample. The sample contained in the special quartz crucible is heated by a tungsten filament at the end of the probe. The probe is provided with a chromel-alumel thermocouple. When the sample is of sufficient quantity, the solid material is placed directly in the crucible. In cases of small samples on paper or Silica Gel chromatograms, the material is extracted with 95% methyl alcohol, introduced into the crucible with a microsyringe and allowed to evaporate under slight vacuum to drive off the solvent. Special care is taken so that the top and outside surface of the crucible is free of sample material after the crucible is introduced into the mass spectrometer. The spectra are taken at room temperature and at three higher temperatures not exceeding 160°C. The lowest volatilization temperature showing good resolution is generally selected for evaluating the spectra. When the tissue extracts have excess amounts of fats and lipids, the solid residue is extracted at room temperature with hexane or petroleum ether,[9] the extracted residue is dried under vacuum and new spectra are recorded at the optium volatilization temperature. The mass spectra are recorded at three different attenuations to evaluate the relative intensities of the mass peaks.

Examples of characteristic mass spectra are shown in Figures 1-3. In Figure 1 are given the clearly defined spectra of Doriden after an acid liver residue was purified by thin layer chromatography and the suspected Doriden was extracted from the Silica Gel with methanol. The spectra of pure Caffeine, shown in Figure 2 is characterized by a strong parent peak at $\frac{m}{e}$ 194, a moderate peak at $\frac{m}{e}$ 165 and a good peak at $\frac{m}{e}$ 137. The mass spectra of caffeine from a paper chromatogram of tissue extract (Fig. 3) is almost identical to the pure drug.

Summary

Mass spectrometry has definite applications for toxicological analyses which cannot be circumvented by other instrumental techniques. It is most useful for confirmation after other analytical testing has indicated possible structures. It is particularly applicable when used in conjunction with purification procedures such as paper, thin layer, gas chromatog-

[7]Legal Medicine, Pathology and Toxicology (Gonzales, Vance, Helpern and Umberger). Chapter 47, pages 1128-1146.

[8]The Visicorder is necessarily a fast recorder and employees light sensitive recording paper which is not permanent and shows all of the blemishes from handling when permanent prints are made.

[9]Relatively few drugs are soluble in hexane or petroleum ether whereas lipids are very soluble. Also, the sensitivity of the method allows considerable loss particularly when the purification gives a sharper drug spectra.

raphy and sublimation. Owing to tissue impurities it is not directly applicable for fundamental structural studies on unknown drugs whose mass fragmentation behaviors have not been previously determined.

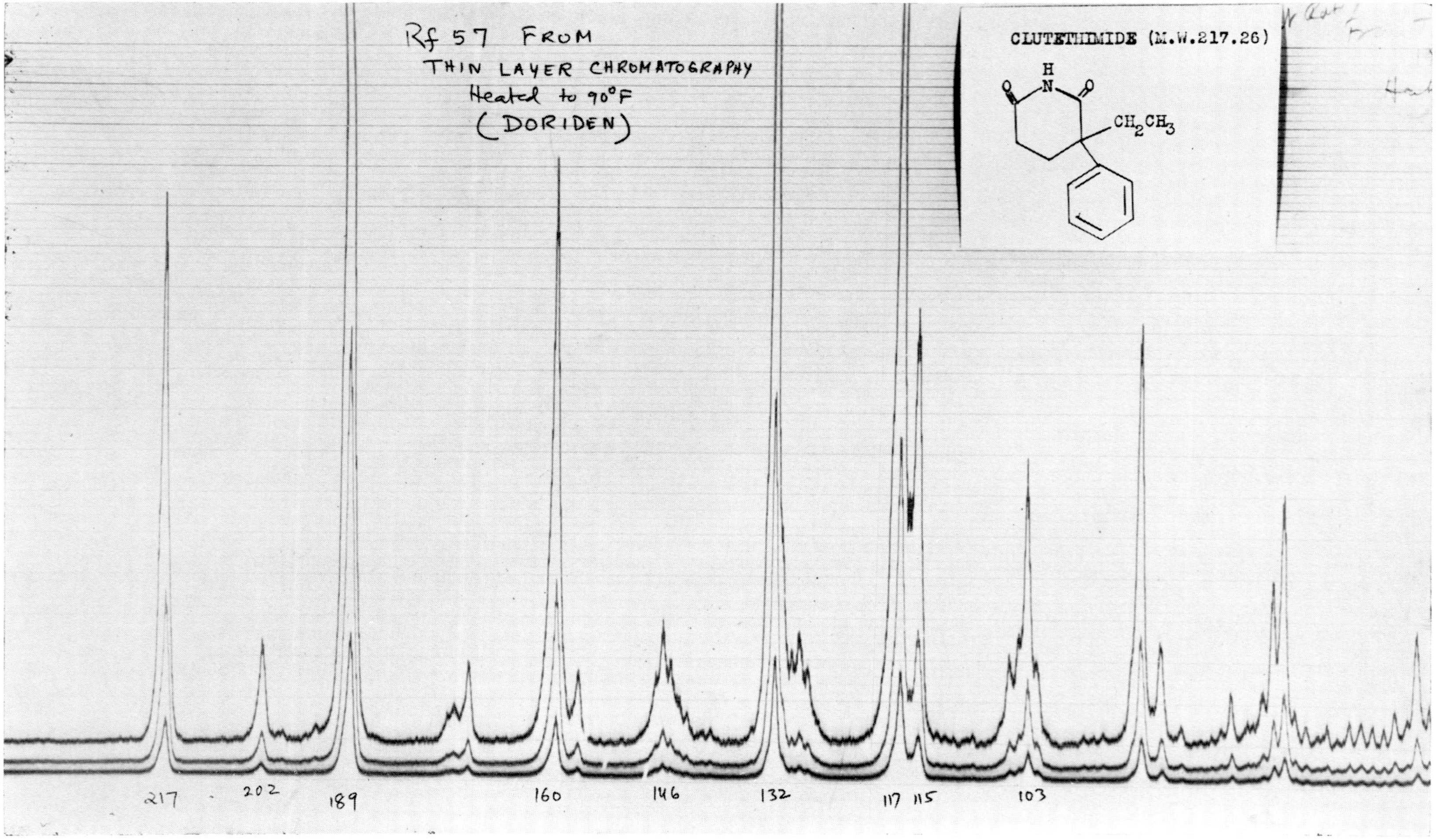
Rf 57 FROM
THIN LAYER CHROMATOGRAPHY
Heated to 90°F
(DORIDEN)
GLUTETHIMIDE (M.W.217.26)
H
N
CH2CH3
217
202
189
160
146
132
117
115
103

Figure 1.

Caffeine
Heated to 90°F
CAFFEINE (M.W.194.19)
CH3
O
CH3
N
N
N
N
CH3
194
165
137
109
82

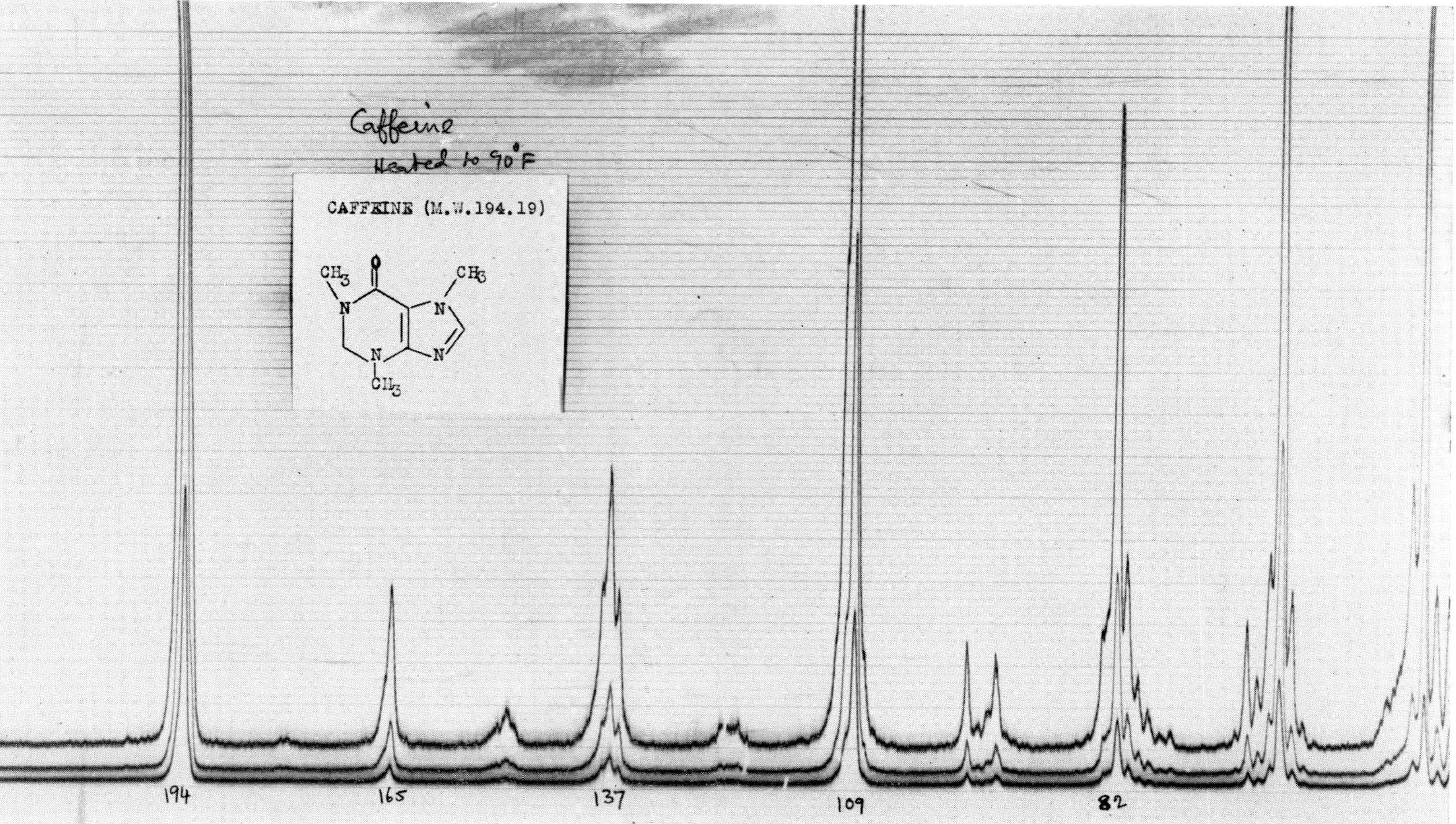

Figure 2.

Rf 67 From
PAPER CHROMATOGRAPHY
Heated to 95°F
CAFFEINE (M.W.194.19)
CH3
CH3
N
N
N
N
CH3
194
165
137
109
82

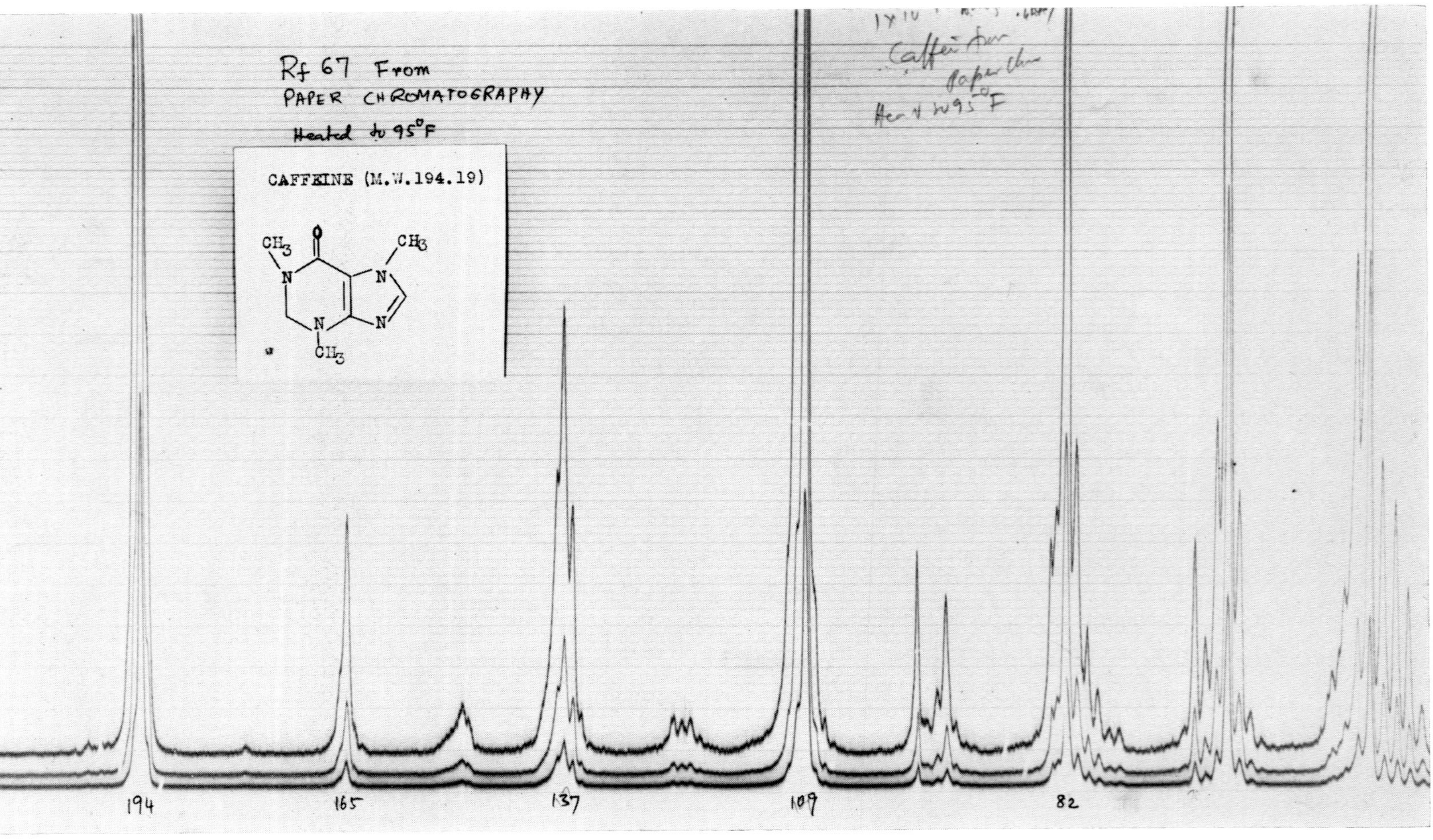

Figure 3.

PART III

SPECIFIC TOXIC AGENTS

Chapter 16

The Toxicity and Side Effects of Antibiotics

JOSEPH F. SADUSK, JR., M.D.

None of the presently available antibiotics are free of an adverse reaction potential. These agents differ among themselves in this respect only by the degree of severity and the particular body system affected. Virtually all body systems may be involved by antibiotics as a group, a fact which is common to all drugs when their potential for harm is considered.

Because of the numerous antibiotics available on the market and the wide spectrum of toxic effects, it is impossible to review such a broad field in the time allocated. Consequently, my remarks will be limited to reactions which are considered serious or life-threatening.

Basically, two types of serious reactions may occur: hypersensitivity reactions, and biological and metabolic alterations. The hypersensitivity reactions are essentially common to most antibiotics. They may vary in type and severity, and range from skin eruptions to anaphylactoid and true anaphylactic reactions, some of which are fatal. The biologic and metabolic alterations in the host revolve around disturbances of the normal microbial flora of the respiratory and gastrointestinal tracts, which may be followed by superinfections of those body systems either with gram-positive or gram-negative microorganisms, depending upon the bacterial spectrum of the antibiotic employed.

Establishing a cause-effect relationship between a drug and an adverse reaction can be extraordinarily difficult. In this respect, antibiotics do not differ from other drugs. The problem is compounded when the incidence of such reactions is very low, such as is the case with some of the hypersensitivity reactions. As a result, the incidence of some of the hypersensitivity reactions may not be determined with accuracy. This is due to the need for studying many thousands of persons at risk with the antibiotic since, while it may not be too difficult to assemble individual reaction cases, the average investigator finds it difficult to determine a significantly large denominator, namely, the number of persons at risk.

Consequently, it will not be possible to relate accurately the incidence of hypersensitivity reactions and the more important biologic and metabolic alterations leading to life-threatening situations, except in a few instances. Indeed, in a recent article concerning adverse effects of antimicrobial drugs, the *Medical Letter* (4) spoke to this point, noting the difficulty of estimating the frequency of such reactions from published reports, and stating that the estimates indicated in their report were based on the personal views of consultants as well as on published reports.

Some of the references (4, 5, 6, 7) noted in this chapter cover the multifarious reactions of the many marketed antibiotics and the reader is referred to these reports for details. Use should be made of the package inserts which accompany the marketed antibiotics for additional details.

The important reactions of the major antibiotics are summarized. If some of the very new antibiotics are not included, such omissions are simply due to the fact that sufficient information is not yet available in the literature.

The following paragraphs outline in alphabetical order those antibiotics causing major types of reactions, or body systems involved. The column of agents to the left lists those antibiotics in which there appears to be established association, or relatively high order of frequency; those on the right pertain to agents causing a lower order of frequency, or in which the association may be controversial.

Allergic Reactions

Cephalothin	Chloramphenicol
Griseofulvin	Erythromycin
Lincomycin	Kanamycin
Novobiocin	Neomycin
Penicillins	Nystatin
Streptomycin	Paromomycin
	Polymyxin B
	Tetracyclines
	Triacetyloleandomycin

Among the antibiotics involved, the penicillins are the most likely to cause allergic reactions. While these reactions are not dose related, they do occur more frequently and are more severe with parenteral administration. Fever, urticaria, maculopapular rash, and serum sickness are the common types of allergic reactions and may be acute or delayed, while anaphylactoid or true anaphylactic reactions are less frequent but carry with them a great potential for death. There is no evidence that the newer penicillins have a lesser potential for acute allergic reactions. And, finally, there is evidence of a cross sensitivity between penicillin and cephalothin, though a quantitative definition of degree is not yet available.

Blood Dyscrasias

Chloramphenicol	Amphotericin B
	Bacitracin (?)
	Cephalothin
	Griseofulvin
	Kanamycin (?)
	Neomycin (?)
	Novobiocin
	Penicillins
	Streptomycin
	Tetracyclines

Many of the antibiotic agents have a potential for adverse effect on the hemapoietic system, including red cells, leukocytes, and platelets. Blood dyscrasias ranging from simple neutropenia and anemia through to agranulocytosis, thrombocytopenia purpura, and aplastic anemia may occur. Among these conditions, the most intensive studies have been devoted to the association of chloramphenicol with aplastic anemia, and two types of bone marrow effect have been reported. First, a reversible type of bone marrow depression has been described, which appears during the course of therapy, is dose related, and is readily reversible upon removal of the drug and sometimes with reduction of dosage. In contrast to this, there is a form of bone marrow depression attributed to chloramphenicol and which seemingly may occur in extraordinarily low frequency weeks or months following therapy, is not dose related, is generally irreversible, and carries with it a high fatality rate. The relationship of these two types of bone depression, if any, has not been defined.

Renal Damage

Amphotericin B
Bacitracin
Kanamycin
Neomycin (Parenteral)
Polymyxin B
Vancomycin
Viomycin
Griseofulvin
Methicillin
Paromomycin (Parenteral)

Some antibiotics are known to produce renal damage, particularly ampotericin B, bacitracin, and polymyxin B. Two agents, namely, neomycin and paromomycin, may cause such effects if administered parenterally; however, only oral dosage is recommended by the manufacturers.

Gastrointestinal Reactions

Erythromycin
Lincomycin
Novobiocin
Nystatin
Tetracyclines
Triacetyloleandomycin

May occur to some extent with most orally administered antibiotics

Nausea, vomiting, and diarrhea occur relatively frequently with most orally administered antibiotics. Generally, these are dose related and are especially found with the tetracyclines, followed next by erythromycin.

Superinfections

Tetracylines — and most broad spectrum antibiotics

While the tetracyclines appear to be the chief offenders in producing superinfections, it must be remembered that most, if not all, of the broad spectrum antibiotics carry this potential. Stomatitis, glossitis, and pruritus ani, caused by superinfection with yeasts, may appear not infrequently. Lower respiratory tract and lower gastrointestinal tract complications of great severity may occur due to superinfection, principally by the staphylococcus aureus. In the latter category, pseudomembraneous enterocolitis carries with it a high mortality.

Hepatotoxicity

Tetracyclines (esp. pregnancy)
Triacetyloleandomycin
Novobiocin
Lincomycin (?)
Amphotericin B

It is well known that excessive doses of the tetracyclines may have a toxic effect upon the liver. Such untoward effects are more likely to occur under conditions of renal impairment interfering with the excretion of the tetracyclines, or when these agents are administered parenterally. In the latter respect, the dangers of parenteral administration of tetracyclines in pregnant women has been emphasized.

Central Nervous System Reactions

Peripheral/Optic Neuritis
Amphotericin B
Chloramphenicol
Kanamycin
Neomycin
Polymyxin B
Vancomycin

8th Nerve Damage
Kanamycin
Neomycin
Paromomycin
Streptomycin
Vancomycin
Viomycin

A number of antibiotics, as presented above, are reported to be associated with peripheral and/or optic neuritis in low frequency. More frequent, however, has been the association of some antibiotics with 8th nerve damage. In the case of neomycin and paromomycin, this association is infrequent when the drug is administered orally as recommended by the manufacturers.

Other Reactions

Tetracyclines	— Staining and deformity of teeth in young children — also in newborn when administered in late pregnancy
Chloramphenicol	— Gray Syndrome in infants

Finally, there are several important reactions, as noted above, which deserve mention. The tetracyclines, when administered during the period of tooth development (including late pregnancy, the neonatal period, and early childhood), may cause discoloration of the teeth with or without deformity. It appears that this is more likely to develop with prolonged tetracycline therapy.

Owing to inadequate mechanisms for the metabolic disposition of chloramphenicol in the newborn infant, the use of this antibiotic in the infant when administered in the ordinarily recommended doses for the adult may lead to a toxic reaction syndrome known as the Gray Syndrome. This condition is characterized by the appearance of abdominal distention with or without vomiting, progressive pallid cyanosis, and vasomotor collapse — sometimes with irregularity of respiration. In most instances, it has been found during treatment instituted within the first 48 hours of life, and the symptoms first appeared after 3 to 4 days of continued treatment with high chloramphenicol dosage. Blood levels of chloramphenicol are found to be unusually high. The process is reversible if appropriate corrective therapy is instituted at an early period.

Large-Scale Studies on Antibiotic Reactions

The brief review which has been presented on the reactions to antibiotics is deficient in its failure to state accurately an incidence, or frequency, of these reactions. As mentioned previously, it is not possible to state such frequencies with any degree of assurance since one must have both an accurate numerator (the number of reactions) and an accurate denominator (the number of persons at risk — or those taking the antibiotic). The fact is, with a few notable exceptions, that this information simply does not exist. Consequently, most authorities must state opinions rather than cite facts. But there are a few large-scale studies which deserve mention and which may clarify a few issues.

The FDA Antibiotic Reaction Study

In 1957, Welch and his co-workers (7) at the Food and Drug Administration reported on the only nationwide study ever made on reactions to antibiotics. But even in this study, no attempt was made to present information on the amount of the reaction-producing antibiotics distributed. Nevertheless, a presentation of their findings may put this reaction matter in true perspective.

This study, limited to antibiotics, was carried out in survey form, encompassing 198,332 of the nation's total of 685,655 hospital beds (28.9%) in 1955, along with interviews of 1,637 physicians throughout the country. Attention was directed primarily to all severe reactions including blood dyscrasias, exfoliative dermatitis, severe angioneurotic edema, severe monilial or fungal infections, and enterocolitis associated with antibiotic medication. The investigation uncovered 2,995 cases for review, of which 1,070 were classified as "severe" and 1,925 cases as "not severe." Of the latter group classified as "not severe," the majority (1,358) were cases of angioneurotic edema and urticaria. The remaining "not severe" cases, in order of frequency, were examples of other dermal lesions, serum sickness type reactions, and local moniliasis. Penicillin was by far the most commonly noted antibiotic in the study and was responsible for 1,616 (84%) of the "not severe" 1,925 cases. Following in order were combined antibiotics (mostly combinations of penicillin with streptomycin or dihydrostreptomycin), the various tetracyclines, novobiocin, erythromycin, streptomycin, chloramphenicol, and neomycin.

Among the 1,070 cases classified as "severe," or life-threatening, the majority were examples of anaphylactoid reactions (809 cases), followed in order by superinfections (107), skin reactions (70), blood dyscrasias (46), and angioneurotic edema with cerebral or respiratory involvement (38).

Of the 809 cases of anaphylactoid shock, 793 were associated with penicillin — 611 due to penicillin alone, and 123 with penicillin-streptomycin/dihydrostreptomycin combinations. Seventy-two, almost 10%, of thes cases died. Of the nonpenicillin anaphylactoid shock cases, nine were due to streptomycin, three to dihydrostreptomycin, three to tetracyclines, and one to chloramphenicol. There were two fatalities in this latter group, one due to streptomycin and one due to dihydrostreptomycin. Age grouping was not significant, ranging from infancy to senior citizen status.

There were 107 cases of severe superinfections, such as enterocolitis and monoliasis with 40 deaths, and these were associated principally with the tetracyclines.

There were 70 cases of severe skin reactions, such as exfoliative dermatitis, anaphylactoid or hemorrhagic purpura, and erythema multiforme, with 70 deaths. These were associated principally with penicillin or penicillin combinations.

There were 46 cases of blood dyscrasias, such as aplastic anemia, granulocytopenia, thrombocytopenic purpura, and leukopenia, with 27 deaths. These were associated principally with chloramphenicol or chloramphenicol combinations.

And, finally, there were 38 cases of angioneurotic edema with respiratory or cerebral involvement and with five deaths, principally associated with penicillin or penicillin combinations.

In sheer numbers and in effort, this study stands out as an outstanding accomplishment in the field of adverse drug reaction evaluation, but, as noted previously, no attempt was made to correlate these data with drug usage. Here again, one is faced with the problem of obtaining incidence figures for a proper view of the risk-to-benefit ratio.

The U. S. Public Health Service Study on Penicillin Reactions

In 1960, Brown (1) reported on the incidence of penicillin reactions observed in patients receiving that agent for venereal disease under treatment conducted in a number of state public health clinics. During such treatment in 1959, he found 206 (9.96/1,000) penicillin reactors among 20,687 cases treated. These 206 cases were broken down as follows:

	Number	*Rate/1,000*
Urticaria	122	5.90
Pruritis, generalized	17	0.82
Angioneurotic edema	5	0.24
Dermatitis medicamentosa	4	0.19
Erythema multiforme	1	0.05
Dermatophytid	1	0.05
TOTAL	150	7.25
Anaphylaxis	19	0.92
Moderate to severe	7	0.34
Mild	12	0.58
Serum sickness	9	0.44
Gastrointestinal	12	0.58
Vertigo, syncope	15	0.73
Chills, fever, headache	9	0.44
Chest pain, dyspnea	2	0.10
Hysteria	1	0.05

In summary of Brown's data, it may be said that he found an overall reaction rate from penicillin of about 1% (1:100), principally consisting of allergic skin manifestations and an anphylactoid reaction rate of about 0.1% (1:1,000) of which about a third – or 0.03% (1:3,000) – were cases of classical anaphylactic shock.

The WHO Penicillin Reaction Review

In the early part of 1968, Idsoe (3) and his group from the World Health Organization reported on their intensive review of the world's literature on penicillin reactions. In brief, they reported the following statistics:

Allergic reactions:	0.7% to 10%
Anaphylactic reactions:	0.004% to 0.015%
	(4:100,000 to 15:100,000)
Fatality rate from anaphylaxis:	0.0015% to 0.002%
	1.5:100,000 to 2:100,000)

In a study of 151 anaphylactic fatalities collected during the course of his study, Idsoe made the following observations:

1. More than half of the fatalities occurred in the 25-64 year age groups.
2. There were no significant sex differences.
3. About 44% of the patients had been treated for infections of the respiratory tract; half of these had bronchitis or pneumonia.
4. In 28%, an allergic diathesis of some type was noted, with 14% of bronchial asthma and 3.3% hay fever type allergy and skin eruptions, including drug allergies.
5. Twenty-five percent had experienced reactions following previous penicillin therapy and, moreover, 36.5% of the 69% of patients who had received penicillin previously, suffered reactions.
6. The type of penicillin preparation was known in 80% of cases. Most fatalities were caused by intermediate-acting and short-acting preparations in contrast to a low number with long-acting preparations and a handful of those receiving oral preparations (2%). On the other hand, this distribution may not be significant since Idsoe considers the distribution of reactions to be in proportion to the consumption of these preparations in medical practice.
7. While the majority of known death-causing doses were essentially within the accepted therapeutic dose range, Idsoe reports an interesting case in which a 41-year old female died in a few minutes after receiving an intradermal test of 4,000 I.V. of penicillin in water. Another fatal case is reported in which a female being treated for syphilis died after an intravenous test dose of 0.01 I.U. of penicillin!
8. Among those patients dying of anaphylactic shock, 81% died following the first administration of penicillin, and 4% after the second administration.
9. The intervals between administration of penicillin and manifestations of symptoms and death was known in 96% and 97% of cases, respectively. In almost 85% of the cases in which these facts were

known, the symptoms appeared within 15 minutes of administration — half of these were said to be "immediate." More than 50% of deaths occurred within 15 minutes of the fatal administration of penicillin. In almost half the cases, symptoms appeared and death occurred within 15 minutes.

The California State Report on Chloramphenicol

During the past few years, there has been much publicity on the association of aplastic anemia with the use of chloramphenicol, leading one to believe that this blood dyscrasia appears rather frequently. Quotations as to incidence have been freely made, usually without reference to the facts.

Indeed, the actual freqeuncy of aplastic anemia appearing after the use of chloramphenicol is not yet known. However, a report made to the California State Assembly and Senate (2) in January, 1967, by the California Medical Association and California State Department of Health, with the assistance of the California Pharmaceutical Association, sheds some light on the occurrence of fatal aplastic anemia following the administration of chloramphenicol.

The study group reviewed 409 death certificates coded to a relevant hematologic disorder from patients dying in California over an 18-month period, January 1, 1963, through June 30, 1964. From this review, they collected 60 cases in which a diagnosis of aplastic anemia appeared to be established. In 40 of these 60 cases, a potentially toxic exposure was not discovered. This constitutes that type of aplastic anemia known as "idiopathic" and which has been thus diagnosed and reported for years.

Among the remaining 20 cases, it was found that a specific toxic exposure, other than chloramphenicol, had occurred prior to the onset of aplastic anemia in 10 of the cases. This left 10 cases for final review.

With regard to these remaining 10 cases (1/6 of the original group of 60), it was found that the deceased patients had received chloramphenicol with or without other drugs prior to the onset of aplastic anemia. In 3 of these 10 cases, the patient had received only chloramphenicol; in the remaining 7 cases the patient also had received one to three potentially toxic agents in addition to chloramphenicol. Indeed, the Committee noted that these agents had been associated with aplastic anemia in the AMA Registry.

However, in calculating rates for the association of chloramphenicol therapy with aplastic anemia, the biostatistician used all 10 cases, even though 7 of these cases had received other agents known to have a potential for producing aplastic anemia. Employing two arbitrarily selected dosage schedules of 7.5 and 4.5 gm, together with the total of 10 cases of aplastic anemia and distribution data for chloramphenicol in California over the 18-month period, the risk of fatal aplastic anemia for patients receiving chloramphenicol was calculated to range from 1:24,200 to 1:40,500, respectively.

On the other hand, if one considers the fact that toxic exposures other than chloramphenicol might have been the causative factors in 7 of the 10 patients, and the calculations are made on the basis of 3 patients receiving chloramphenicol alone, these risk estimates are reduced to one-third, or 1:80,600 to 1:135,000.

Conclusion

When viewed from a unilateral aspect of toxicity alone, the adverse reaction potential from antibiotics is formidable and such an approach could easily lead one to a philosophy of therapeutic nihilism in the treatment of infectious disease. But these reactions are no different than are found with many other drugs, and it is a matter of fact that the use of all drugs carries with it a potential for harm to the patient. For this reason, the doctor must always balance off risk against benefit.

A proper interpretation of risk-to-benefit philosophy for the antibiotics is perhaps best expressed by Goodman and Gilman in their authoritative book *The Pharmacological Basis of Therapeutics.* They say, "The fact that harmful effects may follow the therapeutic or prophylactic use of antibiotics must never discourage the physician from their administration in any situation in which they are definitely indicated. It should, however, make him very careful in their use when they are required, and very hesitant to employ them in instances in which indications for their application are either entirely lacking or, at most, only suggestive. To do otherwise is to run the risk, at times, of converting a simple, benign, and self-limited disease into one that may be serious or even fatal. It must always be kept in mind that the use of any powerful therapeutic agent is accompanied by a calculated risk. The antibiotics are no different; to be concerned with only their potential dangers is no less unrealistic and unwise than to accept them as universally applicable, completely benign, and entirely harmless."

REFERENCES

1. Brown, W. J.: An evaluation of the incidence of reactions to penicillin. Brit. J. Vener. Dis., *36:* 30-33, 1960.
2. California State Senate and Assembly, report by the California Medical Association and the California State Department of Health with the assistance of the California Pharmaceutical Association, January 1967.
3. Idsoe, O., Guthe, T., Willcox, R. R., and DeWeck, A. L.: Nature and extent of penicillin side-reactions, with particular reference to fatalities from anaphylactic shock. Bull. World Health Organization, *38:*159-188, 1968.
4. Medical Letter: Principle toxic, allergic, and other adverse effects of antimicrobial drugs, *10:* 73-76, 1968.
5. Meyler, L.: Side effects of drugs. Excerpta Medical Foundation, 1964, pp. 156-198.
6. New Drugs: American Medical Association, 1967, pp. 1-71.
7. Welch, H., Lewis, C. N., Weinstein, H. I., and Boeckman, B. B.: Severe reactions to antibiotics — a nationwide survey. Antibiotic Med. and Chemotherapy, *4:*80-813, 1957.

Chapter 17

Detection of Enterotoxin

E. P. CASMAN, PH.D. AND JOSEPH C. OLSON, JR., PH.D.

INTRODUCTION

The precipitation of enterotoxin by specific antiserum in a gel and identification of the precipitate with a reference precipitate as developed by Ouchterlony1, 2 is the procedure of choice for the detection of the serologically identified enterotoxins. This chapter is concerned specifically with staphylococcal enterotoxin.

To demonstrate the enterotoxigenicity of the staphylococcus, the enterotoxin is produced in special, well aerated culture medium and its presence in the culture filtrate or supernatant is determined by the geldiffusion precipitation test using unconcentrated, or if indicated, concentrated material. The micro-slide modification by Wadsworth and Crowle[4] of the Ouchterlony procedure is particularly useful because of its sensitivity, speed, simplicity, specificity and economical use of reagents.

For the detection of trace amounts of staphylococcal enterotoxin in foods, the gel-diffusion precipitin test is applied after extracting and separating the enterotoxin from the food constituents and concentrating the enterotoxin to the sensitivity of the gel-diffusion test.

A simple procedure for obtaining well aerated growth of the staphylococcus will be described in detail; the detailed procedure for performing the microslide gel-diffusion test will be presented and the procedure for extracting and concentrating traces of enterotoxin in food will be described.

Production of Enterotoxin

Of the methods described by Casman and Bennett[5] for the production of enterotoxin, cultivation of these staphylococci on semi-solid Brain Heart Infusion Agar of pH 5.3 is simple and does not require the use of special apparatus.

Brain Heart Infusion Broth (Fisher Scientific Co., Baltimore Biological Laboratories) is adjusted to pH 5.3; agar is added to 0.7% concentration and dissolved in the medium by minimal boiling; the medium is distributed in 25 ml quantities in tubes (25 x 200), and autoclaved at 15 lbs steam pressure for *10* minutes. The tubes of sterile medium are emptied aseptically into standard petri dishes (glass or plastic).

A loopful of growth from nutrient agar slants is added to 3 to 5 ml of distilled water. The surface of the semi-solid medium is then inoculated with four drops of this aqueous suspension which should contain approximately 300 million organisms per ml. The turbidity of the suspension is equivalent to No. 1 of the McFarland[6] nephelometer scale. (This turbidity is obtained by mixing one part 1% $BaCl_2$ with 99 parts 1% H_2SO_4.) The drops are spread over the entire surface with a sterile spreader and the plates are incubated under aerobic conditions. Good surface growth is obtained after 48 to 72 hours of incubation at 35 to 37°C, at which time the pH of the culture should have risen to approximately 8.0. The agar and organisms are removed by high speed centrifugation. This is usually accomplished by transferring the contents of the petri dish to a plastic 50-ml centrifuge tube and centrifuging at high speed in the Sorval centrifuge. The supernatant is then examined for the presence of enterotoxin by filling the depots in the slide gel-diffusion assembly as directed below.

THE SLIDE GEL-DIFFUSION TEST

A slight modification of the slide gel-diffusion test as described in detail by Crowle[4] is used. This modification consists of the incorporation of 0.8 percent sodium barbital and 0.1% thimerosal (Merthiolate) in the agar gel and the use of plastic squares in which the distance between the centers of the central and peripheral wells is 4.5 instead of 4.0 mm.

Detailed Description of Preparation and Use of the Slides

A. PREPARATION OF THE SLIDES

a) The slides (3″ x 1″) are cleaned by boiling in a weak detergent solution, rinsed several times in distilled water followed by methanol, ethanol, or acetone. They are air dried and stored in a dust-free container.

b) A double layer of plastic electrician's insulating tape (Homart Plastic Tape ¾″ wide, Sears Roebuck and Co.; Tape Insulation, Electrical, ¾″ wide, Plymouth Rubber Co., Inc., Canton, Massachusetts; or Scotch Electrical Tape, Pressure-Sensitive Adhesive, thickness 0.01 ml, ¾″ wide, St. Paul, Minnesota) is placed on both sides of the middle 2 cm of the clean glass slide. The tape is applied as follows: a piece of tape about 9.5 cm long is started about 0.5 cm from the edge of the under surface of the slide and tightly wrapped around the slide twice. The area between the tapes may be rinsed with 95% ethanol and wiped with clean cheesecloth if soiled during the taping.

c) The upper surface area between the tapes is coated with 0.2% agar in distilled water as follows:

1. The 0.2% agar is melted and held at 55°C in a screw-cap bottle.

2. The slide is held over a beaker placed on a hot plate adjusted to 65 to 85°C (150 to 190°F) and the 0.2% agar is poured or brushed over the slide between the two tapes. Excess agar is allowed to drain off into the beaker. The screw cap bottle containing the 0.2% agar may be kept on the hot plate and the agar collected in the beaker may be used again.

3. The undersurface of the slide is wiped. It is placed on a tray and dried in a dust-free atmosphere (e.g., an incubator). *Note*: If the slides are not clean, the agar will roll off the slide without coating it uniformly.

B. PREPARATION OF THE SLIDE ASSEMBLY

Plastic templates are prepared as described by Crowle[4] except that the distance between the centers of the central and peripheral wells is 4.5 instead of 4.0 mm.

a) A thin film of silicone grease (Dow Corning High Vacuum Grease) is spread on the side of the template that will be placed next to the agar gel (i.e., the side with the smaller holes).

b) Exactly 0.35 ml of melted and cooled (to 55°C) agar (see below) is placed between the tapes.

1. The agar is prepared by adding 1.2 percent Noble Special Agar (Difco 0142-01) to a fluid base prepared as follows:

NaCl	0.85%
Merthiolate	1:10,000 (crystalline-merthiolate is obtained from Eli Lilly & Co.
Sodium barbital	0.8%
pH	7.4
Distilled water	

The agar is melted in the Arnold sterilizer (steamer) and filtered while hot in the steamer through two layers of filter paper.

c) The silicone-coated template is laid immediately on the melted agar and the edges of the bordering tapes. One edge of the template is placed on one of the bordering tapes and the opposite edge is brought to rest on the other bordering tape.

d) The slide is placed in a prepared petri dish (see step C) soon after the agar solidifies and is labelled with the date, number, or any other necessary information.

C. PREPARATION OF PETRI DISHES TO RECEIVE SLIDE ASSEMBLIES

A strip of cotton is placed around the bottom periphery of a 14 cm petri dish and saturated with distilled water. Two or three slide assemblies can be placed in each dish.

D. ADDITION OF REAGENTS

a) A suitable dilution of the anti-enterotoxin is placed in the central well and the homologous reference enterotoxin is placed in one of the upper peripheral wells. The material under examination is placed in a well flanking the well containing the reference enterotoxin.

b) The reference toxins and antitoxins, previously balanced, are used in the tests in concentrations giving a line of precipitation approximately halfway between their respective depots. The dilutions of the reagents are adjusted also to give distinct but faint lines of precipitation for maximal sensitivity.

c) A control slide with only reference toxin and antitoxin is prepared.

d) The wells are filled to convexity with the reagents using a pasteur pipette (prepared by drawing out glass tubing of approximately 7 mm outside diameter) or with a disposable 30 or 40 lambda pipette (obtainable from Kensington Scientific Corp., 1165-67th Street, Oakland, California 94621 or Colab Laboratories, Inc., Chicago Heights, Illinois 60411). Bubbles are removed from all of the wells by probing with a fine glass rod. The rods are made by pulling glass tubing very fine, as for making capillary pipettes, breaking it into appropriate lengths, and melting the ends in a flame. They are inserted into all wells to ensure the removal of trapped air bubbles which may not be visible. The wells are filled and the bubbles removed best against a dark background. The slides are allowed to remain in the covered petri dishes containing moist cotton for 3 days at room temperature before examination.

E. READING THE SLIDE

The template is removed by sliding it to one side, the slide is cleaned by a momentary dip into water and examined against a dark background, holding the slide over a source of light. Lines of precipitation are identified through their coalescence with the reference line of precipitation. Enhancement of the lines of precipitation may be obtained by immersing the slide in 1% cadmium acetate for 5 to 10 minutes or by staining. Such enhancement is necessary when the reagents have been adjusted to give lines of precipitation which are only faintly visible.

F. STAINING OF SLIDES

a) The staining procedure described by Crowle[4] is used when the slide is to be preserved: Any reactant liquid remaining on the slide is rinsed away and the slide is immersed in each of the following baths for 10 minutes: distilled water, distilled water, 0.1% Thiazine-Red-R in 1.0% acetic acid, 1% acetic acid, 1% acetic acid, and 1% acetic acid, containing 1 percent glycerol. After draining excess fluid from the slide and drying in the 35°C incubator, the slide may be stored as a permanent record. Immersion in water may be required for visualization of the lines of precipitation after prolonged storage.

For simple enhancement of the lines of precipitation, the rinsed slide is immersed for a few minutes directly in the Thiazine-Red-R solution and examined.

G. RECOVERY OF SLIDES AND TEMPLATES

a) The slides are cleaned without removing the tape. They are rinsed with tap water and brushed to remove the agar gel. After washing with a washcloth using hot water containing a detergent, they are rinsed in tap water and boiled in a mild detergent for 3 to 5 minutes. They are rinsed in tap water, distilled water, and 95% ethanol and wiped dry with clean cheesecloth. (If the slides cannot be uniformly coated with hot 0.2% agar—see A c) above—–they are not sufficiently clean and must be washed again.)

b) In cleaning the plastic templates, exposure to excessive heat or plastic solvents must be avoided. (Immersion in boiling water may result in warping.)

The templates are washed with hot water containing a moderately strong detergent using a non-abrasive washcloth such as cheesecloth. After rinsing with tapwater, distilled water, and 95% ethanol, they are dried with cheesecloth. Any alcohol trapped in the wells should be tapped out. The templates, and especially the wells must be dry before laying the template on the melted agar.

Detection of Enterotoxin in Food[7]

The procedure described below and in the schematic presentation (Fig. 1) has been found to detect as little as 0.0005 ug enterotoxin A per gm of cheese. Approximately four million pounds of cheese incriminated in a food poisoning outbreak was tested by this procedure recently.[8] It was possible to find enterotoxin A in approximately 62,000 pounds of the cheese. No reports of food poisoning followed the consumption of the released cheese.

EXTRACTION OF FOOD FOR SEROLOGICAL DETECTION OF ENTEROTOXIN

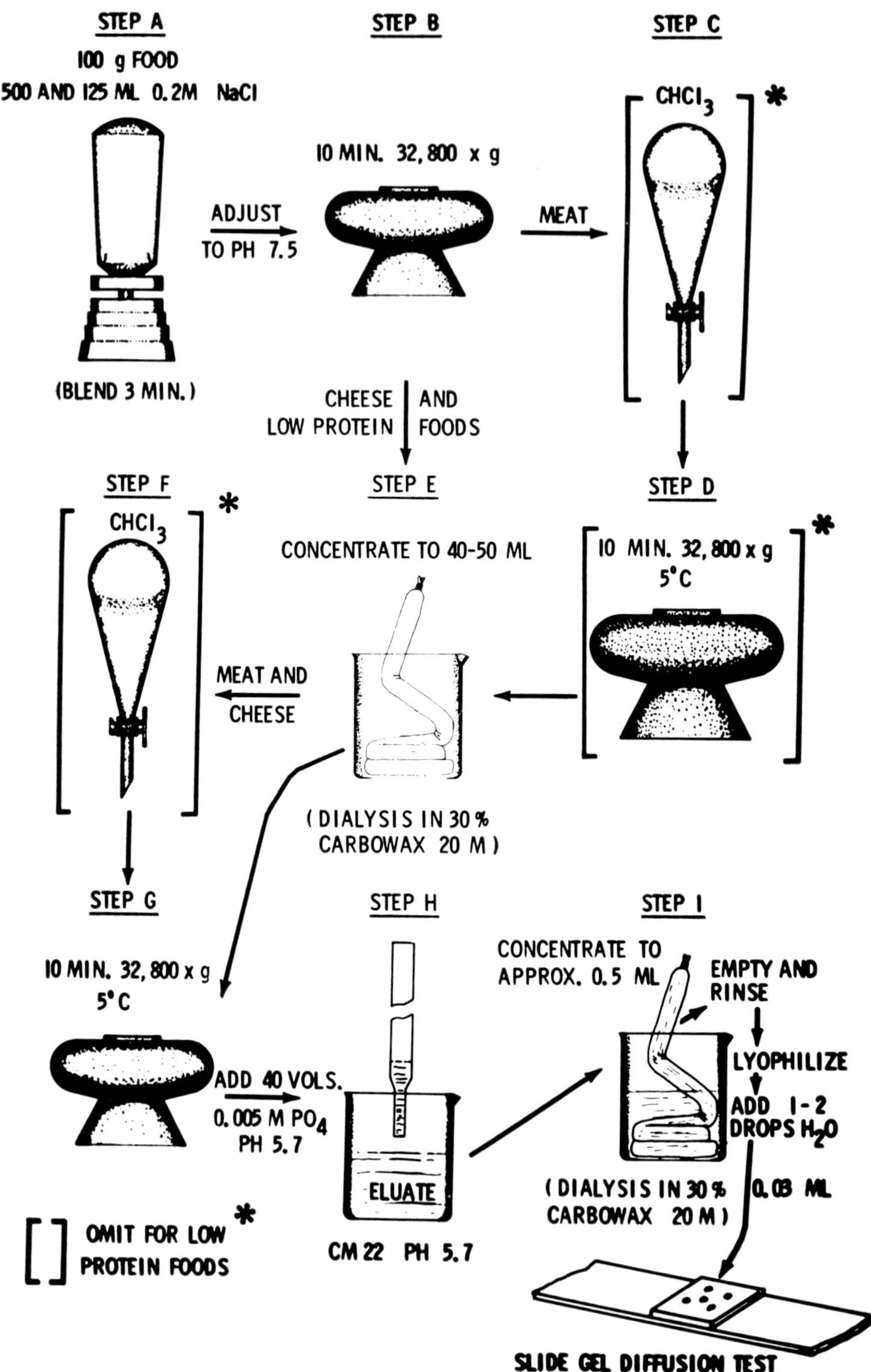

Figure 1.

The successful application of the gel-diffusion precipitation test depends on the efficiency of the procedure for extracting and separating the enterotoxin from the food prior to its specific precipitation with antibody. Two principles are employed for this purpose: selective absorption of the enterotoxin from the food extract onto ion exchangers, and selective removal of food constituents from the food extract, leaving the enterotoxin in solution. Shaking the extract with chloroform, for example, is used to remove excessive amounts of protein from extracts of meat and cheese before using the ion exchanger.

In the schematic presentation in Figure 1, brackets are used to indicate the steps which may be omitted in the examination of low-protein foods such as chicken salad and pastries. In step A, 100 gm of food is blended with 500 ml of 0.2 M NaCl at high speed for 3 minutes. The slurry is adjusted to pH 7.5 and centrifuged at 32,800 G for 10 minutes (Step B). The sediment is extracted with 125 ml of 0.2 M NaCl by blending again for 3 minutes and centrifuging for 10 minutes at 32,800 G. The two extracts are pooled; in the case of meat extracts, they are combined with $\frac{1}{4}$ volume of chloroform (Step C) in a separatory funnel and shaken vigorously 10 times through an arc of 90°. The mixture is centrifuged at 32,800 G at 5°C for 10 minutes (Step D), and the fluid layers are returned to the separatory funnel, leaving any precipitate behind. The chloroform layer is drawn off and discarded. The extract is placed in dialysis tubing and concentrated to 40 to 50 ml by immersion in 30 to 50 percent polyethyleneglycol 20,000 (PEG) (Step E). In the case of meat extracts, it is treated with chloroform a second time (Step F); with cheese, it is treated with chloroform for the first time (Step F). The extract is adjusted to pH 7.4 and centrifuged at 32,800 G for 10 minutes to remove any solids (Step G). It is diluted with 40 volumes of 0.005 M phosphate buffer of pH 5.7, adjusted to pH 5.7 with 0.005 M H_3PO_4 or 0.005 M NaOH, and allowed to percolate at approximately 5°C and at a rate of 1 to 2 ml per minute through a column of 1g of Whatman carboxymethylcellulose (CM_{22}, Reeve Angel and Co., Clifton, New Jersey) equilibrated at pH 5.7 in 100 ml of 0.005 M phosphate buffer (Step H). The column is washed with 100 ml of 0.005 M phosphate buffer, pH 5.7 and the toxin is eluted with 150 ml of 0.2 M NaCl in 0.2 M phosphate buffer, pH 7.4. The eluate is concentrated in PEG to approximately 0.5 ml (Step I). The dialysis sac is emptied of its contents and rinsed with 2.0 ml of distilled water. The washings are added to the concentrate which is then lyophilized. The lyophilized concentrate is dissolved in as little water as possible (usually 0.1 to 0.2 ml) and examined for the presence of enterotoxin by means of the slide gel double diffusion test.

REFERENCES

1. Ouchterlony, O.: Antigen antibody reactions in gels. Acta Pathol. Microbiol. Scand., *25*:507-515, 1949.
2. Ouchterlony, O.: Antigen antibody reactions in gels. IV. Types of reactions in coordinated systems of diffusion. Acta Pathol. Microbiol. Scand., *32*:231-240, 1953.
3. Wadsworth, C. A.: Slide microtechnique for the analysis of immune precipiates in gel. Intern. Arch. Allergy Appl. Immunol., *10*:355-360, 1957.
4. Crowle, A. J.: A simplified micro-double-diffusion agar precipitation technique. J. Lab. Clin. Med., *52*:784-787, 1958.

5. Casman, E. P., and Bennett, R. W.: Culture medium for the production of staphylococcal enterotoxin. A. J. Bacteriol., *86:*18-23, 1963.
6. McFarland, J.: The nephelometer. J.A.M.A., *49:* 1176-1178, 1907.
7. Casman, E. P.: Staphylococcal food poisoning. Health Lab. Science, *4:*199-206, 1967.
8. Zehren, V. L., and Zehren, V. F.: Examination of large quantities of cheese for staphylococcal enterotoxin. Amer. J. Dairy Sci., *51:*634-644, 1968.

Chapter 18

Basic Mechanisms Involved in Intoxication by Organic Phosphate Pesticides

KENNETH P. DuBOIS, PhD.

The organic phosphate insecticides constitute an important group of toxic chemical agents that are used primarily as agricultural insecticides. A few compounds of this class have sufficiently low toxicity to permit their use as household insecticides and for eradication of parasites in domestic animals.

The basic mechanism responsible for the toxicity of organic phosphate insecticides has been well established for more than twenty years as being due to inhibition of acetylcholinesterase. Research on these agents in subsequent years has dealt with the numerous factors which influence the anticholinesterase activity of these compounds. Thus the structural requirements for activity, metabolic activation, reversibility of the enzyme inhibition, and detoxification pathways have been studied in detail in recent years. As a result of the early discovery of the basic mode of action of organic phosphate insecticides and subsequent concentration on the details of their actions and metabolism in various species and under various conditions of exposure, knowledge of the toxicology of this group of compounds is essentially complete.

From a practical standpoint, acute poisoning by all of the organic phosphates results in similar characteristic signs and symptoms which are directly due to elevated acetylcholine levels in the tissues as a consequence of inhibition of the normal enzymatic disposal of acetylcholine. Intoxication by the organic phosphate insecticides always results in the occurrence of at least some symptoms referable to stimulation of structures innervated by the parasymphathetic nervous system. These muscarinic effects of acetylcholine consist of bronchoconstriction, sweating, salivation, and an increase in other glandular secretions, anorexia, nausea, abdominal cramps, vomiting, diarrhea, involuntary defecation, and increased urination. Atropine effectively counteracts these actions of acetylcholine.

The actions of organic phosphate insecticides on skeletal muscle include muscular twitching, muscular fasciculation, and weakness of skeletal muscles including the muscles of respiration. Nearly all of the organic phosphate insecticides are lipid-soluble and gain access to the cholinesterase of the central nervous system. The central effects of these agents include anxiety, restlessness, impairment of memory, speech defects, convulsions, and coma. Atropine is relatively ineffective in counteracting the skeletal muscle and central nervous system effects of these compounds.

From a qualitative standpoint, the signs and symptoms produced by different organic phosphate insecticides in various mammalian species are essentially the same. However, there are appreciable quantitative differences between most of the individual compounds. Thus, the doses of various compounds required to elicit toxic effects differ considerably due to differences in the inherent anticholinesterase activity of the compounds and to differences in rate of metabolism. The time of onset and duration of effects differ from one compound to another. Many of these quantitative differences between organic phosphate insecticides are now explainable on the basis of biochemical reactions which govern the anticholinesterase activity and the fate of organic phosphates in mammalian tissues. It is the purpose of this communication to briefly describe the biochemical reactions which determine the toxicity of organic phosphate insecticides.

Inhibition of Cholinesterase by Organic Phosphate Insecticides

The reaction of greatest importance in in connection with the toxicity of organic phosphate insecticides is the combination of these compounds with the active catalytic site of the cholinesterase molecule. The earliest studies on the mode of action of insecticidal organic phosphates were done in our laboratory in 1947 (4) on a compound called hexaethyl tetraphosphate which had been developed in Germany during World War II as a substitute for nicotine. This compound underwent rapid hydrolysis in aqueous media to yield a potent inhibitor of cholinesterase. Tetraethyl pyrophosphate was considered as the possible active hydrolysis product, and was found (10) to be a strong inhibitor of cholinesterase *in vitro* and *in vivo*. This finding provided the initial demonstration that alkyl-substituted derivatives of pyrophosphoric acid react directly with cholinesterase to inhibit this enzyme. About the same time, it became known that a sulfur-containing organic phosphate with good insecticidal activity, known as parathion, was among the most active insecticidal organic phosphates developed in Germany during World War II. The early work on the mode of action of parathion, which was done in our laboratory in 1949 (5), indicated that it was an inhibitor of cholinesterase *in vitro* and *in vivo*. However as more phosphorothioates related to parathion were studied it became apparent that there was not always a close correlation between their *in vitro* anticholinesterase activity and their toxicity. In 1951, Diggle and Gage (3), followed shortly by other groups (9, 11, 13, 16), presented evidence that highly purified cholinergic phosphorothioates have no anticholinesterase activity *in vitro* but are metabolized to anticholinesterase agents *in vivo*. This activation reaction involves replacement of the sulfur by oxygen through an oxidative mechanism described below to yield the corresponding oxygen analogues which are the actual inhibitors of cholinesterase. Figure 1 shows the chemical structures of parathion and its active metabolite, paraoxon. Included are the structures of a few important phosphorothioate insecticides and their active metabolites which are the actual insecticidal compounds.

The organic phosphates inhibit cholinesterase by reacting with the site in the enzyme molecule with which the ester linkage of acetylcholine normally combines. This is called the esteratic site of the enzyme. In the reaction between the organic phosphate insecticide and cholinesterase, one of the ester groups leaves the molecule and a dialkyl or diaryl derivative of phosphoric acid becomes attached to a serine molecule of the enzyme (1). It is probable that histidine is first phosphorylated and that transphosphorylation to serine then occurs. Through phosphorylation of the active site of the enzyme the normal hydrolysis of acetylcholine is prevented.

With few exceptions, the cholinesterase activity is inhibited very soon after exposure to acutely toxic doses of organic phosphate insecticides regardless of whether or not they have to undergo metabolic activation. Rapid absorption occurs by all routes and maximal enzyme inhibition generally occurs within six hours after exposure. The duration of

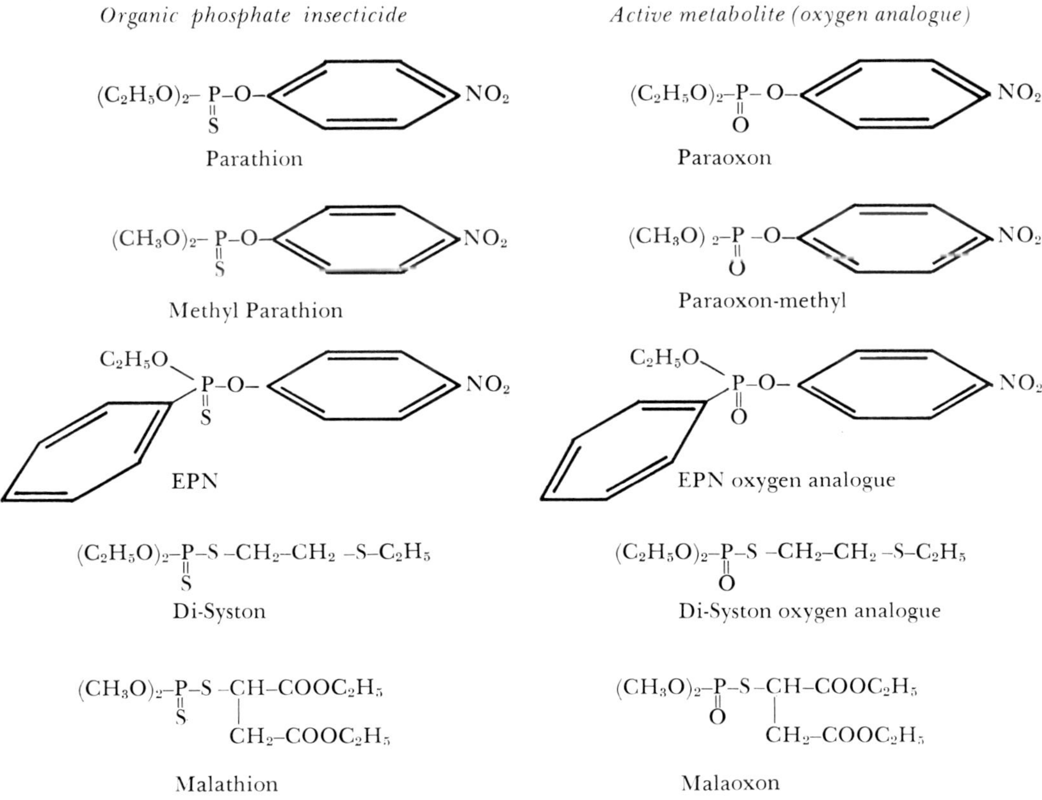

Figure 1. Chemical structures of some organic phosphate insecticides and their oxygen analogues.

inhibition of cholinesterase after exposure to single doses of the organic phosphate insecticides is generally relatively short. Table 1 presents a few examples of the time required for complete reversal of the inhibition of cholinesterase after administration of equivalent fractions (5/8) of the LD_{50} of each compound. The fact that reversal of the inhibition occurs within a few days is an important factor with respect to the length of time that administration of antidotal drugs is necessary in the treatment of accidental poisoning.

TABLE 1: ONSET AND DURATION OF THE ANTICHOLINESTERASE ACTION OF SOME ORGANIC PHOSPHATE PESTICIDES

Organic Phosphate	*Dose*[a] *(mg/kg)*	*Time for Maximum Inhibition of Brain Cholinesterase (Hr.)*	*Time for Complete Reversal of Inhibition (Hr.)*
Di-Syston	1.25	3.0	120
Guthion	3.5	0.5	24
Dylox	140.0	0.25	6
Octamethyl pyrophosphoramide	5.0	2.0	144

[a] All doses represent 5/8 of the acute LD_{50} for female rats.

The rate of regeneration of active cholinesterase after organic phosphate poisoning can be hastened markedly by administration of nucleophilic reagents such as 2-PAM (pyridine-2-aldoxime methiodide). Dephosphorylation of the inhibited enzyme by this mechanism occurs most readily if the nucleophilic reagent is given soon after poisoning. Otherwise, the phosphorylated enzyme gradually undergoes hydrolysis of one of the two esters on the phosphorus atom yielding a monoester which is not removed from the enzyme by 2-PAM.

Inhibition of Aliesterases by Organic Phosphates

It seems worthy of emphasis that the organic phosphates are not specific inhibitors of cholinesterase. They also have the ability to inhibit the non-specific esterases in the liver and serum that are collectively referred to as aliesterases. Since the aliesterases do not have a vital role in normal metabolism, little attention has been given to the fact that these enzymes are more susceptible to inhibition by organic phosphates than cholinesterase. However, in recent years it has become evident that the aliesterases have an important function in the detoxification of ester-type drugs, pesticides, and other chemicals. Inhibition of these enzymes could thus be responsible for potentiation of the toxicity of certain drugs and other chemical agents.

The importance of aliesterase inhibition as a cause of potentiation of toxicity was first recognized in connection with the discovery by Frawley *et al.* (8) that an organic phosphate insecticide, EPN, when given simultaneously with malathion, potentiates the toxicity of the latter compound. The mechanism responsible for this potentiation of toxicity was explained by Murphy and DuBois (14) and Cook *et al.* (2) on the basis that EPN inhibits the aliesterase that catalyzes the rapid detoxification of malathion. More recently, DuBois, Kinoshita, and Frawley (6) conducted a detailed study of the inhibitory action of two organic phosphates, EPN and Delnav, on the aliesterases that hydrolyze diethylsuccinate and tributyrin and the amidase that hydrolyzes acetanilid. Enzyme assays conducted at intervals during a 13-week feeding period demonstrated that all of these esterases were inhibited at dietary levels of the organic phosphates that produce no inhibition of cholinesterase. Thus it seems advisable to consider the inhibitory action of each organic phosphate insecticide on aliesterases in establishing the permitted levels in food as a precaution against potentiation of the toxicity of drugs and other chemicals to which exposure may occur. It should be emphasized that during the recovery period following acute intoxication by organic phosphate insecticides, patients would be expected to be unable to detoxify ester-type drugs at the normal rate and may, therefore, exhibit a marked increase in susceptibility to the toxic effects of some drugs.

Mechanism of the Metabolic Activation of Organic Phosphate Insecticides

The mechanism by which the phosphorothioate insecticides such as parathion, malathion, Systox, Delnav, Guthion, and several others are converted to active anthicholinesterase agents *in vivo* is now well understood. The activation occurs in the liver and consists of the oxidative replacement of sulfur by oxygen. This reaction is catalyzed by an enzyme located in the endoplasmic reticulum or microsome fraction of the liver. Like other microsomal drug metabolizing enzyme systems the desulfuration of phosphorothioates requires reduced triphosphopyridine nucleotide for activity. The conversion of phosphorothioates to their active oxygen analogues may be represented as follows:

$$(R_1O)(R_2O)P(=S)-OR_3 + TPNH + O_2 \xrightarrow[\text{microsomal}]{\text{oxidase}} (R_1O)(R_2O)P(=O)-OR_3 + TPN$$

Studies on factors influencing the rate of conversion of phosphorothioates to their oxygen analogues have demonstrated (15) that this microsomal reaction is subject to the same type of changes in activity as other microsomal drug metabolizing enzymes. Thus, induction of desulfurase can be produced by pretreatment of animals with phenobarbital, methlycholanthrene and other agents known to increase the level of microsomal enzymes. However, stimulation of the activity of the phosphorothioate system does not increase the toxicity of phosphorothioates. One reason is that the desulfurase activity of the liver is normally high enough to convert the phosphorothioates to their oxygen analogues at an extremely rapid rate. Another reason for the failure of increases in desulfurase activity to increase the toxicity is that the detoxification of many organic phosphates is also increased by enzyme inducing agents as indicated below.

Detoxification of Organic Phosphate Insecticides

The detoxification of organic phosphate insecticides has generally been attributed to enzymatic hydrolysis. The oxygen analogues of phosphorothioates such as parathion are hydrolyzed by esterases, and phosphatases specific for various compounds have been identified (12). A carboxyesterase catalyzes the detoxification of malathion and the rapidity of this reaction accounts for the low toxicity of malathion to mammals. It is generally agreed that the organic phosphates which have a direct inhibitory action on cholinesterase, including the oxygen analogues of phosphorothioates, are detoxified by hydrolysis. However, in 1964, Neal and DuBois (17) investigated the mechanism of detoxification of parathion, EPN, and other phosphorothioates. They found that these compounds are detoxified by a microsomal oxidase system. The rate of oxidation to inactive metabolites was much more rapid than hydrolysis. Sex and age differences in susceptibility to parathion and related compounds correlated closely with the rate of microsomal oxidative detoxification. Thus, the greater resistance of male rats as compared with females or with weanling animals of either sex is explainable on the basis of greater activity of the microsomal oxidase detoxification system in the livers of adult male rats. The rate of microsomal detoxification of organic phosphate insecticides is extremely important in governing the toxicity of these compounds. This fact was clearly demonstrated in a recent study by DuBois and Kinoshita (7) in which the toxicity of the important insecticides of the phosphorothioate type was measured in rats pretreated with phenobarbital to induce microsomal enzyme activity. The toxicity of several of the most important insecticides of this class including parathion, Di-Syston, Delnav, EPN, and Ethion was markedly decreased in the phenobarbital-treated animals.

Summary

The basic mechanism responsible for the toxicity of organic phosphate insecticides is the inhibition of acetylcholinesterase of the nervous system with the consequent accumulation of excessive levels of acetylcholine. The organic phosphates readily gain access to the central and peripheral nervous systems and thus produce the nicotinic and muscarinic effects of acetylcholine.

The muscarinic effects are effectively antidoted by atropine. Some organic phosphate insecticides are direct inhibitors of cholinesterase but most of those which are commonly used as insecticides are phosphorothioates, such as parathion, which must be converted to their oxygen analogues in order to inhibit the enzyme. This activation is catalyzed by a desulfuase located in the microsomal fraction of the liver. The toxicity of all phosphorothioates is thus dependent upon the activity of this microsomal enzyme system. Cholinesterase inhibition by organic phosphates involves phosphorylation of the active catalytic center of the enzyme. This is a reversible reaction for the compounds used as insecticides and the reversal can be hastened by nucleophilic agents such as pyridine-2-aldoxime methiodide (2-PAM).

The organic phosphates are not specific for cholinesterase. They also inhibit many other esterases some of which are more susceptible than cholinesterase. The inhibition of aliesterases is not involved in the toxic manifestations of the organic phosphates. However, since other pesticides and some drugs are detoxified by aliesterases, the organic phosphates are capable of potentiating the toxicity of these other substances through inhibition of their normal detoxification. An important example of this type of potentiation is seen in the ability of EPN to potentiate the toxicity of malathion through inhibition of the carboxyesterases that normally detoxify this compound.

The detoxification of organic phosphates involves two enzymatic mechanisms. The pyrophosphates and oxygen analogues of phosphorothioates are detoxified by hydrolysis while the phosphorothioates are detoxified by a microsomal oxidase system. The latter mechanism is the most important because alteration of the activity of microsomal enzymes by inducing agents such as phenobarbital decreases the toxicity of the phosphorothioates.

It is concluded that the toxicity of organic phosphate insecticides is dependent upon the following three enzymatic processes: (a) activation to form the oxygen analogues when the insecticide is a phosphorothioate, (b) reaction of the organic phosphate with cholinesterase resulting in phosphorylation of the esteratic site of the enzyme molecule, and (c) detoxification by hydrolysis or by a microsomal oxidase system.

REFERENCES

1. Cohen, J. A., Oosterbaan, R. A., Jansz, J. S., and Berends, F.: The active site of esterases. J. Cellular Comp. Physiol., *54:*Suppl. 1, 231-244, 1959.
2. Cook, J. W., Blake, J. R., Yip, G., and Williams, M.: Malathionase. I. Activity and inhibition. J. Offic. Agr. Chemists, *41:*399-411, 1958.
3. Diggle, W. M., and Gage, J. C.: Cholinesterase inhibition *in vivo* by O,O-diethyl O-p-nitrophenyl thiophosphate (Parathion, E 605). Biochem. J., *49:*491-494, 1951.
4. DuBois, K. P., and Mangun, G. H.: Effect of hexaethyl tetraphosphate on choline esterase *in vitro* and *in vivo*. Proc. Soc. Exper. Biol. & Med., *64:*137-139, 1947.
5. DuBois, K. P., Doull, J., Salerno, P. R., and Coon, J. M.: Studies on the toxicity and mechanism of action of p-nitrophenyl diethyl thionophosphate (Parathion). J. Pharmacol. Exp. Therapy., *95:*79-91, 1949.
6. DuBois, K. P., Kinoshita, F. K., and Frawley, J. P.: Quantitative measurement of inhibition of aliesterases, acylamidase, and cholinesterase by EPN and Delnav. Toxicol. and Appl. Pharmacol., *12:*273-284, 1968.
7. DuBois, K. P., and Kinoshita, F. K.: Influence of induction of hepatic microsomal enzymes by phenobarbital on toxicity of organic phosphate insecticides. Proc. Soc. Exp. Biol. and Med. *129:*699-702, 1968.
8. Frawley, J. P., Fuyat, H. N., Hagan, E. C., Blake, J. R., and Fitzhugh, O. E.: Marked potentiation in mammalian toxicity from simultaneous administration of two anticholinesterase compounds. J. Pharmacol. Exper. Therap., *121:* 96-106, 1957.
9. Gage, J. C.: A cholinesterase inhibitor derived from O,O-diethyl O-p-nitrophenyl thiophosphate *in vivo*. Biochem. J., *54:*426-430, 1953.
10. Mangun, G. H., and DuBois, K. P.: Toxicity and mechanism of action of tetraethyl pyrophosphate. Fed. Proc., *6:*353, 1947.
11. Metcalf, R. L., and March, R. B.: Reversed-phase paper chromatography of Parathion and related phosphate esters. Science, *117:*527-528, 1953.
12. Mounter, L. A.: Metabolism of organophosphorus anticholinesterase agents. In Handbuch der experimentellen Pharmakologie, Cholinesterases and Anticholinesterase Agents. Ed., George B. Koelle. Springer-Verlag Pub., 1963, pp. 486-504.
13. Murphy, S. D., and DuBois, K. P.: Enzymatic conversion of the dimethoxy ester of benzotriazine dithiophosphoric acid to an anticholinesterase agent. J. Pharmacol. & Exper. Therap., *119:*572-583, 1957.

14. Murphy, S. D., and DuBois, K. P.: Quantitative measurement of inhibition of the enzymatic detoxification of malthion by EPN (ethyl p-nitrophenyl thionobenzenephosphonate). Proc. Soc. Exp. Biol. & Med., *96*:813-818, 1957.
15. Murphy, S. D., and DuBois, K. P.: The influence of various factors on the enzymatic conversion of organic thiophosphates to anticholinesterase agents. J. Pharmacol. & Exper. Therap., *124*: 194-202, 1958.
16. Myers, D. K., Mendel, B., Gersmann, H. R., and Ketelaar, J. A. A.: Oxidation of thiophosphate insecticides in the rat. Nature. *170*:805-807, 1953.
17. Neal, R. A., and DuBois, K. P.: Studies on the mechanism of detoxification of cholinergic phosphorothioates. J. Pharmacol. & Exper. Therap., *148*:185-192, 1964.

Chapter 19A

Detection of Cholinesterase Inhibition

J. DE LA HUERGA, M.D., E. A. PETRUS, M.D. and
J. C. SHERRICK, M.D.

A. The Significance of Cholinesterase Measurements

INTRODUCTION

The widespread agricultural use of the cholinesterase inhibitors as insecticides has made the measurement of cholinesterase in the blood a common and important laboratory determination.

The late Sir Henry Dale (15), discoverer of acetylcholine, postulated that an esterase hydrolyzing acetylcholine must exist to account for the rapid disappearance of acetylcholine from biological systems. In 1926, Loewi and Navratil (30) found such an enzyme in tissue extracts, and in the same year Plattner (39) demonstrated it in the blood. The name "choline esterase" was applied by Stedman, Stedman and Easson (42) (1932), who purified the enzyme from horse plasma.

During the 1940's, work by two groups of investigators (6, 32) showed that the cholinesterase activity of blood was due to the presence of two different enzymes, one in the serum and the other in the erythrocyte. Due to the work of a large number of investigators, these enzymes are now well characterized. The biochemical differences between them are summarized in Table I, which is slightly modified from Augustinsson (10).

In the remainder of this chapter serum cholinesterase will be referred to as SCE and to erythrocyte cholinesterase as ECE.

Mode of Action of Cholinesterases

Various investigators have clarified the mode of action of the cholinesterases (8, 9, 12, 45, 47). Most of the work has been carried out in practically pure preparations of acetylcholinesterase obtained from the electric organ of the electric eel. The molecular weight is about 12 million, and the molecule has on its surface various enzymatic centers (28), each composed of two different sites (8, 45). One has a negative charge, the "anionic site," which binds the positively charged nitrogen of the choline moiety of acetylcholine. The other site is located about 5 angstroms away and is referred to as the "esteratic site." It con-

TABLE I: PROPERTIES OF CHOLINESTERASES

	Group 1	*Group 2*
Nomenclature	Acetylcholinehydrolase 3.1.1.7 Acetylcholinesterase True cholinesterase e (for erythrocyte) Cholinesterase — ECE	Acylcholine acyl-hydrolase 3.1.1.8 Pseudocholinesterase Non-specific cholinesterase s (for serum) Cholinesterase — SCE
Distribution in mammals	Gray matter of nervous system Erythrocytes Motor end plates	Plasma Liver and other organs White matter of nervous system
Substrate specificity	Better for acetyl esters Acetyl-β-methylcholine is hydrolyzed	Butyryl and propionyl esters are hydrolyzed beter than the acetyl esters. Acetyl-β-methylcholine *not* hydrolyzed
Substrate concentration	Optimum at about 0.005 M. Inhibited by higher concentrations	Maximum at about 0.05 M. or higher concentrations
Optimum pH	From about 7.2-8.2	From 7.4-8.5
Molecular weight	About 12×10^6	About 750,000

sits of an acidic group (H) and a basic group (G) (Fig. 1-1). When the enzyme is combined with the substrate, there is a tight fit between the substrate and the enzymatic centers (Fig. 1-2). This combination between the substrate and the enzyme, also referred to as the Michaelis complex, is reversible. How-

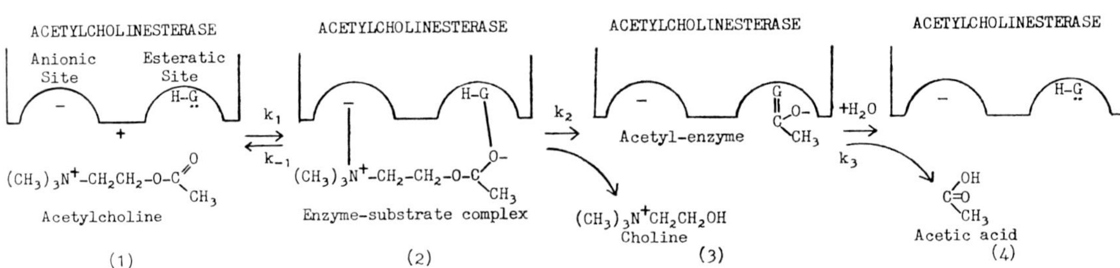

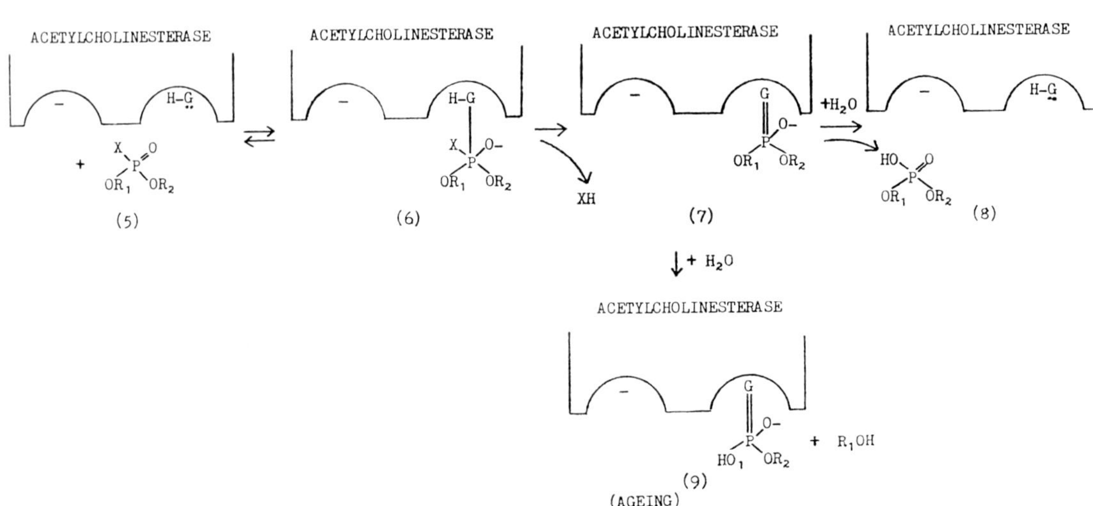

Figure 1. Acetylcholinesterase — Mode of action

ever, the reaction rapidly proceeds to the next step (Fig. 1-3) by which choline is liberated and the acetyl group of the substrate remains attached to the basic group of the esteratic site. This reaction is not reversible. The latter complex is unstable, and is quickly hydrolyzed, thus forming acetic acid and free enzyme, which is available to start a new cycle (Fig. 1-4). Non-choline esters are hydrolyzed by acetylcholinesterase, but at a slower rate. Moreover, other organic esters of choline are also hydrolyzed at a slow rate. These facts indicate that there is not an absolute "true" acetylcholinesterase (9, 10, 28).

In addition to the attachment of substrate to enzyme by the coulombic effects described above, the methyl and methylene groups of the substrate are attracted to the enzyme by van der Waals's dispersion forces (11).

One of the peculiarities of this type of acetylcholinesterase is that the enzyme hydrolyzes the substrate at an optimal concentration of about 0.005 molar (6, 8, 27). The activity decreases with lower or higher substrate concentrations. In the latter case, the excess of substrate may be bound to the free anionic site in reaction 3 (Fig. 1-3), thus acting as an inhibitor by interfering with the next reaction.

The mode of action of serum cholinesterase is different. The presence of the anionic site has been denied. There is no excess substrate inhibition and, as shown in Table I, the enzyme acts on propyl and butyl esters of choline at a higher rate than on acetylcholine (27).

Because of similarity of binding of the acyl esters of choline to that of some of the inhibitors, it is assumed that some of the serine groups in the esteratic site of the enzyme are acylated.

Cholinesterase Inhibitors

Two types of cholinesterase inhibitors will be discussed, the phosphorus esters and the carbamate esters.

Secret investigations in England and Germany shortly before and during World War II showed that the phosphorus esters of organophosphates were poisonous for mammals, and they were investigated for possible use as nerve gases. The German investigators foresaw their uses as insecticides, and at the end of the war large amounts were made for this purpose. Since then they have come into wide use in all agricultural countries.

Animal and human experimentation have shown that the action of the phosphorus esters was similar to that of the well known drug, physostigmine, which acts as a cholinesterase inhibitor, and that the phosphorus esters were even more potent inhibitors. This work was carried out in England in 1941 by Adrian, Feldberg and Kilby (1), but because of its military importance at the time, the reports were kept secret until after the war. Since, then, an intensive amount of work by many groups of investigators has been undertaken to elucidate the action of these inhibitors. The books of Heath (23) and O'Brien (36, 37) are recommended reading for those interested in this subject.

Thousands of phosphorus esters have been synthesized in an effort to find compounds with low toxicity to mammals and high toxicity to insects. The success that has been achieved in this regard is exemplified by such esters as Coral and Ronnel, which may safely be administered to infested mammals without producing toxic effects but which kill worms, mites and ticks.

Orthophosphoric acid has three hydroxyl groups that may be esterified by organic alcohols or phenols, and in some cases one of the hydroxyl groups may also be substituted by an element or by a non-ester radical (phosphonic acid esters). In addition, two molecules of phosphoric acid may combine with loss of one molecule of water to form pyrophosphoric acid which has four esterifiable groups. Table II shows the substitutions that may take place, and one example of each type of derivative.

Mode of Action

The mode of action of the phosphorus esters will be discussed briefly in this chapter. For more extensive discussion, the reader is referred to Chapter 17.

Phosphorus esters are extremely potent cholinesterase inhibitors, some of them at a 10^{-10} molar concentration, by virtue of their binding to the esteratic sites in a manner similar to acetylcholine. The reactions that take place are shown in Figure 1. Reaction 5 and Reaction 6 are similar to Reactions 1 and 2, and are considered to be reversible. However, the reaction proceeds very rapidly to Reaction 7 which is irreversible. The group designated as X in Figure 1-6 represents the fluoride atom of DFP (di-isopropylphosphorofluoride) or one of the esters of the other compounds. These groups are referred to as the "leaving group." Once Reaction 7 has taken place, Reaction 8 is extremely slow, contrary to similar Reaction 3 and the enzyme remains inhibited until the remainder of the organic phosphate group leaves. This may take place in hours or months, so that the phosphorus esters have been considered to be irreversible inhibitors of cholinesterase. The materials liberated in Reaction 8 are monohydrogen diesters of phosphoric acid, which are not inhibitory.

When the enzyme and inhibitor are left standing, some regeneration of the enzyme occurs due to the nucleophilic OH group of water and some of the enzyme REACTIVATES. By adding more potent nucleophilic reagents, pertaining to the hydroxamic acid or oxime reagent (44), such as PAM (pyridine-2-aldoxime methiodate), or 1,2-bis (N-pyridinium-4-aldoxime) propane, or nicotinhydroxamic acid methiodide, the reactivation time can be speeded up to a few minutes or hours. This is INDUCTIVE REACTIVATION. These drugs are being currently used in the treatment of phosphorus ester intoxication.

However, if the enzyme and phosphorus ester are allowed to remain in contact for a longer time, this reactivation is significantly slowed or does not take place. This phenomenon has been referred to as AGING (25). It has been shown that aging is due to the liberation of one of the two esters still bound to the phosphorus atom in Reaction 7, forming a monoester of phosphoric acid-enzyme complex (Figs. 1-9) that is not susceptible to the hydrolysis induced by the nucleophilic agents (26).

Once it became apparent that there was phosphorylization of the enzyme by the phosphorus ester derivatives, studies performed on the enzyme inhibitory complex by using P^{32}-labelled-DFP, then

Table II: Phosphorus Esters with Anticholinesterase Action

Class	Compound	Structure
Phosphate triesters	Paraoxon	C_2H_5O, O, P, C_2H_5O, $OC_6H_4\text{–}4\text{–}NO_2$
Phosphonate diesters	Diisopropyl phosphoro Fluoridate DFP	$\begin{matrix}CH_3\\CH_3\end{matrix}\!>\!\overset{H}{C}O$, O, P, $\begin{matrix}CH_3\\CH_3\end{matrix}\!>\!\overset{H}{C}O$, F
Phosphoroamidate	Ruelene	$CH_3\text{—}O$, O, P, $CH_3\text{—}N(H)$, O, [benzene ring], $C(CH_3)_3$, Cl
Phosphorothionate	Parathion	C_2H_5O, S, P, C_2H_5O, $OC_6H_4\text{–}4\text{–}NO_2$
Phosphorothiolate	Demeton-s	C_2H_5O, O, P, C_2H_5O, $S(CH_2)_2SC_2H_5$
Phosphorodithioate	Malathion	CH_3O, S, P, CH_3O, SCH, $COOC_2H_5$, $CH_2COOC_2H_5$
Pyrophosphate	TEPP	C_2H_5O, O, P—O—P, O, OC_2H_5, C_2H_5O, OC_2H_5

degrading the complex, showed that the P^{32} was bound to serine (13). However, the dissociation constant of serine is such that it is not particularly subject to phosphorylization, while histidine is much more suitable in this regard. Present interpretation of this situation is that histidine is actually first phosphorylated, and that it then passes on the phosphorus to serine by a transphosphorylization reaction. Using horse SCE, the peptide in which the phosphorus is present has been shown to be: phenylalanine-glycine-glutamic acid-phosphorylated serine-alanine-glycine, in this order (13).

The phosphorus esters differ from one another in their inhibition of cholinesterase, and their action is quantitatively different on the different cholinesterases. Moreover, some esters like parathion show a rather weak anticholinesterase activity in vitro. But when administered to animals, they become more potent (ACTIVATION). It has been shown that activation occurs in the liver (18). For instance, parathion (Table II), a weak cholinesterase inhibitor, is converted in the liver to the more potent paraoxon by an oxidative desulfuration. This is a typical example of what has been called "lethal synthesis" by Sir Rudolph Peters (38).

The organic phosphorus esters are themselves substrates for various enzymes. For example, the group of A-esterases of Aldridge (4) can hydrolyze these esters rendering them non-inhibitors of cholinesterase. Phosphatases which are specific for individual esters have been identified; examples are DFPase, Tabunase, Sarinase, etc. (34) These enzymes are of importance in the detoxification of the phosphorus esters. Other types of non-cholinesterases such as Aldridge's B-esterases (3) are also inhibited by the phosphorus esters. In addition, the esterolytic properties of chymotrypsin, trypsin and thrombin are inhibited. These later reactions may diminish somewhat the action of these inhibitors towards cholinesterases.

The Carbamate Esters

Carbamic acid $NH^2\text{-}C\begin{matrix}/\!\!/O \\ \backslash OH\end{matrix}$ forms esters that have potent anticholinesterase action. The best known are physiostigmine and prostigmine, both of which have therapeutic use in clinical medicine. Because these substances are ionized, they cannot penetrate the central nervous systems of insects, and are thus not insecticidal. By synthesizing N-dimethyl derivatives, Swiss investigators were able to produce in 1947 compounds which did not ionize, would penetrate the lipid barriers of the central nervous system, and were potent insecticides. Later on, even more potent derivatives were synthesized. In Table III are examples of the carbamate esters with anticholinesterase activity.

The mode of action on cholinesterase is similar to that of acetylcholine and phosphorus esters. The binding of the carbamate inhibitor is not as firm as that of phosphorus esters, for their action is for the most part reversible, so that the inhibition may be reversed by dialysis or by diluting the enzyme-inhibitor complexes. The actual combinations have been elucidated by Wilson, Hatch and Ginsberg (48) who demonstrated that there is carbamylation of the enzyme similar to acetylation or phosphorylization.

Methods of Determination

Various technics are available for the determination of the cholinesterases. The acid liberated can be used as a measure of the activity of the enzyme. By using a bicarbonate buffer, the acid produced by the enzymatic activity will liberate carbon dioxide, which can be measured in the Warburg apparatus (7). Us-

TABLE III: CARBAMIC ACID DERIVATIVES WITH ANTICHOLINESTERASE ACTION

Ionized, Therapeutic (non-insecticidal)	Physostigmine	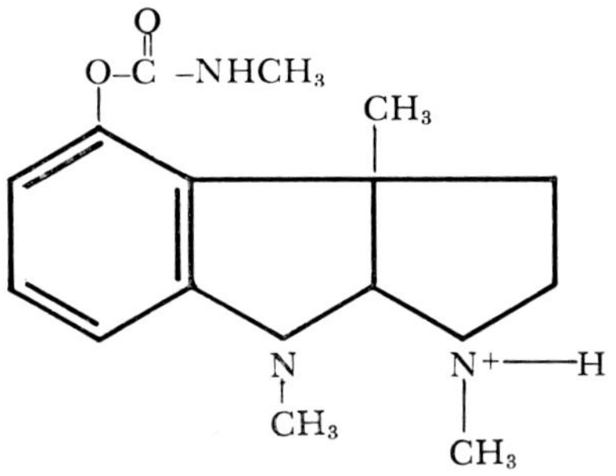 O–C(=O)–NHCH₃; CH₃; N–CH₃; N+—H, CH₃
Heterocyclic N-dimethyl	Isolan	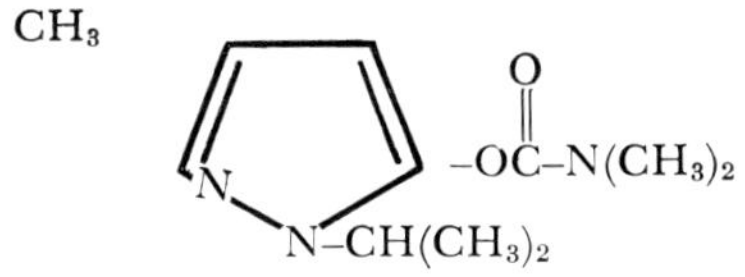 CH₃; N; –OC(=O)–N(CH₃)₂; N–CH(CH₃)₂
Naphtholic N-Monomethyl	Carbaryl	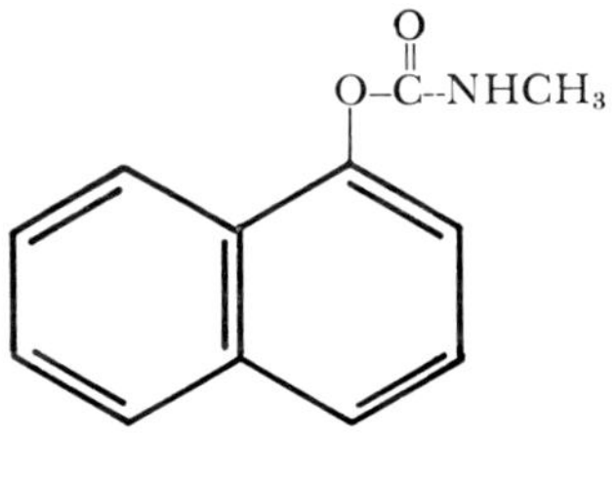 O–C(=O)–NHCH₃
Phenolic N-Monomethyl	Mesurol	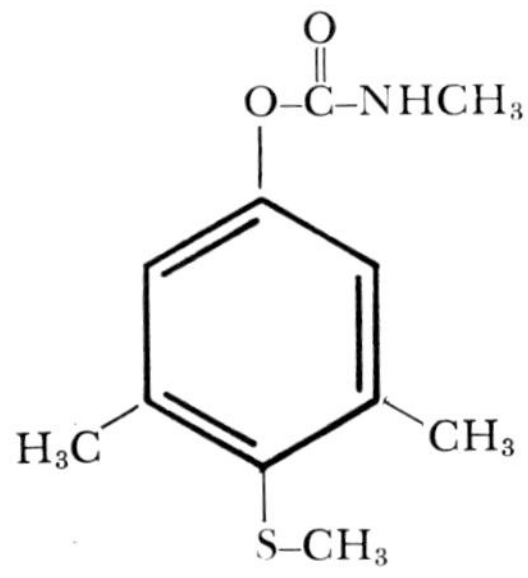 O–C(=O)–NHCH₃; H₃C; CH₃; S–CH₃
Aliphatic Oxime	21149 (Union Carbide)	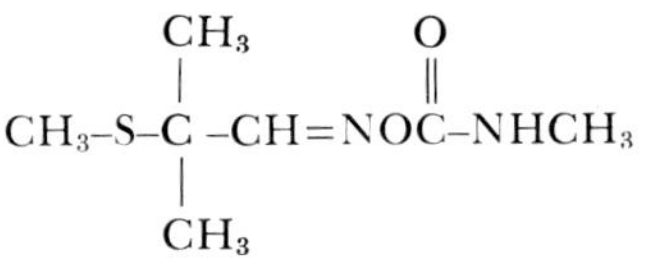 CH_3–S–C(CH_3)(CH_3)–CH=NOC(=O)–NHCH₃

ing dilute buffers, the increase of acidity can be measured by a pH meter (33) or by using acid-base color indicators (41), or better yet, by continuous titration. Use may be made of the fact that benzoylcholine absorbs light at 240 millimicrons, while the hydrolytic products do not. Similarly, another spectrophotometric method has been proposed using O-nitrophenylbutyrate (31), which is colorless, but after enzymatic action, the liberated O-nitrophenol is strongly yellow and absorbs light at about 410 mmc. Some of these methods cannot be applied to ECE because of the high color produced by hemoglobin. Colorimetric methods adapted to the clinical laboratory are also available. Ravin, Tsu and Seligman (40), used carbonaphthoxycholine as substrate. The liberated acyl group is decarboxylated and the napthol thus formed is treated with tetrazotized diorthoanisidine. Hestrin (24) suggested the use of the hydroxamic acid reaction for organic esters. This principle was used in the development of a method by the senior author in 1952 (17), which has been in routine use in our laboratories since that time. For determination of ECE, the method has been modified by including a protein precipitation step and altering the substrate concentration to an optimal level.

Principle

Esters of organic acids like acetylcholine react with alkaline hydroxylamine to form hydroxamates which upon the addition of ferric solutions produce a brown color. The reaction is as follows:

$$CH_3\overset{\overset{O}{\|}}{C}\text{-O-}(CH_2)_2\text{-}N^+(CH_3)_3 + NH_2OH \rightarrow CH_3\overset{\overset{O}{\|}}{C}\text{-NHOH} + CH_2OHCH_2\text{-}N^+(CH_3)_3$$

$$CH_3\overset{\overset{O}{\|}}{C}NHOH + 1/3\,Fe^{3+} \rightarrow CH_3\text{-}\overset{\overset{O\text{---}1/3\,Fe}{\|\quad\diagup}}{C\text{——}NHO}$$

Buffered acetylcholine is added to serum or hemolysate and to a control. After incubation, the difference in color between the control and the sample is a measure of the cholinesterase activity of the sample.

Reagents

1. *Buffer solution.* 18 gm of trishydroxymethylaminomethane (Tris, Tham) are dissolved in about 400 ml of distilled water and 2N hydrochloric acid is added to bring the pH to 8.2. More distilled water is added to make a final volume of 500 ml. This solution keeps well in the refrigerator.

2. *Salt solution.* 4.5 gm. of soduim chloride, 4 gm of magnesium chloride exahydrated, and 0.1 gm of potassium chloride are dissolved in distilled water and the volume made to 100 ml.

3. *Substrate reagent.* 5.7 gm of acetylcholine bromide are dissolved in distilled water, and the volume made to 100 ml. This reagent keeps well when frozen.

4. *Hydroxylamine hydrochloride reagent.* 17% (w/v) aqueous solution. This solution keeps well in the refrigerator.

5. *Sodium hyroxide.* 17% (w/v), aqueous.

6. *Saponin,* 0.01% solution. Aqueous. Keeps well frozen.

7. *Hydrochloric acid solution, 6%.* 30 ml of concentrated hydrochloric acid is made to a volume of 500 ml with distilled water.

8. *Trichloracetic acid solution, 7%.* (w/v) aqueous.

9. *Ferric chloride reagent (ECE).* 7.5 gm of ferric chloride hexahydrate are dissolved in 0.05N hydrochloric acid to make a final volume of 500 ml. This reagent keeps well at room temperature.

10. *Ferric chloride reagent (SCE).* One volume of reagent 9 is diluted with one volume of water. This reagent keeps well at room temperature.

Instrumentation

These methods have been devised for the Coleman Spectrophotometers, and for the Bausch and Lomb Spectronic 20, using the 19 mm cuvettes. Other instruments may be used by modifying the amount of hydrochloric acid and trichloracetic acid to provide readings in the control between 18 and 25% T.

A. SERUM CHOLINESTERASE (SCE) PROCEDURE:

1. Just before starting, two volumes of buffer solution (Reagent 1), one volume of salt solution (Reagent 2), and one volume of substrate (Reagent 3) are mixed and placed in a water bath at 37°C.

2. To test tubes of 18 x 150 mm are transferred the following:

first tube	0.5 ml of distilled water (control)
second tube	0.2 ml of serum
	0.3 ml of water
third tube	0.5 ml of serum

The tubes are placed in the water bath.

3. To all tubes, exactly 2.0 ml of the buffer salt substrate mixture from Step 1 are added. The contents are mixed, and the tubes are allowed to incubate in the 37°C water bath for exactly 60 minutes.

4. About 3 minutes before the end of the incubation period, equal volumes of the hydroxylamine and sodium hyroxide reagent (Reagents 4 and 5) are mixed.

5. At the end of incubation, 2.0 ml of this mixture is added to each tube; the contents are mixed, and the tubes are removed from the water bath and allowed to stand for at least 1 minute.

6. Six ml of hydrochloric acid reagent (Reagent 7) are added to each tube, and the contents are mixed.

7. Exactly 0.5 ml is removed from each tube and transferred to 19 mm cuvettes. 0.5 ml of distilled water is transferred to a cuvette to serve as a colorimetric blank. Then, 10 ml of ferric chloride reagent (Reagent 10) are added to all the cuvettes and the contents are mixed well.

8. With the spectrophotometer at a wave length of 540 mμ, the galvanometer is adjusted to 100%T with the colorimetric blank. Readings are obtained for control and test samples, and the result are obtained from the standard curve or chart prepared as below.

Standardization

Reagent grade acetylcholine bromide crystals are dried in a dessicator over soduim hydroxide pellets for at least 4 days. An aqueous solution is made to contain exactly 1.131 gm/100 ml of solution of this, 2.5, 2.0, 1.5, 1.0 and 0.5 ml are transferred to test tubes and the volume in each tube made to 2.5 ml with distilled water. Without incubating, to all tubes there is added 2.0 ml of the alkaline hydroxylamine mixture, prepared in Step 4 above. The procedure is continued as for the cholinesterase assay, beginning with Step 6. The tubes are considered to represent 625, 500, 375, 250 and 125 micromoles per ml of serum, when 0.2 ml of serum is used for the test, and 0.4 of these values when 0.5 ml of serum is used. The curve is linear in the instruments used. A calibration chart may be prepared from the readings obtained.

Calculation

If the reading obtained for the sample containing 0.2 ml of serum is significantly different from the control, the calculation is performed from this sample. The value in μM/ml found in the chart for this sample is subtracted from the value obtained from the control tube. If the readings do not differ significantly, the values obtained for the sample containing 0.5 ml of serum are used in a similar manner. In this case, the final results obtained are multiplied by 0.4

Normal Values

The results obtained from a series of normal adults varied from 130 to 310 μM/ml of serum. Similar values have been found by Wetstone and Bowers (43), using this method.

B. ERYTHROCYTE CHOLINESTERASE (ECE) PROCEDURE

Blood is collected with heparin or EDTA as anticoagulants. If necessary, blood obtained in a capillary tube may suffice for test. After centrifugation, the plasma is removed and the cells are washed three times with 10 volumes of 0.9% sodium chloride. One volume of packed cells is diluted with 20 volumes of saponin reagent (Reagent 6), and the hemoglobin content determined. It is conveniently performed by diluting 0.2 ml of the hemolysate with 6 ml of Drabkins reagent. Finally, the hemoglobin content is adjusted to have from 2.6 to 3.4 mgm of hemoglobin in the 0.2 ml of hemolysate used. This actual hemoglobin concentration must be recorded.

1. Just before starting 2 volumes of buffer (Reagent 1), 10 volumes of salt solution (Reagent 2), 1 volume of substrate (Reagent 3) and 27 volumes of water are mixed well and placed in a water bath at 37°C.

2. To 18 x 150 mm test tubes are transferred as follows:

first tube	0.5 ml of water (control)
second tube	0.2 ml of hemolysate
	0.3 ml of distilled water
third tube	0.5 ml of hemolysate

The tubes are placed in the water bath for at least 4 minutes.

3. Exactly 2.0 ml of buffer-salt-substrate mixture is added to each tube, and they are allowed to incubate for exactly 60 minutes.

4. Three minutes before the end of the incubation time, the alkaline hydroxylamine is prepared by mixing equal volumes of Reagents 4 and 5. At 60 minutes, 2 ml of this mixture is added to each tube, and the contents are mixed.

5. After at least 1 minute, 10 ml of 7% trichloracetic acid is added to each tube, and the tubes are stoppered and shaken.

6. After at least 1 minute, the contents of the tubes are filtered through retentive filter paper.

7. Five ml of the filtrate from each tube is transferred to 19 mm cuvettes. To another cuvette (blank) 5 ml of distilled water is added. To each cuvette, 3 ml of Reagent 9 (ferric chloride reagent) is added and the contents are mixed. With the spectrophotometer at a wave length of 540 mμ, the galvanometer is adjusted to 100% T with the blank. Readings are obtained from the samples and the control, and the results are obtained from the standard curve or chart prepared as below.

Standardization

Exactly 5 ml of the acetylcholine bromide standard reagent prepared as described in the standardization of SCE is placed in a 50 ml volumetric flask which is filled to the mark with distilled water. The procedure for the standardization of the serum cholinesterase is then followed, with the exception that the technique for ECE is used. Standard tubes contain 12.5, 10, 7.5, 5.0 and 2.5 μM of acetylcholine.

Calculation

If the reading for the sample containing 0.2 ml of hemolysate is significantly different than that of the control, the concentration of the sample is subtracted from that of the control. If the readings do not differ significantly, the difference between the 0.5 ml sample and the control is utilized; in this case, the final result must be multiplied by 0.4. The results divided by the milligrams of hemoglobin found in the cholinesterase activity calculated in μM/mg of hemoglobin. In a similar way, the calculations may be made per volume of packed cells.

Normal Values

The mean value for 352 adults was 1.82 μM of acetylcholine hydrolyzed per mg of hemoglobin per hour at 37°C with a standard deviation of $\pm$ 0.25. A normal distribution was observed; therefore, the range of normal values can be considered to be between 1.30 and 2.30. When the calculations were made in relation to packed erythrocytes, the mean was 520 μM/ml, with a standard deviation of 75 and a normal range of 370 to 670 μM/ml of packed erythrocytes.

Comments on the Methods

The method for the determination of SCE (16), was modified to provide accurate results even when the enzyme activity was very low, as occurs during intoxication by cholinesterase inhibitors. In addition, the method was adapted for ECE by lowering the substrate concentration to 0.005 M, the optimum for this enzyme, and including a protein precipitation step to eliminate the high absorbency produced by hemoglobin. The concentration of the buffer in both procedures is such that even after hydrolysis of the substrate, the pH, which is 8.2 at the beginning of the procedure, does not drop below 7.6, still at the optimal level (12). The substrate concentration is such that it is diminished no more than 50% even by samples which have a high enzyme content, again maintaining optimal conditions for the enzymatic activity (46).

The mean difference of duplicates was 2.6 μM, and 7% of paired determinations were within 7.6 μM, demonstrating the precision of the SCE procedure (43). Similar investigations were carried out for the erythrocyte cholinesterase procedure with similar good precision. (Coefficient of variation, 4.2%.)

When determining these enzymes in normal individuals or in pathological cases with as low as 50% of normal activity, the 0.2 ml aliquot techniques will be adequate. However, in cases of intoxication due to cholinesterase inhibitors, very low values are found, and it may be necessary to use the 0.5 ml aliquot, so that the readings will be significantly different between the control and the sample tubes.

The inhibitory effect of physostigmine and DFP on normal serum and erythrocyte hemolysate were studied. For serum, the pI_{50} for physostigmine was 7.3 and for DFP, 8.8. For the hemolysate, the pI_{50} for physostigmine was 6.8, and for DFP, 5.7. These results are almost identical to those found by Aldridge (2).

Discussion

Since the advent of the phosphorus ester insecticides and their widespread use throughout the world, the determination of the cholinesterase of the blood has become a routine procedure. When persons come in contact with these agents, the small amounts that penetrate the intact skin or mucous membranes have a cumulative effect, and very low levels of cholinesterase may be found without any clinical findings (5, 23). The organic phosphorus compounds include some of the most poisonous substances known. Sarin, for instance, is toxic to human beings at a dose of 0.28 mg/Kg (37). Needless to say, in such cases the individual must be removed from his surroundings, or some other precautionary measure taken. The only way in which to detect this type of exposure to cholinesterase inhibitors is by periodic determination of the blood cholinesterases. In some cases, values as low as 5% of normal have been obtained without clinical evidence of toxicity (23). In such cases, treatment by the so-called "inductive reactivation" agents like PAM is usually considered to be indicated.

The question arises as to which of the two blood cholinesterases should be determined. Most of the phosphorus esters are more potent inhibitors of serum cholinesterase (SCE), but many others act more selectively upon erythrocyte cholinesterase (ECE). In chronic cases of intoxication, this problem is complicated by the fact that the recovery of SCE is much more rapid than that of ECE. With the most potent inhibitors such as Sarin, a slightly better inhibitor for ECE, the recovery is much faster for the serum enzyme. Ten days after a single dose, producing practically complete inhibition of both enzymes, the SCE has recovered about 60% of its activity, while that of ECE is still only about 10% of normal (21). This is in keeping with the *de novo* formation of these enzymes, which takes about 30 days for SCE, and for ECE about 100 days, the life span of the erythrocyte.

Most authors agree that the erythrocyte enzyme has a better correlation with toxicity. As long ago as 1946, Hawkins (22) stated that the inhibition of acetylcholinesterase (erythrocytes) correlated with clinical symptoms, while that of SCE did not. Heath (23) is of the opinion that the measurement of ECE is a fairly reliable indication of the general acetylcholinesterase level in the body, while measurement of SCE may lead to an underestimation of the residual effects of a previous dose. O'Brien agrees that ECE is a good index of intoxication while SCE is less useful (37).

One point that must be taken into consideration is that there is rather wide variation in enzyme levels among normal individuals. It is usually stated that a value of 70% below the average normal value is likely to be of significance. (23)

Regarding the determination of cholinesterase, it must be remembered that even in aqueous solution there is reactivation of the enzyme upon standing, and the amount of this varies according to the inhibitor. In blood this may be of more importance because of other enzymes which may destroy some of the inhibitors. For this reason, the determination should be performed within a reasonable time after the blood sample is obtained.

Finally, it has been recently noted that some phosphorus esters are being used in clinical conditions such as urinary retention, and glaucoma (29), abdominal distension (19) and myasthenia gravis (20). In order to monitor this type of treatment, the periodic determination of the cholinesterases is obviously indicated.

The importance of this type of intoxication can be judged by noting that in California in 1959 there were 121 cases of intoxications in agricultural workers. About 6000 cases were reported in Japan during the six-year period between 1953 and 1959. (35)

The World Health Organization has studied the problem of the safe use of pesticides in public health, and for the past six years has sponsored a program for evaluating new insecticides. A recent report is worth consulting for those with special interest in this subject (58). It points out that the phosphorus esters are best used against insect vectors which have become resistant to chlorinated hydrocarbons such as DDT. The phosphorus esters, although more likely to produce acute toxic states than DDT are not notably persistent, and the danger of permanent widespread contamination of the environment appears small.

Toxic effects on mammals occurs largely through careless use, accidental discharges in industrial wastes, or other accidents. A recent example was seen in the death of 6600 sheep, accidentally subjected to a toxic airborne substance near a testing ground for chemical biological weapons. From accounts of this episode it appears that a phosphorus ester was involved (49, 55). The clinical findings in cases of organophosphorus poisoning include: miosis, sweating, rhinorrhea, salivation, lacrimation, wheezing, cramps and diarrhea, muscle weakness, anxiety and convulsions. The symptoms and signs are in general like those of parasympathetic stimulation. Death may be due to bronchospasm, respiratory paralysis, vasomotor paralysis or depression of the central nervous system.

Treatment is directed at removal of the toxic agent, decontamination of exposed area of skin, and general supportive measures. In addition, atropine in large doses (1-4 mg) is indicated. Reactivation of cholinesterase with oxime drugs may be useful in certain cases of poisoning due to particular compounds. Morphine and tranquillizers must not be given.

Although serum cholinesterase appears to have no known physiological function, it is responsible for hydrolyzing the commonly used muscle relaxant succinylcholine, and certain genetic abnormalities of the enzyme which produce prolonged apnea when this drug is administered during the course of anesthesia or psychiatric shock therapy have been observed in recent years (51-56). By study of the inhibition of SCE activity by dibucaine and fluoride, four genes denoting the type of cholinesterase have been designated as follows:

E_1^n, the normal gene

E_1^a, atypical gene, resistant to dibucaine inhibition

E_1^f, atypical gene, resistant to fluoride inhibition

E_1^s, the "silent gene", indicating complete absence of cholinesterase.

3.8% of individuals are heterozygous for one of the atypical genes, and about 1 of 2500 are abnormally sensitive to succinylcholine. About 1 of 100,000 individuals are homozygous for the "silent gene." These data are for Caucasians; among other races, such as the Eskimo, the "silent gene" may occur in as high as 1.5% of the population (50).

Measurement of serum cholinesterase may be of value in various pathological conditions in addition to its importance in diseases due to toxic agents. The clinicalpathological correlations were thoroughly discussed in a previous seminar (16). Briefly, decreased values were obtained in patients with hepatitis, cirrhosis, malnutrition, malignancy, severe anemia, hyperprexia, infectious diseases, cardiac failure and uremia (56). The determination has been used as a test for cancer (57). High values were found in patients with nephrotic syndrome, possibly related to the high rate of albumin synthesis by the liver.

REFERENCES

1. Adrian, E. D., Feldberg, W., and Kilby, B. A.: The cholinesterase inhibiting action of fluorophosphonates. Brit. J. Pharm., *2:*56-58, 1947.
2. Aldridge, W. N.: The differentiation of true

and pseudo cholinesterase by organo-phosphorus compounds. Biochem. J., *53:*62-67, 1953.

3. Aldridge, W. N.: Serum esterases. 1) Two types of esterase (A and B) hydrolysing p-nitrophenyl acetate, propionate and butyrate, and a method for their determination. Biochem. J., *53:*110-117, 1953.
4. Aldridge, W. N.: Serum esterases. 2) An enzyme hydrolysing diethyl p-nitrophenyl phosphate (E600) and its identity with the A-esterase of mammalian serum. Biochem. J., *53:*117-124, 1953.
5. Aldridge, W. N., and Davies, D. R.: Determination of cholinesterase activity in human blood. Brit. Med. J., *1:*945-947, 1952.
6. Alles, G. A., and Hawes, R. C.: Cholinesterases in the blood of man. J. Biol. Chem., *133:*375-390, 1940.
7. Ammon, R.: Die fermentative Spaltung des Acetylcholins. Pflugers Arch. Ges. Physiol., *233:* 486-491, 1934.
8. Augustinsson, K.: Cholinesterases, a study in comparative enzymology. Acta Physiol. Scand., *15:* Supp. 52, 1-192, 1948.
9. Augustinsson, K.: Assay Methods for Cholinesterases. In: Methods of Biochemical Analysis, Vol. 5. Edited by Glick, David. Interscience Publishers, New York, 1957.
10. Augustinsson, K.: Butyryl- and propionylcholinesterases and related types of the eserine-sensitive esterases. Chap. 31 in, The Enzymes, by Boyer, P., Lardy, H., and Myrback, K. Academic Press, New York, 1960.
11. Bergmann, F., and Segal, R.: The relationship of quaternary ammonium salts to the anionic sites of true and pseudo cholinesterase. Biochem. J., *58:*692-698, 1954.
12. Bergmann, F., Segal, R., Shimoni, A., and Wurzel, M.: The pH-dependence of enzymic ester hydrolysis. Biochem. J., *63:*684-690, 1956.
13. Cohen, J. A., Oosterbaan, R. A., Jansz, J. S., and Berends, F.: The active site of esterases. J. Cellular Comp. Physiol., *54:* Suppl. 1, 231-244, 1959.
14. Colhoun, E. H.: Distribution of choline acetylase in insect conductive tissue. Nature, *182:* 1378, 1958.
15. Dale, H. H.: The action of certain esters and ethers of choline, and their relation to muscarine. J. Pharmacol. Exp. Therap., *6:*147-190, 1914-15.
16. de la Huerga, J., and Volini, F.: Serum cholinesterase. In Sunderman, F. W., and Sunderman, F. W. Jr.: The Laboratory Diagnosis of Liver Diseases. St. Louis, Warren H. Green, Inc., 1968.
17. de la Huerga, J., Yesinick, C., and Popper, H.: Colorimetric method for the determination of serum cholinesterase. Am. J. Clin. Path., *22:* 1126-1133, 1952.
18. Gardiner, J. E., and Kilby, B. A.: Biochemistry of organic phosphorus insecticides. 1) The mammalian metabolism of bis (dimethylamino) phosphonous anhydride (Schradan). Biochem. J., *51:*78-85, 1952.
19. Grob, D., Lilienthal, J. L., Jr., and Harvey, A. M.: The administration of di-isopropyl fluorophosphate (DFP) to man. II. Effect on intestinal motility and use in the treatment of abdominal distention. Bull. Johns Hopkins Hosp. *81:*245-256, 1947.
20. Grob, D., and Harvey, A. M.: Observations on the effects of tetraethyl pyrophosphate (TEPP) in man, and on its use in the treatment of myasthenia gravis. Bull. Johns Hopkins Hosp., *84:* 532-567, 1949.
21. Grob, D., and Harvey, J. C.: Effects in man of the anticholinesterase compound Sarin (Isopropyl Methyl Phosphonofluoridate). J. Clin. Invest., *37:*350-368, 1958.
22. Hawkins, R. D., and Gunter, J. M.: Studies on cholinesterase. The selective inhibition of pseudocholinesterase *in vivo*. Biochem. J., *40:* 192-197, 1946.
23. Heath, D. F.: Organophosphorus Poisons, Anticholinesterases and Related Compounds. Pergamon Press, New York, 1961.
24. Hestrin, S.: The reaction of acetylcholine and other carboxylic derivatives with hydroxylamine and its analytical application. J. Biol. Chem., *180:*249-261, 1949.
25. Hobbiger, F.: Effect of nicotinhydroxamic acid methiodide on human plasma cholinesterase inhibited by organophosphate containing a dialkyphosphato group. Brit. J. Pharmacol., *10:* 356-362, 1955.
26. Jansz, H. S., Brons, D., and Warringa, M. G. P. J.: Chemical nature of the DFP-binding site of pseudocholinesterase. Biochem. Biophys. Acta, *34:*573-575, 1959.
27. Jansz, H. S., and Cohen, J. A.: Pseudocholinesterase from horse serum. I. Purification and properties of the enzume. Biochim. Biophys. Acta, *56:*531-537, 1962.
28. Lawler, H. C.: Turnover time of acetylcholinesterase. J. Biol. Chem., *236:*2296-2301, 1961.
29. Leopold, I. H., and Comroe, J. H., Jr.: Use of di-isopropyl flurophosphate ("DFP") in treatment of glaucoma. Arch. Ophthal. (Chicago), *36:*1-16, 1946.
30. Loewi, O., and Navratil, E.: Uber humorale Ubertragbarkeit der Herznervenwirkung. Pflugers Archiv. Ges. Physiologie, *214:*678-688, 1926.
31. Main, A. R., Miles, K. E., and Braid, D. E.: The determination of human-serum-cholinesterase activity with O-nitrophenyl butyrate. Biochem. J., *78:*769-776, 1961.

32. Mendel, B., and Rudney, H.: Studies on cholinesterase. Biochem. J., *37:*59-63, 1943.
33. Michel, H. C.: An electrometric method for the determination of red blood cell and plasma cholinesterase activity. J. Lab. Clin. Med., *34:* 1564-1568, 1949.
34. Mounter, L. A.: Enzymic hydrolysis of organophosphorus compounds in enzymes. Chap. 32 in, The Enzymes, Vol. 4, by Boyer, P., Lardy, H., and Myrback, K. Academic Press, New York, 1960.
35. Namba, T., and Hiraki, K.: PAM (pyridine-2-aldoxime methiodide) therapy for alkylphosphate poisoning. J.A.M.A., *166:*1834-1839, 1958.
36. O'Brien, R. D.: Toxic Phosphorus Esters. Academic Press, New York, 1960.
37. O'Brien, R. D.: Insecticides; Action and Metabolism. Academic Press, New York, 1967.
38. Peters, R. A.: Biochemistry of some toxic agents. II. Some recent work in the field of fluoroacetate compounds. Bull. Johns Hopkins Hosp., *97:* 21-42, 1955.
39. Plattner, F.: Der Nachweis des Vagusstoffes beim Saugetier. Pflugers Archiv. Ges. Physiol., *214:*112-129, 1926.
40. Ravin, H. A., Tsu, K. C., and Seligman, A. M.: Colorimetric estimation and histochemical demonstration of serum cholinesterase. J. Biol. Chem., *191:*843-857, 1951.
41. Reinhold, J. G., Tourigny, L. G., and Yonan, V. L.: Measurement of serum cholinesterase activity by a photometric indicator method, together with a study of the influence of sex and race. Am. J. Clin. Path., *23:*645-653.
42. Stedman, E., Stedman, E., and Easson, L.: Choline esterase. An enzyme present in the blood serum of the horse. Biochem. J., *26:*2056-2066, 1932.
43. Wetstone, M., and Bowers, G. N.: Serum cholinesterase in Standard Methods of Clinical Chemistry, Vol. 4. pp. 275-276, 1952.
44. Wilson, I. B.: Acetylcholinesterase. XI. Reversibility of tetraethyl pyrophosphate inhibition. J. Biol. Chem., *190:*111-117, 1951.
45. Wilson, I. B.: Acetylcholinesterase, Chap. 30 in, The Enzymes, Vol. 4, by Boyer, P., Lardy, H., and Myrback, K. Academic Press, New York, 1960.
46. Wilson, I. B., and Bergmann, F.: Acetylcholinesterase. VIII Dissociation constants of the active groups. J. Biol. Chem., *186:*683-692, 1950.
47. Wilson, L. B., Bergmann, F., and Nachmansohn, D.: Acetylcholinesterase. X. Mechanism of the catalysis of acylation reactions. J. Biol. Chem., *186:*781-790, 1960.
48. Wilson, I. B., Hatch, M. A., and Ginsburg, S.: Carbamylation of acetylcholinesterase. J. Biol. Chem., *235:*2312-2315, 1960.
49. Boffey, P. M.: Six thousand sheep stricken near CBW center. Science, *159:*1442, 1968.
50. Gutsche, B. B., Scott, E. M., and Wright, R. C.: Hereditary deficiency of pseudocholinesterase in Eskimos. Nature, *215:*322-323, 1967.
51. Kalow, W., and Staron, N.: On distribution and inheritance of atypical forms of human serum cholinesterase, as indicated by dibucaine numbers. Canad. J. Biochem. Physiol., *35:*1305-1320, 1957.
52. Kattamis, C., Davies, D., and Lehmann, H.: The silent serum cholinesterase gene. Acta genet., *17:*299-303, 1967.
53. Leacock, A. M., Campbell, D. J., and McIntyre, J. W. R.: A clinical and biochemical approach to cholinesterase problems in anaesthesia. Can. Anaes. Soc. J., *13:*550-556, 1966.
54. Morrow, A. C., and Motulsky, A. G.: Rapid screening method for the common atypical pseudocholinesterase variant. J. Lab. Clin. Med., *71:*350-356, 1968.
55. Surface, B.: Man's deadliest weapons race. Chicago Daily News, pp 3-4, 7 Oct. 1968.
56. Thompson, J. C., and Whittaker, N.: A study of the pseudocholinesterase in 78 cases of apnoea following Suxamethonium. Acta genet., Basel, *16:*209-222, 1966.
57. Vaccarezza, J. R.: Vaccarezza's Test. Its use in the presumptive diagnosis of cancer. Dis. Chest, *52:*715-719, 1967.
58. World Health Organization: Safe use of pesticides in public health. Wld. Hlth. Org. techn. Rep. Ser. No. 356, 1967.

Chapter 19B

Manometric Method for Measurement of Cholinesterase

KENNETH P. DuBOIS, Ph.D.

INTRODUCTION

The cholinesterase activity of tissues can be accurately measured by a manometric procedure using a conventional Warburg apparatus. The most widely used manometric procedure for cholinesterase was developed in this laboratory in 1947.[1] It has been used extensively in this and other laboratories for studies on the anticholinesterase agents of the organic phosphate series. For research, many investigators prefer this procedure to other more rapid methods because of the accuracy and reproducibility of the results.

PRINCIPLE

The manometric measurement of cholinesterase is based on the reaction between acetic acid liberated during enzymatic hydrolysis of acetylcholine and sodium bicarbonate in the buffer medium according to the following reactions:

$$\text{Acetylcholine} \xrightarrow[\text{H}_2\text{O}]{\text{Cholinesterase}} \text{Choline} + \text{Acetic acid}$$

$$\text{Acetic acid} + \text{Sodium bicarbonate} \longrightarrow \text{Carbonic acid} + \text{Sodium acetate}$$

$$\text{Carbonic acid } (H_2CO_3) \longrightarrow \text{Carbon dioxide} + \text{Water}$$

The liberated carbon dioxide produced by these reactions is measured quantitatively by the pressure change in a closed system. A direct relationship exists between the amount of acetylcholine hydrolyzed and the amount of carbon dioxide liberated. Each micromole of acetylcholine that is hydrolyzed liberates one micromole (22.4 microliters) of carbon dioxide.

REAGENTS

1. *Calcium-free Ringer-bicarbonate buffer* contains 0.025 M sodium bicarbonate, 0.15 M sodium chloride, and 0.04 M magnesium chloride dissolved in redistilled water.

2. *Acetylcholine chloride or bromide* is prepared as a 0.1 M solution in the calcium-free Ringer-bicarbonate buffer. This reagent is prepared freshly in a

quantity of 10 ml immediately before use.

3. *Tissue Preparations.* Undiluted plasma is added to the assay system in the amount of 0.1 ml per Warburg flask. Erythrocytes are washed with the Ringer-bicarbonate buffer and suspended in an equal volume of the buffer. When human erythrocytes are assayed, 0.1 ml of the cell suspension is used containing 50 mg of erythrocytes. Ten percent homogenates of other tissues such as brain are prepared by homogenizing one part of tissue with nine parts of the buffer in a Potter-Elvehjem homogenizer. An amount of homogenate containing 50 mg or 100 mg of tissue is generally used.

SPECIAL APPARATUS

The conventional Warburg apparatus is used for the cholinesterase measurements. Flasks with side-arms are used. The flasks must be calibrated for carbon dioxide evolution measurements. Precalibrated flasks are now available or the calibration can be done by the standard procedure. The apparatus must be equipped with a manifold to permit flushing of a mixture of 5% CO_2 and 95% nitrogen through the flasks to remove air before the measurements are made. A cylinder of commercially available CO_2 and N_2 mixture is used for this purpose.

PROCEDURE

In the side-arm of the Warburg vessel 0.3 ml of 0.1 M acetylcholine.The tissue and enough Ringer-bicarbonate buffer to make a total volume of 2.7 ml are placed in the main compartment of the vessel. The flasks are connected to the Warburg manometers and the air in the system is replaced by passing a mixture of 5% CO_2 and 95% N_2 through the manometer and flask for a period of 5 minutes. The stopcocks are then placed in the flasks and the manometers and flasks are attached to the Warburg bath. The water bath is maintained at 38°C. The flasks are equilibrated to 38°C for a period of 5 minutes. The reaction is then started by tipping the acetylcholine from the side-arm into the main compartment of the Warburg vessel. After another 5 minutes of equilibration, manometer readings of the amount of CO_2 produced by enzymatic hydrolysis of acetylcholine are recorded at 5 minute intervals for 30 minutes.

The results for cholinesterase measurements by this method are usually expressed as microliters of CO_2 produced per 50 mg of tissue per 10 minutes. This value is derived from the manometer scale changes multiplied by the flask constant for CO_2 evolution. The activity can be expressed in terms of micromoles of acetylcholine hydrolyzed since hydrolysis of 1 micromole of acetylcholine will cause liberation of 22.4 microliters of CO_2.

DISCUSSION

The manometric method of measuring cholinesterase activity is a straightforward procedure which utilizes few reagents and consequently the sources of error are few. The availability of the special apparatus and knowledge of its operation are important requirements which cannot always be satisfied in every laboratory. The range of values for the cholinesterase activity of erythrocytes or nervous tissue is generally quite small. However, values for serum cholinesterase may vary considerably from one individual to another. Since the enzyme activity of serum can be influenced by indirect factors such as liver disease, clinical interpretations concerning cholinesterase depression due to insecticide exposure are facilitated by measuring both erythrocyte and plasma cholinesterase.

REFERENCES

1. DuBois, K. P., and Mangun, G. H.: Effect of hexaethyl tetraphosphate on cholinesterase *in vitro* and *in vivo*. Proc. Soc. Exper. Biol. & Med., *64*:137-139, 1947.
2. Umbreit, W. W., Burris, R. H., and Stauffer, J. F.: Calibration of respirometers. In Manometric Techniques, Revised Ed. Burgess Publishing Co., Minneapolis, 1957, pp. 46-63.

Chapter 19C

Electrometric Measurement of Cholinesterase in Serum (Michel Method)

F. WILLIAM SUNDERMAN, M.D., PH.D.

PRINCIPLE

Acetyl cholinesterase enzyme causes the hydrolysis of acetylcholine to acetic acid and choline. The acetic acid which is liberated causes a change in the pH of the buffered medium. This pH change is measured with a glass electrode, and cholinesterase activity is expressed in terms of pH change per hour.

REAGENTS

1. *Buffer* (for serum): 0.006M sodium barbital (1.2371 gm); 0.001M KH_2PO_4 (0.1361 gm); 0.30M NaCl (17.535 gm). For one liter of buffer, dissolve the reagents in about 900 ml of distilled water and add 11.6 ml. of 0.1 N HCl before diluting to volume. The pH of this buffer should be 8.00 at 25°C. As soon as the buffer pH falls below 7.97, a fresh solution should be prepared. (N.B. The potassium dihydrogen phosphate reagent should be anhydrous, of Bureau of Standards quality.)

2. *Acetylcholine Substrate* (for serum): 0.165M acetylcholine (3.0 gm in 100 ml of distilled water). This solution should be stored in the refrigerator and be prepared fresh every two weeks.

PROCEDURE

1. Two-tenths ml of serum is transferred to a 10 ml volumetric flask or calibrated tube. The contents of the flask are diluted to the mark with distilled water.

2. One ml of the diluted serum is transferred to each of two 5 ml beakers.

3. One ml of buffer solution is transferred to each 5 ml beaker, using an Ostwald-Folin blow-out pipet, to insure mixing.

4. The beakers are allowed to equilibrate in a constant-temperature water bath at 25°C for 10 minutes.

5. The initial pH (pH_1) is determined with a pH meter reading to the nearest 0.01 pH unit. Each beaker is immediately replaced in the water bath.

6. Two-tenths ml of the acetyl choline substrate is added to each beaker, at one-minute intervals. A blow-out pipet is employed for this step. The contents of the beaker are mixed thoroughly.

7. The enzymatic reaction is allowed to proceed for exactly one hour after addition of the acetylcholine and then the final pH (pH_2) is determined. In order that the timing is precise, the measure-

ments of pH are made at minute intervals. It is necessary to shake the beaker for a few seconds after the electrodes have been immersed, to establish rapid equilibrium.

CALCULATIONS

Cholinesterase activity is calculated in units of pH change per hour by use of the following formula:

$$\Delta\text{pH per hour} = \left(\frac{\text{pH}_1 - \text{pH}_2}{t_2 - t_1} - b\right) f$$

where

ΔpH = change in pH
pH_1 = initial pH
pH_2 = final pH
t_1 = time of addition of acetylcholine
t_2 = time of reading pH_2
b = non-enzymatic hydrolysis correction corresponding to pH_2 (for table).
f = correction for variations in ΔpH per hour with pH corresponding to pH_2 (from table).

TABLE 1. CORRECTION FACTORS FOR USE IN THE EQUATION

pH_2	*b*	*f*
7.9	0.09	0.98
7.8	0.07	1.00
7.7	0.06	1.01
7.6	0.05	1.02
7.5	0.04	1.02
7.4	0.03	1.01
7.3	0.02	1.01
7.2	0.02	1.00
7.1	0.02	1.00
7.0	0.01	1.00
6.8	0.01	1.00
6.6	0.01	1.01
6.4	0.01	1.02
6.2	0.01	1.04
6.0	0.01	1.09

To express the results in terms of percent activity relative to some normal value, multiply the ΔpH per hour value found for the sample by 100 and divide py the ΔpH per hour value considered to be normal. Where repetitive analyses are performed upon the same individuals, it is preferable to express each result as a percentage of the result of the initial or base-line determination.

REMARKS

The procedure as outlined is applicable only to the measurement of *serum* cholinesterase. For the analysis of erythrocycle cholinesterase slight modification in the concentrations of the buffer and the substrate are required, as well as the use of different values for the "b" and "f" factors. For the detailed procedure for erythrocyte cholinesterase measurement, see the publication of Wolfsie and Winter report the following normal values for erythrocyte cholinesterase:

NORMAL VALUES

Normal mean = 0.91 Δ pH per hour
Standard deviation = $\pm$ 0.14
Normal range = 0.408 to
1.652 Δ pH per hour.

It should be noted that following exposure to organic pyrophosphates the *serum* cholinesterase activity decreases faster and to lower levels than does the *erythrocyte* cholinesterase. Moreover, serum cholinesterase returns to the normal range more rapidly than does erythrocyte cholinesterase. For these reasons, serum cholinesterase measurements provide the best index of acute exposure, while erythrocyte cholinesterase measurements are especially useful in evaluating chronic exposure.

REFERENCES

1. Michel, H.O.: An electrometric method for the determination of red blood cell and plasma cholinesterase activity. J. Lab. Clin. Med., *34:* 1564-1568, 1949.
2. Wolfsie, J.H.: Blood cholinesterase activity. AMA Arch. Industrial Health, *16*:403-410, 1957.
3. Wolfsie, J. H. and Winters, G.D.: Statistical analysis of normal human red blood cell and plasma cholinesterase activity values. AMA Arch. Industrial Hyg. and Occup. Med., *6*:43-49, 1952.

Chapter 20

Neurotoxicity of Some Common Halogenated Hydrocarbons

HAROLD STEVENS, M.D.

Halogenated hydrocarbon, although not a household word, has become a household item. Thanks to the rapidly expanding insecticide industry and the ingenuity of chemists, a vast and growing repertory of these compounds, largely in the form of insecticides, has evolved. However, the ideal insecticide, selectively lethal to the insect, innocuous to the human, has not yet been realized and in spite of the claim that "the development of these effective chemicals has been one of the most spectacular developments in the past decade," (1) an unestimated price will be paid, some of it in human tender. Although incidence of fatal poisoning or of sequelae have been minimized by some, this position has been controverted by others, (2, 3) including Rachel Carsen. Over a 20-year period, 312 cases of poisoning by insecticides have been recorded at Children's Hospital.

These halogenated hydrocarbons which include DDT, chlordane, lindane, aldrin, dieldrin, etc., are chloride-containing organic compounds which have distinguished themselves by their toxicity for numerous species of insects, and also for the similarity of the manifestations of toxicity in humans and other mammals. (1) They are similar also in the following properties: a) Solubility in fats and common organic solvents; insolubility in water. b) Relative chemical stability. c) Similarity as convulsant poisons in warm-blooded animals

The clinical manifestations of halogenated hydrocarbon poisoning is more or less stereotyped and may be found after exposure to the simplest of these compounds, namely, carbon tetrachloride and methylchloride:

Carbon Tetrachloride Poisoning

Industrial poisoning with carbon tetrachloride has markedly diminished while the frequent exposure in a domestic milieu continues to invite a growing risk from accidental poisoning. The increasing ratio of cases of poisoning with carbon tetrachloride in the home largely reflects a systematic program of safeguards initiated by industry, plant, and state authorities. The domestic consumer, however, is often unaware of the lethal nature of carbon tetrachloride and the label on the container gives little or no warning, but rather emphasizes the safety of the product because of its non-inflammable character.

Despite the frequency and importance of effects on the central nervous system there had been no systematic study of the neurological consequences of carbon tetrachloride intoxication until 1953 (4). In a period of five years 15 cases of carbon tetrachloride poisoning were studied by the author. The preponderance of these patients were alcoholic and moreover were drinking alcoholic beverages immediately before, during, or soon after the exposure to carbon tetrachloride. This sinister synergy between alcohol and carbon tetrachloride has been reported frequently, but no satisfactory explanation has yet been found. Alcohol may increase the rate and degree of absorption in the gastrointestinal tract, but reinforcement of toxic effects occurs in animals and humans even when the carbon tetrachloride is inhaled (5).

Neurological involvement was present in seven of the 15 cases. Poisoning occurred in 13 in the home and two in commercial cleaning plants. Of the 13 patients whose poisoning occurred at home, two were children who drank the fluid. two also accidentally drank carbon tetrachloride and the rest were exposed by inhalation; five died. Except for three patients, the poisoning was known to be due to a single exposure. Neurological manifestations began with headache, vertigo, blurred vision, weakness, tremor, paresthesias and lethargy. Confusion, disorientation impaired mental function and coma also developed.

The mechanism of central nervous system involvement in halogenated hydrocarbon poisoning as exemplified by carbon tetrachloride has not been elaborated, but from our experience and the cases recorded in the literature it appears that the nervous system may be affected through three possible mechanisms:

1. Direct toxic effect
   - a) Narcosis
   - b) Encephalomyelitis
   - c) Cerebellar degeneration
   - d) Neuritis
     1. peripheral
     2. optic
2. Hemorrhage
3. Cerebral embolism

In our study, there was evidence of damage to the cerebellum and cerebri. Histological examination of the brain showed scattered small areas of demyelinization with necrosis. Glial nodules were also present. The findings, confirmed by Luse and Wood (6), suggest the same changes produced in rabbits by Biancalani (7) who poisoned dogs and rabbits with carbon tetrachloride, found in the brain a variety of prominent nonspecific changes including glial proliferation, particularly in perivascular areas.

In one autopsy case that was encountered, the cerebellar cortex showed mark disorganization of the mollecular layer with a conspicuous falling out of neuronal elements. These findings have been confirmed by a few others (8, 9).

The treatment of carbon tetrachloride poisoning consists of lavaging the stomach, instilling mineral oil, combating shock and narcosis. Epinephrine and similar drugs are contraindicated. Persistent psychiatric syndromes and peripheral neuritis including optic neuritis have been observed.

Methylchloride

In spite of the known toxic properties of methylchloride and the widespread use of nontoxic agents in modern refrigeration systems, there have continued to be sporadic reports of methylchloride intoxication, mostly in foreign countries (10). The metabolic fate of methylchloride is not definitely known, but it has been inferred that it is broken down to methyl-alcohol and hydrochloric acid, which, on further oxidation, yield formic acid and aldehyde.

Two cases of methylchloride poisoning have been encountered:

Case I. F.M.: A 32-year-old beautician was examined by me in December, 1955. As she rose from the chair to enter the examining room, she fell forward because of sudden development of a complete right foot drop. She had been seated with her right leg crossed over her left in the manner of a right-handed person, and by this minimal and brief compression of the peroneal nerve at the head of the fibula, she had induced a complete foot drop, reflecting the vulnerability of peripheral nerves to halogenated hydrocarbon poisoning. The paralysis resolved over the next two hours.

Her history disclosed that in January, 1953, while seven months pregnant, she returned from her usual work feeling quite well. She prepared dinner and performed other household chores, by which time she felt a bit dizzy, which she attributed to the heat in the apartment and to the closed windows, all of which were stuck and could not be opened. She and her husband retired at the usual hour and both left for work the following morning; however, she felt nauseated, dizzy, and suffered a headache, was unable to perform her duties as a beautician, and left her job to go home. She has amnesia for the subsequent events. Her next recollection is ten days later when she awakened in the George Washington University Hospital. It was subsequently learned that, on the evening prior to admission she seemed to be in a very excited state and her husband appeared to be drunk and dysarthric.

The landlady, out of concern for the couple's welfare, entered the apartment, found the husband in a confused condition and the patient lying in a closet, asleep. She helped the patient to bed, returned to find both quietly in bed asleep, but noted food burning in a pan on a gas range which she turned off, and left. Later in the afternoon, the landlady found the husband undressed in the hall and the patient lying in a pool of blood with a fetus between her legs.

On admission, she was cyanotic and comatose. The following day she was slightly more responsive, speech was slurred, and she showed purposeless jerking movement of her arms and hands. On the third hospital day, there were two generalized grand mal seizures and Dr. Thomas L. Hartman, her physician, prescribed anticonvulsant medication. Five days after the accident the D. C. Health Department toxicologist reported that methylchloride had been found in the apartment from a leak in the central refrigerating system.

She gradually improved, was discharged 20 days after admission with a marked intention tremor, blurred vision, and ataxic gait. She continued to experience positional vertigo. The neurological examination in December, 1955, showed a tense, tremulous, depressed woman with a moderately ataxic gait. There was generalized tremor, worse in the hands and ataxia with the finger-to-nose test, slight ataxia with the heel-to-knee test. Marked hyperhidrosis of the hands was noted.

She continued to suffer from intermittent blurring of vision, insomnia and headache. The electroencephalogram was normal. She remained incapacitated and frustrated over her repeatedly unsuccessful attempts to resume her job and profoundly depressed. In 1965, she committed suicide by ingesting about 100 pentobarbital capsules.

Case II: Her husband had been admitted to another hospital where he improved rapidly. His neurological examination in October, 1956, was negative aside from slight impairment of hearing and slight tremor. He experienced tinnitus in the left ear and noted slight incoordination when attempting to perform skilled acts. Up until one year before the examination, he experienced pain in both legs. Severe incoordination, which he suffered for several months, gradually resolved.

The laboratory findings, reported elsewhere by Hartman and others (10) disclosed that the most significant findings were profound acidosis and transient anemia. The acidosis was manifested clinically by hyperpnea and chemically by the lowered carbon dioxide combining power of the blood; both responded readily to corrective therapy.

These two cases controvert the claim that intoxication by halogen hydrocarbons is trivial and results in no residua. A suit for damages was settled out of court.

Chlordane

Chlordane is a halogenated hydrocarbon insecticide that has been subject to much legal and scientific controversy (11). Its structure, similar to the active principle of cantharides, may be represented as follows:

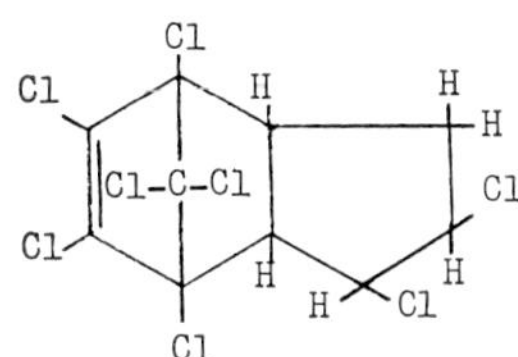

In general, chlordane acts substantially like other chlorinated hydrocarbon insecticides whose sites of action are on the higher motor cortex and cerebellum. It does not affect vital centers in the medulla. It is stored in some form, especially in fat, and seems to disappear fairly rapidly when administration of the insecticide is discontinued. It is one of the most hazardous of the chlorinated hydrocarbon insecticides and is readily absorbed through the unbroken skin. (11) (12) (13) (14). Fumes are given off over an extended period of time and unless readily dissipated, offer a distinct danger to persons who are exposed. This last characteristic is demonstrated by the following case:

D.M.: A 39-year-old woman who was examined in 1960, was exposed to an insecticide "Real Kill"* on May 17, 1956. At this time, she sprayed some clothing placed on the bed in a room where the windows, as well as the door, were all open. After one hour of spraying and carrying the clothes to and from the

*The ingredients of the "Real Kill" moth proofer are: a) Petroleum distilate 38.984% b) Technical chlordane 2.000% c) Phenomercuric lactate 0.016%.

closet in the room, she suddenly lost consciousness. She recalls smelling the insecticide's kerosene-like odor; believed she was unconscious for a period of 5 to 15 minutes. On awakening she became nauseated, vomited and then lethargy was noted. She recalls spraying some of the clothes while she held them in her hand. Her husband, who heard her call out, "I feel faint" before she lost consciousness, carried her to her bedroom and applied artificial respiration for about 10 minutes. He noted that she had no pulse or respiration prior to his ministrations. She revived about ten minutes later, gagged, and vomited her lunch which had consisted of a ham sandwich and milk. She seemed to wander around in a confused state, later burned a steak, became angry and deliberately broke a dish. She later retired at 7:00 p.m., slept until 5:00 the next morning with all her clothes on. She awakened with a headache after she rolled off the bed onto the floor. She did not hit her head. She got up, undressed, put on her pajamas, but did not go back to sleep, remained lethargic and anorexic through the day. Headache continued, but was not localized and she vomited once. She went to church the following morning but was unable to sit through the service. She left, sat in the car until the service was over and while doing so, spit up four or five tablespoons of blood. She was taken home where a physician who was called found her extremely somnolent. Two days later, she "blacked out."

Headache and lethargy persisted and within a period of one year after the exposure, she lost consciousness on three occasions, bruised her knee on one occasion. When examined on March 14, 1960, her husband reported that she had difficulty handling the household accounts and there had been a definite personality change. Previously, she was energetic, perfectionistic, meticulous and had a superior memory. She remained quite disorganized, is frequently unaware of her forgetfulness, but at times feels inadequate and becomes depressed over her predicament. For about one year after the accident, she was unable to organize her household chores or to cook. Ability to plan and prepare meals was gradually returning four years later, but it still required considerable effort to organize and execute her daily routine.

Neurological examination disclosed an unkempt, somewhat obtunded woman who was depressed, tearful, and frequently became quite agitated when discussing her defects. She loudly proclaimed a strong desire to go away, to be hospitalized, etc., states that she feels frustrated because of her inability to plan and execute even ordinary household duties, "and everybody says I am irresponsible." She wrung her hands and cried openly. She displayed poverty of interest and impaired memory. She stated that she has difficulty remembering things, forgets to mail letters and perform routine household duties, forgets where she left off whatever activity she may be engaged in. She often goes to sleep in the chair, on the couch, or even at the table and often after her husband leaves at 8:00 a.m., she may sleep for several hours, sometimes until the children come home at 3:30 p.m. She states that if she is awakened, she is irritable and "infuriated."

Previous to exposure, she had developed considerable skill as a ceramicist, had won two prizes for original pieces, but on trying to resume this pursuit, found that she is unable to finish any project. She used to make all her children's clothing and some of her own clothes, but she is no longer able to plan and prosecute such activity or see them through to final completion.

The electroencephalogram was abnormal; showed no focus.

The patient's impairment is considered to be permanent and the ensuing litigation eventuated in a settlement in the midst of the trial.

SUMMARY

The increasing number and variety of halogenated hydrocarbons expose the domestic consumer to the hazard of poisoning, either accidentally or by ingestion with suicidal intent. Neurotoxicity is a common, but somewhat overlooked consequence of exposure either by ingestion, contact or inhalation.

This group of chemically similar compounds have similar neurotoxic and pathogenic consequences including damage to peripheral nerves, cerebellum and cerebrum. These may be lasting, including psychiatric syndromes.

Concomitant exposure to other drugs or chemicals may enhance the toxic effect of halogenated hydrocarbons, e.g., insecticides may contain toxic organic phosphorus compounds, the effects of which might be mitigated by the oxine compounds which can reverse the combination between the cholinesterase molecule and the inhibitor.

The public should be warned and the physicians informed regarding the danger, mechanism, diagnosis, and treatment of the toxicity from halogenated hydrocarbons.

BIBLIOGRAPHY

1. McGee, L. C.: Chlorinated insecticides: Toxicity for man. Indust. Med. & Surg., *24:*101-109, 1955.
2. Hearings before the House Select Committee to Investigate the Use of Chemicals In Food Products, Part I. U. S. Government Printing Office, 1951, pp. 147-159.
3. Editorial: Health hazards of pesticides. J.A.M.A., *181:*122, 1962.
4. Stevens, H., and Forster, F.: Effect of carbon tetrachloride on the nervous system. Arch. Neurol. & Psychiat., *70:*635, 1953.
5. Geraghty, F., and Rogers, W.: Carbon tetrachloride poisoning with report of a case. West Virginia Med. J., *43:*242, 1947.
6. Luse, S., and Wood, W.: The brain in fatal carbon tetrachloride poisoning. Arch. Neurol., *17:*304, 1967.
7. Biancalani, A.: Experimental research on the alteration of the central nervous system in intoxication by carbon tetrachloride. Rev. Pat. Neurol., *44:*352, 1934.
8. Tanohata, K., and Tagawa, D.: Histopathologic study of central nervous system in experimental carbon tetrachloride poisoning. Nagasaki Igakkai Zassi, *10:*1505, 1932.
9. Cohen, M.: Central nervous system in carbon tetrachloride intoxication. Neurology, *7:*238, 1957.
10. Hartman, T., Wacker, W., and Roll, R.: Methylchloride intoxication. New Engl. J. Med., 253, 552, 1955.
11. Present status of chlordane. J.A.M.A., *158:*1364, 1955. (Council on Pharmacy and Chemistry.)
12. Lensky, P., and Evans, H.: Human poisoning by chlordane. J.A.M.A., *149:*1394, 1952.
13. Ambrose, A., Christensen, H., Robbins, D., and Rather, L.: Toxicological and pharmacological studies on chlordane. A.M.A. Arch. Industrial Hygiene & Occupat. Med., *7:*197, 1953.
14. Heyroth, F.: Chlordane poisoning. J.A.M.A., *150:*715, 1952.

Chapter 21A

Highlights of Fluorocarbon Toxicology

J. WESLEY CLAYTON, JR. PH.D.

INTRODUCTION

Fluorocarbons, organic compounds containing one or more fluorine atoms, combine several desirable properties which derive from their unusual chemical stability. Many fluorocarbons are proving increasingly useful in today's society, a development which necessitates attention to the toxicology of this group.

This may be called the day of exotic chemistry when even the so-called inert gases have been forced into chemical combination by excitation of electrons. Compounds of carbon and fluorine are of this stripe, in that the C-F bond only rarely occurs in nature. Thus, the majority of fluorocarbons are in this sense "unnatural." Once formed, however, fluorocarbons are unusually stable in conventional chemical systems. This high stability is a result of a short interatomic distance between C and F, and the strength of the bond joining the two elements. Contrasted with the C-H bond (rupture eneregy = 93 Kcal) the C-F bond is considerably stronger (rupture energy = 114 Kcal). The presence of even a single F- atom in an organic compound has a profound influence on the properties of the molecule. In organchlorine compounds for example, inclusion of F leads to an increased stability of the C-Cl bond reducing the steric strain thereon caused by the relatively voluminous Cl atom. The accumulation of F- atoms on a carbon chain leads to increasingly higher stability by a progressive shortening of the C-F bonds. For example, the C-F bond length in CCl_3F is 1.348 angstroms, but in CF_4 it is 1.317 angstroms. The latter requires 116 Kcal for rupture while the former needs 112.1 Kcal for this.

In the fluoroalkanes, toxicity generally is inversely related to the chemical stability. The greater the number of fluorine atoms in the fluoroalkane, the lower the toxicity. The presence of a double bond in a fluoroalkene significantly influences the chemical properties of a fluorocarbon. The strong electronegative forces of fluoroalkyl groups joined by a double bond create an area of low electron density making the site susceptible to nucleophilic attack. Accordingly, fluoroalkenes are generally more active than the corresponding fluoroalkane. This point can be illustrated by considering the toxicity of the isomers of C_4F_8.

In Table I are given the acute inhalation toxicity data for rats exposed 4 hours to the particular compound. The

TABLE I: ISOMERS OF C_4F_8 ACUTE INHALATION TOXICITY FOR RATS

4-Hour Exposure	*Approximate Lethal Concentration (ppm)*
F_2C-CF_2 / F_2C-CF_2 (ring)	> 800,000
F_3C-CF = CF-CF_3	6100
$(F_3C)_2$ C = CF_2	0.5

concentrations in parts per million by volume represent the lowest concentration which proved lethal for any of the rats exposed; this concentration is known as the Approximate Lethal Concentration. It is considered a reliable estimate of the LC_{50}.

Fluoropolymers, the third group for consideration in this paper are virtually inert at room temperature. However, because they are resistant to chemical attack and thermal degradation, they are widely used where this resistivity is a desideratum. However, the "breaking point" may be reached and decomposition can occur. It is thus the toxicity of the decomposition products which are of concern with fluoropolymers.

In any discussion of fluorocarbon toxicity, the question immediately arises as to the relative standing of monofluoroacetate and other monofluorinated compounds whose metabolic endpoint is monofluoroacetate. The biochemistry of fluoroacetate toxicity has been well worked out. It is the subject of several reviews (1, 2, and 3). Briefly, this extensive work has shown that the C-F bond of fluoroacetate is not dehalogenated in mammalian systems but passes unchanged into the tricarboxylic acid cycle to fluorocitrate where steric hindrance evidently blocks the enzyme aconitase thus interfering with the conversion to aconitate and resulting in the accumulation of fluorocitrate. This widespread metabolic blockage would seem to be the underlying cause of the high mammalian toxicity of fluoroacetate. However, there is still speculation as to the connection between the metabolic interference and the pharmacologic response. Pattison and Peters (2) propose one idea, namely, citrate accumulation may disturb neural membrane equilibrium of divalent ions producing lower membrane potentials and an excitable system. Whether or not this would explain other phenomena caused by fluoroacetate remains for the results of experimental work.

For the other fluorocarbons covered in this chapter, very little is known at present about the biochemical mechanisms of action. There has been, however, significant progress recently in our knowledge of the toxicology of polyfluorinated compounds; studies on mechanism are sure to follow.

Toxicity of Fluoroalkanes

Acute inhalation toxicity data for three groups of fluoromethanes are shown in Table II. Much of this work was conducted by the Underwriter's Laboratories to investigate fluoroalkanes as refrigerants. The objective of this work was to evaluate the hazard attendant upon the leakage of refrigerant into a kitchen. The historical perspectives of this and other early toxicity work have been reviewed by Clayton (4). This early work could be termed taxonomic toxicology, the assignment of compounds to categories on the basis of lethality.

TABLE II: INHALATION TOXICITY OF FLUOROMETHANES

		EXPOSURE				
Group	*Structure*	*Concentration (%)*	*Time (hr)*	*Fatality*	*Class**	*TLV***
A	$CHCl_3$	2.0	2	Yes	3	50
	$CHCl_2F$	10.0	1	Yes	4-5	1000
	$CHClF_2$	20.0	2	No	5a	(1000)
	CHF_3	20.0	2	No	6***	(1000)
B	CCl	2.0	2	Yes	3	10
	CCl_3F	10.0	2	No	5a	1000
	CCl_2F_2	20.0	2	No	6	1000
	$CClF_3$	20.0	2	No	6***	(1000)
	CF_4	20.0	2	No	6***	(1000)
C	CH_3Cl	2.0	2	Yes	4	100
	CH_2Cl_2	5.0	2	Yes	4-5	500
	$CHCl_2F$	10.0	1	Yes	4-5	1000
	CCl_2F_2	20.0	2	No	6	1000

*Classified according to Underwriters' classification. The higher the value the lower the toxicity.
**TLV, threshold limit value assigned by the American Confernce of Governmental Industrial Hygienists, 1968 values. Figures in parentheses indicate provisional values.
***Based on data from Haskell Laboratory.

As toxicity data became available, a general principle emerged. As with other generalities in biological science, special cases defy the generalization. The data assembled in Table II illustrate the principle that a lower degree of toxicity corresponds to an increasing number of fluorine atoms in the molecule. All three groups in this table reveal this, but the most striking example is evident in group B, which compares CCl_4 with CF_4. The influence of fluorine and its interactions with other atoms in the molecule are also clear. The contrasting toxicities of $CHCl_3$ and $CHCl_2F$ (group A) show that the substitution of even a single F atom for Cl effects a strong lowering of toxicity in the chlorofluoroalkane. To hazard a guess at mechanism, it may be inferred that enhancement of the stability of the Cl atoms by the C-F bond imposes an intractability to enzymatic dehalogenation, with concomitant lower toxicity. Dehalogenation could be an important aspect in the mechanism of fluorocarbon and chlorocarbon toxicity. For example, Slater (5), proposed that CCl_4 is metabolized by homolytic bond scission to a toxic, free radical, which could be responsible for hepatotoxicity. It is plausible that the same mechanism could account for biological activity of other fluoroalkanes, with addition of F resulting in decreased C-Cl bond rupture. Addition of further F atoms in group A shows continued decline in toxicity. Group B provides similar evidence of this stabilizing force of F vis à vis Cl in the methane series. Group C shows another feature relating to the principle under discussion, the interaction of hydrogen, fluorine and chlorine. The substitution of Cl for H appears to lower toxicity; compare CH_3Cl with CH_2Cl_2. However, further chlorination (viz. $CHCl_3$; CCl_4) yields compounds as toxic as CH_3Cl. The replacement of H with F in CH_2Cl_2 and $CHCl_2F$ to give $CHCl_2F$ and CCl_2F_2, respectively, also results in lowered toxicity. Thus, while increasing the Cl complement sometimes decreases toxicity, fluorine is far more effective than chlorine.

Discussing the toxicity of halogenated compounds, Chenoweth and McCarty (6) cite evidence that the fugitive halogen is not the toxic agent. For example, the displacement by enzymatic dehalogenation of Br from CH_3Br results in methylation of methionine and other sulfur containing compounds in vivo, thereby producing toxic effects. In this regard, CH_3Cl is not as active as CH_3Br; as would be anticipated, CH_3F is least active of the three. Thus, toxicologically the order is $CH_3Br > CH_3Cl > CH_3F$. Fluorination evidently imparts a resistance to dehalogenation, thus shielding the toxophoric part of the molecule.

A correspondence of low toxicity with increasing fluorination is disclosed by inhalation experiments with fluoroalkanes of longer chain length. Table III summarizes relevant data on fluoroethanes, several having a chlorine complement, and Table IV depicts, for fluoroethane, the comparative roles of Cl and Br (compare $CH_2Cl\text{-}CF_3$ with $CH_2Br\text{-}CF_3$). In the same table, the relation of H and F is evident from the comparison of $CH_2Cl\text{-}CF_3$ with $CH_2Cl\text{-}CHF_2$ and $CH_2Br\text{-}CF_3$ with $CH_2Br\text{-}CHF_2$.

TABLE III: ACUTE INHALATION TOXICITY OF SEVERAL FLUOROETHANES

Structure	*ALC** *(% by volume)*	*Exposure (hr.)*	*Animal*
$CCl_2F\text{-}CCl_2F$	1.5	4	Rat
$CClF_2\text{-}CCl_3$	1.5	4	Rat
$CCl_2F\text{-}CClF_2$	10	4	Rat
$CClF_2\text{-}CClF_2$	> 20	8	Guinea Pig
$CHCl_2\text{-}CF_3$	3.5**	4	Rat
$CClF_2\text{-}CHF_2$	> 20	2	Guinea Pig
$CClF_2\text{-}CF_3$	> 80***	4	Rat
$CHF_2\text{-}CF_3$	> 10	4	Rat
$CF_3\text{-}CF_3$	> 80***	4	Rat

*ALC, approximate lethal concentration.
**LC_{50}.
***Fluorocarbon, 80%; oxygen, 20%.

TABLE IV: COMPARISON OF BROMINE AND CHLORINE IN THE ACUTE INHALATION TOXICITY OF FLUOROETHANES

Compound	*Lethal Concentration** *(% by volume)*
$CH_2Cl\text{-}CF_3$	25.0
$CH_2Cl\text{-}CHF_2$	7.5
$CH_2Br\text{-}CF_3$	11.7
$CH_2Br\text{-}CHF_2$	4.6

*Mice were exposed for 10 minutes.

Fluoroalkanes affect the central nervous system and the responses in animals to inhaled fluoroalkanes run the gamut from anesthesia to convulsions. Robbins (7) conducted systematic studies on a large number of fluorinated ethanes for the purpose of discovering a safe, nonflammable anesthetic. Emerging from this work was the discovery of halothane, $CF_3\text{-}CHBrCl$. Dishart (8) later examined the anesthetic properties of fluorinated propanes. He showed that compounds with more than four fluorine atoms are poor anesthetics. Not only were high concentrations required to cause signs of anesthesia in mice but these compounds often produced convulsions. For example, Dishart (8) found satisfactory anesthetic effects with $HCF_2\text{-}CF_2\text{-}CH_2Cl$, however with a higher degree of fluorination or decrease in H, as with $HCF_2\text{-}CF_2\text{-}CH_2F$ or with $HCF_2\text{-}CF_2\text{-}CF_2Cl$, mice experienced convulsive seizures and toxic effects were evident. Completely fluorinated compounds are virtually inactive biologically. Inclusion of other halogens changes this.

There have been some reports of the effects of inhalation of fluoroalkanes on humans. Largent (9) reported that 15% by volume of dichlorodifluoromethane can inducc unconsciousness in humans exposed for a few minutes. A concentration of 5% can cause dizziness.

Stopps and McLaughlin (10) studied the responses of humans exposed to trichlorotrifluoroethane, $CCl_2F\text{-}CClF_2$. The plan of their experiments is given in Table V. The battery of tests consisted of two manual dexterity tests, sorting of

TABLE V: HUMAN EXPOSURES TO TRICHLOROTRIFLUOROETHANE TIMETABLE OF EXPERIMENT

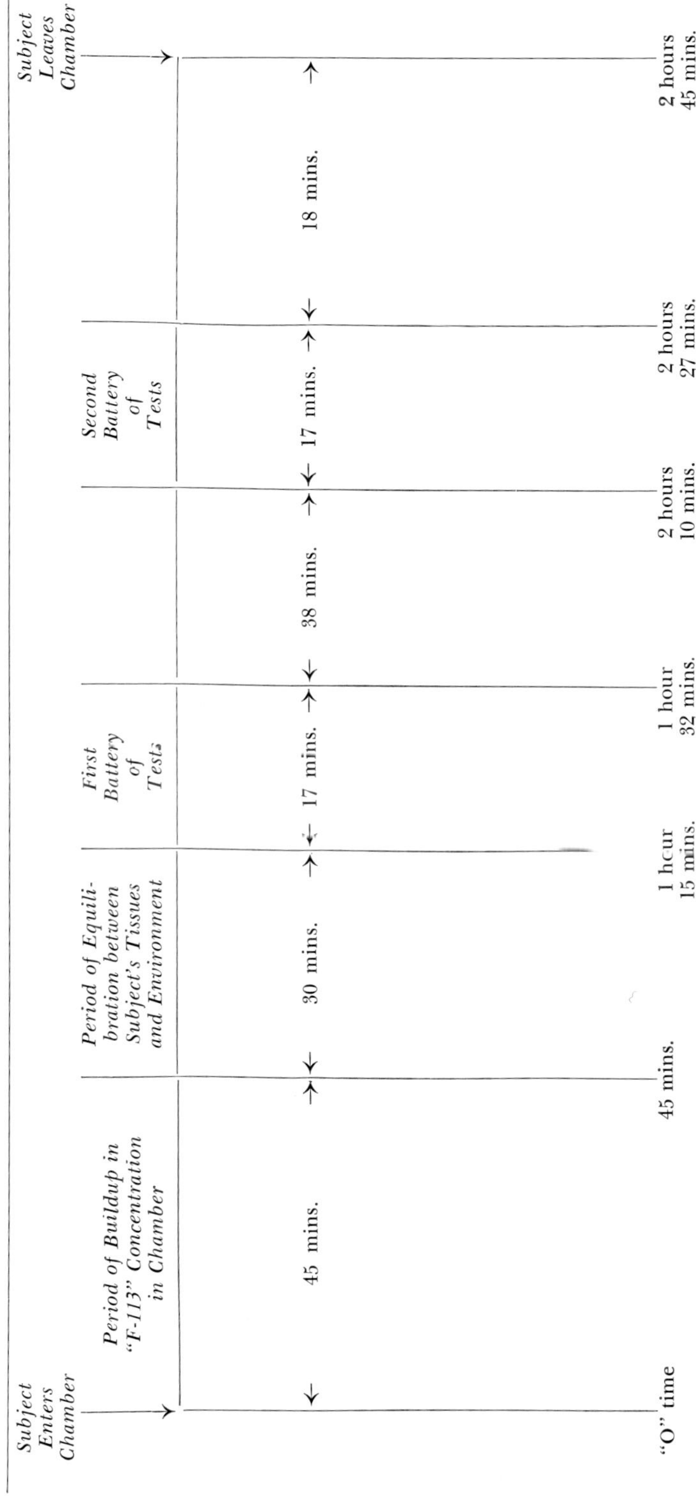

playing cards into suits with and without the auxiliary task of adding a series of three, single digit numbers, and a clerical test in which the subject was asked to code a series of names against a financial balance. In Table VI are recorded the effects observed at the exposure concentrations. Card sorting with the auxiliary task proved a sensitive test in this work. These same authors also investigated the effects on humans of inhaling trichloroethylene. At 500 ppm, there were definite signs of decreased test performance; at 300 ppm the decrement was slight; and at 100 ppm or 200 ppm the scores were within the control range. On the basis of these experiments, it appears that trichloroethylene has a similar effect on psychomotor performance but is an order of magnitude more active in this respect than trichlorotrifluoroethane. Similarly, tetrachloroethylene would appear to be more active than trichlorotrifluoroethane as judged from experiments reported by Rowe, *et al.* (11) and Stewart *et al.* (12).

TABLE VI: EFFECTS ON PSYCHOMOTOR PERFORMANCE BY PERSONS INHALING TRICHLOROTRIFLUOROETHANE

Concentration (ppm)	*(Exposure Time — 2.75 hrs.)* *Performance (Test Results)*	*Subjective Signs*
4500	Reduction in manual dexterity, card sorting and clerical tests.	Loss in ability to concentrate. Tendency to somnolence.
3500	Moderate reduction in test performance.	Same as above.
2500	Slight reduction in test performance.	Same as above.
1500	No effect on test performance.	None reported.

It has been known for some time that certain hydrocarbons, notably cyclopropane among inhalation anesthetics, can make the heart muscle highly reactive to epinephrine, resulting in arrhythmic contractions. Krantz and Rudo (13) note that several halogenated alkenes possess this property, in addition to many straight chain and cyclic hydrocarbons. Perfluorinated compounds studied by these workers were inactive, but the chlorinated ones were active. Among the fluoroalkanes, recent work at Haskell Laboratory has shown that dogs inhaling $CBrF_3$ (5-10% by volume) or CCl_2F-$CClF_2$ (0.5-1.0%) evidenced increased ventricular action after intravenous injection of epinephrine. The degree of cardiac response was directly related to the concentration of the alkane inhaled and the dosage of epinephrine injected.

In summary, the dominant clinical response to inhaled fluoroalkanes is neurological in character, varying from anesthetic to convulsive reactions. When death occurred in animal studies, the principle anatomic finding was pulmonary injury. In humans, early signs of response are dizziness and loss of ability to concentrate, ultimately unconsciousness may occur. The concentrations causing the reaction vary with the compound. In general, fluorocarbons are less active than chlorocarbons. The degree of fluorination appears to be related inversely to the reactions in the central nervous system, as indicated by the clinical signs. In comparison to the chlorinated hydrocarbons, the fluorinated series shows almost no hepatotoxicity, Clayton (4).

The reasons at the cellular level for the low activity of the fluoroalkanes on the liver, especially in compounds where there is a high degree of fluorination, are not apparent from the investigations cited. This remains an important area for further studies in this group. One such attempt is the work of Slater *et al.* (14), who have studied alterations in lipid metabolism and mitochondrial respiratory activity induced in the rat liver by CCl_4 and CCl_3F. Slater has demonstrated that the concentrations of nicotinamide adenine dinucleotides in the rat liver are changed by 1.25 ml of CCl_4 per kg orally (NADP increased; NADPH falls; NAD and NADH are unchanged). These events did not follow dosing with the antihistaminic, Phenergan, which prevents liver necrosis, thus indicating that these features are related in some direct manner with necrogenesis. Slater (15) found that CCl_3F did not produce necrotic livers or the changes in nicotinamide-adenine dinucleotides. Neither was there an escape of beta-glucuronidase with CCl_3F as there was with CCl_4, where increased permeability of the hepatocyte membrane may be inferred by the leakage of various enzymes into the blood. It is known that CCl_4 is dehalogenated and reduced in part to $CHCl_3$. Butler (16) postulated that naturally occurring sulfhydryl compounds may be involved in the reduction of CCl_4 via homolytic cleavage of the C-Cl bond and free radical formation. The resulting deficiency of sulfhydryl compounds may be directly related to hepatocyte damage. In contrast, the fact that CCl_3F did not produce hepatic necrosis in Slater's work (15) may be connected with the stabilizing influence of the C-F bond which makes the C-Cl bonds refractory to homolytic cleavage. Gregory (17) has proposed that halogenated alkanes, notably CCl_4 and $CHCl_3$, interfere *in vivo* with electron transfer reactions. The bonding of exogenous, free radicals (e.g., $Cl_3C^\bullet$) with enzymes could block the normal electron transfer reactions (Fig. 1) to yield an inactivated enzyme (Fig. 2). It may be inferred that fluorocarbons, even those containing chlorine, would not be as easily dehalogenated thus limiting the possibility of free radical formation from homolytic cleavage of the carbon-halogen bond. However, other factors such as rate of uptake, rate of excretion, solubility in cellular lipids and cellular entry need to be investigated for fluoroalkanes before it can be concluded that increased bond stability accounts for the low hepatotoxicity of these compounds.

Summaries of inhalation toxicity data of several fluoroalkenes are found in Tables VII and VIII. A wide range is readily apparent in Table VII; while it may seem that toxicity values in this class are inversely related to the number of fluorine atoms, inadequate knowledge at present obviates any such conclusion. It is more likely that some biological action related to the double bond is predominantly responsible for, for example, the high toxicity of PFIB, rather than its complement of eight fluorine atoms *per se*.

Generally, fluorinated alkenes are less toxic than their chlorinated counterparts. A direct relationship between toxicity and number of chlorine atoms is illustrated by the sequence signifying acute inhalation toxicity: $CCl_2 = CCl_2 >$ $CHCl = CCl_2 > CH_2 = CCl_2 > CH_2 =$ $CHCl$.

Illustrative of fluoroalkenes of relatively low toxicity are $CH_2 = CHF$ and

ENZYMATIC ELECTRON TRANSFER REACTION

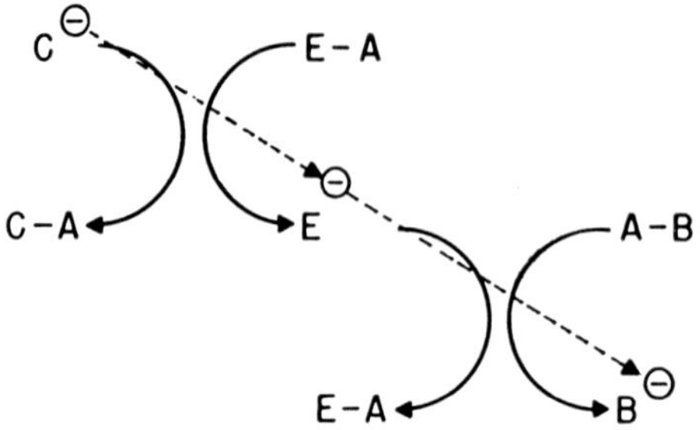

Electron Path: metabolite C ⟶
enzyme E ⟶
metabolite B

E–A = Enzyme with intermediary group

Fig.1

POSTULATED ELECTRON TRANSFER MECHANISM IN CARBON TETRACHLORIDE TOXICITY

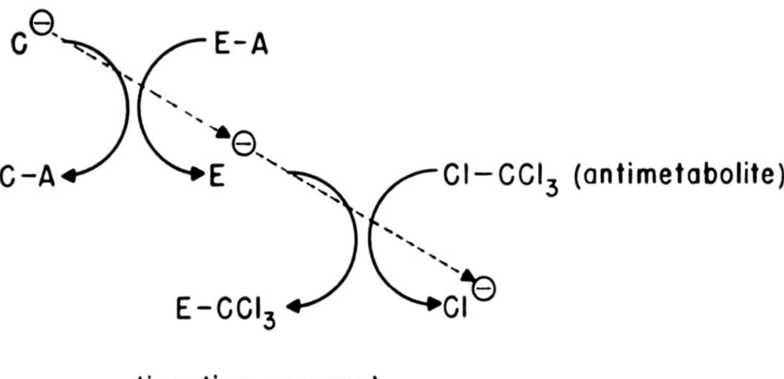

Fig.2

$CH_2 = CF_2$. Lester and Greenberg (18) reported no organ damage to rats exposed to 80% of $CH_2 = CHF$. For $CH_2 = CHF$, Limperos (unpublished data) repeatedly exposed male and female rats to 100,000 ppm, 7 hr per day, 5 days a week for 30 exposures. There were no fatalities; rats gained weight normally and showed no behavioral changes and no tissue changes as evaluated by microscopic examination.

TABLE VII: INHALATION TOXICITY OF SEVERAL FLUOROALKENES

Structure	*No. of F Atoms*	*Acute Toxicity for Rats** *ALC (ppm)*	*LC_{50}*
$CH_2 = CHF$	1	> 800,000**	
$CF_2 = CH_2$	2	128,000	
		> 800,000***	
$CF_2 = CF_2$	4		40,000
CF_3-$CF = CF_2$	6		3,000
$(CF_3)_2 = C = CF_2$	8	0.5, 0.76****	

*Exposures are for 4 hour duration except where noted. ALC, approximate lethal concentration. LC_{50}, lethal concentration for 50% of rats exposed.
**$CH_2 = CHF$, 80%; O_2, 20%; 12.5 hour exposure.
***$CH_2 = CF_2$, 80%; O_2, 20%; 19 hour exposure.
****Exposure at 0.5 ppm, 6 hour; at 0.76 ppm, 4 hour.

Fluoralkenes of moderate to slight toxicity may be exemplified by tetrafluoroethylene (TFE), hexafluoropropylene (HFP) and chlorotrifluoroethylene (CTFE). These compounds are irritating to the respiratory tract in lethal concentrations as judged by animal exposures, but in addition they also can cause kidney injury. Single exposures of rats to varying concentrations of chlorotrifluoroethylene have produced physiological evidence of kidney dysfunction.

TABLE VIII: INHALATION TOXICITY OF SEVERAL HALOGENATED ALKENES

Structure	*No. of Atoms* F	Cl	*Acute Toxicity for Rats** *ALC (ppm)*	*LC_{50}*
$CCl_2 = CH_2$	0	2	32,000	
$CHCl = CCl_2$	0	3	8,000	
$CCl_2 = CCl_2$	0	4	4,000	
$CCl_2 = CF_2$	2	2	1,000	
$CClF = CF_2$	3	1		1,000

*Exposures of 4-hour duration. ALC, approximate lethal concentration. LC_{50}, lethal concentration for 50% of rats exposed.

An increased level of toxicity in the fluoroalkenes is shown by 2,3-dichloro-1,1,1,4,4,4-hexafluorobutene-2 (DCHFB), which was a trace contaminant in halothane anesthetic and suspected of causing postoperative hepatic necrosis. Chenoweth (unpublished data) showed that DCHFB was lethal for rats in a 4-hour exposure at 100 ppm, but that some rats survived 100-ppm exposure of 1- or 2-hour duration. Response of the rats in the lethal exposures was consistent with pulmonary irritation. Pulmonary congestion and edema were observed post mortem. Gross changes in the kidney and liver were also observed. In another study, this author also observed fatalities in rats from severe injury to lungs, liver and kidney on inhaling DCHFB for 4 hours at 50 ppm. In experiments conducted by Cohen *et al.* (19), 85 male rats were exposed to DCHFB for 3-hour periods. Results indicated an LC_{50} of approximately 50 ppm, with 100% fatalities at 105 ppm. Death was from respiratory injury and occurred in 6 to 24 hours at 840 ppm, and was delayed from 4 to 14 days after exposures as low as 52 ppm. The rats exposed to the higher concentrations of DCHFB showed acute hemorrhagic changes in the lungs, while the groups exposed to 105 to 210 ppm showed a healing interstitial pneumonitis and central lobular necrosis of the liver.

Raventós and Lemon (20) have investigated in mice, rats, rabbits, monkeys and dogs the acute inhalation toxicity of several fluoroalkenes which have been found as trace contaminants in halothane. These authors confirm the high order of toxicity of DCHFB (4-hr LC_{50}: rats, 16 ppm; mice, 26 ppm; dogs, 182 ppm; monkeys (3-hr) 90 ppm). In spite of these differences in quantitative toxicity, the pathological changes in the lungs were quite uniform among the various species studied. The pulmonary reaction was evident as dyspnea and cyanosis during or after exposure. Histology disclosed only pulmonary congestion and edema. Unlike the report of hepatotoxicity of DCHFB by Cohen *et al.* (19), Raventós and Lemon (20) observed no significant liver change; renal lesions (small thromboses in glomerular capillaries, vacuolation and degenerative changes in the first part of the proximal tubules and increase in the number of colloid casts) were observed only in a few rats inhaling 330 to 550 ppm for 1 hour.

The reports of Cohen *et al.* (19) and Raventós and Lemon (20) are contradictory in that the former report hepatotoxicity for DCHFB whereas the latter conclude no such change. Also, there are evidently significant differences in toxicity between the *cis* and *trans* isomers of CF_3-CCl = CCl-CF_3 and CF_3-CH = CCl-CF_3. These questions need clarification. On balance, it appears that these fluoroalkenes have a relatively low hepatotoxic potential and as such would seem not to contribute significantly to the above-mentioned postoperative hepatic disease observed in rare cases following halothane anesthesia.

The most toxic of all fluoroalkenes thus far studies is perfluorisobutylene (PFIB). In Table VII are shown the acute inhalation toxicity data of PFIB compared with other fluoroalkenes. PFIB is a potent pulmonary irritant approximately 10 times as toxic as phosgene. Repeated exposures of four male rats to 0.1 ppm PFIB 4 hours a day for 10 days were not lethal. During the exposures, the rats were occasionally restless and had respiratory impairment. The latter was not severe, although it sometimes proceeded to cyanosis, and two rats developed moist rales. There were occasional losses of body weight by two rats during the first week of exposure only, but these were not marked, and the curve of body weights was close to normal. Pathology disclosed no tissue change assignable to PFIB, and the weights of the major organs were not altered by the exposure.

Toxicity of Fluoropolymers

In discussing the toxicity of fluoropolymers, there are two major questions. One pertains to the toxicity of the unheated resin; the other, to the toxicity of the heated polymer. The second has become more important because the high thermal stability of most fluoropolymers, notably polytetrafluoroethylene, means that these are subjected to heating as part of the normal use pattern.

Regarding the first category, tetrafluoroethylene polymer (TFE) and the copolymer of TFE and HFP (FEP resin) have been shown to have a very low order of oral toxicity. In studies at Haskell Laboratory, a dietary level of 25% Teflon TFE resin fed to male and female rats for 90 days was required to elicit even a minimal response. In this 90-day feeding study on three types of Teflon TFE resin, there were no adverse effects on growth rate or behavior of the rats, nor was there microscopic evidence of tissue change. The slight response observed was a shift in the distribution and number of white blood cells and, in one group fed unsintered Teflon 6 TFE resin, an increase in the relative size of the liver, relative to body weight. This was not accompanied by any histological abnormality.

Studies on the toxicity of the pyrolysis products of tetrafluoroethylene (TFE) resins have been conducted at Haskell Laboratory over a period of almost 25 years. Zapp *et al.* (21) reported the inhalation toxicity of pyrolysis products of Teflon 1 and 6 resins, and Clayton *et al.* (22) extended the work to include comparison of steel and glass systems, filtration of effluent materials, and studies on wire insulation materials. A summary of these investigations is included in the reviews published by Clayton (23) and Zapp (24). Recent work has been reported by Waritz and Kwon (25). From these experiments with a variety of mammalian species, it can be concluded that there is little difference in response among rodent-like species. This is true not only from the mortality ratios, but also from the reactions elicited which indicated that the only injury was to the respiratory tract (rapid, shallow respiration, pallor, pulmonary congestion, and edema), with no histological effects on other organs discerned.

Without going into detail about the several fluorocarbon effluents given off by Teflon TFE resin at various temperatures, it has been known for some time that particulate material is an important component toxicologically, Zapp *et al.* (21). Subsequently, it was demonstrated by Clayton *et al.* (22) that there was a positive correlation between the amount of particulate given off by Teflon resin and mortality (Table IX). Waritz and Kwon (25) have confirmed these findings.

Similarly, when the particulate effluent is filtered out, toxicity of the pyrolysis products is strikingly reduced. In early work, rats survived lethal exposure conditions when products from Teflon 6 resin were first passed through cellulose filters (0.1, 2.0, and 5.0 μ pore size). This finding was confirmed by Clayton *et al.* (22), who sufficiently heated Teflon 6 resin to give products lethal for rats

TABLE IX: TOXICITY OF PYROLYSIS PRODUCTS OF TEFLON 6 RESIN IN RELATION TO PARTICULATE EVOLUTION

Sample	*Particulate Evolved in 4-hr,*	*% Mortality, Pyrolysis Temperature*	
No.	*mg/m³*	*300° C*	*350° C*
1	2.8	25	100
2	*	63	—
3	2.0	—	100
4	1.8	—	100
5	*	—	0
6	1.4	—	25
7	0.7	0	6
8	0.6	—	0

*Sample not analyzed.

and passed the effluent through a millipore filter (0.45 μ pore size) located up stream from an exposure chamber containing rats. A striking reduction in mortality resulted, as shown by Table X.

TABLE X: RAT MORTALITY RESULTING FROM EXPOSURES TO FILTERED PYROLYSIS PRODUCTS OF TEFLON 6 (PORE SIZE, 0.45 μ)

No. Rats	*Pyrolysis Temp., °C*	*Mortality* Ratio	*Mortality* % Observed	*Mortality* % Expected*
12	350	0:12	0	100
8	350	0:8	0	100
4	350	0:4	0	100
4	325	0:4	0	38
4	325	0:4	0	38

*On the basis of results obtained in experiments under the same conditions but without the use of filters.

The results of these animal studies demonstrate the low-life hazard involved in the use of Teflon resins. However, there was the proviso that animal experiments did not permit an evaluation of the human reaction of polymer fume fever, the "shakes." As a matter of history, the latter has occurred when TFE resins are heated to 370-430° C in sintering operations or to a maximum of 540° C in burning tobacco with subsequent inhalation of the products of thermal decomposition. Clinically, polymer fume fever is a temporary attack of chills and fever accompanied by an increase in the circulating white blood cells. After the attack, in about 24-48 hours, the symptoms wear off and there are no evident deleterious sequelae. No effects in humans other than polymer fume fever have been clearly attributable to TFE resins.

Polymer fume fever, so far, is unique to resins of tetrafluoroethylene. The first account in the literature was published by Harris (26). The symptoms he recorded are listed in Table XI.

Because of the need to know more about the quantitative aspects of polymer fume fever, Dr. A. M. Kligman in 1962 conducted a study in which human volunteers smoked one or more cigarettes

TABLE XI: SYMPTOMS OF POLYMER FUME FEVER

Symptoms Noted	*Comment*
1. Latent period	Often a few hours
2. Gradual increase in temperature	Does not exceed 104° F
3. Increase in pulse	Generally below 120
4. Increase in respiration rate	
5. Scattered rales in chest	Appears in most severe cases
6. Chest discomfort	Irritation or oppression retrosternally
7. Dry irritating cough	Worsens with chest soreness
8. Shivering attack	
9. Sweating	
10. Mild leucocytosis	First few hours

to which known amounts of a TFE fluorocarbon telomer had been added. The results of smoking a single contaminated cigarette (phase I) are shown in Table XII. The amount of fluorocarbon eliciting a typical polymer fume fever response was 0.40 mg in a single cigarette and 9 of 10 smokers reported typical symptoms. The average maximum body temperature is shown in Table XII. For the group smoking the contaminant level of 0.40 mg, body temperature showed an increase. The change in pulse rate, Table XII, is also suggestive of a change in this group.

TABLE XII: EFFECTS ON HUMANS SMOKING A SINGLE CIGARETTE CONTAINING FLUOROCARBON TELOMER *(Average of 10 Subjects)*

	Body Temp., °F		*Pulse Rate*		
Flurocarbon Telomer, mg	*Before Smoking*	*After Smoking Max.*	*Before Smoking*	*After Smoking Max.*	*Polymer Fume Fever*
0.05	98.2	98.6	77	83	—
0.10	98.1	98.7	81	91	—
0.20	98.1	98.5	77	87	—
0.40*	98.1	100.5	75	99	+

*Average of 9 subjects.

Phase II of this work involved 10 volunteers each smoking up to 10 cigarettes, each of which contained 0.05 mg of added fluorocarbon telomer. Table XIII presents the results, from which it is seen that 4 of the 10 smokers (subjects 2, 3, 7, and 8), after 6 or 8 cigarettes, clearly contracted polymer fume fever, as illustrated by the symptoms and change in pulse and temperature measurements. Four others experienced a slight attack and the remaining two reported no adverse effects. The cumulative amount of resin needed in the four well-defined cases was 0.30-0.40 mg, agreeing well with the 0.40 mg needed on a single cigarette (phase I) to elicit the response. The order of events recorded for phase II differs somewhat from that in phase I. In the latter a cough was reported first by a majority of the subjects, whereas in the former the 4 subjects (2, 3, 7, and 8) reported chills first. It may be that initial respiratory tract irritation was averted in phase II as a result of a lower concentration of irritant substances while the cumulative amount of reactive material was sufficient to produce the febrile com-

TABLE XIII: EFFECTS ON HUMANS SMOKING 10 CIGARETTES EACH CONTAINING 0.05 MG FLUOROCARBON TELOMER

			Temp. Measurements			*Pulse Rate Measurements*					
Subject No.	*Time of Smoking Cigarettes, A.M.-P.M.*	*No. Cigarettes Smoked*	*Before Smoking*	*After First Cigarette, Max.*	*Hr. at Max.*	*Before Smoking*	*After First Cigarette, Max.*	*Hr. at Max.*	*Onset Hr.*	*Clinical Symptoms Reported*	*Return to "Normal," Hr.*
1	9:20-2:55	10	98.6	98.6	3.0	96	88	6.0	—	No adverse symptoms	—
2	9:20-2:10	8	98.4	103.0	6.0	88	112	9.5	5.0	Chills, dizzy, headache, eyes "burning," feverish, malaise, weakness	12.5
3	9:20-11:50 (A.M.)	6	98.6	102.0	5.0	92	100	1.0	3.0	Chills, weakness, malaise, dizzy, legs weak, stiffness in arms and legs	11.5
4	9:20-3:15	10	98.0	99.0	4.0	60	96	4.0	5.0	Slight headache	6.0
5	9:20-3:05	10	98.4	98.4	1.0	84	84	5.0	—	No adverse reaction	—
6	9:20-3:28	10	98.0	98.6	2.5	68	80	9.5	4.5	Slight headache	5.5
7	9:30-12:22	6	98.6	101.2	5.5	96	108	5.5	3.5	Chills, headache, weakness, stomach upset, feverish	7.5
8	9:30-12:15	6	97.6	99.4	5.5	72	124	5.5	3.5	Chills, headache, malaise, leg pains	7.5
9	9:20:3:22	10	97.4	99.2	6.5	60	96	5.5	4.5	Slight headache, slight sotmach and chest pain	11.5
10	9:30-3:20	10	98.0	99.4	2.5	76	112	2.5	2.5	Mouth dry, headache	7.5
Over-all means		8.6	98.2	99.9	4.2	79.2	100.0	5.4	3.9*		8.7*
Means for subjects**		6.5	98.3	101.4	5.5	87.0	111.0	5.4	3.8		9.8

*Mean of 8 values. **2, 3, 7, & 8.

ponent. It is important to relate this difference in symptomatology to the practical situation. The particular sequence of symptoms does not relate specifically to polymer fume fever, e.g., the absence of cough does not preclude a diagnosis of polymer fume fever. The total clinical picture must be considered with reliance on objective measurements of body temperature, pulse rate, and white blood count. In addition, because the symptoms are characteristic of viral infections, it is important to establish whether or not inhalation exposure to a fluorocarbon polymer was involved in the episode. This means an industrial hygiene survey to investigate presumed causative agents.

To elucidate the biomechanism of polymer fume fever, in the usual course of events it would be subjected to laboratory investigation by producing it in experimental animals. By exploring variables of pyrolysis temperature, exposure duration, travel path, and others, and by analyzing the products evolved when polymer fume fever was elicited, the causative agent (s) could be identified and studied, and then a safe exposure level for humans could be estimated. Unfortunately, to date, polymer fume fever has not been reliably produced in experimental animals, although there have been slight changes in the rectal temperature and the number of white blood cells in guinea pigs inhaling pyrolysis products of TFE resin.

REFERENCES

1. Pattison, F. L. M.: Toxic Aliphatic Fluorine Compounds. Elsevier Publishing Company, 1959.
2. Pattison, F. L. M., and Peters, R. A.: Monofluoro Aliphatic Compounds, Handbuch der Experimentellen Pharmakologie, Vol. XX (O. Eichler, A. Farah, H. Herken, and A. D. Welch, eds.) . Springer, Berlin, 1966.
3. Saunders, B. C.: Some Aspects of the Chemistry and Toxic Action of Organic Compounds Containing Phosphorus and Fluorine. Cambridge University Press, 1957.
4. Clayton, J. W.: Fluorocarbon toxicity and biological action. Fluorine Chem. Rev., *1* (2) : 197-252, 1967.
5. Slater, T. F.: Necrogenic action of carbon tetrachloride in the rat: A speculative mechanism based on activation. Nature (Lond.) , *36:*209, 1966.
6. Chenoweth, M. B., and McCarty, L. P.: On the mechanism of the pharmacophoric effect of halogenation. Pharmacol. Rev., *15:*673, 1963.
7. Robbins, B. H.: Preliminary studies on the anesthetic activity of the fluorinated hydrocarbons. J. Pharmacol. Exp. Ther., *86:*197, 1946.
8. Dishart, K. T.: The Synthesis and Evaluation of Some New Fluorinated Inhalation Anesthetics. Paper presented at the Meeting of the American Chemical Society, Chicago, 1961.
9. Largent, E. J., and Largent, K. W.: The hygienic aspects of fluorine and its compounds. Amer. J. Pub. Health, *45:*198, 1955.
10. Stopps, G. J., and McLaughlin, M.: Psychophysiological testing of human subjects exposed to solvent vapor. Amer. Ind. Hyg. Assoc. J., *28:*43, 1967.
11. Rowe, V. K., McCollister, D. D., Spencer, H. C., Adams, E. M., and Irish, D. D.: Vapor toxicity of tetrachloroethylene for laboratory animals and human subjects. AMA Arch. Ind. Hyg., *5:* 566-579, 1952.
12. Stewart, R. D., Gay, H. H., Erley, D. S., Hake, C. L., and Schaffer, A. W.: Human exposure to tetrachloroethylene vapor. AMA Arch. Environ, Health, *2:*516, 1961.
13. Krantz, J. C., and Rudo, F. G.: The Fluorinated Anesthetics, Handbuch der Experimentellen Pharmakologie, Vol. XX, (O. Eichler, A. Farah, H. Herken, and A. D. Welch, eds.) . Springer, Berlin, 1966.
14. Slater, T. F., Straüli, U. D., and Sawyer, B. C.: Changes in liver nucleotide concentrations in experimental liver injury: I. Carbon tetrachloride poisoning. Biochem. J., *93:*260, 1964.
15. Slater, T. F.: A note on the relative toxic activities of tetrachloromethane and trichlorofluoromethane on the rat. Biochem. Pharmacol., *14:* 178, 1965.
16. Butler, T. D.: Reduction of carbon tetrachloride *in vivo* and reduction of carbon tetrachloride and chloroform *in vitro* by tissues and tissue constituents. J. Pharmacol. Exp. Therap., *134:* 311, 1961.
17. Gregory, N. L.: Carbon tetrachloride toxicity and electron capture. Nature (Lond.) , *212:*1460, 1966.

18. Lester, D., and Greenberg, L. A.: Acute and chronic toxicity of some halogenated derivatives of methane and ethane. Arch. Indust. Hyg. & Occupat. Med., 2:335, 1950.
19. Cohen, E. N., Brewer, H. W., Bellville, J. W., and Sher, R.: The chemistry and toxicology of dichlorohexafluorobutene. Anesthesiology, *26:* 140, 1965.
20. Raventós, J., and Lemon, P. G.: The impurities in fluothane: Their biological properties. Brit. J. Anesth., *37:*716, 1965.
21. Zapp, J. A., Limperos, G., and Brinker, K. C.: Toxicity of Pyrolysis Products of "Teflon" Tetrafluoroethylene Resin. Paper presented at the American Industrial Hygiene Association Meeting, Buffalo, N.Y., 1955.
22. Clayton, J. W., Hood, D. B., and Raynsford, G. E.: The Toxicity of Pyrolysis Products of "Teflon" TFE-Fluorocarbon Resins. Paper presented at the American Industrial Hygiene Association Meeting, Chicago, 1959.
23. Clayton, J. W.: The toxicity of fluorocarbons with special reference to chemical constitution. J. Occupat. Med., *4:*262, 1962.
24. Zapp, J. A.: Toxic and health effects of plastics and resins. Arch. Environ. Health, *4:*335, 1962.
25. Waritz, R. S., and Kwon, B. K.: The inhalation toxicity of pyrolysis products of polytetrafluoroethylene heated below 500 degrees centigrade. Am. Indust. Hyg. Assoc. J., *29:*19-26, 1968.
26. Harris, D. K.: Polymer-fume fever. Lancet, *2:* 1008, 1951.

Chapter 21B

Determination of Fluoride in Urine by Fluoride Electrode

FRANKLIN D. GRIFFITH, PH.D. and JOHN R. BARNES, PH.D.

INTRODUCTION

The electrode may be used to determine fluoride content of samples if pH, ionic strength, temperature, and interferring ions are controlled. This procedure uses 0.25 M citrate buffer to control pH, to minimize differences in ionic strength and to chelate interferring ions. Samples and standards are read at room temperature.

PRINCIPLE

Utilizing a crystal through which only fluoride ions can move, the difference in activity between a sample solution and an internal reference solution causes a potential to build up. This potential is measured against a standard calomel reference electrode.

REAGENTS

1. *Sodium Hydroxide, 10 N.* Forty gm of pelleted, reagent grade NaOH are weighed in a tared, 100-ml beaker using a Harvard balance. This is transferred to a 100-ml, glass-stoppered volumetric flask and 25 ml of H_2O are added. After the NaOH has dissolved and cooled to room temperature, H_2O is added to the mark; the solution is transferred to a 4-ounce, polyethylene bottle labeled "10 N. NaOH" and stored at room temperature. This is stable for an indefinite period.

2. *Citrate Buffer,* 0.5 M, pH 7.0. Exactly 96.06 gm of reagent grade citric acid are weighed into a 1-liter beaker (Harvard balance). Five hundred ml of deionized H_2O are added and allowed to cool to room temperature. The pH is adjusted to 7.0 with 10 N NaOH; the solution is transferred quantitatively to a 1-liter, glass-stoppered volumetric flask and diluted to the mark with H_2O. The buffer is transferred to a 32-ounce capacity, polyethylene bottle labeled "Citrate Buffer, 0.5 M, pH 7.0, date prepared" and stored at 4°C. This solution is discarded after one week.

STANDARD SOLUTIONS

1. *Stock Standard.* Three gm of reagent grade NaF are placed in a weighing vessel and dried at 100°C. overnight. The dry powder is cooled to room temperature in a dessicator. Exactly 2.21053 gm are weighed onto a piece of tared, glazed, weighing paper using the analytical balance and transferred quantitatively to a 1-liter, glass-stoppered volumetric flask. Five hundred ml of deionized H_2O

are added; the NaF is dissolved and diluted to the mark with H_2O. The solution is transferred to a 32-ounce polyethylene bottle labeled "Stock Standard" (1 mg F^- per ml) and stored in the refrigerator. This solution is stable for an indefinite period.

2. *Working Standards.* The stock standard is allowed to come to room temperature. Ten ml are transferred to a 100-ml, glass-stoppered volumetric flask, diluted to the mark with H_2O, and transferred to a 4-ounce, polyethylene bottle labeled "Working Standard-1, 100 μg F^- per ml, date prepared." This standard is stored in the refrigerator when not in use and is discarded after one week. "Working Standard-1" is allowed to come to room temperature and other working standards are prepared according to the following table. The indicated amount of "Working Standard-1" is transferred to a glass-stoppered flask of the size indicated and diluted to the mark with H_2O. These standards are prepared immediately before use. Each flask is labeled with the proper standard number and F^- concentration.

Standard No.	*μg F^- per ml*	*Pipet (ml)*	*Flask (ml)*
2	20	2	10
3	10	5	50

The following are prepared from Standard Number 3:

Standard No.	*μg F^- per ml*	*Pipet (ml)*	*Flask (ml)*
4	5	5	10
5	2	2	10
6	1	5	50

The following are prepared from Standard Number 6:

Standard No.	*μg F^- per ml*	*Pipet (ml)*	*Flask (ml)*
7	0.5	5	10
8	0.2	2	10
9	0.1	1	10

SPECIAL APPARATUS

1. Orion® fluoride electrode
2. Orion® microdish
3. Expanded scale pH-conductivity meter
4. Calomel reference electrode (4″)

PROCEDURE

One ml of buffer is pipeted into a labeled, 5-ml beaker. One ml of standard (or fresh urine sample) is added and mixed. Using a disposable pipet and a 2-ml rubber bulb, the solution is transferred to an Orion® microdish and the conductivity is read to the nearest 0.1 millivolt. About 10 minutes are required for the meter to reach its final reading but experience is necessary for recognition of the proper endpoint. The electrodes are rinsed with H_2O and dried with tissue paper between samples.

Conductivity vs μg of F^- per ml is plotted for the standards on K&E semilogarithmetic graph paper No. 47-6010 using the horizontal axis for millivolts and the vertical axis for μg of F^- per ml. A smooth line is drawn through the points using a French curve (K&E 1685-48). Fluoride concentration of the samples is recorded to the nearest 0.1 μg per ml from this curve.

Fluoride content can be read to the nearest 0.01 μg per ml if K&E semilogarithmetic paper No. 46-4970 is used for the standard curve.

DISCUSSION

Heretofore, the analysis of biological samples for fluoride content has been a long, involved procedure requiring a distillation or diffusion step. As a result, the clinical usefulness of the procedures available has been limited. With the development of the fluoride electrode and its increasing acceptance, fluoride analysis can become a useful addition to the services offered by clinical laboratories.

SOURCES OF ERROR

The manufacturer's instructions should be followed closely to avoid problems with air bubbles inside the electrode as well as on the crystal. Also, the distance between the reference and the fluoride electrodes must be kept constant.

If urine samples must be stored, the usual preservation precautions must be observed. E. J. Largent[3] of the Reynolds Metals Company uses 0.4 M citrate buffer with 58 ml per liter of 40 percent formaldehyde added. After adding 40 ml of this solution to 100 ml of fresh urine, no change in F^- concentration was observed over a period of 10 weeks.

The operator must practice the technique before attempting to analyze samples.

RANGE OF VALUES

Singer *et al.*[4] have reported 1.14 ± 0.016 (SD) ppm fluoride in normal human urine by the electrode technique. This laboratory found 0.54 ± 0.33 (SD) ppm in 10 samples from laboratory personnel. The range was 0.18 to 1.08 ppm. These values should not be considered "normal" for all localities because of the wide variation in fluoride intake from area to area. Each laboratory, or locality, should therefore establish its own "normal" values.

REFERENCES

1. Frant, M. S., and Ross, J. W., Jr.: Use of total ionic strength adjustment for electrode determination of fluoride in water supplies. Anal. Chem., *40:*1169-1178, 1968.
2. Gron, P., McCann, H. G., and Brunevold, F.: The direct determination of fluoride in human saliva by a fluoride electrode. Fluoride levels in parotid saliva after ingestion of single doses of sodium fluoride. Arch. Oral Biol., *13:*203-213, 1968.
3. Largent, E. J.: Reynolds Metals Company, Richmond, Virginia. Personal communication.
4. Singer, L., Armstrong, W. D., and Vogel, J. J.: Fluoride determination by electrode potential measurements. Abstracts, 45th General Meeting of the International Association of Dental Research, March, 1967, p. 77.
5. Singer, L., and Armstrong, W. D.: Determination of fluoride in bone with the fluoride elctrode. Ann. Chem., *40:*613-614, 1968.
6. Instruction Manual for Fluoride Electrode Model 94-09. Orion® Research Inc., Cambridge, Mass., 1966.

Chapter 21C

Colorimetric Measurement of Fluorine in Urine

R. DONALD STRAHM, M.S. and
F. WILLIAM SUNDERMAN, M.D., PH.D.

PRINCIPLE

A colorimetric procedure is presented for the measurement of fluorine in urine. Urine is placed in a miniature, disposable, plastic Petri dish containing a fluoride fixative. The sample is acidified and the dish closed with a cover coated on the inner surface with sodium hydroxide. After diffusion for about twenty hours at 50°C, fluorine held in the caustic film is measured colorimetrically with alizarin complexone.

APPARATUS

1. *Diffusion cell.* Disposable plastic Petri dish, 48 mm I.D. by 8 mm.*

2. *Laboratory oven.* Regulated at 50°C.

3. *Vacuum desiccator.* Containing desiccant such as Drierite.

*Millipore Filter Corporation, 38 Ashby Road, Bedford, Massachusetts 01730 Catalog No. PD 10 047 00.

REAGENTS

1. *Silver perchlorate, anhydrous, C.P.* A deliquescent oxidizing agent. (The bottle should be kept tightly closed and the material handled carefully.)

2. *Perchloric acid, 70%.* (This oxidizing agent may cause fire or explosion upon contact with certain organic materials and should be handled carefully.)

3. *Sodium hydroxide (about 0.5N).* Two gm of sodium hydroxide pellets are dissolved in 50 ml of water. The solution is cooled and diluted to 100 ml with ethyl alcohol. The solution is stored in a polyethylene bottle.

4. *Phenolphthalein solution.* Two-tenths of a gm is dissolved in a mixture of 50 ml of ethyl alcohol and 50 ml of water.

5. *Hydrochloric acid (about 0.05N).* One ml of concentrated hydrochloric acid is diluted to 250 ml with water.

6. *Standard sodium fluoride solution, containing 0.5 mg fluorine per 100 ml.* Precisely 0.2210 gm of dried (C.P. grade) sodium fluoride is dissolved in water and diluted to 1 liter in a volumetric flask. A 5-ml aliquot of this solution is diluted to 100 ml in a volumetric flask and stored in a polyethylene bottle.

7. *Cerium nitrate stock solution.* Cerium (cerous) nitrate hexahydrate, 2.98 gm, are dissolved in 500 ml of water.

8. *Alizarin complexone stock solution.* Alizarin complexone** (also called ali-

**Alizarin complexone is obtainable from Hopkins and Williams Ltd., Chadwell Heath, Essex, England, or from Burdick and Jackson Labs, Muskegon, Michigan 49443.

zarin fluorine blue or 3-aminoethylalizarin-N,N-diacetic acid), 0.643 gm, is suspended in 50 ml of water. Concentrated ammonium hydroxide, 0.25 ml, is added and the mixture stirred until dissolved. To this mixture is added 0.25 ml of glacial acetic acid, and the mixture is diluted to 100 ml. This solution is stable for two weeks.

9. *pH 4 buffer.* Sixty gm of sodium acetate trihydrate are dissolved in 500 ml of water. To this solution are added 115 ml of glacial acetic acid and the solution is diluted to 1 liter.

10. *Composite fluoride reagent.* The following solutions are mixed in order with swirling: 330 ml of acetonitrile, 68 ml of the buffer solution, 10 ml of the alizarin complexone solution, 10 ml of the cerium nitrate solution, and 75 ml of water. This reagent is warmed to room temperature, diluted to 500 ml with water, and stored in a polyethylene bottle. Under normal laboratory conditions, this reagent is stable for five days.

11. *Deionized water.* Water used in preparing reagents should be distilled and deionized. All apparatus must be scrupulously clean. It is desirable to rinse glassware well before use with deionized water.

PROCEDURE

Preparation of Diffusion Cell. One-tenth ml of 0.5N sodium hydroxide is placed on the center of the inside top of the plastic Petri dish. Several drops of ethyl alcohol are added so that the sodium hydroxide will spread out over a larger area. The top of the Petri dish is placed in a partially evacuated desiccator and dried overnight. (A number of tops may be prepared at one time and kept in the desiccator until needed.)

Treatment of Urine Sample. One ml of urine is placed on the bottom of the Petri dish. Approximately 0.2 gm of solid silver perchlorate is added. Using a pipet, 2 ml of perchloric acid are cautiously added, and the dish is covered immediately with the prepared top. The dish is then placed in an oven heated to 50°C. and allowed to remain for approximately twenty hours. (The dish must be handled carefully so that none of the solution in the bottom of the unit is splashed onto the top.) After twenty hours, the dish is carefully taken from the oven. The top is removed and water is added to dissolve the alkaline absorbent. The solution is then transferred quantitatively to a 50-ml volumetric flask. A drop of phenolphthalein is added, followed by 0.05N hydrochloric acid dropwise with swirling until the red color just disappears. The residual mixture in the bottom of the Petri dish should be disposed of promptly by washing away with a copious quantity of water.

Development of Color. To the fluoride solution contained in a 50-ml volumetric flask, 15 ml of the composite fluoride reagent are added, and the contents diluted to the mark with water while mixing. After standing for one hour, the absorbance of the solution is measured photometrically at 580 mμ. A blank reading is obtained on a solution containing 15 ml of the composite fluoride reagent diluted to 50 ml with water. The concentration of the fluoride (mg per 100 ml of urine) is estimated by reference to a previously prepared standard curve.

REFERENCES

1. Rowley, R. J., and Farrah, G. H.: Amer. Indust. Hyg. Assoc. J., July-August, 1962, p. 314.
2. Belcher, R., Leonard, M. A., and West, T. S.: J. Chem. Soc., 1959, p. 3577.
3. Yamamura, S. S., Wade, M. A., and Sikes, J. H.: Anal. Chem., *34*:1308, 1962.

Chapter 22

Clinical and Reproductive Dangers Inherent in the Use of Hallucinogenic Agents

CECIL B. JACOBSON, M.D., LUIS ARIAS-BERNAL, M.D., ELIZABETH VOSBECK, M.A., ANA DELRIEGO, D.PHARM., KATHLEEN AHEARN, B.A., and VALERIE MAGYAR, B.A.

INTRODUCTION

Controversy exists over both the somatic and reproductive dangers in the wide use of hallucinogens by a youthful segment of the population of the United States. Reports in the literature (1-4) vary from indications of severe risk to a complete lack of complications. This controversy is further complicated by the fact that some reports have originated in populations with vested interests which tend to prejudice acceptance of their observations. To clarify previously reported genetic effects, the investigators have initiated a prospective study (5) of 50 pregnancies in women who volunteer a history of hallucinogenic use and in whom somatic chromosomal aberrations are demonstrated in serial tissue samples (6, 7). The rationale for utilizing chromosomal aberrations as the standard of clinical assay is supported by previous reports (8-11) implicating their *in vivo* and *in vitro* correlation to LSD-25 exposure. In addition, chromosomal breakage is a visual, quantifiable event that can be photographically scored and coded prints sent to multiple investigators for "blind" confirmation.

Study Population

Pregnant drug users are referred by obstetricians, psychiatrists, adoption agencies, maternity homes, the clergy, and "community volunteer" clinics. The initial screening is by a medical social worker who obtains information concerning the patient's medical, reproductive, and family history, socio-economic condition, drug use, and exposure to proven mutagenic agents (such as irradiation, virus, and selected chemicals) (12-13). All data are kept on a coded record form and confirmed at each subsequent patient contact. When possible, drug use is investigated from samples volunteered by the subject.

Chromosomal study from peripheral blood cultures is initiated at the first interview. If a mutagenic effect is documented in the initial leucocyte cultures, a confirming blood sample and skin biopsy are taken in two weeks. In cases where positive results are shown, the patient is accepted in the study and serial blood and skin samples are scheduled at one month, three month, and six month and thereafter at six month intervals.

Prenatal care, delivery, and post-natal care of this selected population is arranged through private resources, the University Outpatient Clinic, and public agencies. Early monitoring of the fetus is initiated by fetal electrocardiography and aminocentesis. Multiple tissue systems are sampled at the time of delivery with collection from fetal tissue: amnion, cord blood, umbilical cord and circumcision, and maternal tissue: from the episiotomy repair, blood, and skin biopsy.

Pediatric follow-up of the newborn is arranged at the second, sixth, and fourteenth post-natal week and thereafter at three month intervals. During these visits a physical examination, clinical review, and serial peripheral blood and skin samples are collected. Clinical and genetic evaluation plus C. B. C., urinalysis, and gross photography are summarized on study infants each three months. The need for long-term follow-up is emphasized to parents and adoptive agencies and the investigators often meet with prospective adoptive parents for counseling in regards to possible long range complications (14).

Continuing participation in this study by adult patients is encouraged through informal rapport with the investigators and an interest in their medical needs and social development. Group therapy sessions are organized to increase the patient's interest in his own personal development and to foster continued participation with this research group. Little emphasis is needed to these patients as their mutagenic result of prior drug use can have lasting effect on subsequent pregnancies as well as upon their own somatic complications. For this reason, contraceptive assistance is provided when requested.

Chromosomal Analysis

The utilization of the chromosome for the standard of mutagenic assay has both scientific and clinical validity as it is a reliable, visual marker for genetic damage and transfers the genome (genetic complement of a species) to sequential generations. Any variation in number (ploidy) or structure (aberration) in this "basic vehicle of heredity" will constitute a significant genetic change (mutation) to subsequent generations. In that mutagenic studies with ionizing radiation and drugs show DNA change at a fraction of the dose required to cause chromosomal aberrations, it is valid to assume that chromosomal breakage constitutes an underestimate of genetic change (15). This is further substantiated as selective factors exist in sampling and culture techniques and as is evident, the chromosome is the macromolecular vehicle for the gene.

Repairable mutation does not have a sequential generation transmission and appears to be of little biological significance; however, chromosomal breaks that either readhere at the point of breakage (restitution) or to other chromosomal regions (translocation) constitute genetic damage of a significant nature. Translocation to non-homologous chromosomes through the segregation of allelic loci in meiosis results in gene duplication or deletion. In cases of restitution, evidence exists that sufficient molecular change in the DNA occurs to manifest as a perceptible genetic change (point mutation). (16) A self-limiting clinical effect is expected when the mutation occurs in exclusively somatic tissue as only a single generation is affected. However, a more significant change would be expected when gonadal tissue is effected as transmission to sequential generations would produce affected progeny. Thus, the evaluation of the genetic effects of hallucinogenic exposure can be monitored by chromosomal analysis. It is true that this is a small part of the total clinical effect of these drugs, but accounts for the more severe and lasting somatic effects and is the best way to predict risk of clinical complications in subsequent generations. Should such genetic change be documented, both the moral, medical and legal implications in hallucinogenic ingestion would radically change.

The major steps in chromosomal analysis are: tissue cultures to stimulate cellular division, the accumulation of sufficient metaphase spreads via colchicine arrest, hypotonic swelling to disperse the chromosomes, fixation, spreading and staining the cells on a microscope slide, microphotography, and analysis from 8 x 11 photographic prints (17).

CLINICAL SIGNIFICANCE OF CHROMOSOMAL ABERRATIONS

Two levels of mutagenic evaluation have been productive in human research: The cytogenetic study of *somatic tissue* which is basically an assessment of cellular viability and *reproductive fitness* which is the evaluation of the reproductive capacity of gametes and progeny either from gonadal analysis or pedigree analysis.

The cytogenetic study of *somatic tissue* is a valid assay of mutation either in the gamete of fertilization or in exposure to the developing embryo. Mosaics, that is different cell populations showing an identical chromosomal marker (clone), reflect a mutagenic element occurring during embryogenesis which results in a chromosomally mixed fetus (18). The time of mutagenesis can usually be inferred by comparing the relative frequency of aberrant cell clones and studying the different embryologic systems involved. Also, the relative viability of mutant clones may indicate cellular susceptibility towards specific mutagens. Demonstration of genetic change in somatic tissue is clinically significant as it documents the persistence in viable cell mutants throughout multiple cell generations. This viability may result in the premature induction of malignancy or aging.

The major disadvantage of somatic analysis is that the correlative value of mitotic studies to the developing gonad and its meiotic significance in fertilization is in question. An additional difficulty is that multiple cell generations usually occur since the original mutagenic event. This may mask prior mutation as mutant cells are often less viable in tissue culture resulting in an overgrowth of normal cells. Both reservations can be diminished by the *in vivo* study of both mitotic and meiotic tissues (19).

Reproductive studies in man are very difficult owing to the obvious moral and legal implications of anamalous offspring, artificial termination, or selected matings. An additional complication is the long latent period (15 to 25 years) required for the production of subsequent generations. These handicaps can be minimized by cytologic studies of gonadal tissue, inference of gonadal risk from somatic aberrations or *in vitro* study of gametogenesis and early development.

Reproductive fitness in the male is easily studied through testicular biopsy (histologic and cytogenetic study) as well as semen analysis (count, morphology, and viability). In addition, the potential for multiple offspring is possible through artificial insemination. Such studies in the female are complicated since ovarian biopsy is a major surgical procedure and ova recovery, maintenance and fertilization is a new technique. Random pregnancy evaluation are limited but supraovulation and *in vivo* fertilization are of potential promise (20). A marked theoretical difference exists in pre-conceptual exposure to the female as contrasted in the male. Spermatogenesis is a proliferative process, initiated at puberty with continual cellular replenishment. In contrast, oogenesis is a self-consumptive process where all the ova are present in the fetus and a competitive proportion consumed each month. Thus, a marked difference in mutagenic susceptibility exists both in the length of time the gametes are exposed and the probability of selection towards the "fittest gamete." This becomes dramatic in the numerical comparison of fertilization as millions of mature sperm compete, whereas selection in the egg of monovular species is essentially an all-or-none phenomenon.

The correlation of somatic chromosomal damage to meiotic anomalies infers definite reproductive risk. However, mutation of significance to future generations must survive not only meiotic division, but must produce a viable gamete which can withstand the rigors of fertilization and extreme selection until parturition. It is within this spectrum of development and maturation that satisfactory diagnostic methods must be devised.

Clinically, one recognizes the effect of mutation in the *gestational period* as failure to form viable gametes (sterility), impairment of conception or implantation (infertility or irregular menstruation), early embryonic death (abortion), embryonic or fetal damage (teratology), and decreased survival of the offspring (perinatal mortality). In experimental animals, these questions can be investigated by inbreeding (recessive mutants) and experiments where litter size and implantation sites can be studied indicating early reproductive loss (dominant lethals). However, in man other alternatives must be sought. Promising results are obtainable in insemination, superovulation, and *in vitro* fertilization (21). Large numbers and exact control of environmental variables are possible in *in vitro* fertilizations which at present are sacrificed at four days when cytologic markers can be screened from early cleavage stages. At present, only non-human blastocysts have been reimplanted into a properly cycled uterus of a recipient and carried to maturity for morphologic and reproductive analysis (22). Recent developments on the ability to monitor fetal development throughout mid gestation via amniotic fluid aspiration and tissue culture have been reported (23) and allow serial monitoring of an existing pregnancy without fetal complications.

CHROMOSOMAL ANOMALIES IN LSD-25 USERS

A composite of the different types of chromosomal anomalies found in our study of blood and skin cultures is shown in Figure 1. Photocomposite Ia shows the various chromosomal markers (dicentrics, rings, and quadriradial exchanges) that are interpreted as significant genetic change of sequential conse-

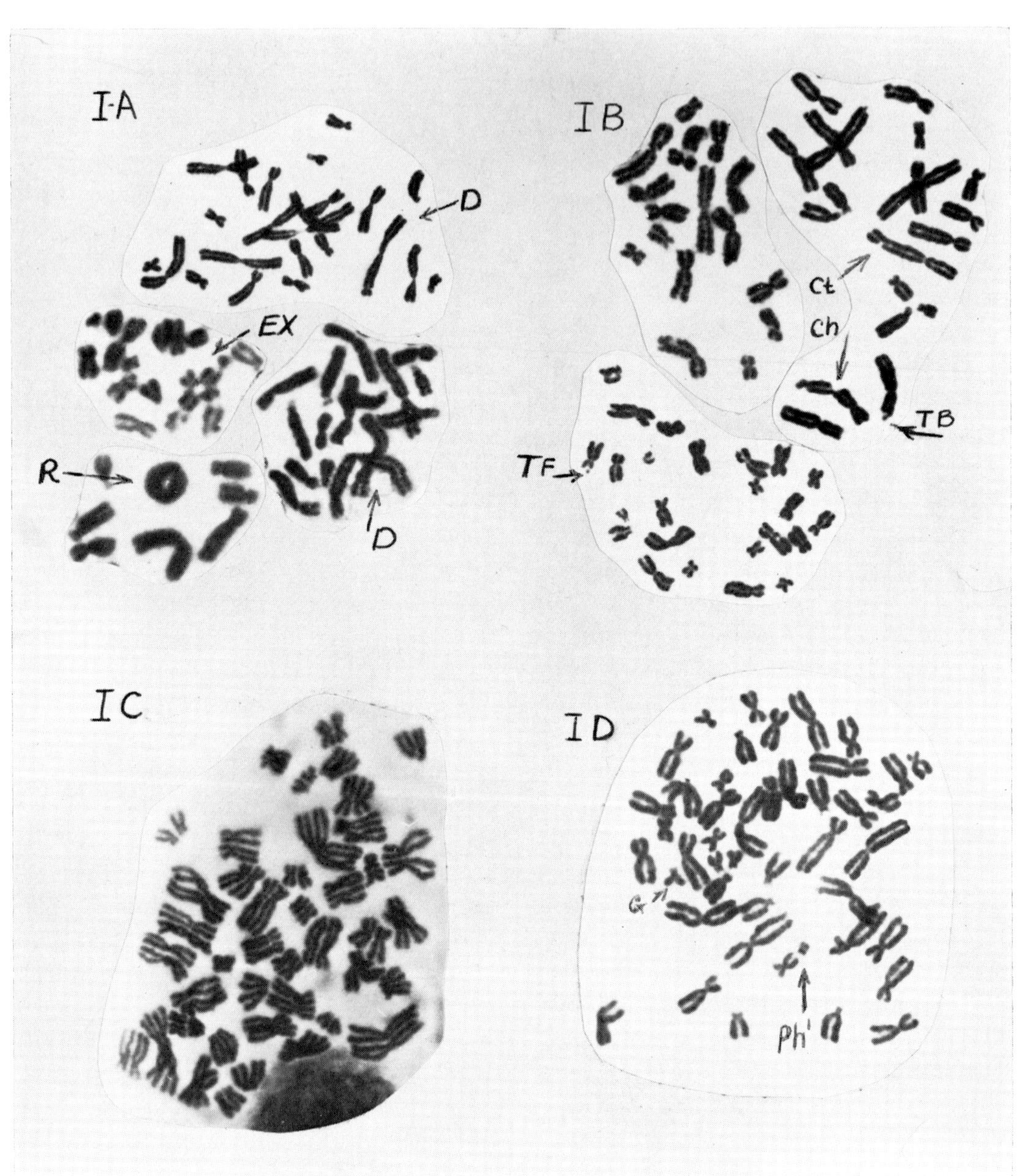

Figure 1. Chromosomal aberrations in LSD users.

Note: Ia. Chromosomal markers: D — Dicentric, R — Ring, Ex — Exchange
Ib. Breakage: Ct — Chromatid, Ch — Chromosome, TB — Telomere Blebs
Ic. Endoreduplication: Replication and pairing of each chromosome
1d. Philadelphia chromosome — ph′ — deleted group G autosome

TABLE I: CLINICAL INTERPRETATION OF CHROMOSOMAL ABERRATIONS
(Note: The Mutagenic level on the top and corresponding clinical significance.)

Mutagenic Level:	*Extreme*	*Severe*	*Moderate*	*Mild*	*Control*
Chromosomal	Quadriradial	Dicentric	Telomere blebs	Ch. gaps	Diploid (46XY)
Aberrations	Exchanges	Rings	Ch. breaks	*****	Note
(Structural Type)	*****	Ch. fragments	Ct. breaks	Random	Satellite assoc.
	Endoreduplication	Ch. deletions	Ct. deletions	Hypodiploidy	2° Constrictions
Normal Incidence	1:10,000	1:1,000	1:50	1:5	4:5
Hyperdiploid	Polyploid	10%	5%	0	0
Hypodiploid	Mosaic	45%	35%	25%	20%
Chromosome (Ch) Breaks	45%	30%	15%	10%	5%
Chromatid (Ct)	65%	50%	35%	35%	15%
Chromosome (Ch) Fragments	20%	15%	10%	5%	0
Chromatid (Ct)	40%	30%	20%	10%	5%
Clinical Significance	Definite	Questionable	Suspect	Borderline	None

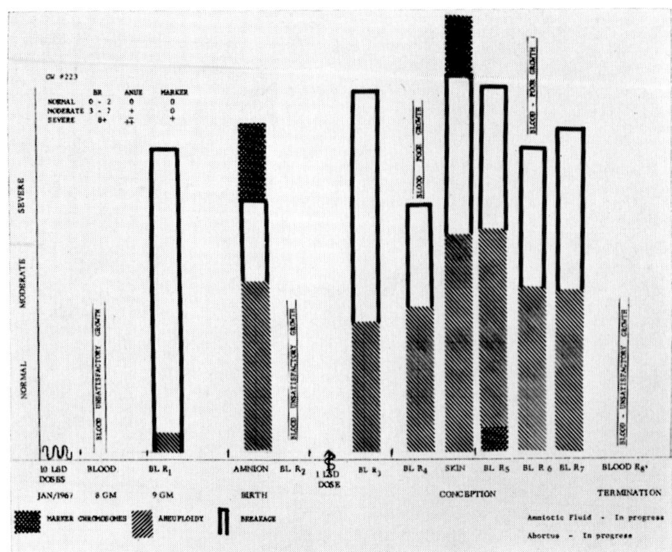

Figure 2. Chromosomal aberrations in LSD mother (GW 223).
Note: Increased markers, aneuploidy and breakage in tissue.

quence. Photocomposite Ib shows single generation breakage, telomere blebs and fragments which will result in either deletion or translocation in subsequent cell division. A severe mitotic anomaly — endoreduplication — as seen in Ic. This anomaly when persistent is interpreted as a pre-malignant anomaly as are the group G deletions (Ph') philadelphia chromosomes as seen in photo Id.

The clinical interpretations of chromosomal aberrations in our patients are seen in Table I. Here an attempt is made to correlate the severity of mutagenic damage to clinical significance for the patient. Definite mutagenic significance is attributed to the chromosomal markers that occur in more than one cell or repeat in subsequent culture. Definite clinical complications are expected in those cases where such chromosomal aberrations persist as the anomaly survives sequential chromosomal replication.

The tabulation of severity of chromosomal aberrations (mutagenic level) of our 370 serial samples is incomplete. However, presentation follows of one of the initial cases (GW 223), a patient whom we have followed for the past 18 months and who has produced both an infant (GW 247) and an abortus (L-5). This was the first pregnancy in a 19-year-old white female who had taken 10 doses of alleged LSD-25 in the three-month period preceeding conception and during the first four weeks of her pregnancy. The tabulation of the severity of mutagenic exposure on 12 serial samples are given in Figure 2. Gradual repair was present until the patient took a single dose of LSD one month prior to conceiving for the second time. The marked increase in markers was evident to the laboratories before the patient was confronted with this increase and confirmed her return to drug usage. Of special interest is the relative high mutagenic level seen in tissue (skin and amnion). This is indicative of both an increased sensitivity and longer repair period. Also, note the high number of culture failures or

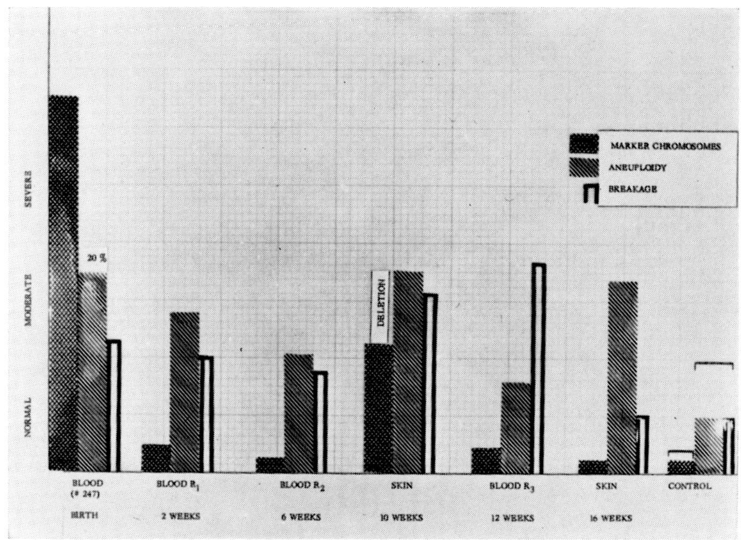

Figure 3. Chromosomal aberrations in LSD baby (GW 247).
Note: The rapid repair within three months.

poor growth (see also Table III). This finding is consistent with other mutagenic assay series in our laboratory and may reflect a true drug effect.

The mutagenic study on her baby (GW 247) is summarized in Figure 3. The same findings are present, i.e., gradual repair when no additional drug exposure is seen and a relative increase in the mutagenic level in tissue, amnion, and skin indicating slower repair. This child has been studied for one year and was released for adoption at six months as both repeat blood and skin culture were within normal limits. No anatomic, clinical, or developmental anomalies have been found in this infant during the first year of life, although many bizarre chromosomal markers were present in the cord blood (20% ph′ and clonal hyperdiploidy).

This picture of severe aberrations in

TABLE II: LSD EMBRYOS
(Note: The marked mutagenesis reflected in embryonic culture and developmental morphology.)

	Aberrations			*Drug Use*		*Embryonic Malformation*
	Markers	*Breakage*	*Aneuploidy*	*Dose*	*Mo/Prior/Concep*	*Visual & Sections*
Embryo # L- 2	0	6	None	1X	2	Exencephalous
Pt. # 264	1	10	50% Hypo			
Embryo # L- 5	3	33	15% Hyper	6X	4	Exencephalous and
Pt. # 283	2	12	25% Hypo			Spina bifida
Embryo # L-20	In process			1X	1/2	No anomaly
Pt. # 223	0	12	30% Hypo	10X	12	
Embryo # L-49	In process			11X	3	Visual encephalocoel
Pt. # 282	0	7	20% Hypo			(Sections in process)
Control	0 - 1	0 - 5	33%	....		Exencephaly 3/1000 (mice)
						Exencephaly 0/284 (human)
						Spina bifida 6/284 (human)

#/20 cells

the cord blood followed by rapid repair after separation from the maternal gestational environment suggests a humeral effect. This has been consistent in the 16 neonates studied to date and has allowed release for adoption in most cases within six months (14).

TABLE III: STUDY POPULATIONS

66 Adults	18 Therapeutic abortions
16 Neonates	2 Missed abortions
8 Pregnant	1 Spontaneous abortion

Two or more successful tissue cultures have been analyzed on each adult, neonate, and abortus.

This genetic repair or minimal mutagenic residual has not been the case in the abortuses studied to date. The abortus of patient 223 was therapeutically terminated at 6 weeks. Though no gross anomaly was found, CNS and cardiac defects were present on serial sections. To date, three other LSD abortuses have shown similar neural tube closure defects (see Table II). In all cases, a midline defect in the occipital region of the neuro-cranium was seen. In addition, other neural tube closure defects were found. On serial embryonic sections, it appears this is a form of exencephaly with failure in the roof of the diencephalon. A complete description of these cases is in preparation; however, in all cases, marked chromosomal anomalies were found in both the abortus cultures and in serial maternal samples.

Description of Population

The study group is summarized in Table III. Orientation is towards pregnancies carried to term and the low frequency of non-therapeutic abortions reflects the average stage of pregnancy (14 weeks) when the patients are referred to the study. The three cases of miscarriage all occurred in the seven patients ascertained early in the first trimester and indicates the increase in pregnancy wastage expected.

A breakdown of the 370 samples processed to date in this study is given in Table IV. This is a partial list of the 520 total samples received as some were isolated samples, failed to grow, or are still in progress. A definite increase in the culture failure rate was noted (normal blood is 95% and abortus tissue approximately 80%). The fact that many poor growing cultures showed mutagenic changes and that matched controls from normal subjects were processed with these failures infers that the poor growth may in fact indicate mutagenic change.

The average age levels of the study patients are given in Table V. The majority of mothers (80%) were 21 years or less and all but three were primagravidas. Paternal study has been attempted; however, the definite establishment of paternity is difficult. This is a vexing

TABLE IV: SERIAL TISSUE SAMPLES

	Blood	*Success Rate*	*Tissue*	*Success Rate*
Adults	202	84%	70	70%
Neonates	47	89%	31	64%
Abortuses	—	—	20	42%
Total	249		121	

*Success is photographic analysis on 20 or more cells.
**No tissue was retrieved on one missed abortion.

TABLE V: AGE DISTRIBUTION OF LSD USERS STUDIED

Age Levels	*Not Pregnant*	*Maternal*	*Paternal*
16 and under	1	3	0
17–18	6	6	4
19–21	8	18	5
22–25	3	6	2
26–30	2	2	2
Over 30	2	—	—
Total	22	35	13

complication as pure paternal exposure would help evaluate maternal humeral influence.

The tabulation of exposure of possible mutagenic significance is given in Table VI. The column "Not Pregnant" refers to pre-conceptual exposure. The estimate of "control" usage is very difficult and valid in comparison only. The additive effect of these compounds is under study; however to date, present data indicates that LSD is the most active in cytogenetic systems.

The extent of LSD usage and time in regards to the pregnancy studied is tabulated in Table VII. Here, the patient is tabulated in both columns if the drug was taken both pre- and post-conceptual. The average dose of 250 μgm is an estimate based on analysis of volunteered samples and inferred from psychedelic reactions to individual batches. It must be emphasized that due to the illicit nature of this drug, precise dosage and purity is highly variable.

Though our study to date infers a

TABLE VII: LSD USE IN 36 PREGNANCIES

*# Exposures**	*# Patients*	*Use Before Pregnancy*	*Use During Pregnancy*
Single dose	7	7	0
2 – 5	9	6	6
6 – 10	6	5	3
11 – 20	9	9	8
20+	5	5	4
Total	36	32	21

*Estimated dose is usually 250 μgm.

severe teratogenetic effect to the human embryo (5), natural selection appears to prevent these anomalies from coming to term. This selection is not complete and isolated cases of chromosomally defective children have been reported (24). In fact, retrospective analysis of maternal investigation in a case of trisomy 21 with marker breakage revealed a mother with both preconceptual exposure to LSD-25 and documented chromosomal breakage and exchanges. (14)

Two major difficulties arise in the evaluation of such cases: (a) the validity of isolated retrospective analysis and (b) the national impact if only a slight increase in defects is seen. The government's interest in this problem is intense (25) and it is encouraging to see support for scientific study in addition to discussion soley of intensified enforcement as present data strongly implicates LSD to be a chemical hallucinogen of marked reproductive detriment.

TABLE VI: ADULT PATIENTS EXPOSED TO POSSIBLE MUTAGENS

	Not Pregnant	*Pregnant*	*Total*	*"Control"*
Prescribed Drugs	14 %	9 %	23 %	30 %
Caffeine	25 %	31 %	56 %	65 %
Nicotene	22 %	32 %	54 %	35 %
Ethanol	5 %	7 %	12 %	50 %
X-ray	11 %	15 %	26 %	15 %
LSD	54 %	46 %	100 %	0 – 1 %
Amphetamines	32 %	31 %	63 %	15 %
Narcotics	10 %	9 %	19 %	0 – 3 %
DMT	6 %	9 %	15 %	0 %
Marijuana	55 %	39 %	94 %	? ? ?

BIBLIOGRAPHY

1. Frosch, W., Robbins, E., and Stern, M.: Untoward reactions to LSD resulting in hospitalization. New Engl. J. Med., *273:*1235, 1965.
2. DeBold, R., and Leaf, R. (ed.): LSD, Man and Society. Ohio, Wesleyan Press, 1967.
3. McGlothin, W., Cohen, S., and McGlothin, M.: Long-lasting effects of LSD on normals. Arch. Gen. Psych., *17:*521, 1967.
4. Hoeffer, A.: D-lysergic acid dethylamide (LSD): A review of its present status. Clin. Pharmacol. Ther., *6:*183-255, Mar-Apr 1965.
5. Jacobson, C. B., and Maryar, V. L.: Genetic evaluation of LSD. Proc. Child. Hosp., Washington, D. C., *24:*5, 152-179, May 1968.
6. Jacobson, C. B.: Cytogenetic techniques. In, Medical Cytogenetics, M. Bartalos and T. Baramki (eds.). Williams and Wilkins, Baltimore, 1967.
7. Jacobson, C. B., and Arias-Bernal, L. F.: Cytogenetic techniques in sexual anomalies. JAMWA, *22:*11, 875-884, 1967.
8. Cohen, M., Back, N., and Marinello, M.: Chromosomal damage in human leukocytes induced by LSD. Science, *159:*749, 1968.
9. Loughman, W., Sargent, T., and Israelstam, D.: Leukocytes of humans exposed to LSD — Lack of chromosomal damage. Science, *158:*508, 1967.
10. Bender, L., and Sanker, D.: Chromosome damage not found in leukocytes of children treated with LSD-25. Science, *159:*749, 1968.
11. Cohen, M., Hirschhorn, K., and Frosch, W.: *In vivo* and *in vitro* chromosomal damage induced by LSD-25. New Engl. J. Med., *277:*1043, 1967.
12. Irwin, S., and Egozcue, J.: Chromosome abnormalities in leukocytes from LSD-25 users. Science, *157:*313, 1967.
13. Kihlman, B. A.: Actions of Chemicals on Dividing Cells. Prentice-Hall, Inc., 1966.
14. Jacobson, C. B., Magyar, V. L., and Berlin, C.: The Perinatal Assessment of a Possible Mutagen LSD-25. Presented November 23, 1968, South Society for Pediatric Research, New Orleans, L. A. (in press).
15. Maio, J. J., and Schildkraut, C. L.: Isolated Mammalian Metaphase Chromosomes. I. General Characteristics of Nucleic Acids and Proteins.
16. Darlington, C. D., and Koller, P. C.: The chemical breakage of chromosomes. Heredity, *1:*187-221, 1947.
17. Jacobson, C. B., and Magyar, V. L.: Reproductive Dangers in LSD Use. Presented at the Multiple Discipline Research Forum, American Medical Association, June 20, 1968.
18. Jacobson, C. B.: The nature of the chromosomal defect in mongolism. Proc. Child. Hosp., Washington, D. C., *22:*2, 43-48, 1967.
19. Petersen, K. D.: Effect of Caffeine on Spermatogenesis in the Rat. Doctoral Thesis, The George Washington University, Washington, D. C., 1968.
20. Jacobson, C. B.: *In vitro* maturation, fertilization and cleavage of human follicular oocytes. South. Med. Assoc., November 19, 1968. S. M. J. (submitted).
21. Jagiello, G., Streptonigrin: Effect on the first meiotic metaphase of the mouse egg. Science, *157:*453-4, July 28, 1967.
22. Pavlok, A.: Development of mouse ova in explanted oviducts: Fertilization, cultivation and transplantation. Science, *157:*1457-8, Sept. 22, 1967.
23. Jacobson, C. B., and Barter, R. H.: Intrauterine diagnosis and management of genetic defects. AJOG, *99:*6, 796-807, 1967.
24. Hirschhorn, K.: Personal communication and discussion at 7th Conference on Mammalian Cytology and Somatic Cell Genetics, Gatlinburg, Tenn., Oct. 23, 1968.
25. Vinson, F. M., Jr.: Report of Proceedings, Comm. on Public Health and Welfare, Comm. on House Interstate and Commerce Committee, Feb. 20, 1968.

Chapter 23

Narcotics, Dangerous Drugs and the Clinical Laboratory

RODNEY F. CARLTON, M. D., and HOWARD QUITTNER, M.D.

A. Habituation as a Social Problem

Widespread publicity has made the public extremely aware of the expansion of drug-taking as a predicament facing our society. It is recognized that the widespread illicit distribution and use of narcotics and dangerous drugs presents an important social and medical problem. The recent extension of this abuse to involve the high school and pre-high school age groups makes this problem more severe.

A booming business has developed to satisfy and enlarge the demand for these psychotropic agents. The sales and marketing of narcotics is lucrative as evidenced by the profit in opium traffic. An original investment of $250.00 for 10 kilograms of crude opium on the illicit market, expands to $250,000.00 from the sale to the addict of the resulting 1 kilogram of refined and diluted product.

The attitude of youth toward the consumption of narcotics and dangerous drugs has changed in the past few years. The use of such drugs, once considered a sign of moral weakness, has developed to the level of a status symbol. It is now the "in thing" to take drugs. Use and possession of these drugs are not hidden from the users' peers but are shown as a badge of merit. In fact, it is not unusual for one who is unable to obtain narcotics, either through lack of funds or lack of contacts with suppliers, to fabricate the possession of the drugs.

This last point is illustrated by the material confiscated from one 13-year-old boy. He had taken a book and cut out the inside to make a concealed compartment. In this, he had placed a syringe and a tube containing a clear liquid substance. This was proudly displayed to his friends with the claim that he was taking "dope." Analysis of the specimen in the tube revealed it to be composed of approximately 16% ethyl alcohol. It was, in fact, the purloined dregs of his father's highball.

Law enforcement related to drug abuse is part of the present day treatment of this social disease. The combination of the increased number of drug arrests and the relatively new element, possession of fake drugs by many youngsters, has placed a heavy burden on the laboratories which analyze the specimens submitted by law enforcement agencies. In many areas of our country, there are no local laboratories for this purpose. The arrests make it manditory that laboratories have available relatively simple and rapid screening tests that will enable an arresting officer to distinguish between sham and real possessors of narcotics or dangerous drugs. In some cases, it is also essential to confirm that the suspect has taken the drug. The presumptive evidence from such tests provides grounds on which to charge the suspect until definitive identification of the material in question is made.

Social diseases such as addiction are a new area of medical practice and require special technics. In the prevention of recurrence of morphine addiction, screening tests of random urine specimens for drug metabolites are an essential facet of the program. In larger communities, the volume of such work is great enough to sustain a whole laboratory effort. Yet, the methods that have been developed are within the capabilities of good general laboratories in every community.

B. Laboratory Diagnosis of Toxicity from Alkaloids

The request for toxicological analysis presents itself from various sources and each source makes a special demand upon the analyst and his aides. While the situation will be described as it relates to the opiates and related drugs, these examples can be generalized to cover all dangerous substances that humans self-administer for essentially non-medical reasons.

The toxicologist supplements the information derived from the autopsy in a case of death due to narcotics by providing qualitative proof of the presence of a potentially lethal agent. The presence of morphine or the quantitation of its level in the tissues of a known addict does not clarify the cause of death. The route of administration, previous exposure, the presence of other drugs, and other causes for variable sensitivity are always significant. The decision as to whether the findings are lethal is based upon much correlated evidence and must always be the subjective opinion of a specialist. The quantitative measurements are most properly the province of the expert, as is the qualitative identification of the offending poison(s). An awareness on the part of all clinical scientists as to the analytical requirements and limitations of the present methods is necessary in order to provide the analyst with sufficient amounts and appropriate types of body tissues and fluids for study. A reference covering the metabolism of dangerous drugs should be part of any pathology library.[27]

Not all cases of poisoning due to dangerous drugs are lethal, and at these times, the clinical laboratory may be called upon to identify the substance. In many situations, the material is unknown, but even if it is known, confirmation is necessary for good treatment. While quantitative values would be reassuring, the knowledge of the causative agent and the relationship between clinical signs and the appropriate treatment are all that is needed for most types of effective therapy. The laboratory approach should be one that provides a reasonably sure qualitative identification in the shortest possible time by the most simple method. Rapid quantitation of narcotics after identification is not practical at this time.

The changing thrust of medical practice in the field of social medicine requires the clinical laboratory to assume a role in the identification of narcotics and dangerous drugs for the various agencies associated with drug abuse. The design of procedures for this purpose is a new facet of laboratory technology.

QUANTITATIVE METHODS

Quantitative methods for the measurement of morphine have been developed to a degree of sensitivity such that one can measure levels in the blood 30 minutes after a 15 mg intramuscular injection.[15] Most methods are not sensitive at this low level but can be readily used for analyses of tissues and body fluids such as bile or urine. The methodology for morphine and its surrogates has been critically reviewed.[8, 30] Colorimetry has been successfully employed by taking advantage of the structure of morphine so that it reacts either as a base, as an amine or as a phenol. Several different nonspecific reagents can be used, the most effective being: silicomolybdic acid,[10] methyl orange,[22] Folin-Ciocalteu reagent,[28, 30] diazotization,[30] α - nitroso β - napthol reaction,[21] or alkaline nitrososalt formation.[9] These colorimetric methods are best performed upon urine.

Other instrumentational procedures can be employed to achieve greater sensitivity with varying increases in the complexity of the methodology and some increase in specificity: ultraviolet spectrophotometry,[12] fluorometry,[15] polarography,[17, 22] and isotope dilution.[1, 19] Successful gas-liquid chromatographic quantitation from biological materials has not yet been reported.

Perhaps the most difficult aspect of analysis is the separation of morphine from biological material. All or part of the morphine exists in the tissues as its conjugate morphine-3-monoglucuronide dihydrate. Prior to analysis, this compound must be converted to free morphine by either acid or glucuronidase hydrolysis. Extraction procedures are generally performed at pH 9, near the isoelectric point of morphine.[12,30] Adsorption has been employed in isolation procedures using ion-exchange resins[23,28] or cation-exchange paper.[7]

Quantitative methods of analysis for other narcotics are not as extensively recorded in the literature as are those for morphine.[27,30] The continual expansion of the abuse of drugs to involve numerous potentially hallucinogenic agents, both old and new, makes any attempt to review these methods futile. Mescaline, harmaline and lysergic acid diethylamide (LSD) can be identified but not quantitated by thin-layer chromatography.[16] LSD can be quantitated by fluorometry.[2]

QUALITATIVE IDENTIFICATION

The use to which qualitative identification is put dictates the degree of specificity of the recognition. The most stringent requirements are for use in medicolegal work. Usually two methods of clear identification suffice. These should be different and scientifically validated. Corroborative methods which are less specific add further support to such findings.

Crystallization and physical characterization are ideal methods but are seldom used because of the difficulty of procedure, the need for special equipment and the large amounts of material required, a seldom encountered circumstance. Ultraviolet spectrophotometric or spectrofluorometric scanning, infrared spectroscopy and gas chromatography offer the best present and future definitive methods for identification. At present, these methods are practical only in specialized laboratories.

Thin-layer chromatography has developed to the point where almost all of the narcotics and dangerous drugs can be easily identified.[16,18] The sensitivity of the method even allows for the qualitative recognition of small amounts of a drug in large scale detection programs covering addicts under treatment.[7,16,18] Paper chromatography has been unwarrantedly neglected in some types of drug examination[11,20] because of the increased sensitivity and speed of thin-layer chromatography. Ionophoresis not only identifies a drug but may also provide enough of the compound for study by other methods.[12] Countercurrent distribution ratios and other comparative solvent studies are too elaborate for any but very specialized laboratories and have now become secondary methods of identification.

The oldest and simplest means for qualitative identification of narcotics and dangerous drugs are crystallography and spot tests. While crystallography is frequently specific, the recognition is subjective and is thus often strongly challenged in medicolegal work. Spot tests are seldom specific and there is always the possibility of previously unrecorded false positive reactions with newly synthesized materials. In addition, the sensitivity of most spot tests is of the order of 5 to 10 micrograms of substance, and they are best done with relatively pure compounds.[8,29] In spite of these disadvantages, spot tests are the best initial procedures for qualitative identification. Their simplicity and speed are unrivalled. They are life-saving in the emergency room and a time-saver in police work.

C. Rapid Screening Tests for the Identification of Narcotics and Dangerous Drugs

INTRODUCTION

Spot tests and crystallography are not necessarily specific methods but they are extremely rapid. They give enough information to allow an arresting officer to "rule in" or "rule out" the presence of a narcotic or dangerous drug in impounded contraband. The tests which follow will provide satisfactory evidence to allow an arresting officer to charge a suspect until definitive identification of the material is possible. These screening procedures will eliminate the confusion resulting from the confiscation of "fake drugs." Modification of the analytical approach provides an emergency room procedure for dangerous drug identification.[5] In addition, through the use of thin-layer chromatography, a simple and rapid screening test for morphine has been developed.[4]

PRINCIPLE

Marquis' and Mecke's tests are empiric in origin but it is probable that the colors produced are the result of free radical formation in the aromatic rings induced by the strong acid in the reagent.[24] The free radicals are modified and possibly stabilized by the presence of side-chains in the drugs and the minor constituents of the reagents. The p-dimethyl aminobenzaldehyde reagent undergoes condensation with indoles such as LSD to form a colored complex. The principles of the other color reactions are unknown.

REAGENTS[3]

1. *Marquis reagent* (must be made up just before use). Eight to ten drops of 40% formaldehyde solution are added to 10 ml of concentrated sulfuric acid, A.C.S.

2. *p-Dimethylaminobenzaldehyde reagent.* (The reagent must be protected from light and must be relatively fresh.)

a. To 12.5 mg of p-dimethylaminobenzaldehyde are added 6.5 ml of concentrated sulfuric acid and 3.5 ml of water.

b. 1% tartaric acid, reagent grade, (w/v).

3. *p-Dimethylaminobenzaldehyde,* paper spot test reagents.[6]

a. *Test paper.* One gm of p-dimethylaminobenzaldehyde is dissolved in 10 ml of ethyl alcohol. One-fourth inch wide strips of Whatman #1 chromatography paper are cut from sheets, immersed in this solution, and removed to dry spontaneously in the air. When dry, the strips are cut into $\frac{1}{4}$ inch squares and stored in a tightly sealed container.

b. 10% ferric chloride, A.C.S., in water (w/v).

c. Absolute methyl alcohol, A.C.S.

d. 50% sulfuric acid (v/v).

4. *Duquenois reagent.* (This reagent is quite stable but should be discarded when it becomes yellow.) To 0.5 gm of vanillin U.S.P., in 20 ml of 95% ethyl alcohol are added 5 drops of acetaldehyde (Eastman).

5. *Dille-Koppanyi reagent* (stored in a brown bottle and refrigerated. This reagent keeps for at least two months).

a. Isopropylamine (Eastman), 5% in methanol (v/v).

b. Cobaltous acetate reagent. One-tenth gm of cobaltous acetate $\cdot 4H_2O$, C.P., are dissolved in 100 ml of absolute methanol. Two-tenths ml of glacial acetic acid are added.

6. *Mecke's reagent.* Exactly 0.25 gm of selenious acid, C.P., are dissolved in 25 ml concentrated sulfuric acid.

7. *Platinic chloride,* 5% in water, (w/v).

8. *Mercuric chloride* 2 percent in 50% ethanol, (w/v).

9. *Colbalt-thiocyanate reagent.*

a. Cobalt chloride, reagent grade, 4% in distilled water (w/v).

b. Potassium thiocyanate, reagent grade, 4% in distilled water (w/v).

Equal parts of a. and b. are mixed immediately before use.

10. *K Bi* I_4 *reagent* (modified).[20] *Solution A:* 260 mg of bismuth subnitrate are dissolved in 100 ml of 33% acetic acid. *Solution B:* 5.72 gm of potassium iodide are dissolved in 100 ml of distilled water. The reagents are stored in brown bottles. Equal parts of A and B are mixed just before use.

11. *Thin layer plates are prepared* in the usual manner with silica gel G but substituting 6 N HCl for water in preparing the slurry.[4]

12. *Solvent system.* Ethyl acetate: methanol: ammonium hyroxide; 85:10:5 (v/v/v). The system is prepared within thirty minutes of use and employed in the chromatography system of choice.

13. *Iodoplatinate spray reagent*

a. 0.5% H_2SO_4

b. 1 ml 10% solution of platinum chloride is added to 25 ml of 4% potassium iodide. This is diluted to 50 ml with distilled water.

14. An *ultraviolet lamp* ("mineralite," Ultraviolet Products, Inc., San Gabriel, California).

It is suggested that the spot test reagents be kept as a set in a box or rack so that the indicated studies can be made quickly and efficiently. It is also advisable to have a small group of known materials that give typical reactions with the various tests: opium powder, meperidine, methamphetamine, an ergot alkaloid, a barbiturate, cocaine, atropine. A complete set would also include a small amount of heroin and marihuana but the possession of these substances is illegal under present federal laws, even for forensic or poison control purposes.

PROCEDURES

Marquis Test (Opium Alkaloids, JB 336, "TWA," "LBJ")

One or two drops of Marquis reagent are added to a small portion of the sample on a spot plate or in a test tube. The immediate production of a purple color indicates the presence of an opium alkaloid. Meperidine slowly produces a yellow color which changes to light green and then to dark green. An orange-brown color is produced by the amphetamines or ergot derivatives. The presence of mescaline is indicated by an immediate green color changing rapidly to a dark brown.

B. P-dimethylaminobenzaldehyde Test (LSD)

1. A portion of the sample is placed in a test tube and 1 ml of water, 1 ml of tartaric acid, and 1 ml of p-dimethylaminobenzaldehyde reagent are added.

2. The tube is mixed and allowed tc stand for 5 to 10 minutes. The formation of a lavender to blue-red color indicates the presence of LSD or other related amines.

C. P-dimethyl Paper Test (LSD)

1. A piece of test paper is placed on a spot plate and a small amount of suspect material is placed on the paper.

2. One drop of ferric chloride solution is added to the well.

3. Sufficient methyl alcohol is dropped on the material to wet the test paper (usually 1 to 2 drops).

4. Sulfuric acid is added dropwise. If effervescence occurs, dropwise addition is continued until it ceases and then two more drops of reagent are added (not to exceed 10 drops).

5. Compounds containing an indole ring produce a pink, purple or blue color on the paper or in the solution within 5 minutes. The less solution used in steps 3 and 4, the more sensitive is the 1 minute reactivity.

D. Duquenois Test. (Marihuana)

1. Approximately 25 to 60 mg (a smaller amount may be used) of the sample are placed in a test tube and 2 ml of Duquenois reagent are added. The mixture is shaken for approximately 1 minute.

2. Two ml of concentrated hydrochloric acid are added and the tube is mixed. Color changes are observed for 3 minutes.

3. Two ml of chloroform are added and the mixture is shaken for 1 minute. If marihuana is present in the sample, the violet shade produced by the acid is transferred to the chloroform layer.

E. Dille-Koppanyi Test (barbituric acid and derivatives)

1. A small amount of sample is placed in a test tube and 2 ml of cobaltous acetate reagent are added and mixed.

2. One ml of isopropylamine solution is added and mixed. A red-blue or purple color indicates barbituric acid or one of its derivatives.

F. Mecke's Test (amphetamines, apomorphine, codeine, mescaline)

A small portion of sample (0.5 mg is sufficient) is placed on a spot plate. Two drops of reagent are added. The resulting colors are observed. The amphetamines will produce a green color which changes rapidly to yellow. A red-orange precipitate usually follows. Apomorphine, codeine and mescaline will produce final green colors.

G. Platinic Chloride Crystallography (heroin, cocaine)

A few crystals of powder or sample are placed on a glass slide and 1 drop of platinic chloride reagent is added. The reaction is observed under the microscope. In the presence of heroin, small "oil droplets" will form after a few minutes; small dark needles will then "grow" from these, finally producing "chestnut burr" formations. Cocaine produces characteristic one-sided barbed-feather crystals.

H. Mercuric Chloride Test (atropine)

Approximately 5 to 10 mg of sample are placed in a test tube and 1 ml of reagent is slowly added dropwise. If a red coloration is produced at once, atropine is present. Homatropine is the only other alkaloid known to give this reaction.

I. Cobalt Thiocyanate Test (cocaine, meperidine, methadon, opiates, promazine)

A small amount of the suspect material is placed in a test tube or on a spot plate and 1 drop of reagent is added. A sky blue color is produced by reaction with cocaine, meperidine or methadon. Other opiates give other shades of blue and promazine gives a green color.

J. Emergency Room Screening[5]

Gastric contents or the first water wash of the stomach is used. Urine is less satisfactory.

1. One third of the washing or gastric contents are taken and acidified with dilute H_2SO_4.

2. This material is extracted with 20 ml of chloroform. The chloroform extract is reserved to test for barbiturates, salicylates, carbromal, chloral hydrate, DDT etc.

3. The aqueous layer is alkalinized with ammonia.

4. 20 ml of chloroform are added and the extraction is repeated. The water layer is discarded.

5. The chloroform is evaporated to near dryness (0.5 ml) on a hot plate.

6. Spot tests. 1 drop of chloroform is placed in each of 3 test tubes and 1 drop is placed on a piece of filter paper.

a. Ultraviolet fluorescence of the filter paper indicates quinine.

b. One drop of $KBiI_4$ reagents is added to tube #1. A pink to orange or brick red precipitate indicates the presence of an alkaloid or a promazine.

c. 1 drop of 10% $FeCl_3$ is added to tube #2. A pink to orange color indicates a promazine.

d. 1 drop of cobalt thiocyanate reagent is added to tube #3. A sky blue color indicates cocaine, meperidine or methadon.

e. Other spot tests may be done if indicated.

K. Detection of Morphine in Urine by Thin-layer Chromatography[4]

1. A prepared acid plate is placed upon a warm hot plate and 100 ul of urine are applied. The heat hastens the drying of the urine thus making the spot smaller.

2. The spotted plate (along with appropriate 4 ug standards of morphine, codeine, quinine, etc.) is placed in an oven at 150° for 90 minutes.

3. After cooling, the plate is developed in the solvent system until the solvent has migrated to about 5 mm from the top of the plate.

4. After drying, the compounds are visualized by spraying and the morphine or other drugs are identified from the standards.

DISCUSSION

Recently, Marquis reagent has been used as a screening procedure for the detection of N-Methyl-3-Piperidyl benzolate hydrochloride (JB 336, "TWA" or "LBJ").[26] The compound gives a rust-brown color which changes to a distinctive blue. At the present time there is no known differentiating field test for the synthetic narcotics with the exception of methadone and meperidine. Mecke's test adds further confirmation to a positive Marquis test. By using known controls the two tests can tentatively identify several different drugs.

The Dille-Koppanyi test is very sensitive and may be performed on a spot plate. One or two mg are enough to give a positive test. The layering out of the colored product on the walls of the well as the methanol evaporates is characteristic of the process. A cloudy solution does not usually interfere with the test. The cloud is due to starch or other insoluble material. If the original substance is colored, the material is added to 2 ml of water and 1 drop of concentrated sulfuric acid, and then extracted into 2 ml of chloroform. The chloroform extract is used in the test. Hydantoins, sulphonamides, pyrimidine, piperdine, and methylprylan also give a purple color, but they are not soluble in chloroform and may be excluded by using extraction as the first step in the test.

The thin-layer method described for morphine eliminates the prior steps of hydrolysis and extraction. The acid in the gel and the heating apparently accomplish the hydrolysis *in situ* on the plate. Codeine usually gives a small morphine spot as well as its own spot. Codeine can be differentiated from morphine by heating the plate to 100°C for 30 minutes before iodoplatinate treatment and then examining under ultraviolet light. Only morphine fluoresces. A phenol spray will differentiate morphine from quinine, a common adulterant.[12,25]

If a considerable amount of unconjugated compound is expected, chromatography on a plain silica gel plate without the heating period will give a positive test as the method is sensitive to 0.5 ug of morphine.

Another very simple method for extracting alkaloids, tranquilizers and barbiturates has been described by Dole, Kim and Eglitis.[7] It employes a cation exchange paper with elution and solvent extraction. A simple, rapid, conventional colorimetric method is also available.[9]

SOURCE OF ERROR

The reactions described are "all or none" phenomena. False negatives should not occur except in the crystallography test for heroin if extremely diluted specimens are used. False positives should not occur. The greater likelihood of confusion will be with closely related compounds present on the illegal drug list of the Bureau of Narcotics and Dangerous Drugs (BNDD) of the United States Department of Justice.

Resumé of Clinical Interpretations

The above screening procedures were selected to give a concise identification of the more commonly abused drugs. However, the large variety of pharmacologic agents and the astounding imagination of "thrill-seekers" and "Hippie-chemists" leaves no chemical free from suspicion. Should investigation suggest that there was use of a variant of the more common drugs or even some drug previously considered as benign, the authors suggest consultation of one of the elaborate lists of qualitative methods[3, 8, 13, 14, 29] for supplementary or expanded approaches. In all identification studies, it is appropriate to run parallel tests using a known sample of the suspect material or a closely related compound as well as a reagent blank.

REFERENCES

1. Adler, T. K., Elliott, H. W., and George, R.: Some factors affecting the biological disposition of small doses of morphine in rats. J. Pharmacol. & Exp. Therap., *120*:475-487, 1957.
2. Axelrod, J., Brady, R. O., Witkof, B., and Evarts, E. E.: The distribution and metabolism of lysergic acid diethylamide. Ann. N. Y Acad. Sci., *66*:435-444, 1957.
3. Butler, W. P., and Mathers, A. P.: Methods of Analysis for Alkaloids, Opiates, Marihuana, Barbiturates and Miscellaneous Drugs. Washington, Internal Revenue Service, Publication No. 341 (Rev. June 1967).
4. Cochin, J.: Analysis for narcotic analgesics and barbiturates in urine by thin-layer chromatographic techniques without previous extraction and concentration. Psychopharm. Bull. *3*:53-60, 1966.
5. Curry, A. S.: Systematic search for an unknown poison. In Stewart, C. P., and Stolman, A. (Eds.); Toxicology, Mechanisms and Analytical Methods, Vol. I. New York, Academic Press, 1960, pp. 276-283.
6. Dechert, D. D.: A rapid identification test kit for materials containing ergot-type alkaloids. Microgram (BNDD), *1*(4):16-17, 1968.
7. Dole, V. P., Kim, W. K., and Eglitis, I.: Extraction of narcotic drugs, tranquilizers, and barbiturates by cation-exchange paper, and detection on a thin-layer chromatogram by a series of reagents. Psychopharm. Bull., *3*:45-48, 1966.
8. Ehrlich-Rogazinsky, S., and Cheronis, N. D.: The identification and determination of morphine. Microchem. J., *7*:336-356, 1963.
9. Feldstein, M., and Klendshoj, N. E.: Rapid spectrophotometric method for the determination of morphine in urine. J. Forens. Sci., *1*:47-56, 1956.
10. Fujimoto, J. M., Way, E. L., and Hine, C. H.: A rapid method for the estimation of morphine. J. Lab. Clin. Med., *44*:627-635, 1954.
11. Goldbaum, L. R., and Kazyak, L.: Identification of alkaloids and other basic drugs by paper partition chromatography. Anal. Chem., *28*:1289-1290, 1956.
12. Goldbaum, L. R., and Williams, M. A.: The identification and determination of micrograms of morphine in biological samples. J. Forens. Sci., *13*:253-261, 1968.
13. Gonzales, T. A., Vance, M., Helpern, M., and Umberger, C. J.: Legal Medicine Pathology and Toxicology, 2nd ed. New York, Appleton-Century-Crofts, 1954, p. 1123-1311.
14. Johnson, C. A., and Thorton-Jones, A. D.: Drug Identification. A Scheme for the Identification of Organic Chemicals Used in Medicine and Pharmacy. London, The Pharmaceutical Press, 1966.
15. Kupferberg, H., Burkhalter, A., and Way, E. L.: A sensitive fluorometric assay for morphine in plasma and brain. J. Pharm. & Exp. Ther., *145*:247-251, 1964.
16. McIsaac, W. M.: Establishment of a new drug addiction program. Psychopharm. Bull., *3*:40-44, 1966.
17. Milthers, K.: Polarographic determination of small amounts of morphine in blood and plasma. Acta pharmacol. et toxicol., *15*:21-28, 1958.
18. Mulé, S. J.: Determination of narcotic analgesics in human biological materials: Application of

ultraviolet spectrophotometry, thin layer and gas liquid chromatography. Anal. Chem., *36:* 1907-1914, 1964.

19. Mulé, S. J., and Woods, L. A.: Distribution of N-C[14]-methyl labeled morphine: I. In central nervous systems of nontolerant and tolerant dogs. J. Pharmacol. & Exper. Therap., *136:*232-241, 1962.
20. Munier, R., and Macheboeuf, M.: Partition chromatography on paper of alkaloids and various biological nitogenous bases. III. Examples of the separation of various alkaloids by the acidified solvent phase technique. Bull. soc. chim. biol., *33:*846, 1951.
21. Ono, M., and Takehashi, K.: The colorimetric determination of morphine by means of α-nitro-β-naphthol. Eisei Shikenjo Hokoku, *82:*50-53, 1964.
22. Paerregaard, P.: A new method for quantitative determination of small amounts of morphine in human urine. Acta pharmacol. et toxicol., *14:* 38-52, 1957.
23. Saunders, L.: Ion-exchange resins. *In* Stewart, C. P., and Stolman, A. (Eds.); Toxicology, Mechanisms and Analytical Methods, Vol. I. New York, Academic Press, 1960, pp. 366-370.
24. Schieser, D. W.: Free radicals in alkaloid color identification tests. J. Pharm. Sci., *53:*909-913, 1964.
25. Schneider, F. H., and Gillis, C. N.: Catecholamine biosynthesis *in vivo:* An application of thin-layer chromatography. Biochem. Pharm., *14:*623-626, 1965.
26. Sperling, A. R., and Koles, J. E.: Communication. Microgram (BNDD), *1* (9):1, 1968.
27. Stolman, A., and Stewart, C. P.: Drugs extractable by organic solvents from aqueous alkaline solution. *In* Stewart, C. P., and Stolman, A. (Eds.); Toxicology, Mechanisms and Analytical Methods, Vol. I. New York, Academic Press, 1960, pp. 120-150.
28. Szerb, J. C., MacLeod, D. P., Moya, F., and McCurdy, D. H.: Determination of morphine in blood and tissues. Arch. Int. Pharmacodyn., *109:*99-107, 1957.
29. Thienes, C. H., and Haley, T. J.: Clinical Toxicology. Philadelphia, Lea & Febiger, 4th ed., 1964.
30. Way, E. L., and Adler, T. K.: The biological disposition of morphine and its surrogates. Bull. Wld. Hlth. Org., *25:*227-262, 1961; and *Ibid., 27:*359-394, 1962.
31. Way, E. L., Kemp, J. W., Young, J. M., and Grassetti, D. R.: The pharmacologic effects of heroin in relationship to its rate of biotransformation. J. Pharmacol. & Exp. Therap., *129:* 144-154, 1960.
32. Woods, L. A., Cochin, J., Fornefeld, E. G., and Seevers, M. H.: Estimation of morphine in biological materials. J. Pharmacol. & Exp. Therap., *111:*64-73, 1954.

Chapter 24

Measurement of Barbiturates and Glutethimide in Serum by Gas Chromatography

JOHN SAVORY, PH.D., and NORRIS O. ROSZEL

INTRODUCTION

In this section is described a modification of the Winsten and Brody[1] method for identification and quantitation of barbiturates and glutethimide (Doriden) in serum.

PRINCIPLE

Drugs are extracted from serum by shaking with chloroform, and an aliquot of the chloroform extract is injected into the gas chromatograph. The drugs are separated and detected in the effluent gas from the chromatographic column by means of a hydrogen flame ionization detector.

REAGENTS

1. *Chloroform,* reagent grade
2. *Barbiturate stock standard solutions,* 50 mg per 100 ml.
Precisely 50 mg of the barbituric acid derivative (U.S.P. grade) are placed into a 100 ml volumetric flask. Sodium hydroxide (0.45 N) is added to the mark. These solutions must be freshly prepared.
3. Barbiturate working standard solutions, 1, 2, and 5 mg per 100 ml. The stock standard solutions are diluted with 0.45 N sodium hydroxide. These solutions must be freshly prepared.
4. *Glutethimide stock standard solution,* 50 mg per 100 ml. Precisely 50 mg of glutethimide (U.S.P. grade) are placed into a 100 ml volumetric flask and absolute ethanol is added to the mark. This solution is stable for one month.
5. *Glutethimide working standard solutions,* 1, 2 and 5 mg per 100 ml. The stock standard solution is diluted with water. These solutions must be freshly prepared.
6. *Stock chloroform solutions of barbiturates and glutethimide,* 50 mg per 100 ml. Precisely 50 mg of the drug (U.S.P. grade) are placed into a 100 ml volumetric flask and chloroform is added to the mark. These solutions are stable for at least one month.
7. *Working chloroform solutions of barbiturates and glutethimide,* 0.5, 1 and 2.5 mg per 100 ml which are equivalent to 1, 2 and 5 mg per 100 ml when related to chloroform extracts of serum. The stock standard solutions are diluted with chloroform. These solutions are stable for at least one week.

SPECIAL APPARATUS

1. *Microsyringes,* 10 ml capacity (Hamilton Co.).

2. *Glass stoppered centrifuged tubes,* 3.0 ml (Ace Glass Co., Inc., Cat. #8379).

3. *Gas chromatograph* – a model 402 gas chromatograph (Hewlett-Packard Company) is used in the authors' laboratory. This gas chromatograph is fitted with a hydrogen flame ionization detector and with a glass chromatographic column (10 feet long and 1/4-inch diameter) packed with 60 to 80 mesh WAW Chromosorb (Applied Science Laboratories, Inc., State College, Pennsylvania) pre-treated with dimethyldisilazane and impregnated with SE-52 (5% w/w). The column temperature is maintained at 175° C with the flash heater at 225° C. The carrier gas is helium with a flow-rate adjusted to 75 ml per minute.

PROCEDURE

1. Into the 3.0 ml centrifuge tubes are added 1.0 ml of serum and 1.0 ml of each of the working aqueous standard solutions.

2. To each tube is added 0.5 ml of chloroform, the glass stopper is inserted and the contents of the tubes are mixed vigorously for one minute.

3. The tubes are centrifuged at 2000 rpm for 5 minutes to achieve a separation of the aqueous and chloroform layers.

GAS CHROMATOGRAPHY MEASUREMENTS

Three microliters of the chloroform solution (lower layer) are injected onto the column of the gas chromatograph. Chloroform emerges from the column after 0.5 minutes to give a large peak returning to the baseline after 1.5 minutes. The areas of all other peaks are determined by measuring the height (h) and the width at the half-height (w); area = h × w. The identities of unknown peaks are established by comparing retention times with retention times of known drugs which have been prepared in chloroform solution and injected into the gas chromatograph. Final confirmation that the retention time of an unknown peak is identical to that of a particular drug is made by spiking the chloroform extract of serum with a sample of the authentic drug and injecting into the gas chromatograph. If the retention times are identical, a geometrical single peak should appear on the chromatogram with an area greater than the unknown peak in the original serum extract.

Calibration curves for barbiturates and glutethimide are linear. Examples of calibration curves for amobarbital and phenobarbital covering the concentration range 1 to 15 mg per 100 ml are illustrated in Figure 1. Thus, the concentration of any of these drugs in serum may be computed as follows:

$$\text{Conc. of drug(mg/100 ml)} = \frac{\text{Serum extract peak area}}{\text{Standard extract peak area}} \times \text{conc. of standard}$$

Discussion

Studies were made of the efficiency of chloroform extraction of barbiturates and glutethimide from serum using the extraction process in the described procedure. Gas chromatogram peak areas obtained from chloroform extracts of aqueous standard solutions of amobarbital and phenobarbital were compared to

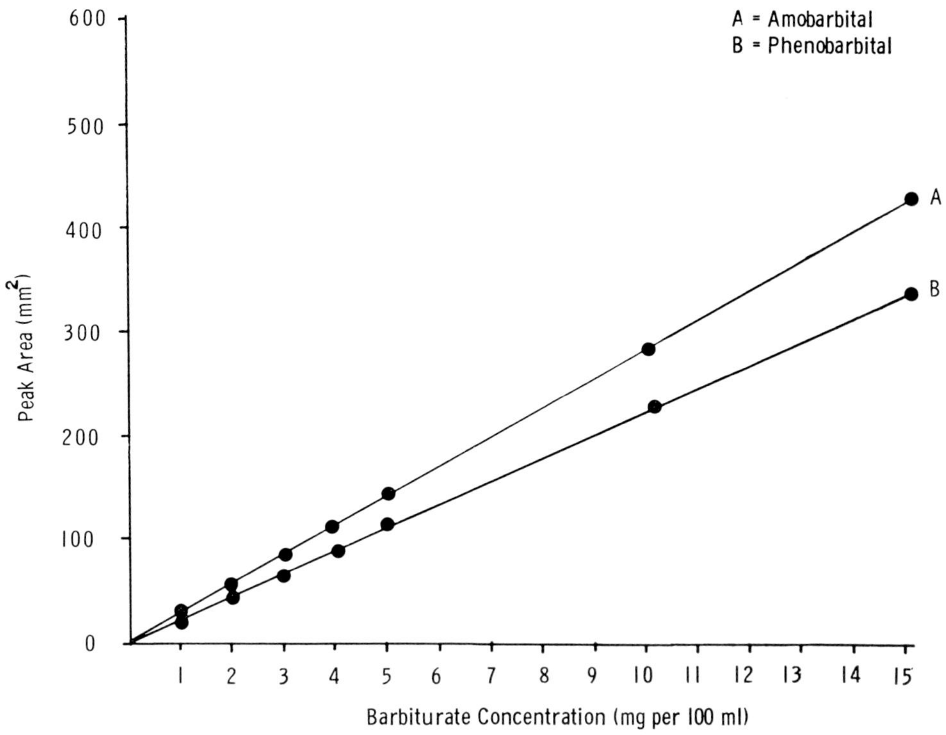

Figure 1. Calibration curves for measurements of amobarbital and phenobarbital.

peak areas from standard chloroform solutions of these two barbiturates. An 80% extraction was obtained over the concentration range of 1 to 10 mg per 100 ml. The present procedure relates gas chromatographic analysis of chloroform extracts of serum to extracts of aqueous standard solutions of barbiturates or glutethimide. Unfortunately, aqueous solutions of barbiturates are relatively unstable and must be prepared daily. Therefore, in most instances it is convenient to use the more stable chloroform solutions of the drugs as standards. Some degree of accuracy is sacrificed when using this method of standardization for the sake of convenience and speed of analysis. If chloroform standards are used, then the calculation for determining the concentration of the drug should involve an additional factor of 1.25 to account for only 80% of the drug being extracted from serum.

Recoveries of amobarbital, phenobarbital and glutethimide added to serum were quantitative and are given in Table I.

The precision of the method was evaluated from the replicate recovery experiments which show a coefficient a variation of approximately 5%.

Using the gas chromatographic conditions in the described procedure, separations of diethylbarbituric acid, amobarbital, pentobarbital, secobarbital, phenobarbital and glutethimide were achieved. The chromatogram obtained from a chloroform solution of a mixture of the barbiturates is illustrated in Figure 2.

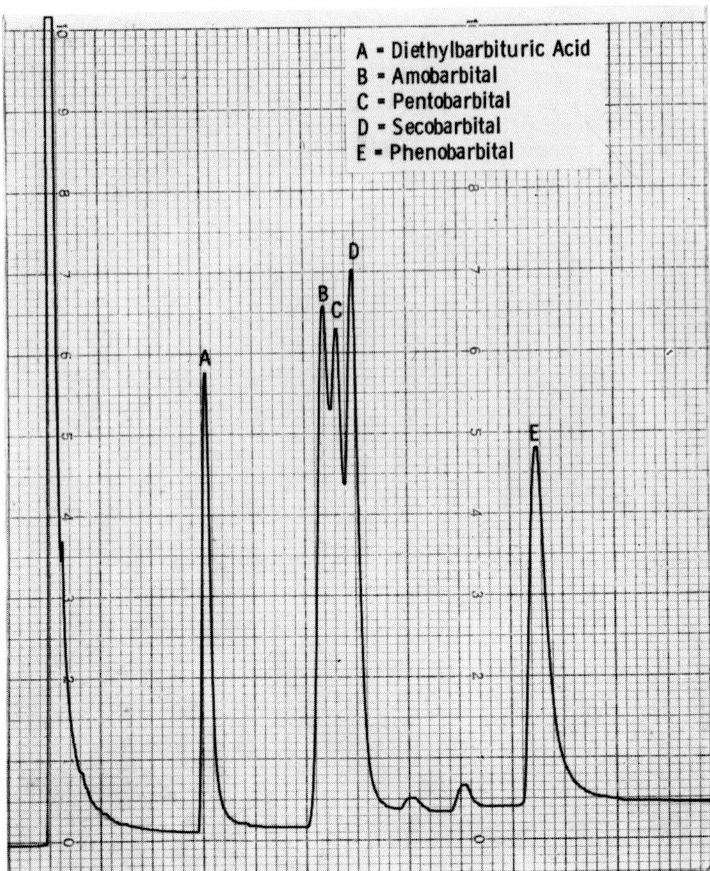

Figure 2. Gas chromatogram of a mixture of barbiturates.

TABLE I: MEASUREMENTS OF THE RECOVERY OF AMOBARBITAL, PHENOBARBITAL, AND GLUTETHIMIDE ADDED TO SERUM

Compound	*Number of Analyses*	*Amount Added (mg per 100 ml)*	*Amount Found* (mg per 100 ml)*	*Recovery* (%)*
Amobarbital	11	6.00	6.00 ± 0.35	101 ± 5.6
Phenobarbital	17	1.51	1.51 ± 0.08	101 ± 5.7
Glutethimide	17	3.50	3.49 ± 0.11	100 ± 3.1

*Mean ± S.D.

Summary

A gas chromatographic procedure for the determination of barbiturates and glutethimide in serum is presented. A chloroform extract of serum is made, an aliquot of the extract injected into the gas chromatograph, and the response of a hydrogen flame ionization detector to the drug is measured. Recoveries of barbiturates and glutethimide added to serum are quantitative. The method can be conveniently used for both qualitative identification and quantitative determination of glutethimide and commonly used barbiturates.

REFERENCE

1. Winsten, S., and Brody, D.: Rapid determination of glutethimide (Doriden) by gas-liquid chromatography. Clin. Chem., *14*:589-594, 1967.

Chapter 25A

Ultraviolet Differential Spectrophotometry for Barbiturates and Salicylates

BENNIE ZAK, PH.D., and LOUIS A. WILLIAMS, B.S.

The difference obtained between two spectra on simultaneously scanning two aliquots of a single concentration of the same compound shifted apart by tautomeric equilibrium or by a change in solvent, pH or oxidation state can be very useful in qualitative and/or quantitative analysis. Several applications of such techniques have been described for ribonucleic acid nucleotides (1), barbiturates (2, 3, 4), thiobarbiturates (5), salicylates (6, 7), alkaloids (8, 9, 10), protein dye binding (11), protein-steroid interactions (12), serum N-acetyl-p-aminophenol (13), salicylate-acetylsalicylate mixtures (14) and indicators (15, 16). Two interesting procedural modifications using ultraviolet spectrophotometry have also been developed for mixtures of barbiturate and salicylate (17, 18).

The ability to screen serum barbiturates as a group is possible because one can easily measure the difference between the two spectra resulting for the two interconvertible forms of the same compound when a spectrophotometric shift is caused by a change in pH. Since both forms of the same compound are simultaneously measured while each is in an individual beam of a ratio-recording spectrophotometer, the response of the photocell can only be due to the absorbance difference between the two chemical species (3). This hypsochromic effect in a spectrophotometric measurement (or bathochromic effect if one happens to shift a spectrum toward the red end of the scale) represents the phenomenon described by some as a type of differential spectroscopy (2, 4, 8). The purpose of this report will be to describe a relatively simple procedure for the determination of barbiturate utilizing this difference between spectra techniques. The change in alkalinity which causes a concommitant change in peak position and intensities and the ratio-recording of this spectrophotometric shift will be described. Since salicylate can be determined by a similar procedure differing only by the pH during the extraction step, its determination and the spectral characteristics of its difference curve will also be discussed. As with barbiturate, some of the problems of interference from other ultraviolet absorbing species present in the serum and extractable under the same conditions can be avoided by the use of the differential characteristics of the ultraviolet spectra of salicylate at two different pH levels. Only substances undergoing a similar hypsochromic effect under the specified conditions could interfere. For example, if salicylate and barbiturate were together and if both were extracted, the 318 nm peak for salicylate would not be interfered with by barbiturates because barbiturates show no differential absorbance characteristics at this wavelength, but the salicylate would distort the differential spectrum of barbiturates (6). Another possibility of the same type is encountered in a procedure for thiobarbiturates. In the determination of surital in the presence of seconal, it has been shown that the 320 nm and 283 nm peaks of surital are not interfered with by seconal because seconal shows no differential absorbance characteristics at these wavelengths though the rest of the surital difference spectrum does interfere with the seconal difference spectrum (5). Some experimental evidence concerning these interferences will be described.

PRINCIPLE

An organic extract of serum is subjected to retrograde extraction into alkaline solution and the latter is then split into 2 equal volumes. To one aliquot is added more alkali while the second aliquot is acidified to pH 10.5 by the addition of ammonium chloride solution (or some other buffer like borate). The lowering of the pH causes a hypsochromic shift of the peak to a shorter wavelength and a hyperchromic effect on the shifted peak since the spectral curve characteristics also change with pH change. The simultaneous recording of the difference between the two spectra is accomplished by means of a two beam ratio-recording spectrophotometer resulting in a spectral curve showing well-defined negative and positive absorbance peaks in the difference spectrum. The choice as to which peak is negative or positive is arbitrary and depends on the placement of either cuvet in the reference beam of the spectrophotometer. If the more alkaline solution is placed in the reference beam, then the 260 nm peak is negative to the base line while the 240 nm peak is positive. If the cuvets are reversed, then the deflections occur in the opposite directions. In either case, the absorbance values obtained will be identical in quantity and will only differ by sign.

REAGENTS

Spectral grade solvents were used for the extraction of barbiturates from serum, although Analytical Reagent grade would be adequate.

1. *Ammonium chloride,* 16% (w/v).
2. *Sodium Hydroxide,* 0.45N.
3. *Chloroform,* spectral grade. Methylene chloride has also been used for this analysis and is preferable if doriden is to be determined on the same sample.
4. *Whatman 41-H paper.*
5. *Stock barbiturate standard.* 100 mg of phenobarbital is dissolved in 100 ml of 0.45N NaOH.
6. *Working barbiturate standard.* 0.1, 0.2, 0.3, 0.4 and 0.5 ml of the stock barbiturate standard are diluted to 10 ml with 0.45N NaOH. Three ml of 0.45N NaOH are added to 5 ml of each standard. Two 3.0 ml aliquots of each aliquot are treated in the same manner as the retrograde extract de-

scribed under procedure. These solutions represent 1, 2, 3, 4 and 5 mg of barbiturate per 100 ml of liquid analyzed for a 5 ml sample aliquot tested.

7. *Stock and working standards* for salicylate are made up in 0.45N NaOH in the same manner as are the phenobarbital standards. These could cover the range of 0-100 mg per 100 ml and would depend on the concentrations expected to be encountered by the analyst.

APPARATUS

1. Extractomatic separatory funnel shaker (Virtis). This equipment is not essential to the procedure but makes the 5 minute extraction step simple to perform and if necessary eight samples can be extracted at one time.
2. Extractomatic funnels (Virtis-100 ml) with teflon stopcocks. This vented extraction funnel fits the equipment above and helps make the extraction process semi-automatic as well as simple.
3. Any automatic, ratio-recording ultraviolet spectrophotometer capable of presenting its information in the logarithmic form. There are several common instruments available which are suitable for the purpose and these include the Beckman DK-2A, the Beckman DBG (or DB) with log recorder and the log converted Coleman-Hitachi 124 with a linear recorder. Other companies such as Unicam, Perkin-Elmer and Cary Instruments also have equipment adequate for carrying out this procedure.

PROCEDURE

1. Serum Barbiturates

Three to five ml of serum, blood or sonicated tissue homogenate are pipetted into 50 ml of spectral grade chloroform contained in a 100 ml extractomatic funnel. The funnel is clamped into the shaking apparatus which is turned on for a period of 5 minutes. On standing, the two layers separate and the chloroform phase (lower) is filtered into a clean and dry separatory funnel. Eight ml of sodium hydroxide (0.45N) are pipetted into the chloroform which is then back extracted on the extraction apparatus for 5 minutes. Although it would seem that such a procedure might be more accurate by using a large aliquot rather than all of the filtered chloroform we have found in practice that careful filtration does not result in enough loss of the organic phase to make this step necessary. However, a user of this procedure might feel safer in taking some exact aliquot. The lower phase is discarded (or saved for a doriden determination) and the upper phase is centrifuged and the remaining chloroform aspirated off. (For this purpose, we have found that a long flat-tipped needle attached to a sink aspirator works well. Pinching the tubing with the aspirator connected provides excellent control of the aspiration rate.) Two 3 ml aliquots of the clear NaOH solution are pipetted into two stoppered silica cuvets. Sodium hydroxide solution (0.5 ml) is added to one cuvet while 0.5 ml of 16 percent NH_4Cl is added to the other cuvet. Two differential techniques are possible for the analyst which yield the same results. In one technique, the zero of the instrument is mechanically displaced by means of the operating range switch on the Beckman DK2A, or DBG, (It is a special attachment on this instrument.) or potentiometrically displaced by the powerful 100% control of the Hitachi 124 spectrophotometer. Such a 100% control can be substituted by wiring it into the DB (DBG) as a replacement potentiometer. In the other technique, if the DBG (or DB) does not have this attachment, the reference beam can be partially blocked by a beam attenuator which is a cuvet sized black metal block with an adjustable opening in the light path of the spectrophotometer. It has a large screw which when turned inward, slowly closes the rectangular opening of the attenuator, changes the ratio of light passed by the two chopped beams of light and thereby causes the pen of the logarithmic recorder to move upscale as it hunts electrical balance. Fine adjustment is then made by means of the 100% control. The zero of the instrument is adjusted to 0.5 absorbance using air beams and the 100 percent control. The more alkaline solution is placed in the sample compartment of the spectrophotometer and the instrument readjusted to 0.5 absorbance if necessary. The differential spectrum of the well-mixed, bubble-free solutions is recorded through the 340 nm — 220 nm portion of the ultraviolet spectrum. The result for barbiturates is a two peak curve showing a positive deflection from the baseline in the 260 nm region and a negative deflection from the baseline in the 240 nm region. A crossover point will be observed in the vicinity of 250 nm which is the isosbestic point of the spectra of the two solutions being measured. The absorbance difference between the 2 peaks at 260 nm and 240 nm (personal communication from L.A. Williams, Clinchem Laboratory, Boston, Mass.) or the reading above baseline of the 260 nm peak is used to determine the concentration of barbiturate. The shape of the difference curve is a qualitative indication of the presence of barbiturate. Thus, one can see that this really is a subtraction step in which the automatic recording instrument plots only the absorbance difference between the pH 13.0 spectrum and the pH 10.5 spectrum. The resultant curve with its flip-flop wave is representative of the barbiturate difference spectrum.

2. Serum salicylates

One ml of 6N HCl is added to 1 ml of serum and the acidified serum is mixed with 50 ml of $CHCl_3$ contained in the extractomatic apparatus. From this point on the procedure is identical to the one described for barbiturates. The differential recording on the aliquots of salicylate at pH 10.5 and 13.0 is made from 340 nm to 220 nm and three peaks are obtained, a positive peak at 318 nm, a negative peak at 283 nm and a second positive peak at 246 nm. Depending on concentrations encountered, any of the three wavelengths could be used for quantitative determinations. The negative peak at 283 nm is the least sensitive and it can be used for high concentrations of barbiturate about 50 mg per 100 ml. The positive peak at 318 nm can be used in the 0-50 mg per 100 ml range while the most sensitive peak at 246 nm is useful in the 0-20 mg per 100 ml range.

Definitions

Some of the terminology used in this report are herewith defined, but one must realize that these effects are relative to each other and this relative character will be described.

Hypsochromic shift, or effect (16).

This is a change in the system which causes a shift in the spectral curve toward a shorter wavelength.

Bathochromic shift, or effect. This is a change in the system which causes a shift in the spectral curve toward a longer wavelength.

Hyperchromic effect. This is a change in the system which causes the solution to have a spectral curve with a higher absorbance reading for the absorption band (20).

Hypochromic effect. This is a change in the system which causes the solution to have a spectral curve with a lower absorbance reading for the absorption band (20).

In case of barbiturate, the change in pH from 13.0 to 10.5 results in a shift in the spectral curve to a shorter wavelength (hypsochromic effect) and an increase in absorbance for the shifted curve (hyperchromic effect). If one were to change the pH from 10.5 to 13.0, then the spectral curve would shift toward the longer wavelength (bathochromic effect) and the absorbance intensity of the peak would be lowered (hypochromic effect). Thus, the relative nature of these effects is easily understood for it depends on which solution you are converting from in the process, or which direction you shift to, towards longer or shorter wavelengths.

Isosbestic point (15, 16). The isosbestic point (point of equal absorbance) is the wavelength at which the spectral curves of the two forms of an interconvertible substance cross each other. The interconversion can take place because of pH change, oxidation-reduction or tautomeric equilibrium. The material scanned would be the same in both cuvets and in the same concentration in both cuvets.

Discussion

The pH system used in this procedure for both salicylate and barbiturate measurements was selected because it shows maximal spectral changes, i.e., the largest hypsochromic shifts and hyperchromic effects leading to the most significant qualitative character for the differential spectrum graphed. Both cuvets contain the same concentration of barbiturate or salicylate and the only distinguishing characteristic of each is the pH difference, 10.5 for one and 13.0 for the other. This is a useful feature, for interference can only occur if another compound was present which exhibited the effect of spectral shifting at the two pH values used. Thus the interference from several extraneous ultraviolet absorbing materials is essentially excluded. The advantage over more conventional manual ultraviolet spectrophotometry is obvious.

Figure 1, upper left quadrant, graphically indicates the basis for the difference spectrum obtained by the use of the described technique. Curve B is the spectrum obtained for phenobarbital at a very alkaline pH in a medium of 0.45N NaOH. When curve C is the resultant spectrum, the same concentration of the barbiturate is looked at spectrophotometrically with the pH of the solution lowered to 10.5 by the addition of 16 percent NH_4Cl. If solution C is placed in the reference beam of a double beam spectrophotometer and solution B in the sample beam, the difference between the two curves can be automatically graphed resulting in curve A. If the two solutions were transposed into the opposite beams, the difference curve would flip over showing a negative peak below the baseline where it had previously shown a positive peak and vice-versa. The point at which the difference curve crosses the zero absorbance line represents the isosbestic point at which curve B crosses curve C. The isosbestic point may also be used for qualitative analysis (7). This zero line would be at 0.50 absorbance on the graph of this quadrant. The upper right quadrant shows the differential absorbance calibration curve covering the range of 0-30 of phenobarbital per ml. This calibration is linear over a rather wide range of concentration. The two lower quadrants show the differential absorption spectra of several representative barbiturates treated as described for phenobarbital and these similar looking difference spectra provide ample evidence of the useful qualitative character of the procedure.

Figure 2, upper left quadrant, shows the percent transmittance-wavelength spectra graphed for several of a number of pH values tested in an effort to obtain the best shift for the differential recording of salicylate Curves 1 and 3 were

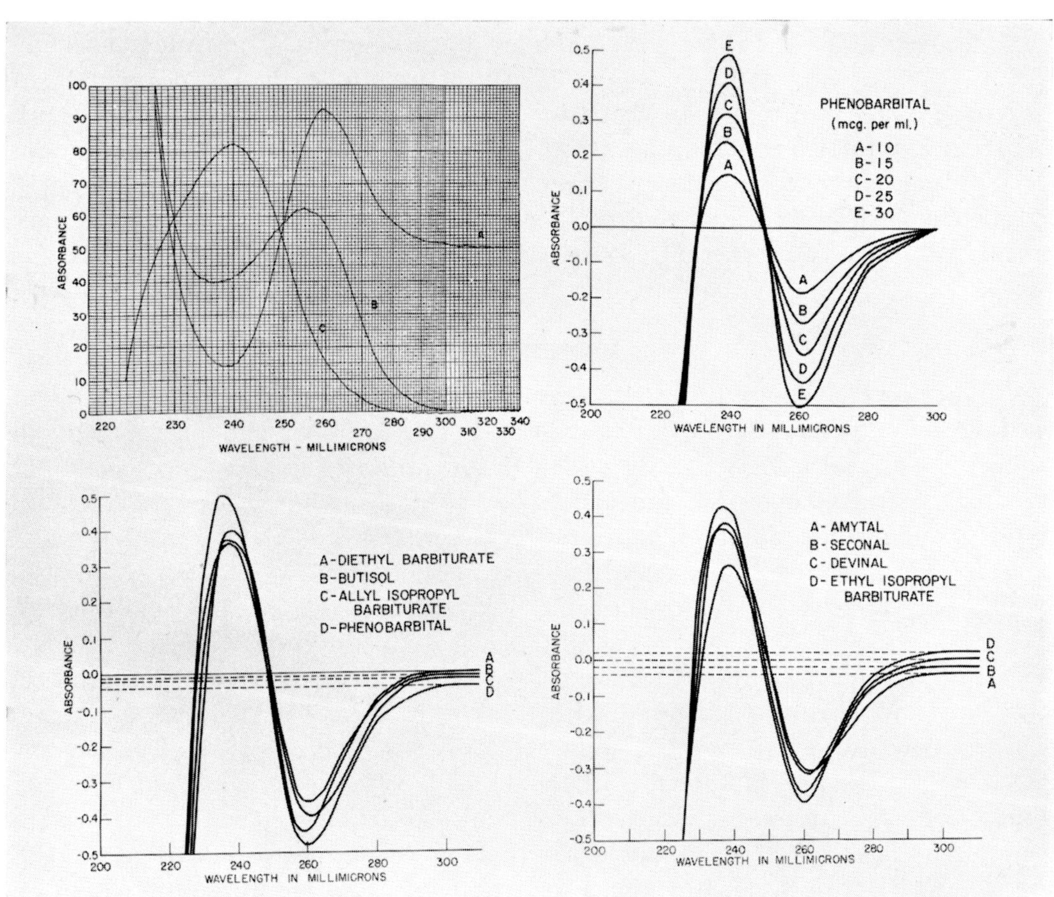

Figure 1. **Upper left** — curve B, normal spectrum (very alkaline), curve C, normal spectrum (pH 10.5) and curve A automatic difference spectrum. **Upper right** — Differential absorbance spectra of various concentrations of phenobarbital. **Lower left and right** — Differential absorbance spectra of several barbiturates. (Reprinted from Reference 2 with permission of the Elsevier Publishing Company).

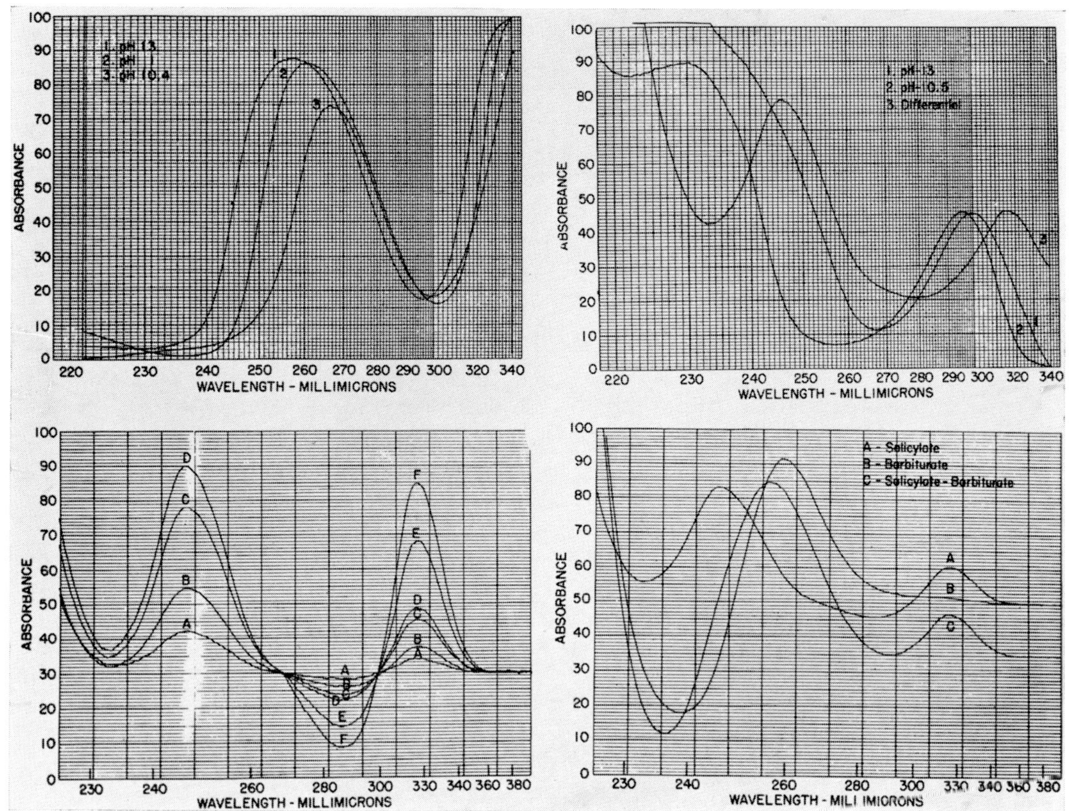

Figure 2. **Upper left** — Wavelength per cent transmittance spectra for salicylate at various pH levels. **Upper right** — Normal and differential spectra of salicylate at pH 10.5 and pH 13.0. **Lower left** — Differential absorbance wavelength graphs of several concentrations of salicylate. **Lower right** — Curve A., salicylate differential spectrum. Curve B. seconal differential spectrum. Curve C. differential spectrum of a mixture of barbiturate and salicylate. (Reprinted from Reference 6 with permission of the C. V. Mosby Company).

selected because they yielded the curves most suited to differential spectroscopy. The upper right quadrant shows the absorbance curves (1 and 2) at the two pH values as well as the differential curve drawn by placing the same concentration solutions of salicylate into the reference and sample compartments of the double beam ratio recording spectrophotometer, then graphing the difference between the two spectra when a hypsochromic or bathochromic shift was caused by the change in pH between the two solutions.

In the lower left quadrant, the calibration difference graphs obtained for several concentrations of salicylate are described. The first positive maximum at 318 nm is useful through the range of 0-50 mg per 100 ml. The much less sensitive minimum at 283 nm could possibly be used for even higher values while the strongest maximum difference was obtained at 246 nm. The use of this peak is accurate and sensitive up to 20 mg per 100 ml.

A mixture of barbiturate and salicylate is graphed as a differential absorption spectrum in the lower right quadrant, curve C. The peak at 318 nm is undistorted for salicylate whereas the other maximum and minimum peaks of either salicylate or barbiturate are shifted and distorted by each other's presence. However, extraction under properly established pH conditions could be established to accomplish differential extraction of salicylate and barbiturate from each other still leaving the residual chloroform phase to contain Doriden after retrograde extraction had been completed.

A special class of barbiturates, the thiobarbiturates used in anaesthesiology, can also be determined by the difference absorbance technique. Since they are commonly used but less commonly determined, the characteristics found for them in the differential procedure will be described.

Figure 3, upper left quadrant, shows the spectra, curves B, obtained for thiamylal (Surital) and thiopental (Pentothal) in 0.45N NaOH while curves C represent the effect of the addition of 16% NH_4Cl to solutions of the same concentrations of the barbiturates. For both compounds, curve A represents the spectrophotometric subtractive results

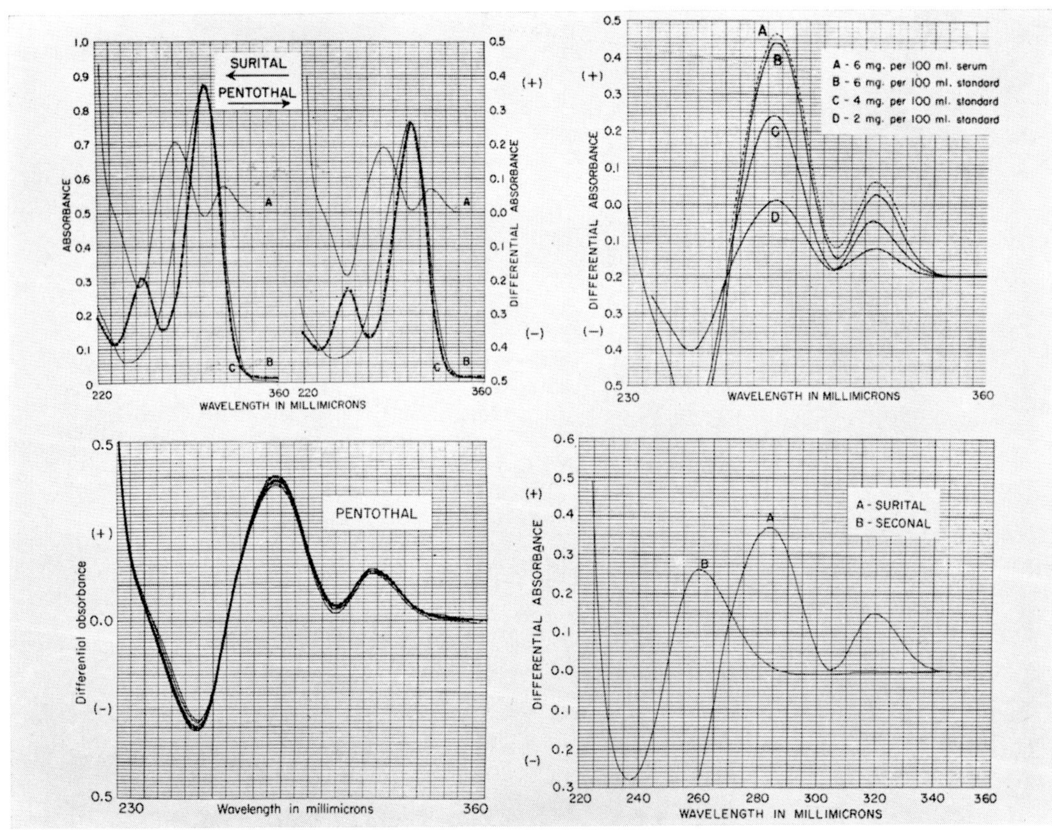

Figure 3. **Upper left** — Normal and differential spectra for thiamylal sodium (Surital) and thiopental sodium (Pentothal) at two different pH values. **Upper right** — Calibration spectra, Curves B, C, and D; and superimposed serum extract spectrum for thiopental sodium, Curve A. **Lower left** — Precision study carried out for thiopental sodium (Pentothal) 3 mg/100 ml showing differential spectra. **Lower right** — Differential spectra of thiamylal sodium (Surital), curve A, and secobarbital (Seconal), curve B.

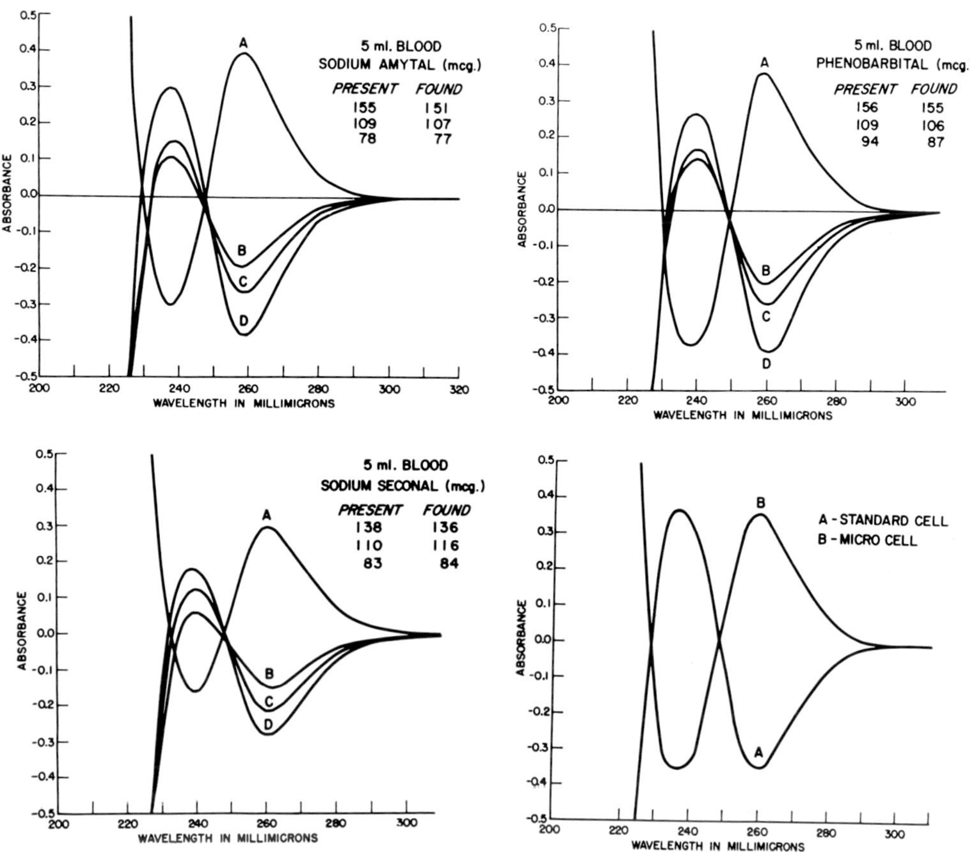

Figure 4. **Upper left, right and lower left** — Recoveries of several concentrations of amytal, phenobarbital and seconal Curves B, C and D added to bloods and a standard flipped over, Curve A. **Lower right** — Differential spectra of barbiturate scanned in macro and micro cuvets. (Used to obtain the recovery data of Reference 2, Table 1.)

showing a differential curve which is somewhat different than the one shown for the barbiturates of Figure 1. Two positve peaks and one negative peak are obtained with these compounds in differential spectrophotometry.

In the upper right quadrant are graphed the differential calibration curves for pentothal covering the range of 0-6 mg per 100 ml. In the same figure, a fortified serum (6 mg per 100 ml) is shown from which the thiobarbiturate was extracted, back extracted and then scanned differentially through the ultraviolet range. Curve A, the resultant spectrum obtained, was shifted up slightly to differentiate it from the 6 mg per 100 ml standard, but it is quite clear that these are superimposable graphs. The lower left quadrant shows the precision obtained for 3 mg per 100 ml pentothal samples in a reprocibility study. The curves were drawn from the analysis of ten artificially fortified serums in the described process and yielded a range of 2.88 mg to 3.14 mg per 100 ml for a 3 mg per 100 ml addition. The lower right quadrant shows the effect on the difference spectrum obtained by the inclusion of a common barbiturate in an interference study. Curve B shows the difference curve obtained for secobarbital while curve A is the difference curve for Surital. There appears to be no interference for the 283 nm peak in the presence of a significant amount of secobarbital.

Figure 4, upper left and right and lower left quadrants show the differential spectra for recovery studies carried out on barbiturate fortified bloods where each value shown was recovered from a different blood specimen. Most of the time, morgue specimens must be blood rather than serum and the values found for amytal, phenobarbital and seconal were determined with the use of this type of specimen. A standard differential spectrum is shown with each of the recovery sets. In the lower right quadrant, two differential spectra are graphed in both a conventional 10 mm cuvet (3 ml volume) and a micro cell. Obviously, the sample size can be decreased by using smaller volume systems throughout the procedure. Although blood was used in this study, as a necessity because this was a medical examiner experiment, we prefer serum or plasma because of the possibility of unequal diffusion across the red cell wall (21) as well as unequal distribution of water between the red blood cell and plasma compartments previously described for ethanol (22).

Quality Control

One area of analysis with respect to toxicological determinations which has seen little exploitation is that of quality control. A proprietary material prepared for this purpose was tested under several conditions of handling. Fifteen vials kept at 4°C were reconstituted at the rate of one each day with 5 ml of distilled water and analyzed for their barbiturate content thirty minutes after the water addition. The results are shown as Group 1 in Table I. Group 2 was another set of vials kept at room temperature throughout the experiment, reconstituted at the rate of one each day for five days and the barbiturate content determined 30 minutes after solubilization with 5.0 ml of distilled water. The third set of five vials, Group 3, were reconstituted with distilled water, kept at room temperature throughout the study and analyzed for barbiturate content at the rate of one per day. Group 4 was a set of five vials whose lyophilized contents were dissolved, refrigerated at 4°C with one vial analyzed each day until all were used up during the experiment. The excellent results indicate that such materials are a distinct advantage for improved analytical control in the determination. Salicylate, bro-

TABLE I: BARBITURATE RECOVERY FROM QUALITY CONTROL SAMPLES[1]

Day	*Group 1*	*Group 2*	*Group 3*	*Group 4*
1	2.0	2.0	—	—
2	2.0	2.0	—	—
3	2.0	2.0	—	—
4	1.9	2.0	—	—
5	2.0	2.0	—	—
6	1.9	—	2.0	—
7	2.0	—	2.0	—
8	2.0	—	2.0	—
9	2.2	—	2.0	—
10	2.2	—	1.9	—
11	2.0	—	—	2.0
12	2.1	—	—	2.1
13	2.2	—	—	2.0
14	2.0	—	—	2.1
15	2.1	—	—	2.0

[1]Lyophilized serums were made up to contain 2.0 mg of barbiturate per 100 ml by the Warner-Chilcott Laboratories, General Diagnostics Division, Morris Plains, New Jersey. Blind determinations carried out by laboratory of Wayne County Medical Examiner (Dr. H. R. Wetherell, Jr.)

mide, doriden and ethanol controls prepared by the same company have also been tested and found to be useful in similar studies.

Another distinct advantage of the automatic differential graphing system over a conventional manual operation is the time saved over plotting a number of points for each aliquot and the numerous though simple calculations entailed in this process (19). Some procedures use 10-11 readings for each of the two solutions (20-22 readings in all) and these many readings must then be subjected to the arithmatic of the calculations (3).

Still another advantage of the procedure is that no blank solutions are required. The two solvents, NaOH and NH_4Cl-NaOH, in the concentrations described, read the same from 340 nm to 230 nm. This enables one to take full advantage of the hypsochromic-hyperchromic effects being measured. The subtraction of one spectrum from the other spectrum is automatic and rapid because of the ratio-recording technique of instrumentation in which the light is rapidly chopped back and forth through the two cuvets to form an effective 2 beam system using a single detector.

Summary

A procedure has been described which is useful for the determination of barbiturates or salicylate. It involves the use of ultraviolet differential spectrophotometry for the simultaneous measurement of two interconvertible forms of the same compound at the same concentration. The response of the photomultiplier results in a specrum which represents the subtraction of the spectral curve of the one form from the spectral curve of the second form to which the compound (barbiturate or salicylate) has been converted by a change in pH. The procedure is simple, relatively rapid and quite reproducible. No separate blanking of the samples is required.

REFERENCES

1. Zak, B., and Weiner, L. M.: Rapid electrophoresis of RNA nucleotides in a dilute agar gel paper medium. J. Chromatog., *13*:255-258, 1964.
2. Williams, L. A., and Zak, B.: Determination of barbiturates by automatic differential spectrophotometry. Clin. Chim. Acta, *4*:170-174, 1959.
3. Goldbaum, L. R.: Determination of barbiturates. Anal. Chem., *24*:1604-1607, 1952.
4. Bush, M. T.: Extraction and identification of barbiturates. Microchem. J., *5*:73-90, 1961.
5. Williams, L. A., Hardy, A. T., Cohen, J. S., and Zak, B.: Ultraviolet differential spectrophotometry of barbiturates. J. Med. Pharm. Chem., *2*:609-615, 1960.
6. Williams, L. A., Linn, R. A., and Zak, B.: Differential ultraviolet spectrophotometric determination of serum salicylates. J. Lab. Clin. Med., *53*: 156-162, 1959.
7. Shane, N. A., and Routh, J. I.: Use of Isosbestic point as a base line in differential spectrophotometry. Anal. Chem., *39*:414, 1967.
8. Goldbaum, L. R., and Williams, M. A.: The identification and determination of micrograms of morphine in biological samples. J. Forensic Sci., *13*:253-261, 1968.
9. Williams, L. A., Brusock, Y. M., and Zak, B.: Rapid elctrophoresis of alkaloids. Anal. Chem., *32*:1883-1885, 1960.
10. Harms, D. R.: Identification of morphine and codeine in the urine by thin-layer chromatography and ultraviolet spectrophotometry. Am. J. Med. Tech., *11*:1-8, 1965.
1. Failing, J. F., Jr., Buckley, M. W., and Zak, B.: A study on an ultramicro and automated procedure for serum proteins. Am. J. Med. Tech., *27*:177-183, 1961.
12. Ryan, M. T.: Examination of steroid protein interaction by ultraviolet difference spectrophotometry. Arch. Biochem. Biophys., *126*:407-417, 1968.

13. Routh, J. I., Shane, N. A., Arredondo, E. G., and Paul, W. D.: Determination of N-acetyl-p-aminophenol in plasma. Clin. Chem., *14*:882-889, 1968.

14. Shane, N. A., and Routh, J. I.: Use of isosbestic point as a base line in differential spectrophotometry. Anal. Chem., *39*:414, 1967.

15. Bauman, R. P.: Absorption Spectroscopy. John Wiley & Sons, Inc., New York, 1962, pp. 419-420.

16. Mellon, M. G.: Analytical Absorption Spectroscopy, Absorptimetry and Colorimetry. John Wiley and Sons, Inc., New York, 1950, pp. 314-318.

17. Guzak, R., and Caraway, W. T.: Simultaneous determination of serum barbiturate and salicylate by ultraviolet absorption spectrophotometry. Am. J. Med. Tech., *29*:231-239, 1963.

18. Bjerre, S., and Porter, C. J.: Simultaneous determination of barbiturates and salicylates by ultraviolet spectrophotometry. Clin. Chem., *11*: 137-154, 1965.

19. Sunshine, I.: Barbiturate in Standard Methods of Clinical Chemistry, Vol. 3, edited by David Seligson. Academic Press, 1961, pp. 46-54.

20. Brode, W. R.: Chemical Spectroscopy, 2nd ed. John Wiley and Sons, Inc., London, 1947, pp. 214-215.

21. Stewart, C. P., and Stolman, A. (Eds.): Toxicology, Mechanisms and Analytical Methods, Vol. 1. New York, Academic Press, 1960, pp. 71-91.

22. Payne, J. P., Hill, D. W., and Wood, D. G. L.: Distribution of ethanol between plasma and erythrocytes in whole blood. Nature, *217*:963-964, 1968.

Chapter 25B

Spectrophotometric Measurement of Bromide in Serum and Urine[1,2]

F. WILLIAM SUNDERMAN, M.D., PH.D., and
J. HENRY WILKINSON, PH.D., D.SC.

Principle

Bromide is measured by a modification of the Barbour, Pilkington, and Sargant method.[3] A colored gold bromide complex is formed by the addition of gold chloride to solutions containing bromide in the presence of excess chloride and hydrogen ions. The resulting color is measured photometrically.

REAGENTS

1. *Sodium chloride solution* (0.5 gm per 100 ml).
2. *Trichloracetic acid* (30 gms per 100 ml).
3. *Gold chloride* 0.5 percent (w/v).
4. *Standard* 128.8 mg of anhydrous sodium bromide are dissolved in 100 ml of water. This solution contains 100 mg bromide per 100 ml. The solution should be discarded if it develops a straw color.

PROCEDURE FOR SERUM

One ml of serum is added to a mixture of 6 ml of the sodium chloride solution and one ml of trichloracetic acid. The precipitated proteins are filtered through a Whatman #40 filter paper. To 4 ml of the filtrate is added 0.5 ml of the gold chloride solution. The solution is then read in a photometer at 470 mμ. The bromide concentration is estimated from a plot of bromide standards using an appropriate factor to correct for dilution.

PROCEDURE FOR URINE

The procedure for the estimation of bromide in urine is similar to that of serum excepting that decolorization is effected by means of activated charcoal.

Approximately 0.8 gm of activated charcoal is added to 8 ml of urine. The urine and charcoal are mixed, allowed to stand for 10 minutes and then filtered.

An aliquot (usually 1 or 2 ml) of the urine filtrate is measured into a tube containing 2 ml of sodium chloride solution and 0.5 ml of trichloracetic acid solution. One-half ml of the gold chloride solution is then added and the volume is adjusted to 5 ml with water. The colored solution is measured photometrically as with serum. With highly colored urine samples, it is desirable to prepare urine blanks.

NORMAL VALUES

The normal range of bromide concentration in serum is 0.5 to 2.5 mg per 100 ml. Bromide intoxication of clinical importance occurs at levels over 50 mg per 100 ml.

REFERENCES

1. Dunlop, M.: Simple colorimetric method for the determination of bromide in urine. J. Clin. Path., *20*:300-301, 1967.
2. Underwood, P. J.: An automated method for the analysis of urinary bromide. Aust. J. Exp. Biol. Med. Sci., *45*:577-580, 1967.
3. Barbour, R. F., Pilkington, F., and Sargant, W.: Bromide intoxication. Brit. Med. Jour., *2*:957-960, 1936.

Chapter 26A

Carbon Monoxide Poisoning: Basic Concepts and Current Clinical-Pathologic Implications

MORRIS F. WIENER, M.D.

INTRODUCTION

No single chemical agent causes more deaths than CO (carbon monoxide) which is mainly a product of civilization and aptly termed the silent killer.[4, 16] Its presence in the fumes of fire, in exhaust gases, in illuminating gases and in tobacco smoke makes it a constant hazard to man. CO, one of the most insidious poisons known, is a colorless, tasteless, non-irritating and almost odorless gas.[5] It is produced by the oxidation or incomplete combustion of any carbonaceous material and hence is a product of many natural, industrial and domestic processes. It is virtually insoluble in water, and water sprays will not remove it from air. It is slightly lighter than air (specific gravity 0.9671:1 at 20°C) and therefore rises above ground level. Human perception of it comes only from its poisoning effect of oxygen-starvation, and practical detection is only by instrument.

Historical

The history of CO gas is entwined with the history of mankind. Awareness of this poison dates back practically from the time fire became known to man. Volcanic gases contain CO, and the mythical gods produced it in their forges. In Ancient Rome, would-be suicides "crossed the bridge of death" in seeking the aid of CO in the fumes of charcoal, and CO was used for punishment at the time of Cicero (106-43 B.C.).

Greek writers of the third century, Erasistratus and Aurelianus, hypothesized that fumes (CO) caused thinness of the air, which in man, obstructed normal breathing and caused insensible disturbance of motion and senses. Indeed, CO actually "obstructs" and prevents respiration at the precellular level.

Ignorance concerning CO poisoning persisted in large areas of Western Europe through the early 18th century and even later despite the advance of knowledge in the natural sciences since antiquity. Many sudden deaths ascribed to the work of the devil in those days were very probably CO poisoning, as in the case of an incident in Jena, Germany, in 1715, in which a student and two farmers died in a hut heated by a kindled wood-fire before the scheduled calling of the spirits at midnight. This created the myth "those who call the devil become victims of the master of darkness." Even with the spreading knowledge of Claude Bernard's observations in 1857 that CO poisoning caused anoxic anoxia, many varied myths regarding this gas persisted into the 20th century. In some European countries, mothers were known to hold their restless children momentarily over the gas-oven to induce sleep.

The greatest single source of CO is now the motor vehicle, increasing in number each year with over 90 million vehicles in the United States in 1967. Every gallon of fuel emits three pounds of CO plus other pollutants into the air. Legal government standards for CO applicable to motor vehicles first became effective in 1968. This is 100 years after the internal combustion engine was recognized as a source of CO, at which time efforts had first been made toward air-pollution control-engineering.

Progressively hazardous pollution of our environment continues with the rapidly growing industrial technology, while we ignore the potentially catastrophic effects of CO. Our conquest of space must not become the only solution of, or escape from, this "cordon malsanitaire." About 169,000,000 lbs of CO from motor vehicles alone are being added daily to the atmospheric aerial garbage. This is equivalent to each urban dweller pouring 30 lbs. of CO into the air of American cities.

Bio-chemical Physiology of Carbon Monoxide, a Chemical Asphyxiant

Carbon monoxide, an otherwise chemically inert gas, rapidly combines with Hb. (hemoglobin) to form COHb (carboxyhemoglobin) which blocks the vital respiratory pigment of the red blood cell from carrying O_2 (oxygen) to the tissues from the lung, and CO_2 (carbon dioxide) to the lung from the tissues. CO is dangerous only to red-blooded mammals who have Hb blood pigment.

Carbon monoxide may also react with other "heme-containing pigments" and enzymes such as myoglobin, cytochrome and certain other pigments found in the brain, the physiologic effects of which are unclear.[51]

The reaction of CO with Hb is reversible, and in many physico-chemical respects, the details of the reversible reaction are very similar to those of the reactions of O_2 with Hb.[20] Hb or blood, when exposed to a gas mixture containing a sufficient pCO (partial pressure of CO), becomes saturated with the gas in the proportion of one molecule of CO to one atom of iron in the Hb molecule, but the pCO required is only about 1/200 to 1/300 of the pO_2 (partial pressure of O_2) for the saturation of Hb with O_2. If exposed to a mixture of the two gases sufficient to saturate the Hb, an equilibrium is eventually reached according to the Haldane equation[23]:

$$\frac{HbCO}{HbO} = M \frac{pCO}{pO_2}$$

The HbCO, HbO_2 represent respectively the number of moles of CO and

O_2 combined with the Hb in one liter of blood (or Hb Solution) and M is a constant. The value of M varies markedly with species, but only slightly, if at all, in different individuals of the same species. In human blood, at 37°C at physiologic pH (7.3), M usually lies within the range of 200 to 250.

The canary has always been considered more "sensitive" to CO than man. This belief is erroneous and is due to the fact that the canary reaches a state of equilibrium with the CO more rapidly than does man; however, this is only true when the concentration is greater than 20 parts CO per 10,000. This counterbalances the lesser affinity of CO for Hb. in the canary, which is 110 against 210 for man. At CO levels of 6 to 12.5 parts per 10,000 the canary will fall from its perch, varying with individual sensitivity. However, in man, unconsciousness will occur at 4 to 5 pp 10,000. Thus the canary is an unreliable indicator of the safety of an environment.[47]

The remarkable affinity of CO for the reactive groups of Hb, which is about 210 times greater than that of O_2 in man, makes it possible for small amounts of CO to immobilize a significant amount of Hb.

Once equilibrium is established between atmosphere and blood CO, a matter of some hours, each ppmCO in the air up to 100ppm will inactivate 1/6 of 1% of Hb. Exposure to the maximum permissible 100ppmCO for 6 to 8 hours will result in 15% COHb saturation. A seemingly inconsequential 0.02% CO can be lethal under certain conditions of temperature, humidity, CO_2 content in the air, anemia and physical activity. The ratio of COHb to HbO in the blood, resulting from breathing air poisoned by CO, depend upon the partial pressures of O_2 and CO, the latter binding equal amounts of Hb. at correspondingly smaller pressures. However, in the presence of CO in the blood, Hb. molecules not combined with CO "cling to O_2 with abnormal tenacity."[23] In other words, CO in the blood displaces the O_2 dissociation curve to the left.[20] The effects of CO in the blood are similar to that of ambient air with low pO_2 in a sense.

Absorption of CO from contaminated air is at first rapid. Increase in the rate of pulmonary ventilation will shorten the time necessary for the CO in the air and blood to reach equilibrium. The amount of CO that can be bound by Hb is usually greater in proportion to the amount in the air due to the high affinity and despite the low pCO. No equilibrium is reached in rapidly fatal cases. The severity of CO poisoning depends upon the concentration, duration of inhalation and rate of pulmonary ventilation.

The bio-chemical exchange of O_2 for the metabolite CO_2 at the cellular level, furthermore, requires the catalytic enzymatic action that is induced by the physico-chemical dissociation of HbO. The COHb, having no such effect, results in the intracellular retention of CO_2 and thereby causes decreased blood-CO_2 content. Although a waste product, CO_2 is vitally important as a stimulant to the respiratory center by increasing the H-ion of the blood. Concurrent with retardation of HbO dissociation, the arterial pO_2 remains unchanged. Since the carotid sinus is stimulated by lowered arterial pO_2, and not by arterial O_2-content, this specific stimulus to increase ventilation is lacking.[20]

The asphyxia caused by CO therefore

differs from suffocation in that the COHb not only interferes with the dissociation of HbO, but also prevents the removal of CO_2 metabolite from the cells.

Histotoxicity of CO is suggested by several observations, such as direct action on the metabolism of porphyrinic pigments. Erythrocytic protoporphyrins and urinary coproporphyrins are increased immediately following CO poisoning.[39a] Rabbits poisoned with CO show an early marked decrease in erythrocytic enzymatic acid phosphatase and later reduced serum phosphatase; increased urinary elimination of iron from bone, liver, spleen muscle and lung are also noted.[39] Studies indicate a diminished elimination of 17-ketosteroids and 17-hydroxycorticosteroids during the period of CO intoxication, and gradual return to normal of the adrenal hormones parallel with clinical improvement.[36] An increase in the globulin fraction of blood serum is described in individuals exposed to occupational risks of CO.[41] Altered plasma protein associated with lower immune response is reported in CO intoxication in dog experiments.[3] Myocardial morphologic, electrocardiographic and functional changes due to CO poisoning are strongly suggested, if not proven, by both animal experiments and clinical experience.[27,37,48,50] Myocardial excitability may be attributed to disturbances of myoglobin and cytochrome C by direct action of the CO. It is erroneous to assume that survivors of acute CO asphyxia may show no chronic pathologic changes.[6]

After 25 minutes of CO anoxia in rats, there followed a significant decrease in brain levels of glutamic acid, glutamine, serine and glycine, and an increase in alanine. These changes are related however, to increased glycolysis and simultaneous depression of aerobic oxidation of glucose in the Kreb cycle. These changes may play a role in the functional brain disorders in anoxia.[46a]

Endogenous CO[20,46] is constantly produced in small amount in man and in other animals as a metabolite resulting from cleavage of the porphyrin rings of hemoglobin molecules. Four molecules of CO are formed from one molecule of Hb. by the splitting of the hemochromogen's tetrapyrole ring. The negligible amount of CO formed circulates as COHb and is deposited in pulmonary alveoli until equilibrium is reached between the CO concentration of the blood and alveolar air. Traces of CO have also been found in green plants. The Pacific Coast kelp, Nereocytis Leutkeana, contains up to 10% CO in the gas in its hollow, 90 foot long stem.

Physiologic Difference Between Anoxia of CO and Anemia[15,20]

The pathologic physiology of carboxyhemoglobin anoxia is in marked contrast to the anoxia of chronic anemia. This is strikingly illustrated in the following instances.

A victim of CO poisoning with 60% COHb saturation leaving 40% Hb available for O_2, lying prone indoors, may regain consciousness and even begin to talk intelligently. He is then allowed to get up with assistance, walk out of doors, where he may again become unconscious. In contrast, a chronically anemic patient with the same net amount of normal Hb of 40% will function with no or minimal difficulty. The explanation for these two different clinical patterns are related to their dissociation curves. The difference between the shape and position of the two dissociation curves explains the fainting and collapse that often occur in CO poisoning, the latter causing a marked lowering of the partial pressure at which O_2 is available for tissue metabolism.

In both cases, the arterial blood contains 8 volume % of O_2 under 100mm Hg as it leaves the lungs (40% of 20 vol % O_2). A minimum of 4 vol % O_2 is required for the blood to unload the O_2 at the cellular level as the blood passes through capillaries to provide the needs of tissues in a body at rest. In other words, despite the presence in the blood of twice the amount of O_2 necessary for normal tissue function, severe anoxemia ensues in the case of CO poisoning. Conversion of 40% or more of Hb to COHb causes a much more serious effect than the loss of the same amount of Hb by anemia.

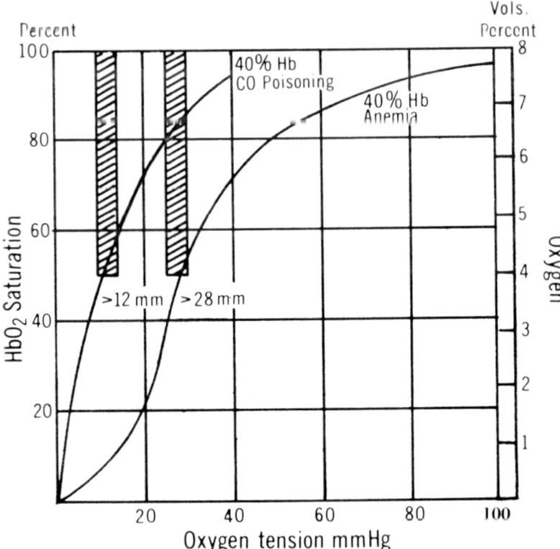

Figure 1. Oxygen dissociation curve of the blood of a case of carbon monoxide poisoning, in which the hemoglobin is 60% saturated with carbon monoxide, contrasted with the curve of a case of severe anemia in which the blood contains but 40% of the normal amount of hemoglobin. In both instances there is, therefore, 40% of the normal oxygen-carrying power. (From Stade and Martin, 1925-1936, p. 89)

In Figure 1, the two hatched columns cross the respective curves at points where unloading of O_2 would take place. It is noted that the dissociation curve is hyperbolic in CO, but sigmoid in anemia.

a) The anemic blood, after delivering 4 vol. % O_2 still contains O_2 under tension of 28 mm Hg.
b) The CO-blood, after delivering the same amount of O_2 to the tissues contains O_2 under the reduced tension of only 12mm Hg.

Referring to Figure 2, only the upper half of the steep portion of the O_2 dis-

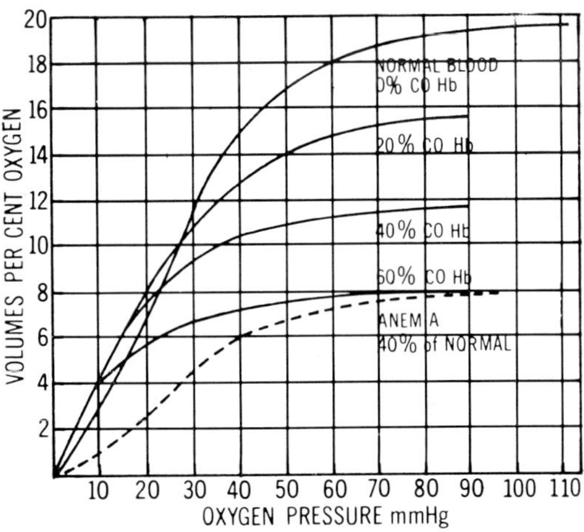

Figure 2. Oxygen dissociation curves of **a**) human blood at pH 7.40 and 38 C, containing various percentages of carboxyhemoglobin, and **b**) of anemic human blood containing only 40 per cent of the normal hemoglobin content.

sociation curve in man is made use of in O_2-unloading; the lower part, corresponding to 10 to 30 mm pO_2, is kept as reserve for exercise or pathologic condition. The O_2 dissociation curves over this low range of pO_2 are much the same for all percentages of COHb within the range of 0 to 40; therefore, the O_2 unloading could be kept up to its usual value by using up more, or even all, of the reserve available from the shape of the dissociation curve. In a normal human subject, at rest or doing light work, conversion of up to one-third of the circulating Hb to COHb does not in fact depress the O_2-uptake of the body appreciably. Above 40% COHb, however, Figures 1 and 2 show that the type of reserve given by the dissociation curve soon becomes exhausted and dangerous anoxemia rapidly develops.

It is recalled that the carotid sinus is sensitive to the arterial pO_2 and not to the arterial O_2-content. Since the pO_2 does not change in CO poisoning (at sea level), there is, therefore, no stimulation of the sinus to provide compensatory increase in heart output or increased ventilation such as occurs when air of low pO_2 is breathed. This lack of such compensation, together with the using up of the dissociation curve, explains the suddenness of collapse if the COHb is raised above the critical level of 40 to 50% saturation. With physical exertion, collapse occurs at lower levels of saturation.

The O_2 dissociation curve of the anemic blood still retains the normal sigmoid shape with its larger available reserve for O_2 uptake by the tissues. Also, the lowered blood viscosity in anemia is more optimum for earlier and larger compensatory increase in circulation than that found in CO poisoning.

The required tension of O_2 to move out of the blood and into the tissues in amounts to prevent anoxia is never less than 15mm Hg ± 5. The shape and position of the O_2 dissociation curve indicate the partial pressure at which O_2 is available for tissue metabolism. Obviously, the anemic patient is better able to function. CO_2 affects HbO in a manner exactly opposite to that of CO by shifting the dissociation curve to the right and thus promoting O_2 release,[23] a basic reason for the use of CO_2 in treating CO poisoning.

Intracellular O_2 tension cannot be measured directly. It is critical when the tension is below that which causes a decrease in tissue respiration. Hypoxia denotes the intracellular O_2 tension below normal but above the critical O_2 tension. Anoxia denotes intracellular tension of O_2 below the critical level. It is assumed that the critical intracellular oxygen tension is the same for all neurons regardless of the mechanisms which causes the anoxia.[8]

Anoxia may be classified according to causative mechanisms into four types:

1. *Anoxic Anoxia:* Due to a reduction in the amount of O_2 available to the body tissues (low oxygen content in air, CO, anethesia, obstruction of air passages).
2. *Anemic Anoxia:* Due to diminshed O_2 carrying capacity of the blood (anemia, blood loss).
3. *Histotoxic Anoxia:* Inability of tissue cells to utilize oxygen (CN inhibiting intracellular oxidative enzymes.)
4. *Stagnant Anoxia:* Due to total or partial arrest of cerebral circulation (cardiac arrest, hanging). This is the most serious form of anoxia because of the additional critical loss of nutritive supply of glucose and the accumulation of lactic acid and and other metabolites.

Oxygen Requirements of the Brain

The source of cerebral energy is the oxidation of glucose. The brain of a normal adult takes up to 9.8mg of glucose from each 100ml of blood, and consumes about 5mg of glucose per 100gm tissue per minute. Amino acids are also involved in brain metabolism.

Cerebral energy requirement varies with circulation and oxygen consumption. The brain, which weighs 2 to 2.5% of the total body weight, receives about 15% of the blood leaving the left ventricle, and its metabolic rate is about 20% of the basal oxygen requirement of the whole body.

There is a rapid fall in cerebral circulation and oxygen utilization from childhood through adolescence, followed by a slower but progressive decrease throughout the remaining life span, indicated as follows:

Age in Years	*Cerebral Blood Flow ml/100gm/minute*	*Oxygen Consumption ml/100gm/minute*
5	104	5.1
45	55	3.5
68	43	2.4

Oxygen consumption decreases along the neuroaxis from cortex to spinal cord. Grey matter has an oxygen consumption about five times that of white matter. The cell body of a single neurone requires 132x$10^{-6}\mu$l O_2 per hour. The glial cell requires less than 12.5 x $10^{-6}\mu$l oxygen per hour.

DIMINISHED OXYGEN METABOLISM OF THE BRAIN

Under physiologic conditions, brain metabolism is constant and remains unchanged during sleep as measured by oxygen consumption of the brain.

A reduction in tissue O_2 consumption, denoted as hypoxidosis, may result from lack of O_2 (hypoxic hypoxidosis), lack of glucose (nutritive hypoxidosis), from inhibition of respiratory enzymes (desenzymatic hypoxidosis, i.e., in beriberi).

During pathologic unconsciousness, the oxygen consumption of the brain is reduced from normal 3.5 ml/100gm/minute to 2±0.1ml/100gm/minute. Such values are seen in diabetic coma, insulin coma, coma after cerebral anoxia, during pentothal anesthesia and during increased intracranial pressure. Lower rates of O_2 consumption are incompatible with survival: the reduction in activity of bulbar centers is followed by cessation of respiration and circulation and leads to complete cerebral anoxia.

PATHOLOGIC PHYSIOLOGY OF CO CEREBRAL ANOXIA

The following indices may be used to describe the vulnerability and severity of the CNS to anoxia,

1. *Survival Time:* Interval between onset of anoxia and disappearance of a given function.
2. *Revival Time:* Longest duration of anoxia compatible with complete recovery.
3. *Recovery Time:* Interval between end of anoxia and reappearance of a given function.
4. *Time to Complete Recovery:* Time lapse to complete recovery.

Revival time is the most important index because it reflects the ability of the neurone to preserve its structure in the absence of oxygen.

The vulnerability of the nervous system to oxygen-lack decreases from cortex to peripheral nerve. The same sequence is fairly reflected in the clinical symptoms and histologic changes caused by acute anoxia.

The EEG is a useful guide to assess recovery of brain damage following anoxia. Post-anoxic EEG abnormalities completely disappear in cats and dogs when the circulatory arrest does not exceed 4 ($\pm$1) minutes. However, when anoxia is confined to the brain the revival time is 7 minutes. Complete EEG recovery, however, does not always imply absence of any CNS lesional change.

The time indices of anoxia are influenced by such factors as type of anoxia age, degree of oxygen-lack, temperature and cardiovascular condition.

With complete or stagnant anoxia, anaerobic energy is necessary for survival because of the rapid exhaustion of oxygen-stores in the cell. Since anaerobic glycolysis is very uneconomical, yielding only one-tenth the energy produced by oxidation of equivalent glucose, the depletion of this basic fuel is rapid, along with the accumulation of CO_2 and lactic acid metabolites. In cat experiments, perfusing the stagnant-anoxic brain with "solution free of both oxygen and glucose" will result in earlier significant improvement in the EEG and in revival and recovery time intervals. It follows therefore that the recovery is slower after stagnant anoxia than after anoxic anoxia.

Age: The new-borne tolerates anoxia more readily than adults. In the human, a viable fetus may be extracted up to 20 minutes after the maternal death. The brain of the new-borne consumes less oxygen for several reasons: 1) lower energy requirements for the CNS; 2) more energy derived from anaerobic metabolism. Tolerance to anoxia decreases as aerobic metabolism becomes dominant.

Degree of Oxygen Lack: The revival and recovery time intervals are prolonged with incomplete stagnant anoxia. In CO anoxic anoxia, the intervals decrease in the presence of anemia.

Heart: The revival time is prolonged if the heart is not involved in the anoxic episode or is supported (massage or adrenalin) in the post-anoxic period.

Temperature: Hypothermia decreases the oxygen requirement and the revival time is increased. Conversely with hyperthermia.

Pathology

Anoxia lasting longer than the revival time causes structural changes. The onset of histologic change depends upon the duration of survival time.

Within one or two days (acute phase), the histopathologic picture is one of congestion, edema, hemorrhage and with little if any cellular damage.

When the survival is longer (subacute and chronic phase), neuronal degeneration and necrosis and encephalomalacia occur in grey matter. Signs of glial repair are noted such as reactive proliferation and scar formation, arteriolar hyalinization, thromboses, and neoangiogenesis.[18]

Carbon monoxide produces characteristic symmetrical areas of necrosis in the globus pallidus, in addition to cortical and subcortical lesions. The basis for the development of the unique selective symmetrical necrosis of the globus pallidus in CO poisoning very probably is related to the peculiar local vascular patterns and the associated hypoxia. The blood supply of this area is sparse and depends entirely upon the long narrow straight end-artery, the anterior choroidal, which probably can undergo spastic contraction, paralytic dilatation, or thrombosis with resulting ischemic necrosis. A specific histotoxic action of CO may also be a factor.

The most sensitive areas affected by CO are the cerebral cortex, corpus striatum, and the visceral motor nuclei, the dorsal sensory areas of the medulla and the Purkinje cells of the cerebellum. Despite good blood supply, the ganglion cells of the cerebral cortex are highly vulnerable to anoxia and readily show hypoxic degeneration; this may relate to their very high O_2 requirement. Coma that persists despite dissipation of the CO is the result of anoxic irreversible degenerative changes in ganglionic cells.

Dutra[17] classified CO brain damage into 4 groups:

1. Absent or minimal gross changes, microscopic evidence of diffuse degeneration of ganglion cells.
2. Necosis of globi palladi, symmetrical and grossly visible, microscopy, diffuse ischemic necrosis. This is a characteristic finding in deaths from delayed CO poisoning.
3. Many and varied size hemorrhages (brain-purpura) and diffuse edema; microscopy, widespread degeneration of ganglia cells.
4. Widespread demyelinization of cerebral white matter and necrosis of globi pallidi. Microscopy shows intense phagocytic activity at sites of demyelinization, and degeneration of cells in cortex and basal ganglia.

The post-mortem findings in the average case of acute CO poisoning are characteristic and offer no problem in diagnosis.[4] The cherry-pink color of viscera, blood and muscle, and the occasional petichiae and a COHb concentration of 50% or more are usually demonstrable.

Difficulties in diagnosis must be recognized in many cases. A pink to red color of skin after death is not pathognomonic of COHb and may be caused by agonal peripheral vascular dilatation or by the body lying in cold. On the other hand, some cases of CO poisoning may actually show pallor of skin due to persistent contraction of peripheral vessels after death despite lethal amounts of COHb with the diagnostic color of viscera, blood and muscle. This acounts for part of the 50% of the cases of CO poisoning, unsuspected prior to autopsy.

In decomposed bodies, the cherry-red color is absent externally, altho visible in tissues and blood, or the characteristic color may be completely absent.

Levels of 20 to 30% COHb are unrecognized at autopsy except by chemical examination. Under some conditions, these apparently low concentrations may actually be found with lethal poisoning. During a 6 hour period in a CO free environment, the saturation level of COHb in a body may decrease from 60 to 20%. If the history is unknown, and a chemical examination is not done, an unrelated, incidental or only predisposing disease such as senility or alcoholism may be wrongly held responsible for the death.

Carbon Monoxide in Peripheral Blood Post-Mortem

Carbon monoxide is not found in significant amounts resulting from putrefaction of the body. Nor can CO be absorbed by heart-blood through exposure of a body to a CO contaminated atmosphere. COHb persists at least several weeks in the blood of victims dying from CO poisoning even after putrefaction.

The laboratory finding of low concentration of COHb in post-mortem blood does not exclude CO poisoning in the presence of symmetrical pallidi necrosis, brain purpura or focal and confluent necrosis in either grey or white matter.

SOURCES OF CO POISONING

Carbon monoxide, a hazard to man from the time of the first fire, is becoming an increasingly ubiquitous poison as a "metabolite" of incomplete combustion incidental to our ever expanding industrialized, motorized, man-machine complex society.

This poisonous gas is found to some extent in all smoke and fumes from burning carbonaceous material as in the internal combustion and diesel engine, garages, furnaces, blasting fuses, explosives, air-craft cabins, weapons, refueling[31] and submarine operations.[2] Gasoline engines emit up to 4% CO, diesel engines about 0.1%.[43]

The most common exposures to CO are from the exhaust of gasoline engines in enclosed spaces. Deaths have even occurred, however, in the open canopy cruiser at sea during a calm.[28]

Carbon monoxide concentrations correlate with traffic density at 99% significance. Residential areas having motor transport have higher concentrations of ambient CO than industrial areas with minimal motor traffic. In cities, automobiles are a major source of CO.[9]

Correlation of Traffic Density to CO Ambient Air

Light traffic	0–5 vehicles/min	up to 1 ppm
Moderate traffic	3–22 vehicles/min	up to 6 ppm
Heavy traffic	16–19 vehicles/min	up to 47 ppm

Traffic control personnel exposed to ambient air containing low concentrations of CO show relatively high COHb content. At the completion of duty at a high traffic street crossing in the Ruhr, 18% COHb was found in the blood of traffic officers.[40] Similarly, between 12 to 40% was reportedly found in some of the Moscow traffic-directing personnel.[52]

The average CO in London streets (1955) was 15 ppm. In the smog of 1956, the CO content rose to 50 ppm. The average pedestrian experiences effects of CO poisoning at a concentration of 50 ppm after exposures of 4 to 8 hours.[43]

During the Suez crisis of 1956 when gasoline was rationed in Great Britain, CO virtually disappeared from the streets of London. When car traffic reappeared 360 ppm CO was recorded. It is fair to assume that concentrations exceeding 500 ppm may be found in calm weather in congested streets of almost any modern city. This is far in excess of the standards adopted by the Department of Health of the State of California where 30 ppm is considered an "adverse" level; exposure to 30 ppm for 8 hours, or 120 ppm for one hour is "serious level of pollution." Normally, in Los Angeles the air contains 10 to 12 parts of CO per million of air. During certain weather conditions, a complex inter-relationship of contaminants in the atmosphere results in the formation of "smog," a photochemical cloud which is known to contain CO, CO_2, SO_2, total sulphur and particulate matter. The physiologic effects of gases, aerosols, and solids so mixed are not presently fully understood.[45]

The role of CO as a cause of car accidents can not be adequately determined unless blood analyses for both CO and alcohol are routinely performed in all cases of fatal accidents or whenever the driver is charged with "failure to drive in a careful and prudent manner."[40a] Police files show that at least 600 CO deaths occur each year in the United States.[5] It can also be assumed that this deceptive gas contributes to a high percentage of the 180,000 or more annual highway accidents caused by drivers who black-out or fall asleep at the wheel.[16] Since the exhaust from the gasoline may produce up to 7% COHb, the level of CO poisoning that may be encountered by a motorist smoking cigarettes should give cause for concern. Heavy smoking per se can give a COHb saturation of 5 to 8%.[25] There is increasing evidence that even low concentrations of CO in the blood, insufficient to cause symptoms, can lead to impaired judgment; the cerebral effects of CO poisoning are extremely varied.[19, 21] Accidents attributed to driver fatigue, drowsiness or inattention, may actually be caused by CO intoxication. The driver in a reported case of a fatal accident was found to have a COHb saturation of 35% caused by the breathing of exhaust gas coming into his car from vehicles ahead in heavy traffic.[40a] Tolerance and response to low concentration CO inhalation is not predictable, and the individual may even act drunk or hilarious. Common early effects of mild CO poisoning are narrowing of the field of vision and drowsiness, two obviously critical factors in causing auto accidents.

Sources of CO within the vehicle are due primarily to engine exhaust and secondarily to combustion of lubricating oils and sources in other vehicles. The CO concentrations are principally affected by changes in the air-fuel ratio.[22] The poison gas enters the interior of the automobile through the breather, manifold, head gaskets, muffler, tail pipe, air-tank and air-operated devices and their connections, fittings and exhausts, and in certain heating and freezing prevention installations.[35] The maximum amounts of CO are produced in automotive exhausts during deceleration, acceleration, and idling at intersections.[25] It is highly improbable that the danger of CO poisoning will ever be completely eliminated in the operation of motor vehicles.

Medico-legal problems involving death by CO poisoning from automobile exhaust fumes can be very perplexing. About half of the fatal poisonings in the United States are attributed to CO, and many chronic sublethal cases remain unrecognized.[34]

Cigarette smoking is a major factor in producing abnormally high levels of COHb among the general population.[13, 25] Smoking 20 cigarettes a day results in the absorption of 200mgm CO, in addition to 3.0mgm of various nitrous oxides (NOs). In any evaluation of the effects of smoking on health, one must consider probable synergism caused by the simultaneous presence of both CO and NOs.[7] The relationship of smoking to pulmonary-cardio-vascular disease is reported in considerable depth by the Surgeon-General's Advisory Committee on Smoking and Health.[49]

Both maternal and fetal bloods show higher CO saturation in smokers than in non-smokers. The placenta is no barrier to the CO in the maternal blood. The more rapidly the mother dies of a lethal concentration of CO the less CO will enter the fetal blood. Neonates of mothers who smoke show decreased carbonic anhydrase, and it takes longer to establish post-natal respiration.[22a, 33, 53]

What Constitutes Harmful Exposure to CO[8,15]

The cerebral effects of exposure to the same concentration of CO are extremely varied in different individuals, depending chiefly on factors that relate to the changing ratio of respiratory volume to blood volume. This ratio, from the viewpoint of CO poisoning, varies according to age, physical activity, metabolic state and pulmonary-cardio vascular condition. Other factors include the presence of anemia and indices such as temperature, humidity, ambient CO_2 and O_2, and air-flow.

Clinically, there is a marked difference between short excessive exposure, and prolonged recurrent mild exposure. Complete recovery usually follows the former with prompt adequate treatment. Sequela of protean variety may follow recurrent exposure with resulting injury or destruction of neurones and other somatic cells including those of the cardio-vascular system.

Sensory losses involving vision and co-ordination may occur at low COHb levels without causing other symptoms.[19, 30] Dark adaptation, light sensitivity, and concentric visual acuity are all adversely affected by small amounts of CO causing 3% COHb saturation.[35] It is shown that 5% COHb depresses visual sensitivity to as great an extent as anoxia at 8,000 to 10,000 feet altitude, while 15% saturation causes an impairment to that of 15,-000 to 19,000 feet altitude.

CO inhalation does not have to produce serious toxic effects to be considered a hazard. Prolonged periods of exposure to 0.01% CO concentrations should not be permitted.[35]

Summary of Effects of CO Concentration in Air

% in Air	*PP/10,000*	*PPM*	*Effect*
0.01	1	100	No symptoms for 2 hours.
0.02	2	200	Possibly mild frontal headache in 2-3 hours.
0.04	4	400	Frontal headaches & nausea after 1-2 hours. Occipital headache — 2-3 hours.
0.06–.07	6–7	600–700	Headache & nausea in 1 hour.
0.08	8	800	Headache, nausea, vertigo in ¾ hour.
0.10–.12	10–12	1,000–1,200	Dangerous after 1 hour.
0.16	16	1,600	Headache, vertigo, nausea in 20 minutes collapse, coma & death in 2 hours.
0.32	32	3,200	Headache, vertigo in 5 min., coma and danger of death in 30 min.
0.64	64	6,400	Headache, vertigo in 1-2 min., coma & danger of death in 10-15 minutes.
2.00	200	20,000	Coma and death in 4 minutes.

High concentrations of CO are found in[4]:

1. Illuminating gas (CO not present in natural gas) .... 6 to 30%
2. Comon conflagration .... 5 to 15%
3. Flue gases and water heaters .. up to 5%
4. Exhaust gas from internal combustion engine .... 2 to 14%

The effects of exposure can be predicted by the "rule of expectancy" suggested by Henderson and Haggard (1921--1922).[26] According to their formula, "T × kCO," where T = time in hours and kCO = concentration of CO in parts per 10,000:

T x kCO = 3, no significant effect
T x kCO = 6, mild effect
T x kCO = 9, marked effect
T x kCO = 15, fatal

Running an auto engine in a single car garage for 5 minutes will create a deadly atmosphere.

The CO from an automotive exhaust lies 5 to 15 feet above the street. Depending upon atmospheric conditions, the concentration will vary, being higher in calm and humid weather.

The American Standards Association has adopted 1:10,000 CO (0.01%) as the maximum permissible concentration for a daily exposure up to 8 hours, or 4:10,000 not exceeding 1 hour daily.[24] A concentration of 10:10,000 (0.1%) CO in air causes a 50% COHb in the blood in 15 minutes and up to 80% in 23 minutes. During exertion, 50% saturation may be reached in 5 minutes. The precise point of saturation that death occurs is not known and is probably influenced by conditional factors. Haldane[23] showed that 20% COHb saturation, the critical point for subjective symptoms in man, results from one hour exposure to a CO concentration of 4:10,000 at rest at normal temperature, or 2.5:10,000 when working hard. Others[44] showed that 2:10,000 produces 15% COHb saturation in 3 hours, 20% in four hours at rest, and the same amount in one half hour doing mild exercise.

The lethal amount of CO depends upon the concentration and rate of inhalation. About 75% COHb saturation may result within two minutes during exertion in a fire, promptly followed by unconsciousness and death. Two deep breaths of 2% CO may cause coma and death in four minutes. Instantaneous unconsciousness from oxygen lack which occurs in conflagration, may occur during exertion in a fire. A concentration of 4.2% oxygen results in a loss of coordination in two minutes with consciousness lasting about seven minutes.

It can be misleading to accept an absolute "threshold" for toxicity of a gas since the minimum toxic concentrations are usually determined in the presence of atmospheric air. In an actual fire, CO is seldom if ever unaccompanied by other toxic gases such as H_2S, NOs and CO_2 which are combustion products of hair, wool and leather. The total toxicity of such mixtures resulting from fire is further increased by low oxygen concentrations and high temperature. Moritz[38] lists the principal causes of fire-deaths as follows, not necessarily in the order of frequency since more than one casual factor may be present in a single case:

1. CO.
2. Anoxemia
3. Combined effects of CO and CO_2.
4. Heat.
5. Shock.
6. Broncho-pulmonary edema secondary to irritants such as acid anhydrides, aldehydes and acids.
7. Toxic gases such as HCN, NOs, fluorides and chlorides.
8. Ventricular fibrillation due to inhalation of hydrocarbons.

SYMPTOMS AND CLINICAL COURSE[8, 15, 42a]

The earliest warning symptom of CO poisoning is mild frontal headache unless the amount of CO is very great. In the latter case, the odorless, tasteless and non-irritating gas rapidly alters the level of consciousness and disturbs the mental, somatomotor and autonomic functions. The alarming cerebral symptoms are caused by the marked hypoxia and rapid decrease in O_2 consumption, the large demand for O_2 by neurones making the brain the most vulnerable organ. Mental and sensory functions, more sensitive to anoxia than are motor functions, are deranged earlier and recover later. Anoxia too brief to cause motor symptoms can impair mental function.

Anoxia changes in the CNS may be reversible with complete restitution of cell function, or irreversible with incomplete recovery and sequela, or incompatible with survival. The degree and duration of oxygen-lack are the critical factors in the resulting hypoxic hypoxidosis.

Mild headache with a sense of pressure may occur in the less fulminant stage, or throbbing may develop with weakness of the knees, dizziness, mental confusion, roaring in the ears, nausea and perhaps vomiting. The next phase is characterized by confusion and/or increasing paralysis, or the victim may appear indifferent, drowsy and drunk. Vomiting and incontinence are soon followed by coma with localized twitchings, or occasionally generalized and resembling an epileptic seizure.

Pulmonary edema is a common feature in acute poisoning; vomiting with altered consciousness may result in aspiration pneumonia.

A wide spectrum of unpredictable neurologic and other protean clinical patterns may develop. Some of the clinical features include apoplectic seizures, difficulty in walking, perservation, confabulation, severe defects in judgment, amnesia, diminished self-control, violent outbursts of temper, secretiveness, religious fervor, loss of libido, Parkinsonism and involutional melancholia. There is no consistent pattern of psychosis characteristic of CO poisoning.

The effects of CO asphyxia on the intellect are classically described by J.S. Haldane based upon experiments on himself.[23] "As the slow onset of anoxemia advances, the senses and the intellect become dulled without the person being aware of it; and if the anoxemia is suddenly relieved by means of oxygen or ordinary air, the corresponding sudden increase in powers of vision, hearing, etc., is an intense surprise. The power of memory is affected early, and is finally almost annulled, so that persons who apparently never lost consciousness can never-the-less remember nothing of what has occurred. Powers of sane judgment are much impaired, and anoxemic persons become subject more-or-less to irrational fixed ideas, and to uncontrolled emotional outbursts. In many respects, the symptoms of anoxemia resemble those of drunkenness, and a man suffering from anoxemia cannot be held responsible for his actions. Without reason, he may begin to laugh, shout, sing, burst in tears or become dangerously violent. He is, however, always quite confident that he himself is perfectly sane and reasonable, though he may notice, for instance, that he cannot walk or write properly, cannot remember what just happened, and cannot properly interpret his visual impressions. When unable even to stand, owing to experimental CO poisoning, or to anoxemia produced by low pressures in a steel chamber, Haldane has always been quite confident of his own sanity, and it was only afterwards that he realized that he could not have been in a rational state of mind."

Incomplete recovery is more likely if rescue is delayed or if pre-existing disease is present, particularly of pulmonary-cardio-vascular type. Elimination of CO from the blood does not necessarily halt or reverse the cyto-pathologic changes, especially those of the CNS which proceed to severe degeneration with progressive and late symptoms of mental impairment, motor and sensory involvement, loss of vision, cardiac disturbances, or apoplexy.

In the average case of CO poisoning, it is rare for the symptoms of excitement followed by depression, apathy, amnesia, intense headache and feeling of shivering to last more than two to three days.

Slow prolonged asphyxia involves basal ganglia and less often the cerebral cortex and peripheral nerves. Mental disorders, such as dulled mentality and loss of memory following severe CO poisoning, have been known for centuries. Haldane considered loss of memory and lack of judgment as definite symptoms of CO asphyxia, both while the victim is under its influence and after recovery.

Chronic CO asphyxia[42a] is now generally accepted as a definite clinical entity resulting from a slow accumulation of effects of damage done day by day by a moderate degree of anoxemia. One of the possible effects is the development of a chronic reversible polycythemia.

The capacity by different individuals to acquire tolerance or develop acclimatization to intermittent, chronic exposure to low concentrations of CO is unpredictable.

Killick in 1936,[29] in experimental studies with human subjects, showed that symptoms of poisoning lessened during successive exposures to the same concentrations of CO. There was no compensatory increase in red blood cells or blood volume to account for the tolerance. Rather, she found that the acclimatization was reflected in the decreased CO blood saturation despite the unchanging concentration of the CO breathed after repeated exposures. The symptoms of the subjects depended upon the percent COHb and not on the percentage of CO in the air breathed. Acclimatization is apparently due to something that happens in the body and not to some change or adaptive mechanism by the blood; this is shown by the fact that specimens of blood taken before and after acclimatization saturate equally *in vitro* with CO.

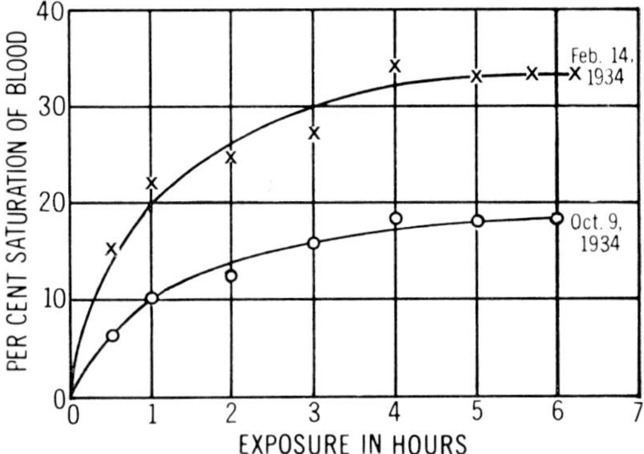

Figure 3. Saturation of the blood during exposure to 0.023 per cent carbon monoxide: X, before acclimatization (Feb. 14, 1934); 0, after acclimitization (Oct. 9, 1934). (Redrawn from Killick, 1936, p. 45.)

Figure 3 shows that: 1) before acclimatization, 20% COHb was reached in one hour when symptoms began to appear. 2) after acclimatization, with intermittent exposure to same concentration of CO, 20% COHb was never reached even in six hours, and no symptoms appeared.

The symptoms experienced depended upon the percentage saturation of the blood CO, and not on the percentage of CO breathed. A possible explanation for such acquired tolerance is the development of increased resistance to the inward diffusion of CO by alveolar cell adaptation.

Roughton[42] has shown that there is no significant loss of CO through the skin, sweat, urine or feces, or by oxidation or other forms of metabolism. Apparent acclimatization to CO may be achieved by the CO combining reversibly with hemoglobin-like pigments outside of the main blood stream; subsequently, as the blood CO content falls, the CO dissociates reversibly from these combinations, diffuses back into the blood and thence into expired air.

Diagnosis of CO Poisoning[4]

1. History of exposure is obviously of cardinal importance.
2. Appearance of victim: Carmine-red tinge most evident on cheeks, tongue, lips and mucous membranes and lower limbs. Some cases appear cyanotic due to blue-red blood distending the capillaries and veins of the face and neck and resembling suffocation.
3. Symptoms may resemble alcoholism.
4. Evidence of anoxemia exaggerated by exertion.
5. Detection of CO in the air or blood. In mild cases of CO poisoning, there are no objective signs or symptoms to suggest the diagnosis unless CO can be detected in the blood. This should be done after the patient has been in the suspected vitiated atmosphere for several hours and before leaving it for the fresh air. Frontal headache begins when blood saturation reaches 18 to 20% COHb.
6. Chronic CO poisoning is frequently incorrectly diagnosed as epilepsy because of neuro-psychiatric symptomotology. There is an apparent individual susceptibility to this type of response to the slower and more insidious form of CO poisoning, with intermittent symptoms and vague relations to the sources of the poison gas. The timing and nature of the seizures, mental changes, and the intermittent symptoms should suggest the diagnosis in individuals exposed to CO from any source.[21]
7. Analysis for CO:[1, 11] The detection and measurement of CO are grouped under chemical and physical methods. The chemical methods are based upon the oxidation of CO in the presence of metallic oxides, by anhydrous iodine liberating iodine gas, by metallic salts, or the formation of complexes. Iodine pentoxide and palladium chloride methods are commonly used. The physical methods involve either an indirect approach by first absorbing the gas, or a direct approach by gas chromatography, which is choice. Other direct methods include refractometry, interferometry, polarography and infrared spectography.

Prognosis[42a]

The incidence of permanent and neurologic disease after CO poisoning is not believed to be as great as once thought. No attempt at prognosis should be considered earlier than a month or two after the incident. Both destructive and reparative process of the brain become stabilized in about two months after poisoning. Although further degeneration is unlikely, the degree of regeneration and recovery is individual and variable, and some continued improvement may be reasonably anticipated.

Recovery of mental functions and the

return of EEG patterns to normal after CO poisoning depend upon the duration of the post-anoxic unconsciousness, age and state of the cardiovascular system.

The duration of post-anoxic unconsciousness cannot be predicted in any case of a victim in a state of deep unconsciousness when admitted to hospitalization. In some patients, the CO remains high in both the blood and tissues with continued anoxia for a variable time. Chemical combination of CO with tissue is suggested by the relatively prolonged delay in the excretion of the last significant increments of the inhaled CO.[8]

Sequelae or delayed symptoms, cerebral or cardiac, may develop 3 to 7 days following acute asphyxiation. Lesions may occur simultaneously in the brain and heart. A definite diagnosis of chronic myocardial disease of CO-origin requires an accurate history of exposure to the gas, presence of symptoms of anoxemia, consistent clinical course, and absence of pre-existing cardiac disease.[6, 27]

Treatment

The imperative in the treatment of CO poisoning is the immediate restoration of the oxygen-carrying power of the hemoglobin as speedily as possible by the prompt elimination of the gas through the same route as that of entry.

This is effected by the quick removal of the victim from the source of CO, and prompt inhalation of a mixture of O_2 and CO_2 (Carbogen).

These measures are based upon the fact that CO does not form a permanent compound with Hb. The combination of CO and Hb is readily reversible in the presence of pure air and excess O_2. The CO is rapidly given off due to its extraordinary rapidity of dilution. The rate of elimination of CO is rapid at first, depending upon the COHb saturation, the rate of pulmonary ventilation, and the condition of the cardio-vascular system.

The victim is kept quiet to minimize the O_2 demand and warm to combat shock as necessary. It must be noted that a gassed person may survive up to 10 minutes after breathing ceases. If breathing is abnormal or absent, artificial respiration must be administered. In order to eliminate the COHb, this should be continued up to four hours in accordance with the following table:

Table showing the approximate time required to eliminate 50% COHb from the blood:

By breathing air	140 minutes
By breathing Oxygen	85 minutes
By breathing air and 5% CO_2	80 minutes
By breathing Oxygen and 5% CO_2	20 minutes

Several unique additional methods of treatment have been reported in isolated cases including prolonged use of intravenous procaine,[14] whole blood transfusions,[28] and hypothermia.[12] Replacement parenteral iron therapy is worthy of clinical investigation in view of the reported appreciable loss of iron from the liver, bone, muscle, spleen and lungs in experimental CO poisoning.[39]

REFERENCES

1. Adams, E. G., and Simmons, N. T.: The determination of CO. J. Appl. Chem. (Lond.) *1* (Suppl. 1): S20-S40, 1951.
2. Alvis, H. J., and Tanner, C. W.: CO toxicity in submarine operations. Arch. Indus. Hyg. & Occupat. Med., *6*:404-406, Nov. 1952.
3. Ambrosio, L., and Mazza, V.: Immunological potency in CO intoxication. Riv. Istituto Sieroterapico Ital (Naples), *34*:399-405, Sept.-Oct. 1959.

4. Anderson, W. A. D.: Pathology. 5th Ed. C. V. Mosby, St. Louis, 1966, p. 47.
5. Barrett, H. M.: CO poisoning. Canad. J. Pub. Health, *25:*430-438, 1934.
6. Beck, H. G., and Suter, G. M.: Role of CO in causation of myocardial disease. J.A.M.A., *110:* 1982-1986, June 11, 1938.
7. Bockhoven, C., and Niessen, H. J.: Amounts of oxides of nitrogen and CO in cigarette smoke, with and without inhalation. Nature, *192:*458-459, Nov. 4, 1961.
8. Bokonjic, Nenad: Stagnant anoxia and CO poisoning. Electroenceph. Clin. Neurophysiol., 1963 Suppl. 21 pp. 2-8.
9. Brief, R. S., *et al.*: Lead, CO and traffic: A correlation study. J. APCA, *10:*384-388, Oct. 1960.
10. Byrom, R. D.: Defense against CO — the silent killer. Eng. & Min. J., *158:*88-89, Oct. 1957.
11. Cier: Detection and measurement of CO. Rev. Corps Santé Militaire (Paris), *14:*338-352, Oct. 1958.
12. Craig, T. V. *et al.*: Hypothermia, its use in CO poisoning. N.E.J.M., *261:*854, 1959.
13. Curphey, T. J., *et al.*: Carboxyhemoglobin in relation to air pollution and smoking. Arch. Environ. Health, *10:*179-185, Feb. 1965.
14. Daneman, E. A.: CO poisoning. Dis. Nervous Sys., *14:*39, 1953.
15. Drinker, C. K.: CO Asphyxia. Oxford Med. Pub., 1938, pp. 18-21.
16. Dunlap, R.: CO, the silent killer. Today's Health. Nov. 1961, pp. 26-27, 67-68, 71-72.
17. Dutra, F. R.: Cerebral residue of acute CO poisoning. Amer. J. Clin. Path., *22:*925, 1952.
18. Eros, G., and Priestman, G.: Cerebral vascular changes in CO poisoning. J. Neuropath. & Exp. Neurol., *1:*158, 1942.
19. Fink, A. I.: CO asphyxia with visual sequelae. Am. J. Ophth., *34:*1024-1027, July 1951.
20. Fenn, W. O., and Rahn, H.: Respiration. Vol. 1, Sec. 3, pp. 778-780, 1964, Am. Physiol. Soc., Washington, D.C.
21. Gilbert, J. G., and Glasser, G. H.: Neurologic manifestations of chronic CO poisoning. NEJM, *261:*1217-1220, Dec. 10, 1959.
22. Hagen, D. F., and Holiday, G. W.: The Effects of Engine Operating and Design Variables on Exhaust Emission. SAE — Paper 486C p. 41, 1962.
22a. Haddon, W., Jr., *et al.*: Smoking and pregnancy: CO in blood during gestation and at term. Ob. Gyn., *18:*262-267, Sept. 1961.
23. Haldane, J. S., and Priestly, J. G.: Respiration. Yale Univ. Press, 1935, pp. 165, 176, 242.
24. Hamilton, A., and Hardy, H. C.: Industrial Toxicology, 2nd Ed. Paul B. Hoeber, 1948, p. 222.
25. Hanson, H. B., and Hastings, A. B.: The effect of smoking on the CO content of the blood. J.A.M.A., *100:*1481, May 13, 1933.
25a. Hajek, F.: How motor vehicles pollute the atmosphere of cities. Silnicmi Doprava (Prague), *12:*4-7, 1964.
26. Henderson, Y., and Haggard, H. W.: Health hazard from automobile exhause gas in city streets, garages and repair shops. J.A.M.A., *81:* 385, 1923.
27. Hayes, J. M., and Hall, G. V.: The myocardial toxicity of CO. Med. J. Australia, June 8, 1964, pp. 865-868.
28. Kaye, S.: CO poisoning. Virginia Med. Monthly, *84:*627, 1957.
29. Killick, E. M.: The nature of acclimatization occurring during repeated exposure of the human subject to atmosphere containing low concentrations of CO. J. Physiol. (Lond.), *107:* 27-44, 1948.
30. Lawther, P. J.: Air Pollution and The Public Health, Smokeless Air. From a lecture to the Royal Society of Arts, 1965, pp. 285-288.
31. Lentz, E. C.: Human factors in "cause undetermined" accidents. Aerospace Med., *36:*214-222, March 1965.
31a. Lewey, F. H., and Drabkin, D. C.: Experiments in chronic CO poisoning in dogs. Amer. J. Med. Sc., *208:*502, 1944.
32. Lewin, L.: CO Poisoning: A manual for physicians, engineers and accident investigators. (German) Julius Springer Verlag, Berlin, 1920. Quoted by A. G. Cooper: CO, A Bibliography. U.S. Dept. of H.E.W., Pub. Health Service, 1966.
33. Mantell, C. D.: Smoking in pregnancy. New Zealand Med. J., *63:*601-603, 1964.
34. McBay, A. J.: CO poisoning. New Eng. J. Med., *272:*252-253, Feb. 4, 1965.
35. McFarland, R. A., and Moore, R. C.: Human factors in highway safety. A review and evaluation. New Eng. J. Med., *256:*890-897, May 9, 1957.
36. Medaglini, E.: Studies on the urinary elimination of 17 ketosteroids and 17 hydroxycorticosteroids in persons affected with chronic intoxication from CO. Rass. Neuropsichiat (Salerno), *16:*55-58, 1962.
37. Middleton, G. D., *et al.*: Delayed and long lasting EKG changes in CO poisoning. Lancet, *1:* 12-14, Jan. 7, 1961.
38. Moritz, Quoted in Fire Gas Research Report, N.F.P.A. No. Q 45-13, 1962.
39. Pecora, L.: Ferrous therapy in acute CO poisoning. Rass. Med. Indust., *33:352-353,* May-Aug., 1964.
39a. Pecora, L., *et al.*: Free erythrocytic Protoporphyrins in Experimental and Clinical CO Poisoning. Folio Med., *40:*213-226, 1957.

40. Portheine, F.: CO and traffic. Arch. of Gewerbepath. u. Gewerbehyg., *13*:253-261, 1954.

40a. Public Health (Johannesburg): Hundreds of motorists killed by CO. Quoted by A. G. Cooper: Bibliography of CO. U.S. Dept. H.E.W., 1966, *63*:30, 32, 1963.

41. Ricci, C., *et al.*: Electrophoretic and immunoelectrophoretic examinations in workers exposed to chronic CO intoxication. Rass. Med. Indust., *33*:414-416, May-Aug., 1964.

42a. Rowan, T., and Coleman, F. C.: CO poisoning: Review of the literature and presentation of a case. J. Forensic Sc., *7*:103-130, Jan. 1962.

42. Roughton, F. J. W., and Root, W. S.: The fate of CO during the recovery from mild CO poisoning in man. Am. J. Phys., *145*:239-252, 1945.

43. Royal Society of Health: Automobiles and air pollution. J.A.M.A., *162*:134, Sept. 8, 1956.

44. Sayers, R. R., *et al.*: Effects of Repeated Daily Exposure of Several Hours to Small Amounts of Automobile Exhaust Gas. U.S. PHSB No. 186, 1929.

45. Schrenk, H. H.: The chemistry of smog. Ind. Hyg. Newsletter, *10*:7-10, 1950.

46. Sjostrand, T.: The formation of CO by the decomposition of hemoglobin *in vivo*. Acta Physiol. Scandinav., *26*:338-344, 1952.

46a. Sklenovsky, A.: Brain levels of free aminoacids in CO anoxia in rats. Activita Nervosa Superior, *6*:272-275, 1964.

47. Spencer, T. D.: The effects of CO on man and canaries. Ann. Occupat. Hyg. (Lond.), *5*:231 240, Oct.-Dec., 1962.

48. Stearns, W. H., *et al.*: The EKG changes found in 22 cases of CO poisoning. Amer. Heart J., *15*: 434-447, 1938.

49. Surgeon General's Advisory Committee: Report on Smoking and Health 1964. U.S.P.H.S.

50. Takahashi, K.: Changes of the heart excitability due to acute CO poisoning. Tohoku J. Exp. Med. (Sendai), *74*:224-233, July 1961.

51. Van Oettingen, W. F.: CO, Its Hazards and The Mechanism of its Action Federal Security Agency, U.S.P.H.S., PHSB No. 290, U.S. Govt. Printing Office, Washington, D.C. 1944, pp. 257.

52. Vasil eva, A. A., and Manita, M. D.: Carboxyhemoglobin in the Blood of Persons Directing City Traffic: USSR Literature on Air Pollution and Related Occupational Diseases. A Survey, Vol. 7, 1962, pp. 290-293, CFSTI-TT-62-11103, U.S. Dept. of Commerce (Quoted by A. G. Cooper: CO Bibliography. U.S. Dept. of HEW 1966.)

53. Woodruff, R. S.: CO poisoning. Med. Sc., *7*:550, April 25, 1960.

Chapter 26B

The Measurement of Carbon Monoxide in Biological Fluids[1,2]

F. LEE RODKEY, PH.D.

INTRODUCTION

Carbon monoxide (CO) is a colorless, odorless gas classified as a chemical asphyxiant. Its major toxic action is produced by combination with the hemoglobin of red blood cells to form carboxyhemoglobin. The reaction with hemoglobin is in competition for the same binding sites which react with oxygen to form oxyhemoglobin. The affinity of human hemoglobin for CO is approximately 220 times that for oxygen (4, 21, 24, 25). Therefore, small concentrations of CO present in air are sufficient to significantly decrease blood transport of oxygen to the tissues, especially the central nervous system, and to cause toxic reactions. Because of the high affinity of hemoglobin for CO and the low solubility of this gas (18), blood is the only biological fluid whose CO content will increase greatly even when death intervenes from carbon monoxide poisoning. Furthermore, essentially all of the CO in blood is combined with hemoglobin even under these extreme conditions.

The most meaningful expresison for evaluation of CO toxicity is carboxyhemoglobin percent saturation (COHb). Existing alevolar CO concentration and the fraction of hemoglobin available for oxygen transport are both related to COHb. Thus it is necessary to determine blood total hemoglobin (active) content as well as CO content. Blood CO content may be estimated directly by spectrophotometric procedures (3, 9, 12, 14) without release of CO from combination with hemoglobin. However, the sensitivity of this analysis is limited by the presence of oxyhemoglobin usually present in much higher concentration. Blood CO content may also be measured by releasing the CO from combination with hemoglobin and determining the amount of CO gasometrically (22, 23, 28), by its reaction with palladium chloride (1), by infrared absorption (5, 11), by Hopcalite oxidation (26), or by gas chromatography (2, 8, 15).

PRINCIPLE

Carbon monoxide of blood is released by hemolysis and reaction with $K_3Fe(CN)_6$ into the gas space of a closed reaction vessel. Helium carrier gas is

[1]Supported by the Bureau of Medicine and Surgery, Navy Department Research Tasks MR005.04-0103 and M4306.07-1002.

[2]The opinions or assertions contained herein are those of the author and are not to be construed as official or reflecting the views of the Navy Depart- ment or the naval service at large.

used to sweep the entire gas phase of the reaction vessel over a column of 5A molecular sieve to separate CO from all other blood gases. The column effluent is mixed with hydrogen and passed over hot nickel to catalytically reduce CO to methane. Methane, derived from blood CO, is detected by hydrogen flame ionization. Response of the flame ionization detector is directly proportional to the amount of CO originally present. A stable solution of carboxyhemoglobin is used to determine the sensitivity of the detector.

Total hemoglobin is determined as cyanmethemoglobin at 540 nm by use of the extinction coefficient given by Drabkin and Austin (10). Because of the slow reaction of carboxyhemoglobin with Drabkin's reagent (19, 27) a reaction time of 3 hours is used with samples containing appreciable COHb.

REAGENTS

1. *Sterox, 10% (v/v).* Dilute 10 ml of Sterox SE (Aloe Scientific Co.) to 100 ml with distilled water.

2. *Potassium Ferricyanide, 10% (w/v).* Dissolve 1 gm of $K_3Fe(CN)_6$ in 10 ml of distilled water. Prepare fresh weekly. The Sterox and ferricyanide reagents are placed in bottles equipped with droppers to deliver about 20 drops per ml.

3. *Borate buffer, pH 8.2-8.4.* Dissolve 6.18 gm of H_3BO_3 in 55 ml of 0.20 N NaOH and dilute to 500 ml with water.

4. *Carboxyhemoglobin standard.* The carboxyhemoglobin standard must have an accurately known CO content in the range of 7-10 volumes percent. It is prepared and standardized as follows:

Preparation. Dilute approximately 10 ml of freshly drawn heparinized human blood with 5 volumes of 0.9% (w/v) NaCl solution and recover the cells by centrifugation. Resuspend the cells in 25 ml of 0.9% NaCl and centrifuge to obtain the washed, packed red cells with a minimum volume of saline. For each volume of packed cells, add 0.1 volume of 10% Sterox and 3 volumes of pH 8.2 borate buffer. Mix by inversion and allow 5 minutes for complete hemolysis. Centrifuge and carefully decant the clear hemoglobin solution. Transfer about 15 ml of the solution to a lightly oiled 100 ml glass syringe equipped with a 3-way stopcock and expel all air. Add approximately 35 ml of 100% CO to the syringe and rotate horizontally for 15 minutes to saturate the solution with CO. Expel the excess CO from the syringe and add about 80 ml of 100% N_2. Rotate the syringe for 15 minutes to remove dissolved CO from the carboxyhemoglobin solution. Expel all gas from the syringe and store the solution anaerobically in a lightly oiled glass syringe at refrigerator temperature, 4°C, when not in use.

Standardization. The CO content of the solution prepared in this manner may be determined, with equal accuracy, by the gasometric procedure of Sendroy and Liu (23) or by spectrophotometric measurement of HbCO. For the Spectrophotometric measurement, the HbCO solution is accurately diluted about 1:100 with 0.1% (w/v) K_2CO_3 and the absorbance measured in a 1 cm curvette at 540 nm. The concentration of CO in the fully saturated, oxygen-free solution is calculated from the equation.

$$\text{CO content (vol\%)} = \frac{\text{A} \times \text{dilution} \times 2.24}{14.95}$$

where A is the measured absorbance of the diluted sample at 540 nm and 14.95 is the millimolar absorptivity of HbCO at this wavelength. Since the millimolar absorptivities of HbCO and HbO_2 are the same at 540 nm, it is essential for the spectrophotometric standardization that saturation of Hb with CO be complete and that dissolved CO be removed without dissociation of HbCO or exposure to air. Gasometric and spectrophotometric measurements have both been used to show that solutions prepared in this manner and stored at 4°C maintain constant CO content for more than 8 months.

APPARATUS

Gas Chromatograph. A schematic diagram of the chromatographic system is presented in Figure 1. Helium is used both as carrier gas (50 ml/min) and to

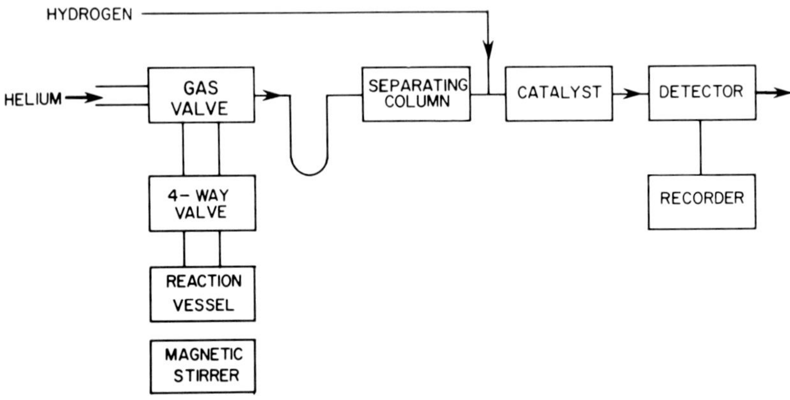

Figure 1. Arrangement of components for gas chromatographic measurement of blood CO.

purge the reaction vessel (50 ml/min). A glass U tube (7mm I.D. × 20 cm length) containing a layer of Ascarite between two layers of Drierite is installed between the gas valve and the separating column for removal of CO_2 and water. The separating column ($\frac{1}{4}$" x 6 feet stainless steel packed with 30-80 mesh 5A molecular sieve) is kept at 100°C.

The effluent of the column is mixed with hydrogen (20-30 ml/min) and the combined gas mixture passed through a $\frac{1}{8}$" x 4" column of nickel catalyst on firebrick prepared according to Porter and Volman (17). The nickel catalyst is maintained at 300°C by means of heating tape or other resistance wire with power supplied from a variable transformer. The gas mixture emerging from the catalyst is discharged into the jet of the flame ionization detector. Response of the detector is monitored with a recorder equipped with a disc integrator to evaluate the area under the chromatogram peak.

Reaction vessel. Release of CO from blood and its transfer to the separating column is carried out by use of the vessel illustrated in Fig. 2. This system was designed to replace the standard gas sample loop of the chromatograph (20). The magnet and reagents are placed in the reaction tube (C) which is then seated on the brass body (B) with silicone grease and held in place by a copper basket and springs. The vessel is purged with helium through the 4-way valve positioned as shown. The helium filled tube is then isolated by turning the key of the 4-way valve. Blood or HbCO solution (0.1 ml) is injected through the centrally located silicone-rubber injection port directly into the reagents by use of a microsyringe. At the end of a predetermined reaction period the 4-way valve and the gas valve of the chromatograph are positioned to pass the carrier gas stream through the reaction vessel and onto the separating column. A sweep-out period of 3 minutes is used after which the gas valve of the chromatograph is positioned to by-pass the reaction vessel. The reaction tube is removed and prepared for the next analysis during the time required for separation on the column.

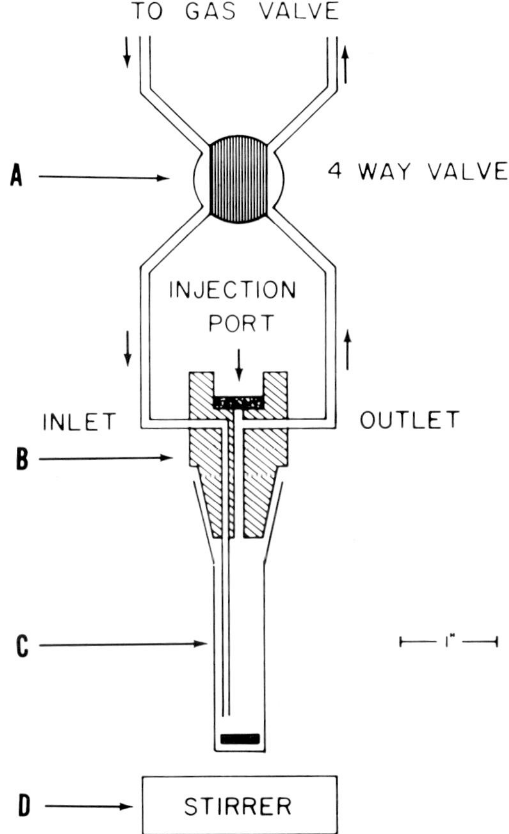

Figure 2. Reaction vessel for liberation of gases from aqueous solutions prior to chromatographic analysis. See text for details of use.

PROCEDURE AND CALCULATIONS

Add 4 drops of 10% $K_3Fe(CN)_6$, 2 drops of 10% Sterox, and a plastic or glass covered stirring bar to a clean reaction tube. Seat the reaction tube in place, start the magnetic stirrer and purge the reaction vessel with helium for 3 minutes. Turn the key on the 4-way valve to isolate the helium filled reaction vessel and inject 0.1 ml of blood directly into the reagents. Allow the blood and ferricyanide to react for 5 minutes. Turn the valve on the chromatograph and then the 4-way valve to pass the carrier gas stream through the reaction vessel onto the separating column for 3 minutes. Turn the valve on the chromatograph so the carrier stream does not pass through the reaction vessel. With the conditions described the CO peak on the chromatogram will begin to appear about 3 minutes after the carrier gas was started through the reaction vessel.

The area under the chromatogram CO peak (observed area x attenuation) is directly proportional to the CO concentration. The area is measured and compared with the area obtained when exactly the same volume of standard HbCO solution is analyzed by the same procedure. The CO content of blood is calculated from the equation

$$CO_B = A_B \times Attn_B \times \frac{CO_S}{A_S \times Attn_S}$$

where A is the observed area, Attn. is the recorder attenuation used, and the subscripts B and S refer to blood and standard, respectively. The operating conditions are most nearly reproduced when equal volumes of blood and standard HbCO solution are compared. If the volumes differ, appropriate changes are made in this calculation to reflect the actual volumes used.

The COHb percent saturation is calculated from the CO content and the CO capacity. CO capacity is taken as 1.34 times the hemoglobin concentration in grams %

$$COHb\ \% = \frac{CO\ content}{CO\ capacity} \times 100$$

DISCUSSION

Separation of CO from other blood gases on the 5A molecular sieve column permits accurate estimation of the CO content with minimal interference from other components. Although the gradual accumulation of water and CO_2 on the column decreases its separating efficiency, the column may be regenerated by heating at 250°C for 48 hours while maintaining a low carrier gas flow. Reduction of CO to methane for detection by flame ionization provides an increase in sensitivity of several orders of magnitude over conventional thermal detectors. The extent of CO reduction by nickel at 300°C is essentially complete and remains constant for long periods of time. There is, however, a gradual decrease in catalyst efficiency after several months when samples containing oxygen are analyzed. The catalyst is replaced if linear response is no longer obtained when different volumes of HbCO standard are measured.

A coefficient of variation (S.D. × 100/mean) for this procedure of ± 1.5% was obtained for HbCO solutions and blood containing from 10.0 to 0.10 volumes % CO. This represents the range of reproducibility of both sample volume measurement and chromatogram area estimation. These two factors determine the over-all accuracy of the procedure since they are greater than the uncertainty in standardization of the reference HbCO solution.

SOURCES OF ERROR

Failure to achieve complete hemolysis of the erythrocytes will result in incomplete release of CO because $K_3Fe(CN)_6$ does not enter the red cell rapidly Low results will also be obtained if the reaction time of hemoglobin with $K_3Fe(CN)_6$ is insufficient to liberate all CO.

Extreme care should be taken to keep all conditions of analysis uniform between sample and standard. These include volume measurement, reaction time, and sweep-out of the reaction vessel as well as the routine operating conditions of the gas chromatograph.

The principal source of error in blood analysis is failure to completely mix the blood sample before an aliquot is removed for analysis. The stability of the base line of the flame ionization detector establishes the lower limit of detection to be about 0.002 volumes % CO with a 0.10 ml sample. Assuming a variability of ± 1% for both the total hemoglobin and CO content measurements, the calculated percent COHb saturation is uncertain by about ± 0.04%.

RANGE OF VALUES

The most important factor affecting blood COHb saturation is the degree of CO contamination of the inspired air. This contamination varies by several fold depending upon weather conditions, traffic flow — especially in urban areas — and industrial contamination. Specific pollution of an individual's inspired air by smoking or riding in a closed automobile with faulty exhaust system is important. It must be remembered, however, that changes in COHb depend not only on the degree of inspired air contamination, but also on the exposure time. Patients who have an increased rate of erythrocyte destruction show elevated COHb as a result of increased endogenous CO production from heme catabolism (6, 7). Patients receiving oxygen therapy have decreased COHb.

It is not practical to establish a definitive "normal" value for COHb without reference to the steady state level of CO in their inspired air. A group of 34 nonsmoking hospital patients without evidence of increased erythrocyte destruction had COHb of 0.85 ± 0.26% (range 0.43-1.50). A group of 17 normal adult non-smoking males who were not hospitalized but whose blood was analyzed during the same period showed COHb of 0.88 ± 0.21%.

A similar group of 34 smokers in the hospital without evidence of abnomal heme catabolism had COHb levels of 3.97 ± 1.88%, while a group of 19 normal males who smoked but were not hospitalized had 4.66 ± 1.68% COHb. The high standard deviations for the smokers reflects the wide range of values for all smokers from 1.53 to 10.1%. Variations in individual smoking habits and the time of blood sampling with respect to the last smoking experience are responsible for the extreme range of values obtained.

CLINICAL INTERPRETATION

The blood COHb for normal nonsmokers will be under 2% when atmospheric contaminations is below 5 ppm CO. Values in excess of this may result from increased endogenous CO formation or from atmospheric contamination. Blood COHb may be as high as 10% for smokers who are otherwise normal even though the general atmospheric contamination is acceptably low. The relatively small changes in COHb due to differences in endogenous CO production are meaningless with smokers because of the wide range of saturations observed. Severe acute CO exposure or contamination from extremely heavy smoking is indicated if COHb is in excess of 10%.

Removal of CO from blood is accomplished by displacing the CO from hemoglobin with oxygen. Since the relative affinity of hemoglobin for these two gases is completely independent of pH, the two most effective methods, for CO removal are: a) an increase in alveolar ventilation and b) an increase in oxygen partial pressure of the inspired air. The most convenient procedure of accomplishment both effects simultaneously is to have the patient breathe 5% CO_2 in oxygen. Hyperbaric oxygen at 2.5 atmospheres was shown by Pitts and Pace (16) to significantly increase the rate of CO elimination in man. The combined effect of respiratory stimulation and moderate increase in oxygen by 5% CO_2 in oxygen is an effective procedure. In addition, it is more convenient and less hazardous since the erythrocyte destruction caused by oxygen at high pressure (13) is minimized.

REFERENCES

1. Allen, T. H., and Root, W. S.: An improved palladium chloride method for the determination of carbon monoxide in blood. J Biol Chem., *216:*319-323, 1955.
2. Ayres, S. M. Criscitiello, A., and Giannelli, S. Jr.: Determination of blood carbon monoxide content by gas chromatography. J. Appl. Physiol., *21:*1368-1370, 1966.
3. Brückner, J., and Desmond, F. B.: A Spectrophotometrical method for the estimation of carbon monoxide hemoglobin in blood. Clin. Chim. Acta, *3:*173-178, 1958.
4. Carlston, A., Holgren, A., Linroth, K., Sjöstrand, T., and Ström, G.: Relationship between low values of alveolar carbon monoxide and carboxyhemoglobin percentage in human blood. Acta Physiol. Scand., *31:*62-74, 1954.
5. Coburn, R. F., Danielson, G. K., Blakemore, W. S., and Forster, R. E., II: Carbon monoxide in blood: Analytical method and sources of error. J. Appl Physiol., *19:*510-515, 1964.
6. Coburn, R. F., Williams, W. J., and Kahn, S. B.: Endogenous carbon monoxide production in patients with hemolytic anemia. J. Clin. Invest., *45:*460-468, 1966.
7. Coburn, R. F., Williams, W. J., Kahn, S. B., and Forster, R. E.: Endogenous carbon monoxide production in patients with hemolytic anemia. J. Clin. Invest., *42:*924, 1963.
8. Collison, H. A., Rodkey, F. L., and O'Neal, J. D.: Determination of carbon monoxide in blood by gas chromatography. Clin. Chem., *14:*162-171, 1968.
9. Commins, B. T., and Lawther, P. J.: A sensitive method for the determination of carboxyhemoglobin in a finger prick sample of blood. Brit. J. Indust. Med., *22:*139-143, 1965.
10. Drabkin, D. L., and Austin, J. H.: Spectrophotometric studies II. Preparation from washed blood cells; nitric oxide hemoglobin and sulfhemoglobin. J. Biol. Chem., *112:*51-65, 1935.
11. Gaensler, E. A., Cadigan, J. B., Jr., Ellicott, M. F., and Jones, R. H.: A new method for rapid precise determination of carbon monoxide in blood. J. Lab. Clin. Med., *49:*945-957, 1957.
12. Horecker, B. L., and Brackett, F. S.: A rapid spectrophotometric method for the determination of methemoglobin and carbonylhemoglobin in blood. J. Biol. Chem., *152:*669-677, 1944.
13. Kann, H. E., Jr.,Mengel, C. E., Clancy, W. T., and Timms, R.: Effects of in vivo hyperoxia on Erythrocytes. VI. Hemolysis occurring after exposure to oxygen under high pressure. J. Lab. Clin. Med., *70:*150-157, 1967.
14. Klendshoj, N. C., Feldstein, M., and Sprague, A. L.: The spectrophotometric determination of carbon monoxide. J. Biol. Chem., *183:*297-303, 1950.
15. McCredie, R. M., and Jose, A. D.: Analysis of blood carbon monoxide and oxygen by gas chromatography. J. Appl. Physiol., *22:*863-866, 1967.
16. Pitts, G. C., and Pace, N. O.: The effect of oxygen at 2.5 atmospheres on the rate of elimination of carbon monoxide in man. Naval Medical Research Report, project NM001.056.01.14, 1949.
17. Porter, K., and Volman, D. H.: Flame ionization detection of carbon monoxide for gas chromatographic analysis. Anal. Chem., *34:*748-749, 1962.
18. Power, G. G.: Solubility of O_2 and CO in blood and pulmonary and placental tissue. J. Appl. Physiol., *24:*468-474, 1968.
19. Rodkey, F. L.: Kinetic aspects of cyanmethemoglobin formation from carboxyhemoglobin. Clin. Chem., *13:*2-5, 1967.
20. Rodkey, F. L., and Collison, H. A.: A reaction vessel for use in gas chromatographic analysis of aqueous solutions. Application for blood carbon monoxide determination. Naval Medical Research Report MR005.04.0002. Report No. 16, 1967.
21. Rodkey, F. L., O'Neal, J. D., and Collison, H. A.: Oxygen and carbon monoxide equilibria of human adult hemoglobin at atmospheric and elevated pressure. Blood. *33:*57-65, 1969.
22. Roughton, F. J. W., and Root, W. S.: The estimation of small amounts of carbon monoxide in blood. J. Biol. Chem., *160:*123-133, 1945.

23. Sendroy, J., Jr., and Liu, S. H.: Gasometric determination of oxygen and carbon monoxide in blood. J. Biol. Chem., *89:*133-152, 1930.
24. Sendroy, J., Jr., Liu, S. H., and Van Slyke, D. D.: The gasometric estimation of the relative affinity constant for carbon monoxide and oxygen in whole blood at 38°. Am. J. Physiol., *90:*511, 1929.
25. Sendroy, J., Jr., and O'Neal, J. D.: Relative affinity constant for carbon monoxide and oxygen in blood. Fed. Proc., *14:*134, 1955.
26. Siösteen, S. M., and Sjöstrand, T.: A method for determination of low concentration of carbon monoxide in the blood and the relation between the CO concentration in the blood and that in the alveolar air. Acta Physiol. Scand., *22:*129-136, 1951.
27. Taylor, J. D., and Miller, J. D. M.: A source of error in the cyanmethemoglobin method of determination of hemoglobin concentration in blood containing carbon monoxide. Am. J. Clin. Path., *43:*265-271, 1965.
28. Van Slyke, D. D., Hiller, A., Weisiger, J. R., and Cruz, W. O.: Determination of carbon monoxide in blood and of total and active hemoglobin by carbon monoxide capacity. Inactive hemoglobin and methemoglobin contents of normal human blood. J. Biol. Chem., *166:*121-148, 1946.

Chapter 27

Laboratory Detection of Cyanide Poisoning

ALFRED H. FREE, PH.D. and HELEN M. FREE, B.S.

INTRODUCTION

Homocides, suicides, and accidental poisoning involving cyanides account for 79 to 245 deaths per year in the United States (4). Cyanide is a poison which has been known since ancient times. Ancient Egyptians extracted the poison from peach seeds, and the Romans used almond extracts as a source of poison for suicides. Prussic acid or hydrogen cyanide was discovered by the famous Swedish chemist, Karl Wilhelm Scheele, in 1782. Scheele's biographers have indicated their amazement in the fact that he described not only the odor of hydrogen cyanide but also its taste and, at the same time, was unaware of its poisonous nature (10). Some accounts ascribe Scheele's death to a laboratory accident in which a flask containing cyanide was broken (12).

Cyanide has appeared as a poison in several famous homocides, one of these being the plot by Prince Youssoupoff to poison the Mad Monk, Rasputin, who was a famous figure in the Russian political scene just prior to the Revolution. Rasputin was invited to a banquet and fed cakes and wine containing cyanide. He showed no effect from ingestion of this material and so his enemies were forced to shoot him (8).

Cyanide, either as hydrogen cyanide or sodium or potassium cyanide, is very famous as a poison. Although many laymen think of it as the most poisonous of all poisons, there are a number of substances which are effective in smaller quantities than cyanide. It is regarded as one of the most rapid-acting (12). Within the past century, cyanide has been used in many interesting ways. It was employed as a poison war gas. The British and French used it in World War I in retaliation to the German use of chlorine. Cyanide was quite ineffective. Hydrogen cyanide has been used for the execution of criminals in the USA. It was employed in the gas chambers in which millions of political prisoners were murdered during World War II. It is used extensively in the fumigation of houses, ships, and railway cars. It is unique as a component of certain analytical chemical systems. It is employed in plating processes. Most surprising is the usage of a 0.1% solution of cyanide which is injected intravenously as a stimulus for the respiratory center.

Cyanide is known in several forms.

Hydrogen cyanide, HCN, is a liquid which boils at room temperature so it also exists as a gas. Soluble salts such as sodium cyanide and potassium cyanide are quite common as are the insoluble salts such as magnesium or calcium cyanide. Hydrogen cyanide can also be released from many organic cyanide compounds. The cyanide content of tissues of those who have died of cyanide poisoning ranges from 0.3 to 2 mg per 100 gms of tissue or per 100 ml of blood. Measurements for cyanide described in this chapter will include a spot test for cyanide and a quantitative colorimetric method for measurement of cyanide. There are many different types of spot tests for cyanide detection in tissue or blood and these have been reviewed by Gettler and Baine (5). We have chosen to present the copper-guaiac test along with the quantitative method proposed by Baar (1).

PRINCIPLE

The methods used either for qualitative identification of cyanide or for the quantitative measurements involve a preliminary separation of the cyanide from the sample. The separated cyanide then reacts with a reagent to give a qualitative or a quantitative measurement.

1. *Qualitative Method:* This method consists of using tartaric acid to release hydrogen cyanide from the sample in a closed system. A paper impregnated with 10% guaiac and moistened with 0.1% copper sulfate solution is suspended in the closed system and hydrogen cyanide gas, if present, turns the paper blue.
2. *Quantitative Method:* This system uses a modified Cavett flask or a Conway diffusion dish to absorb hydrogen cyanide which has been released by acid from the blood. The cyanide is absorbed in dilute alkali and is then subjected to a color reaction. The intensity of color is proportional to the amount of cyanide.

REAGENTS

1. *Qualitative Test*
   a. Guaiac paper — filter paper is impregnated with a 10% alcoholic solution of gum guaiac and allowed to dry in air.
   b. 0.1% copper sulfate — 100 mg of $CuSO_4 \cdot 5H_2O$ are dissolved in 100 ml of distilled water.
2. *Quantitative Method*
   a. Pyrazolone Reagent — (prepared fresh daily). 240 mg of 3-methyl-1-phenyl-2-pyrazolin-5-one are dissolved in 100 ml of water at 75°C. (This requires about 1½ hours.) 20 mg of 4,4′-bis-(3-methyl-1-phenyl-2-pyrazolin-5-one) are dissolved in 20 ml of pyridine. These solutions are mixed just before use.
   b. 0.1N NaOH — 4 gm sodium hydroxide are dissolved in 1 liter of water or appropriate dilution is made from concentrated sodium hydroxide.
   c. 1M NaH_2PO_4 — 120 gm anhydrous sodium dihydrogen phosphate are dissolved in 1 liter of water.
   d. 15% H_2SO_4 — 15 ml of concentrated sulfuric acid are slowly added to 85 ml of water.
   e. 0.1% Chloramine T — this solution is refrigerated. Just before use, 1 volume of this solution is mixed with 3 volumes of 1M NaH_2PO_4. The solution is cooled to about 5°C.
   f. n-butanol

STANDARD SOLUTIONS

For either the qualitative test or the quantitative method, 500 mg of potassium cyanide are dissolved in 1 liter of 0.1N sodium hydroxide and suitable dilutions of this stock solution are prepared in water prior to use.

SPECIAL APPARATUS

1. *Diffusion Flask:* For diffusion of cyanide in the Baar method, a modified Cavett flask is made by gluing a small cup on the floor of the flask. The cup is prepared by sawing off the bottom of a 15 mm diameter polystyrene specimen tube to measure 5 mm high. A slot 1.5 mm wide is cut into the wall of the cup before mounting it in the flask. The capacity of the cup is about 0.5 ml.
2. Other specialized equipment includes a centrifuge and a spectrophotometer for measuring absorbance at 615 nm with a 1 cm light path.

PROCEDURE

1. *Qualitative Test:* The tissue or blood to be tested is placed in the bottom of a small flask. The material is acidified with tartaric acid and above the mixture is suspended a strip of freshly prepared copper sulfate-guaiac paper. The flask is stoppered and warmed slightly and allowed to stand for ½ hour. If a blue-green color does not develop on the paper, this excludes the presence of cyanide. The appearance of a blue-green color on the paper is not completely specific for cyanide and in such cases further confirmatory tests should be done.
2. *Quantitative Test:* 1.2 ml of 0.1N NaOH are placed into the diffusion cup of the Cavett flask. With the flask tilted at about a 25° angle, 4 ml of water and 2 ml of blood containing 2 mg of EDTA as anticoagulant are pipetted onto the floor of the flask. 0.5 ml of 15% H_2SO_4 is pipetted into the modified cup on the floor of the flask and the ground glass stopper is replaced and the flask returned to its upright position. The springs are attached to the flask and it is tilted and tapped gently to allow the acid to flow out of the slit in the modified cup. The flask is rotated on a flat surface to mix the contents about 30 seconds later and diffusion is allowed to proceed for 2 hours.

   After diffusion, 1 ml is removed from the diffusion cup (NaOH plus diffused cyanide) and placed into a tube, cooled to 5°C and 0.2 ml of buffered Chloramine T solution is added and mixed. After 2 minutes, 3 ml of pyrazolone reagent are added rapidly and mixed. Color is allowed to develop for 45 minutes then extracted into 2 ml of n-butanol. After centrifuging, the absorbance of the butanol layer is measured at 615 nm against n-butanol. Concentration of cyanide is calculated from a calibration curve prepared using dilutions of potassium cyanide.

DISCUSSION

The critical nature of acute cyanide intoxication is such that prompt action is required. Effective means of treating cyanide poisoning have been described (2, 11). Usually, the circumstances surrounding a specific incident are most meaningful in helping establish the likelihood of acute cyanide intoxication. Cyanide has a characteristic odor which can be recognized even at very low concentrations. However, approximately one out of four individuals have a genetic inability to recognize the odor of cyanide. It is most important to be able to identify cyanide in blood or tissues or gastric residues in cases of suspected acute intoxication which have medicolegal implications. Hydrogen cyanide is metabolized by the body and, accordingly, it will disappear from the blood. It is ordinarily destroyed by preservative fluids which contain formaldehyde. Cyanide also disappears from decomposed or putrefied tissue.

Since cyanide is metabolized rapidly, the recognition of chronic intoxication cannot clearly be established. Marginal levels of cyanide in the blood in cases of suspected chronic intoxication are so low and so evanescent that there is no general agreement with regard to chronic cyanide intoxication. The human body has a metabolic mechanism for efficient conversion of small quantities of cyanide into thiocyanate. Accordingly, the first step in investigating the possibilities of chronic cyanide intoxication is to establish whether thiocyanate is increased in the blood, urine or saliva. Such elevated levels exist in persons who smoke, this being a consequence of the high level of cyanide in cigarette and other tobacco smoke.

SOURCES OF ERROR

The identification or measurement of cyanide is not part of the "routine" of a typical clinical laboratory. Accordingly, it can be anticipated that much more effort will need to be expended in order to avoid errors. Personnel may forget or confuse the steps in the procedure; reagents may deteriorate; miscalculation of the results may occur. In order to minimize errors in a procedure such as that for cyanide which is used infrequently, it is important to make extensive use of blanks, knowns or recoveries, and standards.

Cyanide is rapidly metabolized and, accordingly, it will promptly disappear from blood or tissue in a living organism. Similarly, small quantities will rapidly disappear from unpreserved or putrefied specimens. In contrast, if the quantity of cyanide is large, it may be recognized in gastric contents recovered several weeks after death. Formalin, which may be used in embalming or preserving fluids, causes decomposition and disappearance of cyanide.

One of the important mechanisms of recognizing cyanide poisoning is the identification of the characteristic odor. However, one out of four people possess a genetic defect which prevents recognition of this odor.

RANGE OF VALUES

There is no significant level of cyanide in normal blood or urine as determined by current-day methodology. Following ingestion of cyanide or inhalation of hydrogen cyanide gas, blood or tissue levels in fatal cases ranging from 0.3 mg per 100 gm to 2 mg have been reported (5, 10) . Data on blood levels of surviving cases have also been reported and it is surprising on first consideration that there is a considerable overlap in values. These variations may, in part, be due to differences in resistance of the subjects, difference in the handling of samples, differences in the methodology of measurement, and possibly due to an occasional laboratory error. One report (6) indicates a level of cyanide in blood in a case which survived which is so tremendously greater than other values that one can only speculate as to the basis for such a value.

The very high level of toxicity of cyanide and its extremely rapid action provide the basis for finding a large proportion such as 70 to 90% of an ingested dose of cyanide in the gastro-intestinal tract (5).

RESUME OF CLINICAL INTERPRETATIONS

The extremely rapid action of cyanide tends to minimize the utility of laboratory tests as an aid to diagnosis prior to treatment. The laboratory detection or measurement of cyanide is of great importance in confirming or aiding in the definition of cyanide poisoning, particularly in cases having medico-legal implications. The situations surrounding specific cases of cyanide intoxication are quite varied. There is a great variation in resistance of different individuals to cyanide intoxication. Also, the effects of rapid treatment procedures which may be applied prior to obtaining specimens for study are not standardized or readily defined. All of these factors make it extremely difficult to relate results of laboratory measurements to the clinical situation. In fact, a general knowledge of the circumstances of a specific case, along with an understanding of the nature of cyanide intoxication and data from laboratory measurements, enables the clinician or the toxicologist to provide maximal utilization of laboratory findings.

Table I presents levels of hydrogen cyanide in air which are regarded as safe as well as those which are toxic (7). It will be seen that there is a direct relationship between the level of cyanide in inspired air and the time required to produce acute intoxication. The tremendously high level of cyanide in cigarette smoke (14) is a surprising value which accounts for the fact that smokers have high levels of the detoxification product, thiocyanate, in blood, urine, and saliva.

TABLE I: RELATION OF CYANIDE IN AIR TO TOXIC ACTION

	Parts Per Million
Maximal safe level in air	10 ppm.
Mild symptoms of intoxication	20 ppm.
Death after several hours	50 ppm.
Death in 30-60 minutes	100 ppm.
Death in a few minutes	500 ppm.
Cigaret smoke	1,600 ppm.

Low levels of cyanide are converted by rhoadanese into thiocyanate. This conversion accounts for the fact that cyanide does not have a cumulative effect in the body. The thiocyanate appears in the blood and is excreted in the urine. The salivary glands have an ability to concentrate thiocyanate with the result that saliva may contain concentrations that are as much as ten times as great as the concentrations found in the blood. In cases of suspected chronic cyanide intoxication, tests for thiocyanate on saliva (9) or urine (3) can be informative. If the person being studied is a smoker, the level of thiocyanate is so great that it obscures the picture as to whether any additional chronic intoxication is involved.

Sodium nitroprusside, as an inorganic compound, and a large number of organic compounds owe their toxicity to the fact that they yield cyanide in the body. Sunderman and Kincaid (13) have described the toxicity of acetone cyanohydrin and ethylene cyanohydrin, and Polson and Tattersall have reviewed a case of nitroprusside intoxication (10).

If one considers the fact that cyanide is well known as a potent poison, that it is widely available for commercial applications in engraving, plating, and photography, that it is widely employed in fumigation processes, that it is a reagent on the shelf of most chemistry laboratories; it is surprising that more deaths as a result of accidents, suicides, and homocides are not ascribed to cyanide. There is no clear-cut basis for the low incidence of cyanide intoxication, but it can in part be ascribed to the fact that most people have a healthy respect for the poisonous nature of cyanide and this is reflected in handling practices.

REFERENCES

1. Baar, S.: The micro determination of cyanide: its application to the analysis of whole blood. Analyst, *91:*268-272, 1966.
2. Bain, J. T. B., and Knowles, E. L.: Successful treatment of cyanide poisoning. Brit Med. J., *2:*763, 1967.
3. Djuric, D., Raicevic, P., and Konstantinovic, I.: Excretion of thiocyanates in urine of smokers. Arch. Environ. Health, *5:*12-15, 1962.
4. Editorial: Recovery from Cyanide poisoning. J. A. M. A., *140:*541, 1949.
5. Gettler, A. O., and Baine, J. O.: The toxicology of cyanide. Amer. J. Med. Sci., *195:*182-198, 1938.
6. Liebowitz, D., and Schwartz, H.: Cyanide poisoning—a case with recovery. Amer. J. Clin. Path., *18:*965-970, 1948.
7. Lockett, S.: *Clinical Toxicology*. London, Henry Kimpton, 1957, pp. 198-199.
8. Mellan, I., and Mellan, E.: *Dictionary of Poisons*. New York, Philosophical Library, 1956, pp. 65-67.
9. Monekosso, G. L., Jantjie, V. V., and Williams, H.: Starch-iodic-acid paper in predicting plasma-thiocyanate concentrations. Lancet, *2:*1330-1331, 1967.
10. Polson, C. J., and Tattersall, R. N.: *Clinical Toxicology*. Philadelphia, J. B. Lippincott, 1959, pp. 107-128.
11. Rose, C. L., Worth, R. M., Kikuchi, K., and Chen, K. K.: Cobalt salts in acute cyanide poisoning. Proc. Soc. Expt. Biol. Med., *120:*780-782, 1965.
12. Sollman, T.: *A Manual of Pharmacology*, 8th ed. Philadelphia, W. B. Saunders, 1957, pp. 982-990.
13. Sunderman, F. W., and Kincaid, J. F.: Toxicity studies of acetone cyanohydrin and ethylene cyanohydrin. J. Ind. Hyg. and Occup. Med., *8:*371-376, 1953.
14. Terry, L. L.: Smoking and Health. Public Health Service Publication No. 1103. Report of the Advisory Committee to the Surgeon General of the Public Health Service, 1964, p. 60.

Chapter 28

Diazomethane Poisoning

F. WILLIAM SUNDERMAN, M.D., PH.D.

INTRODUCTION

The toxicity of diazomethane has long been underestimated and until recently has received comparatively scant treatment in the medical literature. Most of the early references regarding the symptoms produced by exposure to the gas had been confined almost exclusively to brief statements in the chemical literature. The compound was first described in 1894 by von Pechmann[1] who indicated that it was extremely poisonous, causing air hunger and chest pains. In a publication in 1895, von Pechmann[2] stated that he had been delayed in making further studies with the compound owing to the poisonous effect that the gas produced in him. Corroborating von Pechmann's observations, Bamberger and Renauld[3] reported in 1895 that they had also experienced toxic effects in experimenting with the gas and that their symptoms were essentially dizziness and tinnitus.

According to Gottstein, Schlossmann and Teleky,[4] skin exposure to diazomethane produces denudation of the skin and mucous membranes. These authors claim that the action of diazomethane is similar to that of dimethyl sulphate. Loring[5] also note that the vapors from the ether solution of the gas are irritating to the skin and render the fingers so tender that it is difficult to pick up a pin.

Arndt and Amende[6] in 1930 reported that two persons developed chest pains, fever and severe asthmatic symptoms about 5 hours after exposure to mere traces of the gas. Arndt[7] described diazomethane as being "an especially insidious poison." He stated that "a person may work with it carelessly for some time without noticing effects. This leads, however, to a supersensitivity so that it is almost impossible to work carefully with diazomethane without being subjected to attacks of asthma and fever."

The toxicity of diazomethane has been attributed by Flury and Zernik[8] to the intracellular formation of formaldehyde. Diazomethane reacts slowly with water to form methyl alcohol and liberate nitrogen. Formaldehyde, in turn, is formed by the oxidation of methyl alcohol. The possibilities of liberation *in vivo* of methyl alcohol or of the reaction of diazomethane with carboxylic compounds to form toxic methyl esters may be considered; on the other hand, the deleterious effects of diazomethane may be primarily due to the strongly irritant action of the gas on the respiratory system.

$$CH_2N_2 + H_2O \longrightarrow CH_3OH + N_2$$
$$RCOOH + CH_2N_2 \longrightarrow RCOOCH_3 + N_2$$

PHYSICAL AND CHEMICAL PROPERTIES

In addition to the toxicity of diazomethane, the explosive nature of this compound represents a special hazard. Staudinger and Kupfer[9] reported that either in the gaseous or liquid state diazomethane explodes with flashes. Even at —80°C. Steacie[10] found that liquid diazomethane detonated. Other investigators[11, 12, 13] also directed attention to the explosive nature of this compound. It has been the general experience, however, that explosions do not occur when diazomethane is prepared and contained in solvents such as ether or benzene.

At ordinary temperatures, diazomethane, or azimethylene, is an unstable, yellow, odorless gas having the following characteristics:

Formula	CH_2N_2
Mol. wt.	42.04
m.p.	—145°C.
b.p.	—23°C.

The gas is soluble in benzene or ether. Dissolved in these solvents it has proved to be a valuable agent in the synthesis of organic compounds, since it yields products of methylation quantitatively at room temperature and without the use of other reagents. Owing to the expense of preparation, diazomethane has not found widespread commercial application. However, as a laboratory reagent, the use of this compound has increased to such an extent that methods for its preparation have been included in elementary manuals of organic chemistry. It is normally prepared by von Pechmann's original method, i.e., from methyl nitrosourethan and sodium methoxide. Alternate methods of preparation include the treatment of nitrosomethylurea with potassium hydroxide and the reaction of potassium hydroxide with a chloroform solution of hydrazine.

CASE REPORTS

The first clinical report of poisoning from diazomethane was published by Sunderman *et al.*[14] in 1938. Sunderman and coworkers directed special attention to the dangers of exposure by inhalation. Subsequently, six additional cases of acute diazomethane poisoning, including one death, have been reported in the medical literature. In all cases, symptoms of intoxication included irritating cough, fever, and malaise, varying in intensity to the degree and duration of exposure. The victims were all chemists or laboratory workers. A tabulation of the cases of diazomethane poisoning is given in Table I.

TABLE 1: CASE REPORTS OF DIAZOMETHANE POISONING

Date of Report	*Author(s)*	*Symptoms of Intoxication*
1938	Sunderman,	Violet paroxysms of coughing, chest pain, pulmonary edema
1949	Le Winn[15] *et al.*[14]	Fulminating pneumonia, moderate cyanosis, progressive shock, death
1951	Braun[16]	Cough, expectoration, tremor, respiratory insufficiency, asthma, allergy
1952	Berg[17]	Paroxysmal dyspnea, hepatic enlargement, hemolysis
1964	Lewis[18]	Fatigue, flushing of skin, cough, chest pain, severe headache
1965	Vyskocil, *et al.*[19]	Irritating cough, asthma, chest discomfort, fever
1966	Hanusch, *et al.*[20]	Cough, asthma, vomiting, dyspnea

STUDIES ON EXPERIMENTAL ANIMALS

A number of studies regarding the effects of diazomethane on experimental animals have been reported. A concentration of 175 ppm for 10 minutes caused hemorrhage, emphysema and edema of the lungs in cats, with death in three days.[8] Exposed guinea pigs showed symptoms of severe respiratory tract irritation and pulmonary edema.[14] Chronic exposure of rabbits to an atmosphere containing 2 to 12 mg diazomethane per liter resulted in bronchopneumonia followed by death.[21]

Diazomethane has been shown by Schoental[22] to be a lung carcinogen. Exposure by inhalation may induce lung adenoma and carcinoma in mice and rats. Skin application and subcutaneous injection, as well as inhalation of the compound have been shown to cause tumor development in experimental animals.[22]

It is noteworthy that in the metabolism of the carcinogens, dimethylnitrosamine and cycasin, one of the intermediary products is diazomethane (Fig. 1).[23]

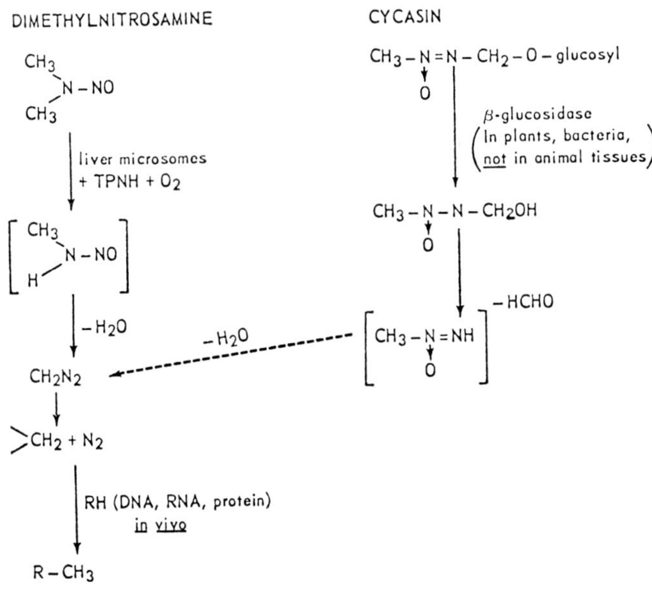

Figure 1. Dimethylnitrosamine and cycasin.

SUMMARY

In view of the known hazards of working with diazomethane, it should be handled as an extremely toxic chemical. The first exposure to the gas may not produce any noteworthy initial reactions; however, subsequent exposures may produce extremely severe ones. The pulmonary symptoms may be explained either on the basis of a true allergic sensitivity after repeated exposure to the gas, and particularly in individuals of allergic heredity; or on the basis of a powerful irritant action of the gas on the mucous membranes. To support the former possibility is the statement by Ardnt[7] that individuals who had first handled the gas with relative impunity later experienced symptoms on even the slightest exposure. Sunderman's patient gave a clear-cut familial history of asthma and the patient himself reported that at times he had suffered mildly from hay fever.

The only explanation for the pulmonary lesions observed after primary exposure in experimental animals appears to be that of a direct irritant action.

REFERENCES

1. Peckmann, H. V.: Ueber diazomethan. Ber. Dtsch. Chem. Ges. *27:*1888-94, 1894.
2. Peckmann, H. V.: Ueber diazomethan. Ber. Dtsch. Chem. Ges. *28:*855-61, 1895.
3. Bamberger, E., and Renauld, E.: Eine neue bildungsweise des diazomethans. Ber. Dtsch. Chem. Ges. *28:*1682-5, 1895.
4. Gottstein, F., Schlossman, A., and Teleky, L.: *Handbuch der Sozialen Hygiene u. Gesundheitsfürsorge.* Vol. II. Gewerbehygiene und Gewerbekrankheiten. J. Springer—Berlin, 1926. 816 ppm
5. Loring, F. H.: Diazomethane. Chem. News *115:* 225, 1917.
6. Arndt, F., and Amende, J.: Preparation of diazomethane. Ztschr. f. Angew. Chem. *13:*111 6, 1930.
7. Arndt, F.: Diazomethane. Organic Syntheses *15:*3-5, 1935.
8. Flury, F., and Zernik, F.: *Shadliche Gase, Dampfe, Nebel, Rauch- und Staubarten.* J. Springer—Berlin, 1931. 637 pp.
9. Staudinger, H., and Kupfer, O.: Uber reaktionen des methylens. III. Diazomethan. Ber. Dtsch. Chem. Ges. *45:*501-9, 1912.
10. Steacie, E. W. R.: The thermal decomposition of diabomethane. J. Phys. Chem. *35:*1493-5, 1931.
11. Boersch, H.: Determination of the structure of simple molecules by electron interference. Monatschr. f. Chem. *65:*311-32, 1935.
12. Kirkbride, F. W., and Norrish, R. G. W.: Primary photochemical processes. II Absorption, spectrum and photochemical decomposition of diazomethane. J. Chem. Soc. *1933:*119-26. 1933.
13. Meerwein, H., and Burneleit, W.: Action of diazomethane on ketones in the presence of catalysts. Ber. Dtsch. Chem. Ges. *61B:*1840-7, 1928.
14. Sunderman, F. W., Connor, R., and Fields, H.: Diazomethane poisoning. First clinical case report. Am. J. Med. Sci. *195:* (4) 469-73, 1938.
15. Le Winn, E. B.: Diazomethane poisoning: Report of a fatal case with autopsy. Am. J. Med. Sci. *218:*556-62, 1949.
16. Braun, H.: Üeber diazomethanvergiftungen unter besonderer Berucksichtitung eines in der medizinischen poliklinik der universitat München beobachteten falles. Med. Monatsschr. *5:* 284-6, 1951.
17. Berg, V.: Ueber diazomethanvergiftungen. Zb. Arbeitsmed. und Arbeitsschutz, *2:*132-5, 1952.
18. Lewis, C. E.: Diazomethane poisoning; Report of a case suggesting sensitization reaction. J. Occup. Med., *6:*91-2, 1964.
19. Vyskocil, J., Sklensky, B., and Klimova, M.: Clinical study of the toxic effect of diazomethane. Pracovni Lekar., *17:* (10) 452-4, 1965.
20. Hanusch, A. W., Schafer, H., and Hanusch, A.: Diazomethan-Intoxikation. Zbl. Arbeitsmed. und Arbeitsschutz, *16:* (9) 261-6, 1966.
21. Vyskocil, J., Sklensky, B., and Dluhos, M.: Toxic effect of diazomethane. Pracvoni Lekar, *18:* (1) 10-13, 1966.
22. Schoental, R.: Carcinogenic action of diazomethane and of nitroso-N-methyl urethane. Nature, *188:*420-1, 1960.
23. Miller, J. A.: Comments on chemistry of cycads. Fed. Proc., *23:*1361-2, 1964.

Chapter 29

Toxicity from Exposure to Solvents

W. WALTER OPPELT, M.D.

In this chapter, some factors relating to the toxicity to the human being of commonly used industrial solvents will be summarized. A few examples in each of the following groups of solvents will be discussed: aromatic hydrocarbons, cyclic hydrocarbons, technical hydrocarbons, halogenated hydrocarbons, ketones and glycols. Finally, brief consideration will be given to a modern social problem, that of glue sniffing, and an attempt will be made to relate this to our knowledge of solvent toxicity. To the reader, *Toxicity and Metabolism of Industrial Solvents* (3) by Browning is suggested as a useful source book.

AROMATIC HYDROCARBONS

This exceedingly important group of industrial solvents is usually derived from coal and petroleum and is characterized by its simplest, and most important member, benzene (Fig. 1). The structure of benzene is now generally agreed to be a hexagon, consisting of carbon atoms separated by alternating double bonds. Other members of this group, which we will consider in some detail, include toluene, xylene and ethyl benzene.

Benzene

It is initially important to differentiate between benz*ene* (also caled benzol) and benz*ine*. The former is, of course, the well-known aromatic hydrocarbon, whereas the latter is a totally unrelated mixture of volatile aliphatic hydrocarbons derived from petroleum distillation. Much confusion in the literature has resulted from the failure to differentiate between these two chemicals.

Benzene is a colorless liquid, somewhat lighter than water (SG of 0.884) which is used extensively in the manufacture of rubber, plastics, paints, linoleum, glues, floor waxes, watches, cameras, etc. Potential exposure to this solvent is therefore common, and often, unsuspected.

Several methods involving colorimetric or ultraviolet spectroscopic techniques (5, 6, 13) are available for estimating benzene in air, fluids and tissues.

Benzene may be absorbed through the skin, the respiratory epithelium or the gastrointestinal tract. Because of its high lipid solubility, it is widely distributed in body tissues and tends to concentrate in tissues with high fat contents.

Excretion of the unchanged agent occurs mainly through the lungs, whereas metabolites are excreted in the urine. It is estimated that after a high dose, approximately 40% of the ingested benzene is excreted unchanged through the lungs and the rest is metabolized (22).

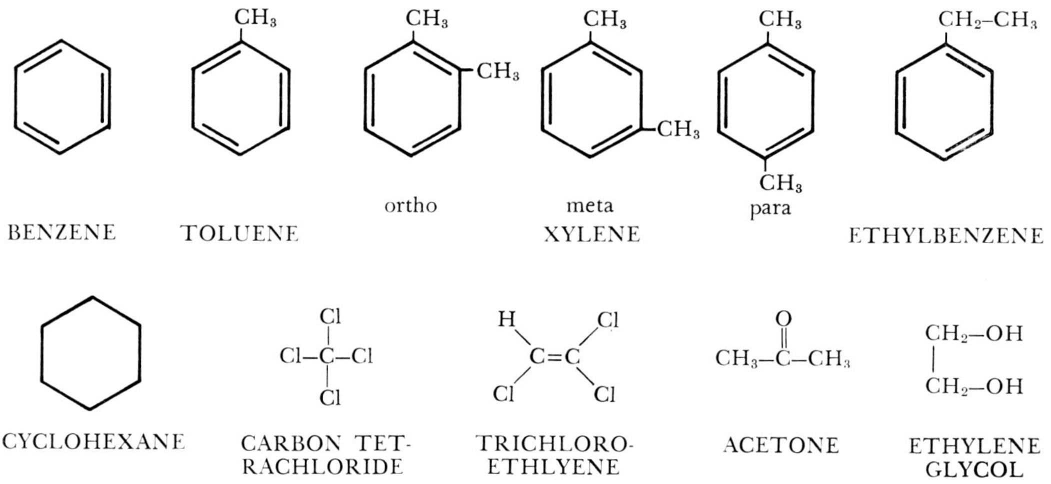

BENZENE TOLUENE ortho meta para XYLENE ETHYLBENZENE

CH_3 CH_3 CH_3 CH_3 CH_3 CH_3 CH_3 CH_2-CH_3

CYCLOHEXANE CARBON TETRACHLORIDE TRICHLOROETHLYENE ACETONE ETHYLENE GLYCOL

CCl_4 $ClHC=CCl_2$ $CH_3-CO-CH_3$ CH_2-OH / CH_2-OH

Figure 1.

The major metabolite is phenol; minor metabolites include conjugated phenols, quinol, catechols, hydroxyquinol, phenylmercapturic acid and trans-transmuconic acid. As the major urinary metabolite is phenol, monitoring its urinary concentration is the easiest method to check for benzene exposure. The phenols are also thought to be responsible for the major toxicity observed after benzene inhalation or ingestion.

The toxicity of benzene might be divided into the acute and chronic form. Acute, lethal toxicity, occurring if one inhales 20,000 ppm for 5 minutes, manifests itself by convulsions, paralysis and unconsciousness. Non-fatal cases may recover from unconsciousness or show only euphoria, giddiness, headache, nausea, violent excitement and ataxia. There is great variation in individual susceptibility. The major changes noted at autopsy include hyperemia of various organs, petechial hemorrhages and prominent benzene odor of all organs.

The major manifestation of chronic benzene toxicity is a general depression of the bone marrow which may be followed by the development of leukemia. There is wide variation of susceptibility among victims. It is generally agreed that women are more susceptible than men (17). Symptoms early in the exposure history are either absent or non-specific. They may include non-specific dermatitis, nausea, fatigue and headaches. Later on, symptoms are those related to leucopenia, anemia and thrombocytopenia. A selective neuopenia, with a relative lymphocytosis, is usually the earliest blood abnormality noted after chronic benzene exposure. This is followed by eosinophilia and basophilia, a normocytic or macrocytic anemia and thrombocytopenia. Bone marrow examinations may show anything from mild hypoplasia to complete aplasia. If removal from exposure occurs early, there is recovery of the marrow, while late cases progress to death because of permanent marrow aplasia. No consistently effective treatment has been described. It is now generally agreed that there is some association between benzene exposure and leukemia in humans. It is not a common association, and various types of leukemia have been seen. There is usually a 10-year or longer history of exposure and frequently leukemia develops only after a long bout of aplastic anemia.

It is possible that chronic benzene exposure causes mild liver toxicity, although most authorities believe that these abnormalities are secondary to the marrow abnormalities and infection which seem to be always present in such cases.

Because of the serious nature of chronic benzene toxicity, considerable efforts are being made to decrease the use of this solvent and to substitute less toxic agents such as toluene, xylene or isopropyl benzene. As the agent is so widely used, chronic exposure may occur in most unexpected places. For example, it is not generally realized that gasoline may contain from 1.5% to 10% benzene and that more safe solvents, such as commercial toluene and xylene, may contain significant quantities of benzene, as a contaminant.

Toluene

Toluene is methyl benzene and has physical properties somewhat similar to benzene (Fig. 1). As commercially produced, it may contain various quantities of benzene, ranging from 15% in Germany in 1954, to 0.3%, which is the current amount in "pure" toluene in this country. It is also produced from petroleum or coal and is used as a solvent for gums, fats and resins, as a thinner of various paint products, as a constituent of motor fuels, in glues and in the rubber and plastics industry.

It may be determined by ultraviolet spectroscopy (13, 19), colorimetry (7) or, indirectly, by its major metabolite, hippuric acid, which appears in the urine.

Toluene is well-absorbed from the respiratory mucosa or the gastrointestinal tract, but is poorly absorbed through the skin. After ingestion, 18% is excreted unchanged by exhalation (11). Most of the remainder is oxidized to benzoic acid, which in turn, is conjugated with glycine and excreted as hippuric acid by the kidney (11).

It is widely distributed in the body, but is found in highest concentration in brain, adrenals and bone marrow (9).

Acute toxicity in humans is characterized by ataxia, acute dermatitis and an irritative pneumonitis. Unconsciousness is rare. It is questionable whether there is significant toxicity to the human who is chronically exposed to low concentrations of toluene. The possibility of liver damage had been raised (12) but later studies (23) could not confirm either liver enlargement or abnormal liver function tests in exposed workers when they were compared to a control group. Again, most evidence points to the absence of hematopoietic toxicity in exposed workers (2). It thus appears that toluene is considerably safer than benzene and that the severe marrow toxicity noted with benzene is specific and unique among hydrocarbons (11).

Xylene

Xylene, being dimethyl benzene, has three isomers: ortho-, meta-, and paraxylene. (Fig. 1). Commercial xylene, which is also called xylol, is a mixture of these three isomers. The material is a colorless liquid with an aromatic odor. There are significant differences in the physical properties between the three isomers (3).

Xylene is derived from coal tar and is used in the printing, leather, rubber and paint industry as a de-greasing agent and a constituent of aviation fuel, and as a starting agent and intermediate in the manufacture of phthalic and terephthalic acids which, in turn, are used in the manufacture of plastics and synthetic textiles.

It may be estimated by spectrophotometric methods similar to those described for benzene and toluene (19).

After ingestion, a small amount is exhaled unchanged and the major portion of the agent is metabolized by oxidation of its methyl groups to form toluic acid. This may either be directly excreted by the kidney or first conjugated with glucoronic acid, glycine or sulfuric acid (31).

There does not seem to be significant central nervous system toxicity secondary to xylene. Irritation of the eyes, dermatitis and irritative bronchitis are the most prominent symptoms of acute heavy exposure. Although several cases of marrow hypoplasia have been described secondary to xylol exposure (1, 18), it is difficult to blame these abnormalities on xylene, as exposure to other agents, especially benzene, was usually involved. It is possible that occasional slight liver and kidney toxicity may result from xylene exposure. All in all, though, xylene seems to be quite nontoxic to the human.

Ethylbenzene

This solvent (Fig. 1) is produced by the alkylation of benzene and finds its prime use in the manufacture of styrene, as a paint thinner, and as an "antiknock" constituent of motor fuels.

It is estimated by the same methods as xylene.

Hydroxylation to methylphenyl carbinol is seen and hippuric acid is another metabolic procedure (11).

In high concentrations, it may be a narcotic to animals. In humans, irritations of eyes and skin have been the only reported toxic manifestations.

CYCLIC HYDROCARBONS

Cyclohexane is the only important member of this group of solvents. Its structure is smilar to benzene, except that the ring is fully saturated (Fig. 1). It is a liquid with similar odor and physical characteristics as benzene. It is usually produced by the catalytic hydrogenation of benzene and is used in the rubber, chemical and perfume industry. There are no specific analytical techniques for its estimation and nothing is known about its distribution in the body. It is metabolized to cyclohexanol, which, in turn, is conjugated with glucoronic acid (8). Some of the ingested dose is exhaled unchanged. It is most likely quite harmless to humans. Some of the cases of so-called cyclohexane intoxication which have been reported are probably due to benzene, which is a very common contaminant of commercial cyclohexane.

TECHNICAL HYDROCARBONS

Technical hydrocarbons are mixtures of hydrocarbons which are derived from petroleum. These mixtures include paraffins, olefins, cyclic hydrocarbons aromatic hydrocarbons, acetylenes, etc. Commercially, these hydrocarbons are known as gasoline, benz*ine,* petroleum spirits, white spirits, etc. *Gasoline* is obviously the most important member of this group from the point of view of exposure to humans. The composition of gasolines may include significant quantities of benz*ene,* however, this is not the case in modern, American gasolines.

Gasolines are mainly absorbed through the respiratory tract; skin absorption apparently does not occur to a significant extent. If the material is taken by mouth, gastrointestinal absorption is rapid. As far as is known, the various components are excreted unchanged by exhalation. (Of course, any aromatic hydrocarbon would be metabolized, as indicated earlier.)

Acute intoxication due to inhalation is followed by giddiness, a feeling of "drunkenness," not dissimilar from alcoholic intoxication. There may be nausea, vomiting, diarrhea; and unconsciousness and death occurs when very high concentrations are inhaled or ingested. Chronic exposure to gasoline is sometimes followed by dermatitis (bullous lesions, pigmentation or depigmentation, or a picture resembling pellagra), slight anemia or leucopenia (this may be due to benzene contamination), nausea, anorexia and weight loss, and certain neurological disturbances. These may include drowsiness, apathy, forgetfulness, neuropathies, weakness, tremors and loss of smell. Again, the neurological picture may be very similar to that seen in chronic alcoholism.

Habituation to gasoline may occur. In the past, gasoline sniffing was practiced by some adolescents. This has lost popularity and has been replaced by glue sniffing, marijuana smoking, etc. Gasoline is apparently sniffed for the acute central nervous system effect which resembles acute alcoholic intoxication.

HALOGENATED HYDROCARBONS

This group includes a large number of compounds, which are usually rather simple, aliphatic, saturated or non-saturated hydrocarbons, containing varying numbers of halogen atoms, frequently chloride. They all have a narcotic effect and therefore, some of them are used as anesthetic agents. Many have potential for renal and liver injury. We will only discuss two members of this group, carbon tetrachloride and trichloroethylene, as these have extensive industrial usage and have been important agents in causing human toxicity.

Carbon Tetrachloride

A name more descriptive of the chemical structure of this liquid is tetrachloromethane (Fig. 1). It is a heavy, clear, colorless liquid with an odor similar to chloroform. It is generally produced by the chlorination of methane. In the past, it found great use as a dry cleaner and in fire extinguishers. Presently, safer agents are used for these two applications, as a great number of people were severely intoxicated when the agent was used for these purposes. Rather recent government regulations (i.e., the Coast Guard) forbid the use of this agent in fire extinguishers. However, older fire extinguishers still in use may contain carbon tetrachloride. In Europe, it is still used as a fumigant for grain and is widely used in industry in the manufacture of Freon 12, DDT, rubber, paint and for the extraction of oils and fats.

A relatively simple method, based on absorption on silica gel with subsequent hydrolysis, has been found useful in estimating carbon tetrachloride (7). Infra-red spectrophotometry is used to determine the agent in blood and tissues (29).

The solvent is readily absorbed from respiratory and gastrointestinal tract. It seems to be concentrated in marrow and fat (21) and is also found in brain, pancreas and liver. Most of the agent is exhaled unchanged, although unidentified metabolites are found in the urine (21).

Toxicity is mainly confined to the central nervous system, the liver and kidneys. In addition to carbon tetrachloride toxicity per se, phosgene may be liberated when the agent is used near a flame (i.e., when extinguishing a fire), thus increasing the toxic hazard of carbon tetrachloride.

Acute exposure to high concentrations may lead to rapid unconsciousness and death. If rapid death does not occur, survival is complicated by the effect of the agent on liver and kidneys. Within 48 hours, signs of severe hepatocellular disease, with jaundice, elevated SGOT levels and BSP retention, may occur. This may progress to fatal hepatic coma. Within hours after heavy exposure, oliguria, followed by anuria, may be seen. This seems to be due to renal tubular toxicity and the anuria is similar to that described after acute tubular necrosis of any etiology. Treatment of the liver and renal failure is purely supportive. If recovery occurs, all evidence of renal and liver damage may disappear within a year or two (16). Cardiac and gastrointestinal complications have been described but these are usually secondary to liver and kidney injury. The severe toxicity, described above, is most often seen after acute, heavy exposure, either by inhalation or ingestion. It is unclear whether prolonged exposure to low concentrations of the agent results in recognizable liver and kidney damage.

Trichloroethylene (Fig. 1)

This is a very effective solvent which, in addition, is non-flammable. It has therefore found wide application in industry where it is used in rubber, paint and leather manufacture, as well as a degreasing agent and a dry-cleaning fluid. It has also been used as a surgical or obstetrical anesthetic.

It is produced by thermal decomposition of pentachloroethane. It is estimated by methods similar to those described for carbon tetrachloride (7). In addition, methods based on the Fujiwara reactions are also useful, especially when estimating it in blood or tissues (4).

Trichloroethylene is rapidly absorbed from the gastrointestinal or the respiratory tract and is extensively metabolized. The metabolic pathway involves the formation of the intermediate, chloral hydrate, which in turn, is converted to trichloroacetic acid and trichloroethanol (30). Attempts have been made to correlate toxicity of trochloroethylene to the level of the metabolites present, however, the correlation is poor. Similarly, poor correlation is obtained when exposure to the solvent is quantitated by the levels of the metabolites in the urine.

The major toxicity of trichloroethylene is due to its narcotic effect. Large doses, either by ingestion or inhalation, may cause deep coma, associated with cardiovascular collapse and consequent renal injury. With supportive treatment, many even deeply comatose patients, may survive without significant final liver or renal injury. There is real disagreement as to the toxic potential of chronic exposure to trichloroethylene. Everyone agrees that the hazard is not great. Mucous membrane and respiratory tract irritation has been described, as has anemia and mild evidence of liver injury. It was not clear, however, whether trichloroethylene could be blamed for the liver and marrow abnormalities. There have been reports of trigeminal and optic nerve injury (26) and a few mysterious, sudden deaths have been associated with exposure. Habituation to the solvent, presumably because of the narcotic effects, is occasionally seen. All in all, it is quite evident that trichloroethylene is much safer than carbon tetrachloride.

KETONES

Ketones are widely used industrial general solvents which, on the whole, are not very toxic to the human. The most familiar ketone is acetone and this will be the only member of this group which we will consider.

Acetone

The structure of acetone is described better by its synonym, dimethyl ketone (Fig. 1). It is a volatile, flammable, pungent liquid with a low boiling point. It is a good solvent for various fats and oils, and, in addition, is miscible with water. This, of course, leads to its use as a dryer of laboratory glassware, where we all have encountered this material. It is produced by destructive distillation of wood, distillation of calcium acetate, fermentation of corn products or by catalytic oxidation of isopropyl alcohol or natural gas.

It is used in the chemical, rubber, varnish, plastic and dyeing industries and is commonly encountered by the average housewife as it is used as a nail polish remover.

Variations of the bisulphite method can be used to estimate acetone, both in air and in blood and tissues (14).

Acetone is well-absorbed from the respiratory tract, but not in significant quantities from the intact skin.

It is largely excreted unchanged by exhalation (31) and small amounts are oxidized.

Acute intoxication with large amounts of acetone may produce narcosis or unconsciousness, although few such cases have been recorded. When this does occur, there is also evidence of mild, temporary liver and kidney injury. Chronic exposure to even high doses of acetone may, at the most, produce a feeling of faintness, some irritation of the conjuntivae, headaches and respiratory irritation. There is no evidence of liver, kidney or marrow toxicity in such cases.

GLYCOLS

Among the glycols, I only want to discuss ethylene glycol because of its wide use as an antifreeze agent and its toxic hazard to humans.

Ethylene Glycol

Ethylene glycol, also called glycol alcohol (Fig. 1), is a clear, colorless liquid with a sweet, not unpleasant taste, with high boiling point (197 C) and a low freezing point. These properties, in addition to its water miscibility and non-corrosiveness, make it an excellent radiator coolant and antifreeze. In addition, it is used as an industrial solvent for dyes, as a vehicle for food extracts and flavorings, and as a component of skin lotions.

It is produced by various chemical processes, involving ethylene bromide, chlorohydrin or ethyleneoxide.

It may be determined by a colorimetric technique after oxidation with periodate (28). The material is well-absorbed from the gastrointestinal tract, but most likely, not from the skin. As it is a rather non-volatile solvent, absorption from the respiratory mucosa is not a problem, unless the material is heated to boiling.

Oxidation to oxalic acid is the major metabolic change that occurs in the body (31). There may be intermediates in this oxidation and some of these have been isolated from the urine of some animals.

It is likely that the oxalic acid is responsible for the nephrotoxic effect of ethylene glycol.

Ethylene glycol is thought to be responsible for 40-60 deaths annually in the United States (15). Ingestion occurs accidentally when the material is thought to be alcohol, or purposely, when it is taken in as an alcohol substitute. The fatal dose is thought to be about 100 ml. In fatal cases, initial symptoms resemble alcoholic intoxication which is followed by coma, pulmonary edema, respiratory failure and death within 72 hours. If death does not occur acutely, severe renal damage, typically acute tubular necrosis with anuria, becomes manifest within 24 hours (10). In such cases, the urine, in addition to the usual findings of acute tubular necrosis, shows many oxalate crystals. With vigorous management, including hemodialysis, survival and recovery of renal function may occur (10). The pathologic lesion in the kidney consists of typical acute tubular necrosis, however, in addition, many oxalate crystals are deposited throughout the parenchyma (24). Chronic intoxication is usually only seen when there is exposure to ethylene glycol vapors, such as might occur when the material is heated. The symptoms here include brief periods of unconsciousness and nystagmus.

In acute intoxication with ethylene glycol, supportive measures, including standard techniques for the treatment of anuria due to acute tubular necrosis, are most worthwhile, as the renal lesion is reversible. Another interesting approach is the administration, acutely, of ethyl alcohol (25). This is associated with increased excretion of unchanged ethylene glycol and therefore, with decreased formation of the metabolite, oxalic acid. This is thought to be due to the enzyme, liver alcohol dehydrogenase, which uses both ethyl alcohol and ethylene glycol as a substrate. Ethyl alcohol has a greater affinity for this enzyme and competitive inhibition of ethylene glycol oxidation results.

GLUE SNIFFING

Consideration may be directed to a current fad of adolescents, glue sniffing. This phenomena, seen in junior high and high school boys, has recently gained popularity and has been of concern to teachers and educators. Various plastic and household cements, particularly those used for polystyrene plastics, are used. The glue is put onto a rag or into a paper bag and the fumes are inhaled. A feeling of exhilaration, euphoria and excitement sometimes results, somewhat similar to that seen after alcohol ingestion. With high doses, drowsiness, hallucinations, diplopia and tinnitus are seen. Some tolerance to these effects develops, as does habituation. Therefore, chronic users may sniff a dozen or more tubes of glue per day. The volatile components of these glues are toluene, acetone and isopropanol and, to a lesser degree, hexane, benzene, xylene, carbon tetrochloride, chloroform and butyl or ethyl acetate. Toxicity noted in chronic users mainly involves anorexia, weight loss, mucous membrane irritation, bad breath and general maladjustment (the latter not due to the glue). Aplastic anemia has been reported (27), however, a study of liver and renal function suggests that there is no toxicity secondary to glue sniffing (20). All in all, other than the psychological factors, there does not seem to be a great hazard to glue sniffing. The reason for this is that the major volatile components of such glue, namely toluene and acetone, are rather non-toxic and that exposure usually is temporary and that the doses inhaled are generally small.

REFERENCES

1. Appuhn, E., and Goldeck, H.: Fruh-und Spatschaden der Blutbildung durch Benzol und seine Homologen. Arch. Gewerbepathol. Gewerbehyg., *15:*399, 1957.
2. Banfer, W.: Untersuchungen uber Einwirkung von Reintoluol auf das Blutbild von Drucker und Hilfsarbeitern im Tiefdruck. Zentr. Arbeitsmed. Arbeitsschutz., *11:*35, 1961.
3. Browning, E.: Toxicity and Metabolism of Industrial Solvents. Elsevier Publishing Co., New York, 1965.
4. Conway, E. J.: Microdiffusion Analysis and Volumetric Error, 4th Ed. Crosby Lockwood, London, 1957, p. 324.
5. Dolin, B. H.: Determination of benzene in presence of toluene, xylene and other substances. Industr. Hyg. Bull., *22:*373. Industr. Eng. Chem. Anal. Ed., *15:*242, 1943.
6. Elkins, H. B.: The Chemistry of Industrial Toxicology, 2nd ed. Wiley & Sons, New York, 1959, p. 410.
7. Elkins, H. B.: The Chemistry of Industrial Toxicology. Chapman & Hall Ltd., London, 1959.
8. Elliot, T. H., Parke, D. V., and Williams, R. T.: The metabolism of cyclo (14C) hexane and its derivatives. Biochem. J., *72:*193, 1959.
9. Fabre, R., Truhaut, R., Laham, S. and Peron, M.: Recherches toxicologiques sur les Solvants de Remplacement de Benzene. Arch Malad. Profess., *16:*197, 195.
10. Friedmann, E. A., Greenberg, J. B., Merrill, J. P., and Dammin, G. J.: Consequences of ethylene glycol poisoning. Am. J. Med., *32:*891, 1962.
11. Gerarde, H. W.: Toxicology and Biochemistry of Aromatic Hydrocarbons. Elsevier, Amsterdam, 1960.
12. Greenburg, L., Mayers, M. R., Heiman, H., and Moskowitz, S.: The effects of exposure to toluene in industry. J. A. M. A., *118:*573, 1942.
13. Guertin, D. L., and Gerarde, H. W.: Toxicological studies on hydrocarbons. A method for the quantitative determination of benzene and certain alkyl benzenes in blood. Arch. Ind. Hlth., *20:*262, 1959.
14. Haggard, A. W., Greenberg, L. A., and Turner, J. M.: The physiological principles governing the action of acetone, together with determination of toxicity. J. Ind. Hyg. Toxicol., *26:*133, 1944.
15. Haggerty, R. J.: Toxic hazards: Deaths from permanent antifreeze ingestion. New Eng. J. Med., *261:*1296, 1959.
16. Hamburger, J.: Petite Encyclopedie Medicale. Flammarion, Paris, 1958.
17. Hirokawa, T.: Quelques Observations sur l'Intoxication Benzenique. Arch. Malad. Profess., *21:*46, 1960.
18. Lob, M.: L'Intoxication chronique au Toluol et au Xylol et ses Repercussions sur les Organes hemopoietiques. Schweiz. Med. Wøchschr., *82:*1125, 1952.
19. Maffet, P. S., Doherty, T. F., Monkman, J. L.: A direct method for the collection and determination of micro-amounts of benzene and toluene in air. Am. Ind. Hyg. Assoc. Quart., *17:*186, 1956.
20. Massengale, O. N., Glaser, H. H., Lelieure, R. E. Dodds, J. B., and Klock, M. E.: Physical and psychological factors in glue sniffing. New Eng. J. Med., *269:*1340, 1963.
21. McCollister, D. D., W. H. Beamer, G. J. Atchison, and Spencer, H. C.: Absorption, distribution and elimination of radioactive CCl_4 by monkeys. J. Pharmacol., *102:*112, 1951.
22. Parke, D. V., and Williams, R. T.: The Metabolism of Benzene. Biochem J., *46:*236, 1953.
23. Parmeggiani, L., and Sassi, C.: Sul Rischio Professionale da Toluolo Med. Lavoro., *45:*574, 1954.
24. Patscheider, H., and Hetzel, H.: Histologische Befunde bei einem Fall akuter Vergifung durch Athylenglykol. Arch. Toxikol., *19:*143, 1961.
25. Peterson, D. I., Peterson, J. E., Hardinge, M. G., and Wacker, W. E. C.: Experimental treatment of ethylene glycol poisoning. J. A. M. A., *186:*955, 1963.
26. Plessner, W.: Uber Trigeminuserkrankung infolge von Tri-vergiftung. Neurol. Zentr., *34:* 916, 1915.
27. Powers, D.: Aplastic anemia secondary to glue sniffing. New Eng. J. Med., *273:*700, 1965.
28. Rowe, V. K., McCollister, D. D., Spencer, H. C., Oyen, F., Hollingsworth, R. L., and Drill, V. A.: Toxicology of mono-, di- and tripropylene glycol methyl ethers. Arch. Ind. Hyg., *9:*509, 1954.
29. Stewart, R. D., Torkelson, T. R., Hake, C. L., and Erley, D. S.: Infrared analysis of CCl_4 and ethanol in blood. J. Lab. Clin. Med., *56:* 148, 1960.
30. Uhl, G., and Haag, T. P.: Perorale Vergiftung mt Trichlorathylen und ihr chemischen Nachweis. Arch. Toxikol., *17:*197, 1958.
31. Williams, R. T.: Detoxication Mechanisms. Chapman & Hall, London, 1959.

Chapter 30A

The Laboratory and Clinical Diagnosis of Ethanol Intoxication

ROBERT E. JONES, JR., M.D., KENDALL K. KANE, M.D., and LEO R. GOLDBAUM, PH.D.,

Recent emphasis in the United States and abroad on preventing injuries and fatalities on the highways due to driving while intoxicated has required many laboratories to perform accurate, routine blood alcohol determinations for local law enforcement agencies. Convictions based on blood alcohol levels (BAL) are becoming numerous and states are beginning to change laws and enforce old statutes dealing with "drunk" driving.[3] Utah is the first state in the United States to establish the presumptive level of intoxication at 80 mg% but seven other states have established 100 mg% as the presumptive level. The usual presumptive level is 150 mg%. Forty-two states had chemical test laws by October 1967.[5] Even though the Supreme Court of the United States has apparently cleared the way for compulsory test laws,[14] no state as yet has enacted such a law as in some foreign countries.[9]

The clinical pathologist will be directly involved when his laboratory is requested to perform blood alcohol levels, as will the clinician when he must evaluate individuals who are suspected of driving while intoxicated. State law enforcement laboratories may be available to many but in some areas local laboratories are requested to perform these tests.

Alcoholic intoxication can be determined in various ways. Body fluids or breath can be analyzed for ethanol content.[6, 11] Clinical testing of suspects can be attempted by law enforcement officers or physicians. Sobriety testing is performed frequently by law enforcement officers at the site of the apprehension. The type of test and its interpretation are usually left to each officer; however, most conform to several basic techniques.[13] The reliability of clinical examinations even by physicians is questionable and chemical testing is becoming more popular.

Opportunity has recently been provided to evaluate a large number of individuals, apprehended by law enforcement officers, for driving while intoxicated. A standard sobriety test was performed by a physician and the concentration of blood alcohol was determined in the laboratory.

Experience with sobriety testing is as follows: Opinions of physicians and quantitative sobriety scores consistently fail to predict the degree of intoxication and in many cases the diagnosis of intoxication or sobriety is wrong. Shapiro reports that 3% of motorists examined by police surgeons in Denmark were thought to be clinically intoxicated but chemical test proved they had no ethanol in their blood.[15] In the authors' study of 149 patients, 10 (6.7%) with blood alcohol levels over 100 mg per 100 ml were thought to be unintoxicated by the examining physician. Eight of this group had the lowest possible quantitative sobriety score with blood alcohols ranging from 107 to 165 mg per 100 ml. In evaluation of sobriety testing, the following observations were studied on each patient and various degrees of involvement given numerical values: Narcosis, attitude, actions, clothing, balance, walk, speech, alcoholic breath, color, and eyes. In Figure 1, is shown a comparison of sobriety scores with blood alcohol levels. The lowest score obtainable is 6.7 and highest 30.0. There is no predictable range until the blood alcohol reaches 100 mg per 100 ml. A low score only suggest a level of less than 100 mg per 100 ml.

Alcoholic breath and walk, two commonly used observations, were evaluated

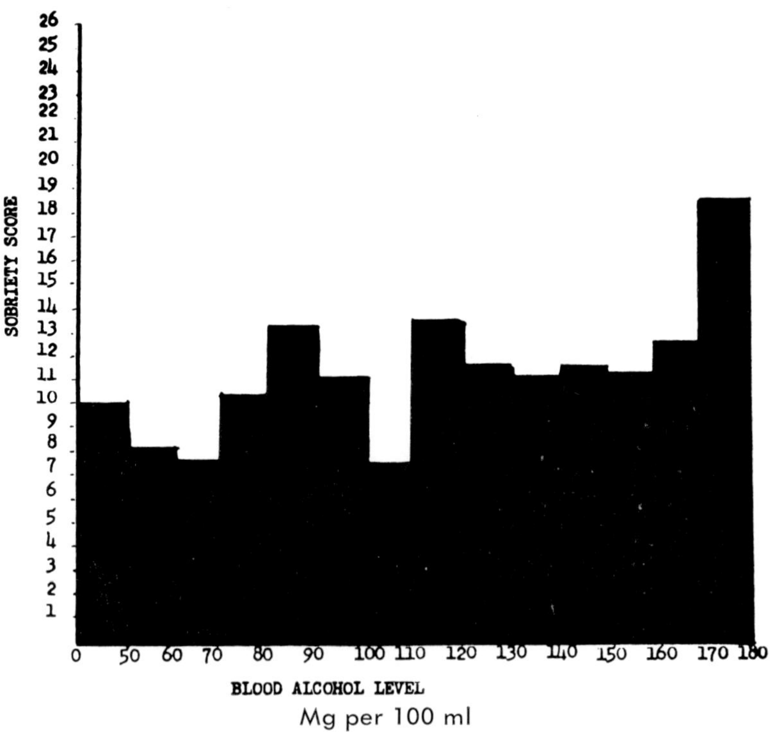

Figure 1. Comparison of blood alcohol levels and average sobriety scores in 149 individuals.

and compared with blood alcohol levels (Table 1). Individuals with blood alcohol levels over 100 mg per 100 ml usually have alcoholic breath but 10 to 14 percent may not. The validity of the old standby test of walking a straight line should also be questioned since an amazing 56% of individuals with concentration of blood alcohol over 150 mg per 100 ml had "normal" walks. From

TABLE I

Blood Alcohol Level In Mg per 100 ml	*No Alcoholic Breath* *Total Evaluated*	*Number*	%	*Normal Walk* *Total Evaluated*	*Number*	%
150	56	6	10%	52	29	56%
100-149	49	7	14%	46	29	63%
50-99	20	10	50%	21	17	80%
5-50	22	11	50%	22	15	70%

these results, it appears that opinions of physicians regarding ethanol intoxication are variable and should not be used as proof of intoxication. Chemical tests are more reliable.

Routine laboratory tests for blood alcohol are quite good and most utilize two basic principles. The reduction of dichromate or permanganate in an acid solution by ethanol is used in many different procedures that differ only in apparatus and technique. A routine procedure of this type is that of Leifheit which is used in many military hospital laboratories.[10] Alcohol is volatilized in a closed system in an autoclave. Dichromate in a strong acid solution (H_2SO_4) is reduced to a green chromium salt. The intensity of the color is proportional to the concentration. No special equipment is needed.

PROCEDURE

REAGENT ANSTIE'S REAGENT

Potassium dichromate ($K_2Cr_2O_7$) 3.7 gm
Sulfuric acid (H_2SO_4) (Concentrated) 280.0 ml
Distilled water q. s. to 500.0 ml

Dissolve the potassium dichromate in 150 ml of distilled water. Add the sulfuric acid slowly with constant stirring. Dilute to 500 ml with distilled water.

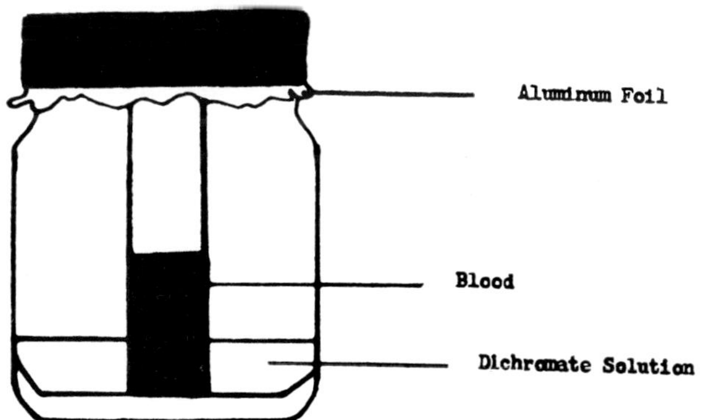

Figure 2. Microdiffusion apparatus for Leifheit blood alcohol method.

TECHNIQUE

1. To two screw-cap, round, widemouth specimen bottles are added 10 ml of Anstie's reagent. The microdiffusion apparatus for this procedure is shown in Figure 2.
2. To two 9 ml specimen vials, labeled "U" and "B" (with diamond marking pencil) are added solutions as follows:

Unknown (U)	Blank (B)
2 ml whole blood	2 ml dist. H_2O

3. The specimen vials are placed, uncovered, in widemouth, 84 ml

specimen bottles containing the Anstie's reagent and the outside container is labeled to avoid error.

4. The mouth of the 84 ml container is covered with aluminum foil.
5. The caps on these containers are screwed on tightly.
6. The bottles are placed in an autoclave at 15 pounds pressure for 30 minutes.
7. The autoclave is allowed to cool before releasing pressure.
8. The screw caps, foil, are removed and the smaller vials are discarded.
9. The Anstie's reagent is poured into cuvets labeled "unknown" and "blank."
10. The optical density of the solutions is read at a wavelength of 600 mu

Calculations

The alcohol concentration is determined from a calibrated curve.

Standardization Procedure

1. The use of a calibration curve is preferred to a single standard owing to the difficulty of working with a volatile compound such as alcohol.

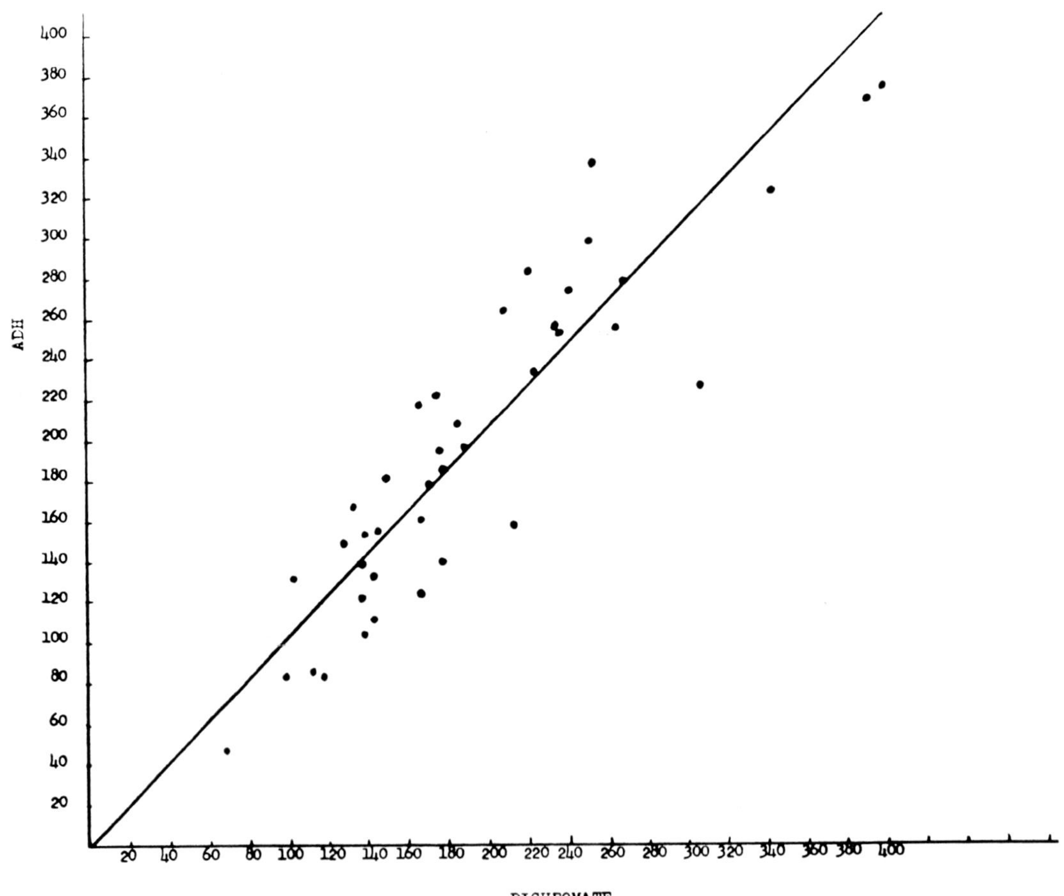

Mg per 100 ml

Figure 3. Comparison of alcohol dehydrogenase and dichromate reduction method on 40 blood samples processed as routine tests in two different laboratories.

2. Five screw-capped bottles and vials are set up in duplicate. The following amounts of standard 2% ethanol solution and distilled water are added to the vials:
3. To each bottle are added 10 ml Anstie's reagent and the procedure is followed as previously described.
4. A graph is prepared of optical density versus concentration.

ml 2% ethanol	ml distilled water	mg ethanol per ml
0.0	2.0	control
0.1	1.9	1.0
0.2	1.8	2.0
0.3	1.7	3.0
0.4	1.6	4.0

Enzymatic Method for the Measurement of Ethyl Alcohol in Biological Fluids

INTRODUCTION

In 1951, two groups of investigators independently reported an enzymatic method for blood alcohol determination.[2,4] The method is simple, accurate, and quite specific. Other primary and secondary aliphatic alcohols react to a much lesser degree, but methanol and acetone do not.[16]

PRINCIPLE

Ethanol is converted to acetaldehyde in the presence of ADH (alcohol dehydrogenase) and DPN, which is reduced to DPNH. The reaction is driven to the right by removal of acetaldehyde by semicarbazide. The reaction continues until the ethanol is exhausted. The amount of DPNH produced is equimolar to the amount of ethanol originally present. The DPNH produced is measured by the increase in O.D. at 340 mu.

REAGENTS

1. *Perchloric Acid, 2%*. 2.85 ml of 70% perchloric acid is made up to 100 ml with distilled water. Glassware should be thoroughly flushed with water after wetting with perchloric acid since it may be explosive on drying. However, the dilute solution could not be induced to explode in this laboratory by heating or by percussion.

2. *DPN-ADH Single Determination Vial.* Stable in freezer in dessicator box.

3. *Pyrophosphate Buffer, pH 9.2.* Contains semicarbazide and glycine. Keep tightly closed in refrigerator.

Reagents 2 and 3, as well as Ethanol Control, are available from Sigma Chemical Company, 3500 DeKalb Street, St. Louis, Mo. 63118, as Sigma Kit No. 330-UV.

STANDARD SOLUTIONS

One ml of absolute ethanol weighs 0.798 gm. One ml of alcohol is diluted to 20 ml with water. One-half (0.5) ml of this solution is then rediluted to 20 ml with water. The resulting standard contains 100 mg ethanol per 100 ml.[1] Working standards are subject to loss of ethanol by evaporation, while absolute alcohol absorbs atmospheric moisture. Standards should be remade frequently from freshly opened absolute alcohol. Working Ethanol Standard, as stated above, is available from Sigma.

SPECIAL APPARATUS

Ultraviolet spectrophotometer.

PROCEDURE

1. The following is pipetted into a centrifuge tube:
   2.0 ml 2% perchloric acid
   0.5 ml blood or other fluid

Any lumps are broken up with a small glass rod. The contents are mixed well. The tube is stoppered and centrifuged for five minutes at 3000 rpm.

2. The following is pipetted into a DPN-ADH vial:
   3.0 ml pyrophosphate buffer

The vial is capped and shaken well. The contents are poured carefully and completely into a cuvet with a 10 mm light path. The spectrophotometer is set at 340 mu. The "Initial O.D." is read and *recorded,* using water as a blank.

3. Twenty microliters of supernatant from the centrifuge tube are pipetted into the cuvet. The cuvet is mixed by inversion. Optical density values are noted at intervals until a plateau "Maximum O.D." is reached. Approximately 30 minutes are required for completion of the reaction. A standard should be run with the unknowns.

Calculation: Maximum O.D. — Initial O.D. = Change of O.D.

$$\text{Conc. of Unknown} = \frac{\text{Change of O.D. of Unknown}}{\text{Change of O.D. of Standard}} \times \text{Conc. of Standard}$$

DISCUSSION

Whole blood is conventionally used for Blood Alcohol determination. Potassium oxalate and citrate may be used as anticoagulants; other anticoagulants have not been investigated. Serum or plasma may be used, but values average 1.18 times the whole blood values. This is apparently due to the higher water content of serum and plasma as compared to whole blood.[12] The enzymatic method may be used for analysis of other body fluids and tissue extracts.

Whole blood specimens stored in stoppered tubes in the refrigerator showed no significant change in alcohol values after 9-10 months.[7] Alcohol may slowly diffuse through rubber stoppers; polyethylene stoppers are preferred for storage.

Perchloric acid serves to deproteinize the specimen. The size of the aliquot of deproteinized specimen transferred to the cuvet may be adjusted to give an optimal O.D. range for the range of alcohol values anticipated. The 20 microliter aliquot chosen here permits determinations of the entire clinical spectrum to 500 mg per 100 ml with a Maximum O.D. of less than 1.0. The method is linear to at least O.D. = 1.0.

SOURCES OF ERROR

Alcohol must never be used to prep the skin or to rinse needles and glassware used in this determination. The reagents must be protected from contamination by alcohol vapor. E.g., an open bottle of buffer solution will absorb appreciable ethanol overnight if kept in a refrigerator with an alcoholic solution.[16] Standards must be protected from evaporation of alcohol. Absolute alcohol must be handled promptly and protected against absorption of atmospheric moisture. Heavy metal contamination must be guarded against as it will impair enzyme activity. Use of flouride as anticoagulant should be avoided until further investigated.

RANGE OF VALUES

Blood alcohol values are negligible in the absence of ethanol ingestion or other exposure.[8]

RESUME OF CLINICAL INTERPRETATIONS

Objective impairment of driving ability is observed at threshold blood alcohol levels of 35 to 40 mg per 100 ml. Values below 50 mg per 100 ml are considered "not under the influence" by the courts in most states. Values of 150 mg per 100 ml and above are prima facie evidence of "under the influence." Most persons are obviously intoxicated in this range. Values of 500 to 600 mg per 100 ml are associated with alcoholic coma and death.[8]

Alcohol is eliminated from the body at the rate of 10 mg per kg per hour. This is about 10 ml of ethanol per hour for a 150 pound man. The rate of elimination is independent of the blood alcohol level.[8]

REFERENCES

1. Annino, J. S.: *Clinical Chemistry, Principles and Procedures,* 3rd ed. Little, Brown and Co., Boston, 1964, p. 349.
2. Bonnichsen, R., and Theorell, H.: An enzymatic method for the microdetermination of ethanol. Scand. J. Clin. & Lab. Invest., *3:*58-62, 1951.
3. Bowles, P. E.: The Medicolegal Implication of the New Implied Consent Law and the "Driving Under the Influence" Statute in Virginia. Medicoleg. Bull., *168:*1-5, April 1967.
4. Bucher, T., and Redetzki, H.: Eine spezifische photometrische Bestimmung von Athylalkohol auf fermentativem. Wege. Klin. Wchnschr., *29:* 615-616, 1951.
5. Donigan, R. L.: Annual Report of Subcommittee on Legal Matters of the National Safety Council (Committee on Alcohol and Drugs), October 1967.
6. Freedman, T. D., and Dubowski, K. M.: Chemical testing procedures for the determination of ethyl alcohol. J. A. M. A., *170:*47-71, 1959.
7. Glendening, B. L., and Waugh, T. C.: The stability of ordinary blood alcohol samples held various periods of time under different conditions. J. Forensic Sci., *10:*192-200, 1965.
8. Harger, R. N.: Ethyl alcohol. In Toxicology: Mechanisms and Analytical Methods, C. P. Stewart and A. Stolman, Eds. Academic Press, New York, 1961, Vol. II., pp. 85-151.
9. Kaselow, J.: Norway has the answer to drunken driving. This Week, February 24, pp. 4-6, 1963.
10. Leifheit, H.: Air Force Manual. No. 160-49, Ch. 9:3-5.
11. Manual on Alcohol. American Society of Clinical Pathologists Workshop Manual.
12. Payne, J. P., Hill, D. W., and Wood, D. G.: Distribution of ethanol between plasma and erythrocytes in whole blood. Nature (London), *217:*963-964, March 9, 1968.
13. Personal Communication, South Carolina Highway Patrol.
14. Schmerber vs. California, 384. J. S. 787, 86 Sup. Ct. 1826, June 20, 1966.
15. Shapiro, H. A.: Medical practitioners and clinical examinations. J. Forensic Med., *11:*129-130, 1964.
16. Stiles, D., Batsakis, J. G., Kremers, B., and Briere, R. O.: The evaluation of ethanol measurements with alcohol dehydrogenase. Am. J. Clin. Path., *46:*608-611, 1966.

Chapter 30B

Gas Chromatographic Method for the Measurement of Ethyl Alcohol

LEO R. GOLDBAUM, PH.D.

INTRODUCTION

Gas chromatographic methods for the determination of ethanol now are used in most forensic laboratories.[1] Various methods for sample preparation are used, such as extraction, distillation, and direct injection of sample. The latter procedure can be a direct injection into the gas chromatograph of the sample itself or an air sample above the specimen. The procedure to be described uses a direct injection of an air sample above the specimen.[2]

PRINCIPLE

Harger and co-workers[3] have demonstrated the feasibility of determining the alcohol concentration in the liquid phase from the analysis of an air sample. They have investigated the partition of alcohol between water, blood, urine, and air. The concentration of alcohol in the air phase is independent of the volume of the solution, but it is influenced primarily by temperature and salt concentration. For alcohol, the partition ratio between blood and air at 37°C. is approximately 2,000 to 1. For most volatile compounds present in biological samples, the concentration in the air phase is low; however, the capability of the gas chromatography to rapidly analyze compounds in part per billion concentrations makes this technique ideally suited for the analysis of the equilibrated air above the sample. Because of the low concentration of water vapor in the injection samples, there is no interference with the analysis of volatile compounds utilizing the argon ionization detector.

SYRINGES

Hypak B. D. disposable syringes (2.5 ml). These syringes have been found to be as satisfactory as the more expensive Hamilton syringes. Their low cost enables the analyst to use many syringes and discharge the contaminated ones.

STANDARDS

1. Standards are prepared by adding known amounts of ethanol to blood containing the same amount of anticoagulant present in the unknown. A suggested procedure is that of Glendening *et al.*[4]

Standards are prepared from fresh bovine blood collected at the slaughter house in pint jars containing 4.7 gm of sodium fluoride. Shake thoroughly.

Prepare a 2.00% alcohol solution w/v by adding 2.53 ml of absolute ethanol to about 90 ml of blood with shaking and make to 100 ml.

Since the Kansas law is based on per cent by weight the following standards are made by adding the following amounts of 2.00% alcohol-blood w/v into a tared polyethylene bottle and adding sufficient blank blood to equal 100 gm net total (w/v standards would substitute 100 ml of 100 gm).

Percent EtOH Standard (w/w)	*ml of 2.00 w/v blood-alcohol*
0.04%	2.0
0.08%	4.0
0.16%	8.0
0.24%	12.0
0.32%	16.0
0.40%	20.0

After preparation, standards are divided, put in small glass bottles and stored in a refrigerator. One set of standards may be used several times and are stable at least 3 months.

2. Aqueous standards of a mixture of volatile compounds such as acetaldehyde (0.04 mg per 100 ml), formaldehyde (0.33 mg per 100 ml), acetone (0.19 mg per 100 ml), methanal (0.79 mg per 100 ml), ethanol (0.79 mg per 100 ml), isopropanol (0.79 mg per 100 ml).

SPECIAL APPARATUS AND OPERATING CONDITIONS

The apparatus is Gas Chromatograph equipped with a Beta Ionization microdetector Rd 226 or Sr 90. (A Hydrogen Flame detector also can be used.) The chromatographic column is a borosilicate coiled glass tube of 3 mm internal diameter, 6 ft. in length, and packed with a 42 to 60 mesh, C-22 firebrick impregnated with 28 gm of liquid to 100 gm of firebrick. The liquid used for impregnation was a mixture of 15 parts by weight of flavol 8N8 (2, 2′ (2-ethylhexamido) diethyl di (2 ethlyhexoate), 10 parts diiosodecyl phthalate and 3 parts polythylene glycol 600. This column material is available commercially from Beckman Instruments Inc., Fullerton, California 92634. The column was pre-conditioned for 4 hours at 120°C. For injecting samples into the column, a two-way surgical stopcock is attached with a 19 gauge needle penetrating the half-hole silicone rubber stopper of the sample injection port of the instrument. This prevents damage to the stopper caused by repeated injections. The stopcock is turned to the closed position after the injection. The sample is injected with a gas-tight Hypak disposable syringe.

The operating conditions for the determination of volatile compounds were: Column temperature 95° ± 5°C.; flash temperature 105°C.; detector temperature 150°C.; the high voltage, 1.2 kv; the relative gain (1×10^{-8} amps).

PROCEDURE

The samples should be collected in containers stoppered with a puncture-type rubber cap. A recommended container for blood is the vacu-tube containing fluoride as a preservative. The air space above the specimen should be at least 10 ml. Approximately 1 to 2 ml of blood is collected.

1. The unknown specimens and the standards are placed in a water bath until their temperatures are at the temperatures of bath (25°C.). An air-tight syringe is filled with 1 ml of air and the needle of the syringe is inserted through the puncture-type rubber cap of the sample container. The barrel of the syringe is moved up and down a few times to obtain an equilibrated air sample of 1 ml. The needle is disengaged from the syringe and the syringe is attached to the

two-way stopcock on the injection port of the chromatograph. The two-way stopcock is opened and the sample is injected into the flash portion of the column. The two-way stopcock then is closed. The air sample, which appears as a negative peak, marks the point from which the retention times are determined.

2. Before analyzing the unknowns, 1 ml of equilibrated air above the standard containing volatile compounds is injected to establish the resolution of these volatiles and 1 ml of equilibrated air above a blood standard containing 0.2 mg per ml is injected to establish the sensitivity of the instrument.

When only ethanol is to be determined, successive 1 ml of equilibrated air samples of the unknowns are injected immediately after the appearance of the ethanol peak from the preceding injection. For those blood samples which show the presence of a significant ethanol peak, a repeat injection is made. This is immediately followed by an injection of air from a blood standard of similar concentration.

When the concentration of ethanol is greater than 1.5 mg per ml, the electrometer is set at a lower voltage. This provides for linearity at the high concentrations.

DISCUSSION

1. This gas chromatographic procedure has the advantage of easily and rapidly analyzing samples for ethanol and other volatile compounds.

2. The presence of contaminants such as formalin, fuels and products of putrefaction are readily detected. Acetaldehyde, acetone, methanal, and isopropanol are determined as well as separated. Ethanol can be quantitated in the presence of these compounds.

3. There is only one easily measured sample — air. The volume of the blood sample has no significant effect on the results. This eliminates errors due to pipetting, contamination, and mislabeling.

4. The quantity of sample removed for analysis is extremely small, enabling the analyst to make many replicate determinations. The small sample is available for quantitative analysis by some other method.

5. The chromatograph provides a permanent record of each of the samples analyzed.

SOURCES OF ERROR

The use of equilibrated air samples depends on comparing standards at the same temperature and salt concentration as the unknown. The instrument must be leak proof and care taken in transferring the air sample into the gas chromatograph. It is best to use a blood standard with an ethanol concentration nearest the unknown. Blood standards should be carefully prepared and stored. Normally present volatile compounds do not have the sample retention time as ethanol.

RANGE OF VALUES

The method can detect concentrations as low as 0.1 mg per ml. For high ethanol concentration greater than 2.0 mg per ml use lower voltage.

REFERENCES

1. Anders, M. W., and Mannering, G. J.: Application of Gas Chromatography to Toxicology. In, Progress in Chemical Toxicology, Vol. III, Stolman, A. (Ed.). Academic Press, New York, 1967, pp. 161-175.

2. Goldbaum, L. R., Domanski, T. J., and Schloegel, E. L. Analysis of biological specimens for volatile compounds by gas chromatography. J. Forensic Sci., *9*:63-71, 1964.
3. Harger, R. N., Raney, B. B., Bridwell, E. G., and Kitchel, M. F.: The partition ratio of alcohol between air and water, urine and blood; Estimation and identification of alcohol in these liquids from analysis of air equilibrated with them. J. Biol. Chem., *183*:197-213, 1950.
4. Glendening, B. L., and Harvey, R. A.: Presented at the Twentieth Annual Meeting of the American Academy of Forensic Sciences. Chicago, February 24, 1968.

Chapter 31

Measurement of Ethyl Alcohol in Breath

KURT M. DUBOWSKI, PH.D.†

INTRODUCTION

Procedures for the identification and estimation of ethanol in human body fluids and tissues were first described approximately 100 years ago (1). There has since been a steady increase in the frequency of their use and in their medicolegal and clinical importance, paralleled by a concomitant proliferation of methods. Alcohol* determinations have been the most commonly performed forensic chemical examination for the past 50 years, the great majority being performed in order to establish the absence, or presence and extent, of alcoholic influence in motor vehicle operators and in victims of traffic accidents, homicide, and other forms of trauma. While the relation of alcohol to vehicular accidents and traffic deaths is widely recognized and documented in such vivid terms as "... the use of alcohol by drivers and pedestrians leads to some 25,000 deaths and a total of at least 800,000 crashes in the United States each year..." (2), the equally great or perhaps greater impact of alcohol on the causes and severity of non-traffic forms of trauma is much less fully appreciated (3).

More than 300 analytical methods for alcohol have been published, including about 2 dozen procedures for analysis of alcohol in breath. Most methods for the determination of alcohol in biological materials include several common elements: (1) Sampling, including collection and processing of exhaled breath, body liquids, or tissues and measurement of the aliquot to be analyzed; (2) separation of alcohol from the biological matrix; and (3) quantitation of the separated alcohol. Some methods include a fourth step, (4) identification of ethanol and/or possible interfering substances. The majority of procedures depend on two important properties of ethanol — its volatility or vapor pressure (59.02 mm Hg at 25° C.) and its easy oxidizability. These properties and other biological and laboratory considerations dictate a predilection for analysis of ethanol in breath as the method of choice for forensic and clinical applications in living and conscious subjects.

†"Supported in part by PHS Research Grant No. GM 16211-01 from the National Institute of General Medical Sciences."

*The unmodified word *alcohol* in this chapter refers to *ethanol*, C_2H_5OH, also commonly called ethyl alcohol.

Breath Alcohol Analysis

CHARACTERISTICS AND APPLICATIONS

The great majority of alcohol determinations of human body materials are performed in connection with the investigation of alleged traffic offenses, chiefly on motor vehicle operators suspected of driving under the influence of alcohol. While theoretically analysis of any body fluid would suffice for the direct or indirect determination of the blood alcohol concentration under strictly controlled conditions, the indirect determination of the blood alcohol concentration by breath alcohol analysis has proven to have certain special advantages in these situations. Conventional methods for alcohol analysis in body liquids (blood, urine, saliva, etc.) require relatively elaborate laboratory facilities frequently not in operation or otherwise unavailable at the time these problems arise; and often require longer to perform than it is practical to wait for decisions based upon the analysis results. Geographic inaccessibility of such laboratory facilities or even of personnel qualified to obtain blood specimens are a frequent factor in traffic law enforcement, particularly in county and state highway patrol operations in our larger states and in areas of low population density.

In practice, because of the requirements for minimal physical facilities and technical proficiency combined with adequate reliability and practicability, such techniques are limited to analysis of breath. Breath alcohol analyses all share the following characteristic advantages:

1. A breath alcohol analysis result, usually expressed in terms of the blood alcohol concentration, is obtained within a few minutes of the start of the analysis.
2. Breath as the analyzed material accurately reflects the actual pulmonary arterial plasma alcohol concentration at the time of the test, without lag or overrun; and is often obtainable nearer the time in issue than other materials.
3. When breath obtained at the time of the analysis is the specimen, the problem of positively identifying the specimen donor, and most of the collection, identification, preservation, transportation and evidentiary safeguard problems common to other body materials are eliminated, together with the need for specially qualified collection personnel, special collection facilities and containers.
4. Since breath analysis eliminates certain difficult steps of the tissue and liquid alcohol analyses, requirements for technical background and skill of the analyst are greatly reduced, and adequate supervision considerably simplified.
5. Required test facilities can be minmal and are usually limited to the self-contained breath alcohol apparatus. Therefore, costs per test after acquisition of the necessary equipment are generally much lower than for comparable laboratory analysis of body liquids or tissues.
6. There is usually less objection by the tested subject to collection of a breath sample for alcohol analysis than to the body penetration required to obtain a blood specimen, and generally less cooperation and considerably less time are required

than for collection of suitable saliva or urine specimens.

7. Multiple, replicate, and serial alcohol determinations at frequent brief intervals are practical, because of the rapidity and relative simplicity of breath analyses and the rapid non-traumatic sampling of breath specimens; allowing accurate determination of the directional trend of the blood alcohol curve, and many experimental analyses on a given subject.

Breath alcohol analyses also embody a few inherent limitations:

1. It is difficult to preserve entire breath specimens in practice, for later replicate or independent confirmatory analysis, although the alcohol from a measured volume of breath can be collected and preserved for later analysis.
2. Some cooperation is required from the tested subject for collection of an adequate breath specimen, the extent varying with the nature of the required breath sample (alveolar air, re-breathed air) and the collection apparatus (balloon, sample chamber of apparatus, etc.).
3. Most breath alcohol methods are inapplicable to unconscious or completely uncooperative subjects.
4. A period of approximately 15 minutes after the last ingestion of alcohol (or regurgitation) must elapse before breath alcohol analysis, to insure complete absorption of any residual mouth alcohol.

These characteristics of breath alcohol tests make them highly useful as rapid and simple screening tests. Under properly controlled conditions, which include suitable methods and equipment, proper training and continuing expert supervision of competent operators, and adequate expert control of equipment, reagents and procedures (4, 5), quantitative breath analyses are also capable of yielding accurate measurements of breath alcohol, acceptable as an index of the concentration of blood alcohol which is regarded as adequate for clinical and legal purposes (6-11). The human physiological characteristics (blood composition, body temperature, respiratory action, etc.) normally vary within sufficiently narrow limits to permit full realization of this technical potential (7, 10, 12, 13).

GENERAL PRINCIPLES OF BREATH ALCOHOL ANALYSIS

Since the first application of breath alcohol analysis to medical purposes in the United States by Bogen in 1927 (14), a number of breath alcohol analysis methods and devices have been developed, falling into three functional categories:

1. Laboratory alcohol determinations, performed on laboratory-collected breath specimens, or on those collected in the field with breath screening-and-collecting equipment, yielding definitive blood alcohol concentration results.
2. Breath alcohol determinations employing portable apparatus and yielding definitive blood alcohol concentration results.
3. Semi-quantitative breath alcohol screening tests employing portable apparatus or disposable single-test units, yielding only approximate blood alcohol concentration results.

Breath alcohol analysis depends upon the fundamental principle that the distribution of alcohol between circulating pulmonary blood plasma and alveolar air occurs by simple diffusion and, like that of other volatile substances, obeys Henry's Law* (10, 15-18) meaning that a physiological distribution equilibrium exists, and that consequently for a given temperature a constant ratio exists between the concentrations of alcohol in the blood and in alveolar air.

There is general agreement that the mean value of the Ostwald partition ratio of blood alcohol concentration to last-phase air concentration at the average temperature of exhaled air, 34° C, is 2100:1; i.e., 2100 ml of alveolar air (saturated with water and at 34° C) contain the same quantity of alcohol as 1 ml of circulating pulmonary arterial blood (8, 13, 19-22).

In practice, alveolar air in the classical physiological sense is neither required nor employed for breath alcohol analysis. Hundreds of correlation studies of blood alcohol concentrations, in the post-absorptive state, with breath alcohol analysis results obtained with apparatus calibrated on the basis of the 2100:1 ratio have verified that samples of so-called last phase or "deep-lung" air (the terminal portion of a prolonged uninterrupted exhalation approximately 400 ml or more in volume) and re-breathed air are identical to actual alveolar air with respect to alcohol concentration.

The breath alcohol methods determine the quantity of alcohol in a known volume of breath, or measure the breath volume containing a fixed known quantity of alcohol, in either instance yielding a breath alcohol concentration, generally expressed in milligrams of alcohol per liter of breath, as collected. From the blood alcohol/alveolar air alcohol ratio of 2100:1 and knowledge of the alveolar (or last-phase) air content of the analyzed breath sample, the corresponding blood alcohol concentration is then readily calculated. Alcohol quantitation is accomplished by the same 10 general principles generally applied in analysis of body liquids or tissues for alcohol; most commonly by controlled oxidation with potassium dichromate in acid solution.

A key element in each breath alcohol method is the procedure employed for determination of the quantity of deep lung air actually analyzed for its alcohol content. The following methods have been employed:

1. Last-phase or "deep-lung" air equivalent in alcohol concentration to true alveolar air is collected, as by mechanically trapping the final portion of a prolonged expiration (volume greater than 400 ml); and is analyzed directly.
2. Re-breathed ("venous") air, which is identical in alcohol concentration to alveolar air (22, 23), is obtained by having the subject re-breathe ordinary expired air four or five times with the nostrils closed, and is analyzed directly.
3. Mixed expired air is collected and analyzed for alcohol and carbon dioxide content. The proportion of alveolar air in the sample is estimated from its carbon dioxide concentration; on the basis of the assumption that the alveolar air of normal individuals contains about

*Henry's Law: "The mass of gas dissolved by a given volume of solvent, at constant temperature, is proportional to the pressure of the gas with which it is in equilibrium," whence

$$\frac{\text{Concentration of gas in liquid phase}}{\text{Concentration of gas in gaseous phase}} = \text{constant}$$

at a definite temperature.

5.5% carbon dioxide by volume (17, 24, 25) while atmospheric air contains only approximately 0.03 volumes per cent CO_2.

4. Mixed expired air is collected and analyzed for alcohol only. As screening methods for the estimation of the approximate blood alcohol concentration, some "volumetric" tests assume that ordinary expired breath normally contains about 58 to 63% alveolar air, and hence employ an equivalence factor of approximately 3200 ml of ordinary mixed expired breath measured at 25° C as containing the same quantity of alcohol as 1 ml of blood (23, 25).

PHYSIOLOGICAL CONSIDERATIONS

Temperature Effects. The blood/alveolar air ratio is temperature dependent and the partition coefficient at the alveolar interface would be expected to vary with different body temperatures. Based on the partition ratio data for air and blood given by Harger *et al.* (16), theoretically an increase between 34° C and 37° C in blood and alveolar breath temperature *at the interface* would tend to increase the calculated blood alcohol concentration by about 6.5% per degree C over the actual concentration. While the pulmonary capillary-alveolar temper ature probably does not fluctuate widely in healthy adults, it does vary within a range of about ± 0.7° C from the mean temperature even in a given subject over short periods (26). However, the distribution of alcohol between blood and breath is a complex phenomenon involving not only the equilibrium diffusion process at the alveolar interface, but also sequential distributions of alcohol between the various components of respiratory tract air and exchanges of the water-soluble alcohol in the several breath components with the walls of the respiratory dead space (27). These processes attenuate the theoretical variations attributable to temperature quite effectively. Thus, while breath alcohol concentrations in various segments of a prolonged expiration do increase somewhat during expiration, the increase is not generally linearly correlated with the observed increase in breath temperature (28). The factors more likely to cause variation in the blood/breath alcohol ratio are differential rates of equilibration at different points in the respiratory tract, the length of time available for equilibration to take place (including the respiratory rate), and individual differences in breathing habits (8, 28, 29). Standardized sampling of last-phase or "deep-lung" air specimens, in such a manner that a continuous exhalation against moderate pressure resulting in discard of the initial two-thirds of the sample is required of the subject, will eliminate most of these potential sources of variation in non-febrile subjects.

Alveolar Carbon Dioxide Content. Those breath alcohol procedures which utilize the alcohol/carbon dioxide ratio assume uniformity of four biologic relationships, as pointed out by Greenberg (8), Harger (23), and Smith (30), among others: (a) That the CO_2 concentration in alveolar air is uniformly 5.5% by volume; (b) that the ratio of alcohol to carbon dioxide is identical for alveolar air and air from other parts of the respiratory tract; (c) that the ratio of alcohol to carbon dioxide is therefore identical in alveolar air and in mixed expired air; (d) that the ratio of alcohol between alveolar air and pulmonary blood is a constant 1:2100.

The alveolar carbon dioxide content varies somewhat in normal individuals and averages about 13% less for women than for men (31). The mean for women in a study of 100 subjects was indeed found to be 5.50 volumes percent; however, the mean for men was 6.33 volumes percent with respective ranges of 3.25 to 7.30 for women and 3.90 to 7.60 for men (31). Further substantial deviations from the subject's own normal mean alveolar CO_2 content can result from marked hyperventilation and metabolic alkalosis (7). Breath alcohol devices dependent on the alcohol/carbon dioxide ratio are therefore being supplanted by those employing "deep-lung" air.

CALIBRATION AND TESTING OF BREATH ALCOHOL APPARATUS

The several types of commercial breath alcohol apparatus incorporate either instrument scales reading directly in blood alcohol concentration, or provide calibration tables yielding blood alcohol concentrations from the observed variables (e.g., breath volume analyzed, etc.). The accuracy of predictions of blood alcohol concentration by these means can, of course, be checked by direct analysis of a simultaneously obtained blood sample, keeping in mind the limitations of the referee method, and arterial-venous-capillary blood differences during and after active alcohol absorption from the gastro-intestinal tract.

Methods and apparatus have been developed for calibration and testing of breath alcohol instruments, employing mixtures of ethyl alcohol in air or other gases. Careful experimental work has established considerable independently confirmed data on the Ostwald partition ratio of alcohol between air and water at various temperatures (16, 21, 32). Using this information, one can easily prepare various known concentrations of alcohol in air by equilibrating air with aqueous alcohol solutions of known concentration at known temperatures. A simple equilibrator consists essentially of a closed metal, glass, or plastic cylinder bearing an air inlet tube terminating in a porous gas-dispersion disk or cylinder, a thermometer, and an air outlet tube connected to a liquid trap. Room air is forced through a 5 cm layer of alcohol solution by means of an atomizer bulb, in a flow of very small air bubbles, thus attaining complete alcohol distribution equilibrium in one passage; the resulting alcohol concentration of the effluent air being controlled by the concentration of alcohol in the solution and by the temperature. Constant-temperature maintained devices of this type are commercially available, usually with the alcohol solution maintained at 34° C, as so-called alcoholic breath simulators (33). Their use considerably simplifies the necessary calculations, increasing the practicability of calibration and facilitating system checks with each breath alcohol analysis.

Analysis of an adequate number of such known air-alcohol mixtures in a breath alcohol apparatus will yield the necessary information for preparation of calibration scales or calibration tables. The original and continuing validity of these or of factory pre-calibrations can be readily confirmed whenever desired by analysis of one or more air-alcohol samples.

EXAMPLE OF CALIBRATION CHECK WITH EQUILIBRATOR

1. The mean Ostwald alcohol partition ratio constant for the air-water system, $k_{A/W}$*, is 0.000217 at 25.0° C (16). Hence, 1 liter of air equilibrated at 25° C with water containing 4.0 mg of ethanol per ml will contain (1000 × 4.0 × 0.000217 =) 0.868 mg alcohol.
2. 2100 ml of this air, warmed to 34° C, will contain $(2.1 \times \frac{(273 + 25)^\circ}{(273 + 34)^\circ} \times 0.868 =)$ 1.769 mg alcohol.
3. A person whose "deep-lung" air contains the same alcohol concentration, 1.769 mg/2100 ml, will have a *blood* alcohol concentration of (1.76 mg/ml =) 0.17% W/V, according to the established blood/alveolar air ratio of 2100:1 at 34° C.
4. Analysis of the above air-alcohol mixture in a properly calibrated breath alcohol apparatus should, therefore, yield the theoretical blood alcohol concentration reading of 0.17% W/V.

The Breath Alcohol Tests

Experimental methods for breath alcohol analysis have been used for many years; Subbotin (34) determined breath alcohol in rabbits in 1871, Anstie (35) reported the results of human breath alcohol analyses in 1874, Bodländer (36) in 1883, and Strassmann (37) in 1891. More recently, breath alcohol determination methods have been reported by Bogen (14) in 1927, Liljestrand and Linde (18) in 1930, Harger (38) in 1931, Haggard and Greenberg (39) in 1934), Harger, Lamb and Hulpieu (25) in 1938, Schawerin (40) in 1939, Greenberg and Keator (41) in 1941, Jetter, Moore and Forrester (42) in 1941, Harger, Forney, and Barnes (23) in 1950, Seifert and Günther (43) in 1951, Kobayashi and Kitagawa (44) in 1953, Grosskopf and Scheibe (45) in 1953, Borkenstein (46) in 1954, Harger, Forney and Baker (22) in 1956, Forrester (47) in 1960, Kitagawa and Wright (48, 49) in 1962, Forrester (50) in 1964, and by others.

RELIABILITY OF BREATH ALCOHOL ANALYSIS

Correlation Between Blood Alcohol Concentrations Obtained by Direct Blood Analysis and from Breath Analysis

The validity of breath alcohol analysis for the determination of the blood alcohol concentration depends upon two components: The analytical reliability of the breath alcohol analysis itself, and the constancy to the required extent of the human physiological variables affecting the formulae for conversion of the breath alcohol concentration to blood alcohol concentration. Both factors can be tested by examining statistically in an appropriately large series the closeness with which breath alcohol analyses predict actual blood alcohol concentrations. Consequently, the correlation between breath analysis-derived blood alcohol concentrations and those obtained by direct blood analysis has been universally

*Ostwald partition ratio coefficient,

$$k_{A/W} = \frac{\text{Wt. of alcohol per unit volume of air}}{\text{Wt. of alcohol per unit volume of water}}$$

considered as a measure of the reliability of breath alcohol analyses for the indirect determination of blood alcohol concentrations, and has been extensively studied.

In evaluating such studies, the physiological and technical variables inherent in *blood* alcohol analysis as well as those attending breath alcohol analysis must be recognized and considered. Analytically, the blood alcohol methods are subject to considerable variation in reliability, with the chemical accuracy, precision, and specificity of some methods for the determination of blood alcohol being far inferior to those of reliable methods for the determination of breath alcohol (7, 10, 51). Consequently, the reliability characteristics of the referee blood alcohol method must be known and considered in comparing the results of simultaneous blood and breath alcohol analyses. Any consequential difference in collection times of the blood and breath specimens should also be considered, particularly in the light of the usual experimental conditions which sometimes preclude complete alcohol distribution equilibrium (52). These external variables, of course, are absent in correlation studies of the results of simultaneous breath alcohol analyses by different systems or apparatus, provided the samples analyzed are aliquots of a single breath specimen.

Only those findings of such investigations which apply to breath alcohol analysis with the Breathalyzer will be summarized here. Several major studies deserve mention in this connection.

In 1957, Chastain (6) reported the results of breath alcohol determinations on 36 subjects arrested for drunkenness or driving while intoxicated, performed essentially simultaneously with withdrawal of blood specimens which were analyzed by the method of Dubowski and Withrow (53). Differences found between the results were as follows:

Breathalyzer (46) (34 tests):

Mean absolute difference = 0.013% W/W
Difference range .... = +0.031 to —0.034% W/W

Also in 1957, a report of a detailed and extensive practical experimental study of alcoholic impairment of driving performance was issued from the Royal Canadian Mounted Police Crime Detection Laboratories (54). Included therein were the results of 247 venous blood alcohol analyses from 66 subjects, performed by the Smith desiccation method (55), compared with the same number of breath alcohol analyses. Findings were as follows:

Breathalyzer (46) (253 tests):

Mean absolute difference = 0.012% W/V
Difference range .... = +0.025 to —0.043% W/V

The study was further described by Coldwell and Smith (56) who concluded that from 0.5 to 2.5 hours after consumption of alcohol and over a venous blood alcohol concentration range from 0.04 to 0.17% W/V, the magnitude of the difference between Breathalyzer-derived and directly determined blood alcohol concentrations was independent of the alcohol concentration, and that the Breathalyzer model used by them estimated the venous blood alcohol concentration within ± 0.012 per cent W/V of the existing level in more than 95% of the cases.

In 1959, Drew, Colquhoun, and Long (57) reported a study on the effects of small amounts of alcohol, during which they had occasion to evaluate breath alcohol analyses. They reported the following results in comparison with direct capillary blood analysis by a modified Cavett method (58):

Breathalyzer (46) (103 tests):

Standard deviation of the differences = 0.012% W/V
95% confidence limits .... = ±0.024% W/V

The authors concluded that blood alcohol concentrations obtained by Breathalyzer analysis were in close agreement with those obtained by direct blood analysis, and that differences between the concentrations so obtained will be less than ± 0.025% W/V 95 times in 100.

In 1962, Fox *et al.* (12), using a specially modified Breathalyzer and careful control of physiological factors, reported a comparison of the results of direct blood alcohol determination on 16 samples in triplicate by the Smith desiccation method (55) with Breathalyzer results. With blood samples up to 0.12% W/V, the standard deviation of the differences was 0.002% W/V, and the mean difference "very close to zero" after correction of bias.

A study by Scroggie (59) reported in 1962 included data pertaining to correlation of Breathalyzer results with those of direct analysis of 357 cubital vein specimens from 155 different subjects, each obtained within 5 minutes of the collection of the breath sample, and analyzed by the Kozelka and Hine (61) method. In approximately 85% of the paired results, agreement within ± 0.025% W/V was obtained; the mean deviation was –0.012% W/V (for Breathalyzer results vs. blood analysis), while the maximum differences were –0.067% W/V and +0.028% W/V.

Begg, Hill, and Nickolls (62) in 1962 also reported an extensive comparison study of direct blood alcohol determinations and Breathalyzer results. An overall correlation of 0.956 was obtained between direct blood analysis by a modified Cavett method (64) of 104 blood specimens from 18 subjects ranging from 0.03 to 0.18% W/V, and the mean of the results of 2 consecutive Breathalyzer analyses obtained 7 minutes apart. The standard deviation of the Breathalyzer analyses was 0.007% W/V, and the authors concluded that 95% of Breathalyzer results would be expected to lie within 0.018% W/V of the "true" value and 99% of such results within 0.023% W/V of the "true" value.

A meticulously controlled study of breath-blood blood correlations and of Breathalyzer analysis results has been reported by Fox and associates (65), employing refined Breathalyzer instruments and procedures (12) and analyzing the blood specimens by the Smith desiccation method (55). They reported that, with correction for slope and intercept of individual subject blood alcohol curves, a direct blood-alcohol determination was "very predictable from a given breath determination, with a standard error of estimate of 0.0055%," and concluded that this value implied "that about 95% of all breath readings will be correct to within 0.01% or 0.011% when compared to a blood determination taken at the same time." These investigators also found mean differences of Breathalyzer test results from the target values of equilibrator-produced standard alcohol-in-air specimens of +0.00278% W/V, +0.00433% W/V, and +0.00692% W/V, respectively, for nominal target values of 0.05% W/V, 0.10% W/V, and 0.15% W/V expressed as the corresponding blood alcohol concentrations.

Britt and Borkenstein (66) reported the results of 96 successive determinations, with a standard model Breathalyzer, of alcohol-in-air mixtures equivalent to a nominal blood alcohol target value of 0.100% W/V produced with a Simulator* maintained at 34° C. A minimum standard deviation of 0.00132% W/V was computed at the 0.100% W/V nominal blood alcohol value level for theoretical conditions, and an observed standard deviation of 0.00260% W/V was found in actual practice. In a similar project, these authors found a minimum standard deviation of 0.00124% W/V for a comparable set of analyses on Simulator-derived alcohol-in-air mixtures nominally equivalent to 0.200% W/V blood alcohol values.

Specificity of Breath Alcohol Analyses

The specificity of breath alcohol analysis methods is an important consideration, since the nature of most of these tests precludes analytically establishing the absence of interferants — volatile reducing substances which like ethyl alcohol diffuse from the blood into the alveolar air, and some of which can reduce the commonly employed oxidizing reagents. The major reagents employed for alcohol quantitation in breath have been iodine pentoxide, potassium dichromate in sulfuric acid solution, and potassium permanganate in sulfuric acid. Potassium dichromate in acid solution is known to react with aldehydes, ether, methyl alcohol, etc. In general, low concentrations of acetone cause no interference under the reaction conditions employed in breath tests, and food-derived odoriferous flavor substances cause none.

Theoretically, there are hundreds of compounds which could react with the breath analysis reagents in vitro, to produce false-positive apparent ethyl alcohol concentrations or false elevations of a true alcohol level. However, in actual practice, four factors combine to minimize the possibility of unsuspected chemical interference in tests of alcohol-free subjects: (1) Since the instruments are designed solely for analysis of breath samples, the reagents can only come into contact with volatile substances capable of appearing *in the breath* of living and conscious persons. (2) The reaction conditions of time, temperature, sample volumes, and concentrations further sharply reduce the number of such volatile substances which can react in these systems. (3) Most of the potential interfering substances have highly characteristic odors in the breath which are readily recognized. (4) The actual potential interferants are also intoxicants and their presence in the blood (and hence in the breath) in concentrations sufficient to yield significant apparent blood alcohol levels is associated with severe intoxication. Consequently, a marked discrepancy between the apparent blood ethyl alcohol level in such intoxications and the actual subject state usually exists when chemical interference with breath-alcohol test is present.

Under these conditions, the potassium dichromate reagent employed in the Breathalyzer system can be affected by the following substances: acetaldehyde, ethyl ether, isopropyl alcohol, methanol, paraldehyde, and tetrachlorethylene (68). However, presence of most of these compounds in the breath of a tested subject is obvious from their odor and, in most instances, from the difference in their reaction rates compared to ethyl alcohol (67). Acetone in concentrations which can appear in the breath of living persons does not give an apparent ethyl

*The "Alcoholic Breath Simulator" is a temperature-controlled equilibrator.

alcohol result exceeding the blank value (67), and various volatile food and beverage flavor substances other than alcohol appearing in the breath (garlic, onion, etc.) do not cause changes in the reagent. Tobacco smoke in the breath can cause some reduction of the potassium dichromate, but is excluded as a possible source of error by proper sampling and analysis technique. Ingestion of alcohol-containing medications, can, of course, affect the test results, although the resulting true blood alcohol levels will usually be very low and without toxicological significance. Paraldehyde, a common sedative, appears in the breath after ingestion and does react with the dichromate reagent but is readily detected by its breath odor.

The entire interference problem is somewhat academic because in actual practice under the conditions under which breath tests are employed, predominantly in traffic law enforcement, substances chemically capable of interfering are generally not present in concentrations yielding marked false apparent alcohol levels. Conversely, the possible presence of food odors, halitosis, and similar conditions will not prevent complete reaction of alcohol with the breath test reagents; nor will masking of beverage odors on the breath, as by chlorophyllin, affect the alcohol content of the breath or the breath alcohol tests (13).

True reactions with alcohol in expired breath from sources other than the alveolar air (eructation, regurgitation, vomiting) will, of course, vitiate the breath alcohol results, but these actions can be detected by observation of the test subject, and their effects obviated by the subject's rinsing out his mouth with water.

Measurement of Ethyl Alcohol in Breath with the Breathalyzer

While many methods for breath-alcohol analysis have been described and several different instruments are presently available commercially, this presentation is necessarily restricted to breath-alcohol analysis with the most widely employed instrument — the Breathalyzer — by space and time limitations.

PRINCIPLE

The Breathalyzer (Fig. 1) (Manufacturer: Stephenson Company of Bangor Punta, Red Bank, N. J. 07701) was developed by Borkenstein (46) and utilizes potassium dichromate in sulfuric acid solution as the reagent for oxidizing alcohol in last-phase or "deep-lung" air. Ethanol is oxidized as formula below. The reaction is accompanied by a color change from the yellow of the potassium dichromate to the green of the chromic sulfate, and is catalyzed by the presence of silver nitrate in the reagent.

The operation consists of four principal phases (Fig. 2): (1) Flushing of the apparatus with room air; (2) collecting a measured volume of last-phase breath (52.5 ml at 34° C); (3) passing the

$$\underset{\text{(yellow)}}{2K_2Cr_2O_7} + 8H_2SO_4 + 3C_2H_5OH \longrightarrow \underset{\text{(green)}}{2Cr_2(SO_4)_3} + 2K_2SO_4 + 3CH_3COOH + 11H_2O \qquad \text{(I)}$$

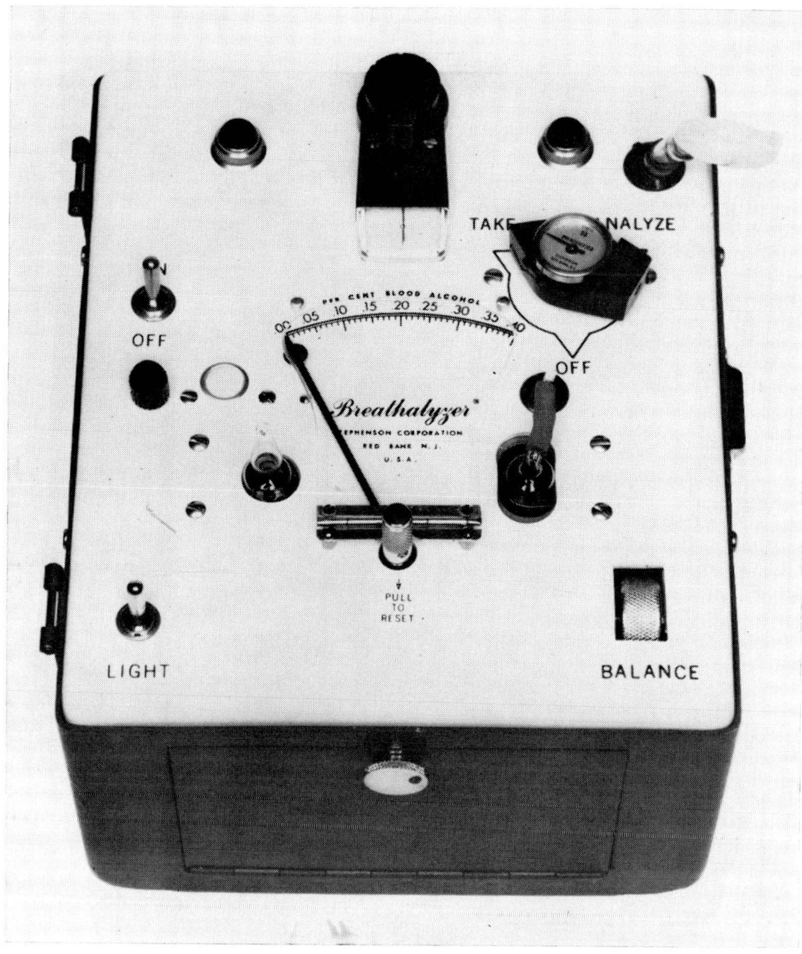

Figure 1. The Breathalyzer.

breath sample through potassium dichromate-sulfuric acid solution in an ampul-cuvette and allowing oxidation to proceed; and (4) measuring the resulting color change of the reagent with an integral photoelectric filter photometer. The increased light transmittance through the test ampul, resulting from the color change from the yellow of the dichromate to the green of the chromic sulfate, is measured with a balanced electrical circuit from two matched photovoltaic cells, using the Bunsen principle. A sensitive galvanometer serves as the electrical balance and end point detector. A light bulb is mounted on a movable carriage between the ampuls, and the distance the light must be moved to re-establish the original photometric balance between light transmittance through the ampuls prior to analysis is registered by the movement of a coupled pointer across a linear scale calibrated directly in blood alcohol concentration from 0 to 0.40% W/V, on the basis of the 2100:1 blood-breath ratio.

In sample collection, (Phase 2, above) the subject blows forcefully through a retractable heated plastic intake tube into the bottom of the heated sample

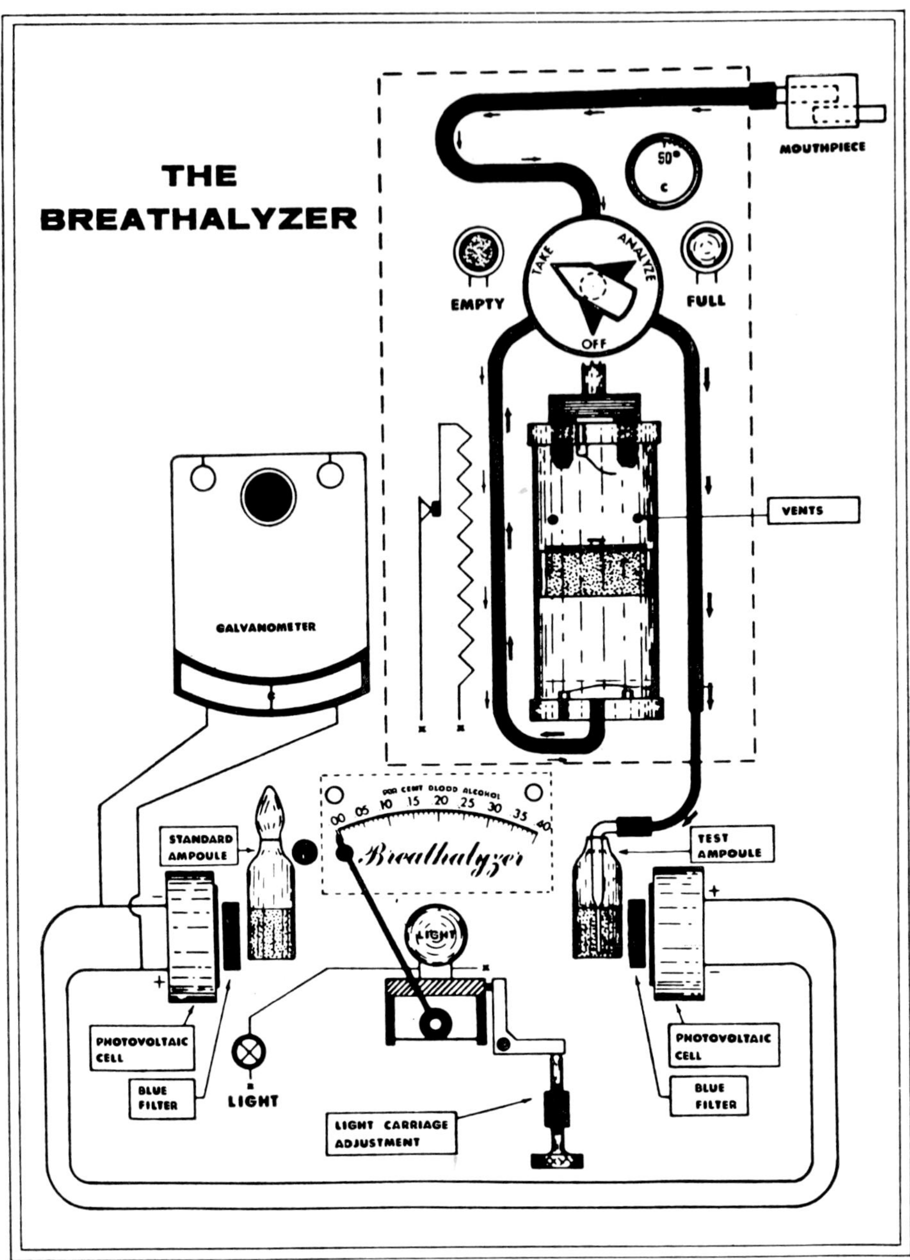

Figure 2. Schematic diagram of the Breathalyzer.

chamber. With the control valve in the "TAKE" position, the breath raises a metal piston in the sample cylinder until it clears the vents near the top of the chamber, permitting the first portion of the sample to escape. When blowing stops, the piston drops just sufficiently to cover the vents, being held in position by magnets aligned with fixed pole pieces in the top of the sample chamber, thus retaining the final portion (last phase) of the prolonged expiration. The sample chamber contains 56.5 ml since (1) the breath sample temperature is raised from

34° to 45-50° C with a resultant volume increase from 52.5 ml to about 55.2 ml, and (2) the delivery tube and bubbler remain full of breath after the test, requiring approximately 1.3 ml of sample.

In the reaction phase (Phase 3 above), the control valve is turned to the "ANALYZE" position, which disaligns the magnet with the fixed pole pieces and permits the piston to descend under its own weight. This forces the sample through the glass bubbler tube into the ampul in about 30 seconds, in a constant stream of fine bubbles. Any alcohol present is absorbed by the sulfuric acid solution from the escaping sample and is then quantitatively oxidized to acetic acid in the ensuing 90 seconds, with a corresponding reduction of the yellow dichromate ions to the green chromic ion. The reaction is exothermic, and the resultant convection and mixing by the bubble train produce sufficient mixing to effect homogeneity of the final mixture. The test ampul contains 3.0 ml of 0.025% W/V potassium dichromate + 0.025% W/V silver nitrate in 50% V/V sulfuric acid. From equation I, it follows that 0.176 mg of ethanol is required to reduce completely the 0.75 mg of potassium dichromate in the test ampul. This quantity of alcohol in a 52.5 ml last-phase breath sample (= 7.04 mg/2100 ml breath) coresponds to a blood alcohol concentration of 0.70% W/V which, therefore, represents the maximum range of the ampul.

In the measurement phase (Phase 4 above), any decrease in yellow color results in the decreased absorbance of light at 450 nm by the ampul solution, compared to initial conditions. Prior to the start of the analysis, the "Test" ampul is balanced photometrically against another "Reference"' ampul, the light source being moved back and forth mechanically with a rack and pinion adjustment until the null meter centers, indicating identical electrical outputs from the two matched photovoltaic cells (and hence equal illumination upon each cell). The blood-alcohol scale pointer is then aligned with the base line (or zero point) of the scale. After the analysis, the light is again turned on. If any oxidation-reduction has occurred, the yellow color will have decreased in intensity through conversion of the dichromate to chromate ion. There is consequently an increase in the transmittance of blue light (obtained through a 440-450 nm photometric glass filter) to the "Test" photocell, compared with the "Reference" photocell and with initial conditions, producing a change in the null meter. The light source is moved toward the "Reference" ampul until photometric balance is again established as indicated by the centering of the null meter. The distance the light is moved to restore photometric balance is directly related to the quantity of alcohol in the breath sample and results in a proportionate movement of the coupled pointer over the linear scale calibrated in per cent W/V blood alcohol concentration.

The photometric system of the Breathalyzer is unusual because the scale is linear rather than logarithmic and the reading is independent of the absolute concentration of the reagent. As noted, the color change in the system is quantitative and proportional to the quantity of alcohol reacting with the reagent solution. The resultant *increase* in blue light transmittance proceeds logarithmically in accordance with the Beer-Lambert relationship, shown by the solid curve in Figure 3 which shows the changes in blue light transmittance (at 450 nm)

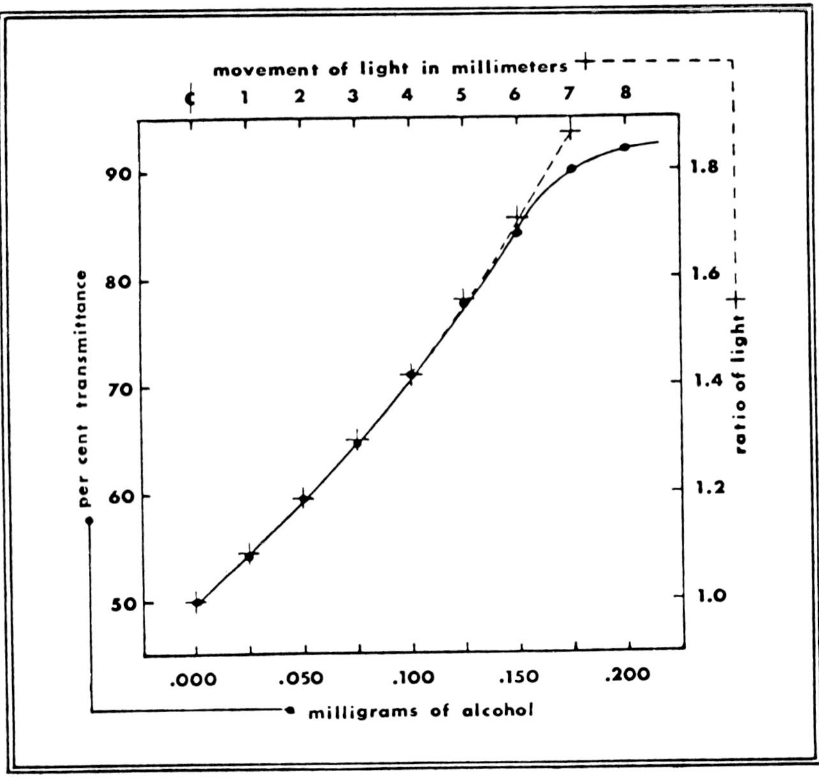

Figure 3. Breathalyzer calibration curves (left and bottom scales). Effect of light source movement upon the light ratio at the photocells (right and top Scales).

caused by addition of known quantities of alcohol. (The figures of the abscissa represent 1/40 of the blood alcohol values per ml since the Breathalyzer analyzes 52.5 ml of last-phase breath or 1/40 of 2100 ml of breath, the volume equivalent in alcohol content to 1 ml of blood.) The movement of the light closer to or farther away from either ampul and photocell changes the intensity of illumination on each according to the Inverse Square Law, a change which progresses geometrically. A linear movement of the light source therefore causes a logarithmic change in the ratio of light falling on the two ampuls and photocells, represented by the dotted curve in Figure 3. The two curves are congruent to well above the 0.1 mg point which represents full scale on the Breathalyzer; i.e., a blood alcohol concentration of 0.40% W/V. As illustrated in Figure 3, the logarithmic response of the photometer in effect cancels out the logarithmic increase in blue light transmittance of the "Test" ampul solution. Therefore, the distance the light source must be moved to restore photometric balance after the test is directly (linearly) proportional to the quantity of alcohol which has reacted with the reagent solution and is registered in terms of blood alcohol concentration on the linear scale of the Breathalyzer. The measurements are made with the galvometer in the electrical null-balance position, which is also the mechanical zero point of the galvanometer. Thus, when the photocells are receiving the same amount of light, the position of the light source between the ampuls is a function of the relative transmittance of light at 450 nm by the "Test" solution. The initial and final scale readings therefore reflect only the relative change in the concentration of potassium dichromate and are not affected by the absolute concentration of potassium dichromate (provided it suffices for the immediate test completed), by ageing of the light source, or by line voltage fluctuations resulting in instantaneous light intensity changes.

A single complete analysis requires about 6 minutes, and the initial warmup of the instrument requires about 20 minutes.

Operation of the Breathalyzer is generally controlled by use of the Alcoholic Breath Simulator (Fig. 4), an equilibrator device maintained at 34° C ± 0.2°. This unit contains 500 ml of a dilute ethanol solution appropriately selected to yield alcohol-in-air mixtures equivalent to last-phase breath specimens from subjects with blood alcohol concentrations in the 0.05 to 0.30% W/V range (as outlined under "Calibration and Testing of Breath Alcohol Apparatus"). For example, equilibration of air with an ethanol solution containing 1.21 mg ethanol per ml, at 34° C, will yield a gas mixture equivalent in alcohol content to last-phase breath of a subject with an 0.10% W/V (= 1.0 mg ethanol/ml blood) blood alcohol concentration; i.e., the gas mixture contains 1.0 mg ethanol/2100 ml gas mixture (= 0.476 mg ethanol/liter).

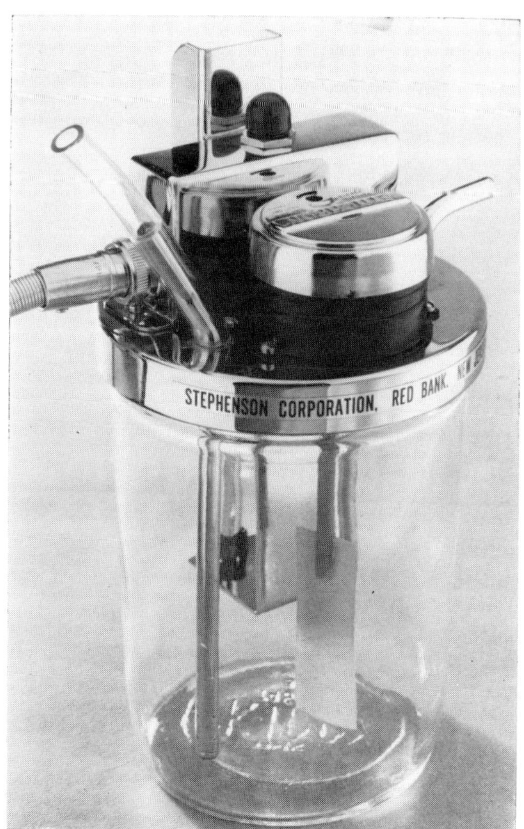

Figure 4. The alcoholic breath simulator.

REAGENTS

1. Breathalyzer Reagent: 3.0 ml of 0.025% W/V potassium dichromate ($K_2Cr_2O_7$) + 0.025% W/V silver nitrate ($AgNO_3$) in 50% V/V sulfuric acid (H_2SO_4).

REFERENCE SOLUTIONS

1. Ethanol Reference Solution, Stock: 60.5 g/liter. Exactly 77.0 ml of absolute reagent-grade ethanol (measured at 25° C) are placed in a 1-liter volumetric flask and diluted to volume with distilled-demineralized water with the usual volumetric technique. The stock solution, when stored in glass at 4° C, is stable for 1 year.
2. Ethanol Reference Solution, Dilute, for Simulator Use: Into a 500 ml volumetric flask are placed the number of milliliters of Stock Ethanol Reference Solution corresponding to the equivalent nominal blood alcohol concentration desired (expressed in % W/V) × 100.

(Thus, to check a breath alcohol apparatus calibrated according to the 2100:1 relation at 0.10% W/V blood alcohol, place 10.0 ml of Stock Ethanol Reference Solution into the volumetric flask.) Dilute to volume with distilled-demineralized water using volumetric technique. Stable about 1-2 weeks at room temperature in closed glass containers.

SPECIAL APPARATUS

1. Breathalyzer, Model 900 (Stephenson Company of Bangor Punta, Red Bank, N. J. 07701).
2. Alcoholic Breath Simulator, Model 6000 (Stephenson Company of Bangor Punta, Red Bank, N. J. 07701).

In addition to the Breathalyzer apparatus in its self-contained aluminum carrying case, the following expendable materials are required for each test: (1) Two Breathalyzer reagent ampuls (one ampul serves as a photometric standard and is reusable; the ampuls also serve as photometer cuvettes); (2) a glass capillary bubbler tube for delivering the breath sample into the reagent ampul, and (3) a plastic mouthpiece-saliva trap.

PROCEDURE (69)
(See Figure 5)

A. Preparation of the Instrument for Operation

1. The On-Off switch is turned on, and the galvanometer is unlocked and mechanically centered. The instrument is permitted to warm up until the sample chamber thermometer indicates 50±3°C.
2. A comparison ampul is "gauged" and inserted into the "Reference" ampul holder (Left Side).
3. A reagent ampul is cleaned, "gauged," and fitted with a new

BREATHALYZER OPERATIONAL CHECK LIST

Name of subject .... **Date** ....

Time (of test) .... **Blood Alcohol 0.** ....% **Ampul Control No.** ....

Operator .... **Witness** ....

Instrument .... **No.** ....

V

PREPARATION 1. ☐ Throw SWITCH to "ON", wait until THERMOMETER shows 50±3°C.
2. ☐ Gauge TEST AMPUL, open, insert BUBBLER and connect to OUTLET.

PURGE 3. ☐ Turn to TAKE, flush out, turn to ANALYZE.
4, ☐ When RED empty signal appears, wait 1½ minutes, turn on LIGHT, BALANCE.

ANALYSIS 5. ☐ Set BLOOD ALCOHOL POINTER on START line.
6. ☐ Turn to TAKE, take breath sample, turn to ANALYZE, (record time)
7. ☐ When RED empty signal appears, wait 1½ minutes, turn on LIGHT BALANCE.

Record answer, dispose of test ampul, TURN CONTROL KNOB to "OFF"

Figure 5. Operational check list.

glass bubbler tube with the rubber delivery tube sleeve attached. The ampul is placed into the "Test" ampul holder (Right Side) and the delivery tube connected to the outlet.

B. Purging, Sampling, and Analysis

1. With the Control Handle in the "TAKE" position, the sample chamber is flushed repeatedly with room air by means of an atomizer bulb protected with a silica gel entrance filter. The Control Handle is turned to the "ANALYZE" position and the cylinder allowed to empty until the "EMPTY" light appears. After 90 seconds, the source light is turned on and photometric balance restored (if necessary) by turning the Balance Adjustment Wheel until the galvanometer is nulled. The scale pointer is then aligned with the zero mark.
2. With the Control Handle in the "TAKE" position, and a new mouthpiece inserted into the Sample Tube, the Sample Tube is extended and the subject is instructed to retain his breath momentarily and then to blow vigorously and continuously into the mouthpiece as long as possible after the "FULL" signal light appears. (If the sample appears unsatisfactory, another breath specimen is similarly obtained without apparatus change.)
3. The Control Handle is moved to the "ANALYZE" position and the specimen permitted to bubble through the ampul until the "EMPTY" light appears. After 90 seconds, the light source is turned on and photometric balance restored by adjustment of the Balance Adjustment Wheel.
4. The analysis result, expressed in % W/V blood alcohol concentration, is now indicated on the instrument scale.

C. Recording of Results and Securing of the Instrument

1. The analysis result is either entered into an appropriate record book or, optionally, may be recorded on a printed scale overlay by stamping the pointer impression on the facsimile scale.
2. An appropriately filled-out "Operational Check List" is marked during the analysis as each step is carried out (Fig. 5).
3. The test ampul, bubbler and mouthpiece are discarded, with due caution for the corrosive ampul content. The Control Handle is moved to the "OFF" position and the on-off switch turned to off.

D. Routine Instrument and Performance Testing (69, 70)

1. Prior to first use of the instrument and at regular intervals thereafter (preferably weekly), the following visual and instrumental checks should be performed and any indicated preventive maintenance or corrective adjustments or repairs carried out.
2. A visual inspection of the entire instrument is carried out. The panel, ampul holders and breath intake and delivery tubes are cleaned as required. All screws, nuts, and electrical connections are checked to insure tightness.
3. Sample chamber temperature is

checked with the built-in thermometer. After the instrument is first turned on, the sample chamber temperature should rise to 50° C ± 3° in about 20 minutes, at ordinary ambient temperature. The thermostat is adjusted, if necessary.

4. The output of the sample chamber is checked after the instrument has reached stable operating temperature, with an output gauge or comparable device. Appropriate Charles' Law* temperature corrections must be applied unless both chamber and output gauge are at the same temperature. For example, 52.5 ml of breath or other gas originally collected at 34° C will occupy

$$\left[\ 52.5 \times \frac{273 + 50^{\circ}\mathrm{K}}{273 + 34^{\circ}\mathrm{K}} = \right] 55.2 \text{ ml}$$

at 50° C; and at 25° C room temperature the corresponding chamber output of *sample* should be

$$\left[\ 52.5 \times \frac{273 + 25^{\circ}\mathrm{K}}{273 + 50^{\circ}\mathrm{K}} = \right] 50.9 \text{ ml.}$$

With additional allowance for dead space displacement the measured output volume should be 56.5 ± 1.5 ml, with both sample chamber and output gauge at 25° C. The delivery time (between "Full" light and "Empty" light indications) should be 25-35 seconds and remain constant for a given instrument.

5. Optical system balance is checked by centering the light source between the photocells to yield a vertical light beam through the central pin hole in the panel, inserting two optically clean sealed reagent ampuls bearing the same control number, and noting whether the galvanometer needle swings more than 0.25 inch from its mechanical null initially or upon right-left reversal of the ampuls in their holders. If necessary, the shutter screw assemblies are adjusted to achieve photometric balance. Thereafter, photometer backlash is checked, with the sealed matched ampuls in place, by nulling the galvanometer with source light on, setting the scale pointer to 0.20% W/V on the blood alcohol scale, and successively adjusting the balance wheel several times to return the pointer to 0.00% W/V and to the galvanometer null balance point. The final pointer position should remain 0.20% W/V within ± 0.005% W/V per pointer excursion. The same check is repeated at a 0.40% W/V scale position; the same variation limits should apply.

6. Finally, overall operations of the system (including instrument performance, reagent characteristics, and operator performance) is checked by performing one or more complete control analyses of Simulator produced alcohol-in-air reference specimens. The results should coincide within ± 0.01% W/V with the predicted target values. Target values of approximately 0.10% W/V and 0.20% W/V are generally most appropriate for this purpose, and the corresponding alcohol reference solutions are prepared as described under "Reference Solutions."

*Charles' Law: The volume of a gas, at a constant pressure, varies directly with the absolute temperature.

DISCUSSION

Instrumental Considerations

Since the Breathalyzer scale is linear and the result is independent of the absolute concentration of the reagent, it is possible to perform repeated analyses of the same or different samples using a single ampul, with separate zero restoration between analyses, within the overall reaction capacity or range of up to 0.176 mg of ethanol (corresponding to 0.70% W/V expressed as blood alcohol). Recommended practice is, therefore, to perform successive analyses of: a) a sample of room air as a "blank" determination; b) one or more breath specimens, and c) a control specimen such as a Simulator-produced alcohol-in-air mixture with a single reagent ampul. This routine permits replicate specimen analysis in most instances at generally encountered breath alcohol concentrations, and duplicates a well-controlled laboratory analysis scheme of blank, sample, and control specimen analysis.

The sampling system including the sample chamber, valve, intake, and delivery tubes is maintained at approximately 50° C to prevent condensation of water vapor from the breath which could, in turn, cause absorption of alcohol from the breath specimen and binding of the close-tolerance sample chamber piston. The last-phase collection technique facilitates obtaining breath which is substantially alveolar with respect to alcohol content (i.e., in alcohol-equilibrium with pulmonary arterial blood plasma) from untrained subjects with a minimum of cooperation. However, obtaining a suitable breath specimen is a key step in the procedure and requires specific attention and care.

While dichromate oxidation procedures inherently are not specific for ethanol, the reaction system employed in the Breathalyzer is characterized by considerable selectivity for ethanol and further identification of the reducing substance present is readily possible in positive tests, by a very simple technique. The number of potential chemical interferants capable of appearing in the breath of living subjects *and* capable of reacting under the conditions of the Breathalyzer analysis is limited as already noted above. For several such substances, the rate of reaction in this system differs markedly from that of ethanol which is essentially completely oxidized in 90 seconds. With ethanol, variations in reaction time (to reading) of −15 to +60 seconds do not significantly alter the results (67). However, ethyl ether, methanol, isobutanol, and n-butanol for example, react much more slowly in equal concentrations than ethanol and a second reading at 3 minutes will reveal substantially higher results than obtained at the initial 1.5 minute reading, in contrast to the ethanol results which remain unchanged (67). Acetone in physiologically significant concentrations does not yield results exceeding the blank values.

Necessary Safeguards

Since breath alcohol analysis is a rather simple procedure which can be competently performed after limited training of personnel, rather elaborate safeguard systems have been proposed to maintain the reliability of the analysis and the validity of its evidentiary value for forensic purposes (4, 71, 72, 5). These recommendations uniformly include proposals for standardized minimal training of breath alcohol test operator and supervisor personnel and for administrative and procedural safeguards. The latter minimally include: 1) observation of the subject for at least 15 minutes prior to collection of the breath specimen, during which period the subject must not have ingested alcoholic beverages or other fluids, regurgitated, vomited, eaten, or smoked; 2) a blank analysis; 3) analysis of a suitable reference or control sample, such as air equilibrated with a reference solution of known alcohol content at known temperature accompanying each subject breath analysis (4, 71, 72, 5). At least duplicate analyses of breath specimens are strongly recommended by many authorities (4, 71, 72) and adequate and appropriate expert scientific supervision is always required. Under such conditions, even non-laboratory personnel can consistently achieve satisfactory results in routine breath alcohol analysis as judged by the coincidence of the results with those obtained by careful direct analysis of *simultaneously* obtained blood specimens (73).

Remote Sampling

It is often convenient and desirable to collect breath specimens for quantitative alcohol analysis at times and locations different from those of the analysis. Early apparatus and procedures for such purposes relied chiefly upon determination of the alcohol/carbon dioxide ratio in mixed expired breath which had been passed through a chemical train that absorbed alcohol and water vapor with one reagent and carbon dioxide with another. The recognized shortcomings of such schemes, including the considerable and unpredictable variation of alveolar CO_2 content from any population average, have led to more recent attempts to collect and preserve entire breath specimens in original form, or to remove and retain the alcohol from a volumetrically measured last-phase breath specimen. Harger and associates (22) briefly reviewed the major trends in collecting and storing of breath samples for alcohol analysis. These include storage of breath in flexible rubber, aluminum, polyethylene, polyvinyl chloride, and Saran bags; and absorption of ethanol from measured samples of breath with anhydrous magnesium perchlorate, anhydrous calcium chloride, silica gel, sulfuric acid, and water. Harger and associates (22) reported the least alcohol loss, 15% at the end of 20 hours, from flexible aluminum bags; and Salem and associates (74) found that an improved Saran breath container showed alcohol losses of less than 7% after 62 hours.

The DPC Intoximeter (50) is a heated breath sampling device, which can serve both as a temporary storage unit and to obtain a fixed breath volume the alcohol from which is then absorbed in a suitable chemical column. Laboratory analysis of such collected alcohol specimens can then be carried out by any suitable procedure, including oxidation procedures and gas-liquid or gas-solid chromatography upon the separated alcohol which is usually recovered by distillation or aeration. A current apparatus development for remote sampling of breath and subsequent analysis of the alcohol by means of the Breathalyzer (or other appropriate analytical scheme) is illustrated in Figure 6 (75). The smaller device on the left is a Breathalyzer Remote Collection Unit* which is based on the sampling module of the Model 900 Breathalyzer and collects a 52.5 ml (at 34° C) last-phase breath sample in a heated sample cylinder. A valve permits holding the specimen or its discharge through a narrow column of finely di-

*Stephenson Company of Bangor Punta, Red Bank, N. J. 07701.

vided anhydrous calcium chloride (contained in a 7 mm diameter borosilicate glass tube) which quantitatively removes and retains any ethanol and water vapor present. The larger device on the right is a Transfer Unit* in which the calcium chloride column can be subjected to a flow of air, free of volatile substances and heated to 150° C, for a period of up to 5 minutes, which suffices to recover any alcohol present. The effluent from the Transfer Unit can be analyzed for alcohol content with the Breathalyzer by direct introduction into the "Test" reagent ampul, or by any other appropriate procedure such as gas chromatography. Since the breath sample collected in the Remote Collection Unit is 52.5 ml, like that in the Model 900 Breathalyzer, the results of the analysis can be obtained directly from its blood alcohol concentration scale without calculations.

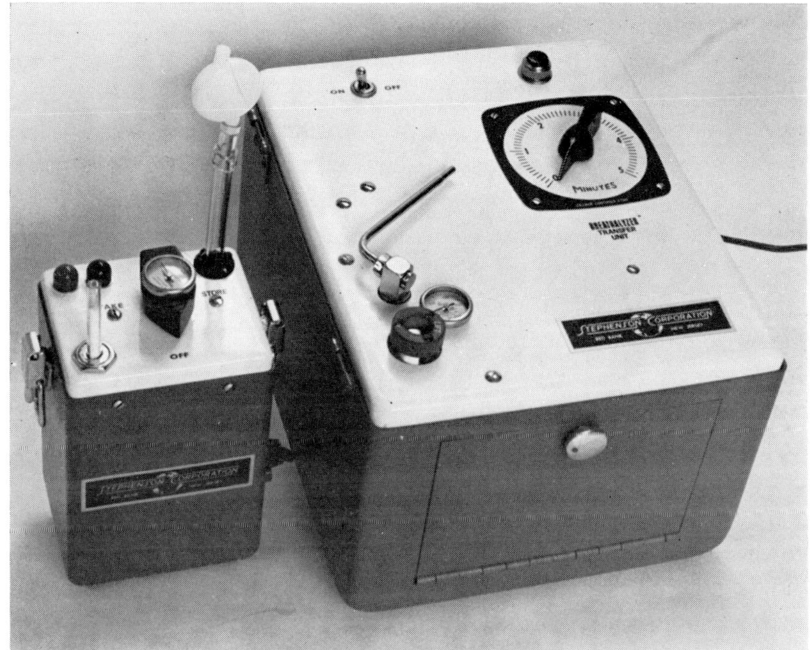

Figure 6. Breathalyzer remote collection unit (left) and transfer unit (right).

SOURCES OF ERROR

Significant errors in the breath analysis procedure are limited essentially to those arising from physiological factors since the instrumental design and procedural safeguards virtually exclude undetected aberrations. Failure to obtain a true last-phase ("deep-lung") air sample essentially alveolar with respect to alcohol can cause spuriously low blood-alcohol values. The Henry's Law relation is temperature dependent, and body temperatures significantly above normal (as in fever) can result in spuriously high values since the physiological 2100:1 blood/breath ratio for alcohol applies to normal body temperatures. Theoretically, a 1° C temperature increase above normal at the interface (alveolar/capillary surface) would tend to increase the blood alcohol concentration calculated on the basis of an assumed 2100:1 ratio by about 6.5% over the actual concentration (16, 23). In actual practice, some attenuation of the higher breath alcohol concentration tends to occur because of alcohol redistribution phenomena in the upper respiratory tract. Presence of mouth alcohol from undetected regurgitation, vomiting, or eructation while the stomach still contains alcohol would, of course, vitiate the result. In addition to the normal period of 15 minutes of continuous observation prior to sampling to assure absence of these complications, duplicate analyses of separate breath specimens provide a secure means of avoiding undetected difficulty from this source. Substantially identical results (within ±0.01% W/V) on duplicate specimen analyses experimentally establish absence of such sources of error.

The instrumental and analytical features of the system are such that undetected mechanical or chemical problems will either have no effect upon the result or result in lower than actual values. Thus, variations in the reagent sulfuric acid concentration of ± 10%, in reaction time of –15 to +60 seconds, and in reaction temperature of –5 to +25°C do not significantly alter the results (67). The absolute concentration of potassium dichromate in the Test ampul has no effect upon the result, provided some dichromate remains after completion of the analysis. If insufficient potassium dichromate is present (as from inadvertent repeated analyses beyond the ampul capacity) the result is low. Absence of the catalyst could also give low results because of incomplete reaction within the 90-second period. Chemical interference phenomena and their detection and avoidance have been covered. Incomplete collection of breath specimens is obviated by the design of the sampling system, and undetected leakage or loss of the specimen prior to its delivery into the test ampul results in spuriously low values. The reagent ampul should contain 3.0 ml of reagent with a tolerance of –0.00 and +0.08 ml and its external diameter should be between 0.625 inch and 0.650 inch. A reagent volume consequentially less than 3.0 ml will cause spuriously high results while a substantially greater volume yields low results. The gauging process described under "Procedure" establishes that the ampul diameter is within the specified limits and that the reagent meniscus is at or above the gauge shoulder, thus eliminating these potential sources of error.

The entire analysis is unusually secure with respect to analytical reliability because the reference or control analysis by means of the Simulator, equilibrator or comparable device reveals experimentally at the time of a subject analysis whether any potential sources of error are operative. Coincidence of the control result with the target value effectively confirms their absence. Clearly, meticulous preparation and careful storage of the reference solutions for Simulator use is fundamental to their value. These dilute solutions deteriorate with storage and, of course, decrease in concentration with continued use. They should therefore be replaced after one week's use or after 25 Simulator analyses (whichever occurs earlier).

RANGE OF VALUES

The controversy over the existence of "normal" body ethanol concentrations, if any, in the blood and other fluids and tissues is long and tedious (76). It is generally agreed that "endogenous" alcohol in human blood, when present, exists at concentrations from 0 to 0.15 mg/100 ml (= 0 to 0.00015% W/V). Breath alcohol analysis with the Breathalyzer in abstaining subjects therefore yields no demonstrable alcohol value, and the results of such analyses are therefore equal to those of reagent blanks. Since this breath alcohol analysis requires some cooperation from the subject, its use as described is generally limited to specimens from conscious persons which normally limits the maximal blood alcohol values encountered to those below 0.40% W/V). (Procedural modifications for breath alcohol estimations on rebreathed air from unconscious subjects have been attempted.)

RÉSUMÉ OF CLINICAL INTERPRETATIONS

In Table I are correlated blood alcohol concentrations with the usually recognized stages of acute alcoholic influence, and with the corresponding clinical signs and symptoms. The deliberate overlap between the stages reflects the existence of some variation in these ef-

TABLE I

STAGES OF ACUTE ALCOHOLIC INFLUENCE/INTOXICATION

ETHYL ALCOHOL LEVEL, Per Cent W/V		STAGE OF ALCOHOLIC INFLUENCE	CLINICAL SIGNS/SYMPTOMS
Blood	Urine		
0.01-0.05	0.01-0.07	Sobriety	No apparent influence Behavior nearly normal by ordinary observation Slight changes detectable by special tests
0.03-0.12	0.04-0.16	Euphoria	Mild euphoria, sociability, talkativeness Increased self-confidence; decreased inhibitions Diminution of attention, judgment, and control Loss of efficiency in finer performance tests
0.09-0.25	0.12-0.34	Excitement	Emotional instability; decreased inhibitions Loss of critical judgment Impairment of memory and comprehension Decreased sensitory response; increased reaction time Some muscular incoordination
0.18-0.30	0.24-0.41	Confusion	Disorientation, mental confusion; dizziness Exaggerated emotional states (fear, anger, grief, etc.) Disturbance of sensation (diplopia, etc.) and of perception of color, form, motion, dimensions Decreased pain sense Impaired balance; muscular incoordination; staggering gait, slurred speech
0.27-0.40	0.37-0.54	Stupor	Apathy; general inertia, approaching paralysis Markedly decreased response to stimuli Marked muscular incoordination; inability to stand or walk Vomiting; incontinence of urine and feces Impaired consciousness; sleep or stupor
0.35-0.50	0.47-0.67	Coma	Complete unconsciousness; coma; anesthesia Depressed or abolished reflexes Subnormal temperature Incontinence of urine and feces Embarrassment of circulation and respiration Possible death
0.45+	0.60+	Death	Death from respiratory paralysis

fects among individuals, a recognized biological phenomenon. At blood alcohol concentrations below 0.03 and 0.05% W/V, existence of alcoholic influence is generally not detectable clinically, although impairment in central nervous system functions and performance can be demonstrated at concentrations as low as 0.01% W/V by sophisticated procedures.

Since various activities differ in their requirements for judgment and other physical and mental fitness and performance capabilities, the extent of impairment by alcohol which constitutes unfitness for safe performance also necessarily varies with the activity, task and total circumstances. Consequently different blood alcohol concentrations should be employed as criteria of the presence or absence of alcoholic influence to the extent of unfitness for different activities.

ACKNOWLEDGMENT

Figures 1, 4, 5, and 6 are used through the courtesy of Stephenson Company of Bangor Punta, Red Bank, New Jersey; and Figures 2 and 3 are used through the courtesy of Professor R. F. Borkenstein, Department of Police Administration, Indiana University, Bloomington, Indiana.

REFERENCES

1. Dubowski, K. M.: Some major developments related to chemical tests for intoxication. Police, *2*:54-56, 1957.
2. Alcohol and Highway Safety. A Report to the Congress from the Secretary of Transportation. Washington, U. S. Department of Transportation, August 1968.
3. Alcohol and Accidental Injury. Conference Proceedings, U. S. Department of Health, Education, and Welfare, Washington, U. S. Government Printing Office, 1966.
4. Dubowski, K. M.: Necessary scientific safeguards in breath alcohol analysis. J. Forensic Sci., *5*:422-433, 1960.
5. Recommendations of the Ad Hoc Committee on Testing and Training of the Committee on Alcohol and Drugs. Chicago, National Safety Council Committee on Alcohol and Drugs, August 1968.
6. Chastain, J. D.: A correlation study of blood alcohol levels as determined by Alcometer, Breathalyzer, and direct blood analysis, includblood-urine ratio. Austin, Texas Department of Public Safety, 1957.
7. Dubowski, K. M.: Alcohol determination—some physiological and metabolic considerations, in Alcohol and Traffic Safety, ed. by B. H. Fox and J. H. Fox. Public Health Service Publication No. 1043. Washington, U. S. Government Printing Office, 1963, pp. 91-115.
8. Greenberg, L. A.: Physiological factors affecting breath samples. J. Forensic Sci., *5*:411-418, 1960.
9. Report of the Commission on "Driving While Under the Influence of Drink or a Drug." Dublin, The Stationery Office, 1963, p. 117.
10. Smith, H. W.: Methods for determining alcohol. In, Methods of Forensic Science, Vol. 4, ed. by A. S. Curry. London, Interscience Publishers, Inc., 1965, pp. 1-97.
11. The Medico-Legal Investigation of the Drinking Driver—Report of a Special Committee of the British Medical Association. London, Britis Medical Association, 1965.
12. Fox, B. H., Lower, J., and Fox, M. W.: Measurement and reduction of some sources of variation in a breath instrument. In Alcohol and Road Traffic, op. cit. (60), pp. 261-271.
13. Greenberg, L. A., and Lester, D.: Alcohol breath tests and breath deodorization by chlorophyll derivatives. Quart. J. Stud. on Alcohol, *15*:16-20, 1954.
14. Bogen, E.: Drunkenness, quantitative study of acute alcoholic intoxication. J.A.M.A., *89*:1508-1510, 1927.
15. Cushny, A. R.: On the exhalation of drugs by the lungs. J. Physiol., *40*:17-27, 1910.
16. Harger, R. N., Raney, B. B., Bridwell, E. G., and Kitchel, M. F.: Partition ratio of alcohol between air and water, urine and blood; estimation and identification of alcohol in these liquids from anaylsis of air equilibrated with them. J. Biol. Chem., *183*:197-213, 1950.
17. Jetter, W. W., and Forrester, G. C.: Perchlorate method for determining the concentration of alcohol in expired air as a medicolegal test. Arch. Path., *32*:828-842, 1941.
18. Liljestrand, C., and Linde, P.: Über die Ausscheidung des Alkohols mit der Expirationsluft. Skand. Arch. Physiol., *60*:273-298, 1930.
19. Committee on Tests for Intoxication, National Safety Council: Evaluating Chemical Tests for Intoxication. Chicago, National Safety Council, 1953.

20. Elbel, H., and Schleyer, F.: Blutalkohol, 2nd ed. Stuttgart, Georg Thieme Verlag, 1956, p. 40.
21. Grosskopf, K.: Die Atemalkohol-bestimmung als analytische Aufgabe. Angew. Chemie, *66:* 295-297, 1954.
22. Harger, R. N., Forney, R. B., and Baker, R. S.: Estimation of the level of blood alcohol from analysis of breath, II. Use of rebreathed air. Quart. J. Stud. on Alcohol, *17:*1-18, 1956.
23. Harger, R. N., Forney, R. B., and Barnes, H. B.: Estimation of level of blood alcohol from analysis of breath. J. Lab. & Clin. Med., *36:* 306-318, 1950.
24. Fitzgerald, M. P., and Haldane, J. S.: The normal alveolar carbonic acid pressures in man. J. Physiol., *32:*486-494, 1905.
25. Harger, R. N., Lamb, E. B., and Hulpieu, H. R.: Rapid chemical test for intoxication employing breath; new reagent for alcohol and procedure for estimating concentration of alcohol in body from ratio of alcohol to carbon dioxide in breath. J.A.M.A., *110:*779-785, 1938.
26. Edwards, A. W. T., Velasquez, T., and Farhi, L. E.: Determination of alveolar capillary temperature. J. Appl. Physiol., *18:*107-113, 1963.
27. Forster, R. E.: Breathing tests for alcohol. J.A.M.A., *190:*85, 1964.
28. Legge, D.: The influence of breath temperature on assessments of blood alcohol level by breath analysis. Quart. J. Studies on Alc., *26:* 371-377, 1965.
29. Wright, B.M.: Influence of breath temperature on blood alcohol determination by breath analysis. Quart. J. Studies on Alc., *27:*112-114, 1966.
30. Smith, J. C.: The avoidance of biologic variables in breath tests for alcohol in blood. Am. J. Clin. Path., *32:*34-40, 1959.
31. Dubowski, K. M.: Unpublished observations, 1964.
32. Harger, R. N.: Ethyl alcohol. In, Toxicology —Mechanisms and Analytical Methods, Vol. II, ed. by C. P. Stewart and A. Stolman. New York, Academic Press, Inc., 1961, pp. 85-151.
33. Borkenstein, R. F.: Breath Tests to Determine Alcoholic Influence. Red Bank, Stephenson Corporation, 1963, pp. 33-34.
34. Subbotin, V.: Z. Biol., *7:*361, 1871.
35. Anstie, F. E.: Final experiments on the elimination of alcohol from the body. Practitioner, *13:*15, 1874.
36. Bodländer, G.: Die Ausscheidung aufgenommenen Weingeistes aus dem Körper. Arch. ges. Physiol., *32:*398-426, 1883.
37. Strassmann, F.: Untersuchungen über den Nahrwert und die Ausscheidung des Alkohols. Arch. ges. Physiol., *49:*315- , 1891.
38. Harger, R. N.: Science News. Science, *73:*10, 1931.
39. Haggard, H. W., and Greenberg, L. A.: Studies on absorption, distribution, and elimination of ethyl alcohol. I. Quantitative determination of ethyl alcohol in air, blood and urine by means of iodine pentoxide. J. Pharmacol. & Exper. Therap., *52:*137-49, 1934; II. The excretion of alcohol in urine and expired air; and the distribution of alcohol between air and water, blood, and urine. J. Pharmacol. & Exper. Therap., *52:*150-66, 1934.
40. Schawerin, V. M.: Klin. Med. U.S.S.R., *17:*86, 1938.
41. Greenberg, L. A., and Keator, F. W.: Portable automatic apparatus for indirect determination of the concentration of alcohol in the blood. Quart. J. Stud. on Alc., *2:*57-72, 1941.
42. Jetter, W. W., Moore, M., and Forrester, G. C.: Studies in alcohol. IV. A new method for the determination of breath alcohol. Am. J. Clin. Path., *11:*75-89, 1941.
43. Seifert, P., and Günther, H.: Alkoholintoxikation und Atemalkohol. Arch. exp. Path. u. Pharmakol., *213:*37-43, 1951.
44. Kobayashi, Y.: Gas analysis by detector tubes. VII. Rapid method for ethyl alcohol. J. Chem. Soc. Japan, *56:*526-7, 1953.
45. Grosskopf, K.: Technical analysis of gases and liquids by chromometric gas analysis. Angew. Chem., *63:*306-311, 1951.
46. Borkenstein, R. F., and Smith, H. W.: The Breathalyzer and its application. Medicine, Science and the Law, 1:13-22, 1961.
47. Forrester, G. C.: Training Manual—The Photo-electric Intoximeter. Niagara Falls, The Intoximeter Association, 1960.
48. Kitagawa, T., and Wright, B. M.: A quantitative detector-tube method for breath-alcohol estimation. Brit. Med. J., *2:*652-653, 1962.
49. Wright, B. M.: Breath alcohol analysis. In Alcohol and Road Traffic. op. cit. (63), pp. 251-257.
50. Forrester, G. C.: Manual for the DPC Intoximeter. St. Louis, Intoximeters-Midwestern, 1964.
51. Dubowski, K. M.: Some practical laboratory aspects of forensic alcohol determination. Proc. Iowa Acad. Science, *63:*364-390, 1956.
52. Forney, R. B., Hughes, F. W., Harger, R. N., and Richards, A. B.: Alcohol distribution in the vascular system. Quart. J. Studies on Alc., *25:*205-217, 1964.
53. Dubowski, K. M., and Withrow, J. R.: A photometric microdetermination method for ethyl alcohol in biological materials. Proc. Am. Academy Forensic Sci., *2:*323-37, 1952.
54. Report on Impaired Driving Tests, ed. by B. B. Coldwell. Ottawa, Queen's Printer, 1957.

55. Smith, H. W.: The specificity of the desiccation method for determining alcohol in biological fluids. J. Lab. Clin. Med., *38:*762-766, 1951.
56. Coldwell, B. B., and Smith, H. W.: Alcohol levels in body fluids after ingestion of distilled spirits. Can. J. Biochem. Physiol., *37:*43-52, 1959.
57. Drew, G. C., Colquhoun, W. P., and Long, H. A.: Effect of Small Doses of Alcohol on a Skill Resembling Driving. Med. Res. Council Memorandum 38. London, H. M. Stationery Office, 1959.
58. Kent-Jones, D. W., and Taylor, G.: Determination of alcohol in blood and urine. Analyst, *79:*121-136, 1954.
59. Scroggie, J. G.: Some aspects of recent Australian research in breath tests for alcohol. In, Alcohol and Road Traffic. op. cit. (60), pp. 272-276.
60. Alcohol and Road Traffic. Proceedings of the Third International Conference on Alcohol and Road Traffic, London, 1962. London, British Medical Association, 1963.
61. Kozelka, F. L., and Hine, C. H.: Method for determination of ethyl alcohol for medicolegal purposes. Ind. Eng. Chem., Anal. Ed., *13:*905-907, 1941.
62. Begg, T. B., Hill, I. D., and Nickolls, L. C.: A statistically-planned comparison of blood and breath alcohol levels. In, Alcohol and Road Traffic. op. cit. (60), pp. 277-280.
63. Alcohol and Road Traffic. Proceedings of the Second International Conference on Alcohol and Road Traffic, Toronto, 1953. Toronto, Garden City Press Co-Operative, 1955.
64. Nickolls, L. C.: Analyst, *85:*840, 1960.
65. Fox, B. H., Hallett, R. A., Makowski, W., Schnall, A. M., and Pelch, A.: Refined comparison of blood- and breath-alcohol measures and variability of breaths around trend of decline. In, Alcohol and Traffic Safety: Proceedings of the Fourth International Conference on Alcohol and Traffic Safety, ed. by R. N. Harger. Bloomington, Indiana University, 1966, pp. 128-139.
66. Britt, B. J., and Borkenstein, R. F.: Reproducibility of Breathalyzer tests using an alcoholic breath simulator. In, Alcohol and Traffic Safety: Proceedings of the Fourth International Conference on Alcohol and Traffic Safety, ed. by R. N. Harger. Bloomington, Indiana University, 1966, pp. 140-143.
67. Coldwell, B. B., and Grant, G. L.: Study of some factors affecting the accuracy of the Breathalyzer. J. Forensic Sci., *8:*149-162, 1963.
68. Dubowski, K. M.: Specificity of breath-alcohol analyses. J.A.M.A., *189:*1039, 1964.
69. Breathalyzer Model 900 Instruction Manual. Red Bank, Stephenson Company of Bangor Punta, 1968.
70. Breathalyzer Model 900 Service Manual. Red Bank, Stephenson Company of Bangor Punta, 1968.
71. Smith, H. W., and Lucas, D. M.: The development of a large scale breath testing programme in Ontario. In Proceedings of the Third International Conference on Alcohol and Road Traffic, op. cit. (60), pp. 189-196.
72. Smith, W. C., Harding, D. M., Biasotti, A. A., Finkle, B. S., and Bradford, L. W.: Breathalyzer experiences under the operational conditions recommended by the California Association of Criminalists. J. Forensic Science Society, *9:*58-64, 1969.
73. Howes, J. R., Hallett, R. A., and Lucas, D. M.: A study of the accuracy of the Breathalyzer as operated by police personnel. J. Forensic Sci., *12:*444-453, 1967.
74. Salem, H., Lucas, G. H. W., and Lucas, D. M.: Saran plastic bags as containers for breath samples. Canad. M. A. J., *82:*682-683, 1960.
75. Borkenstein, R. F.: Personal Communication, Jan. 1968.
76. Harger, R. N., and Forney, R. B. :Aliphatic Alcohols. In, Progress in Chemical Toxicology, Vol. 2, ed. by a Stolman. New York, Academic Press, Inc., 1967, pp. 1-61.

Chapter 32A

Methyl Alcohol Poisoning

IRENE E. ROECKEL, M.D., and
WILMIER M. TALBERT, JR., M.D.

Methyl alcohol poisoning may occur in epidemic form (3, 10) or as sporadic cases (2, 6, 7, 8, 11, 12, 17). Epidemics, such as the one recently seen in Kentucky (10), may be associated with a high mortality. Eight of eighteen patients died (44%) and the mortality could have been even higher had not gas chromatography been used to identify the victims in an asymptomatic stage so that peritoneal dialysis could be instituted. Epidemic methanol poisoning is the result of the wholesale distribution of methanol usually from a single source.

Sporadic cases of methanol intoxication are due to accidental or willful ingestion of methanol and are difficult, if not impossible, to recognize in the early stages without chemical analysis of the blood or urine. Gas chromatography of biological materials provides a rapid method of screening of intoxicated people to identify the sporadic case of methanol poisoning. Since the epidemic, which popularized gas chromatographic analysis for methanol in our laboratory, there were 130 blood samples tested during a 12-month period. Ten of these patients had significant methanol levels in their blood (from 5 to 93 mg per 100 ml) indicating that the sporadic case is not rare. An additional 9 cases revealed significant amounts of isopropyl alcohol and 43 patients were positive for ethyl alcohol.

CLINICAL CHARACTERISTICS

The ingestion of methanol may lead to an anesthetic death with levels above 400 mg per 100 ml (7, 10). This mechanism of death is not basically different from that due to ethyl alcohol at similar blood levels. Usually, however, methyl alcohol poisoning is attributable to the effects of the metabolic end products of methyl alcohol metabolism, namely formaldehyde and formic acid (13, 15, 16, 18, 19). It is important to realize that there is a 12 to 36 hour asymptomatic phase (3, 10) after the ingestion of methyl alcohol during which time the body is converting the methyl alcohol to the acidic end product. The loss of the buffer reserve is manifested by a falling concentration of serum bicarbonate and serum pH (3, 5, 9, 10, 13, 14). When this happens, the classical signs of methyl alcohol intoxication occur. These include coma with cerebral edema, often progressing to massive hemorrhage (7). Pancreatitis manifested by elevated serum amylase during life has been described almost invariably in autopsy reports (3). Visual disturbances (3, 14, 15), often leading to blindness, have been popularized in the literature and are even appreciated as being related to methyl alcohol by the lay population. Visual disturbances, however, are a late and irregular manifestation of methyl alcohol poisoning (10).

LABORATORY DIAGNOSIS

Physical signs and symptoms consistent with methanol intoxication are, of course, common in the emergency room population. An alcoholic odor to the breath, added to any sign or symptom suggestive of methanol poisoning, is probably sufficient justification for a determination of the blood methanol. Our recent experience in the Kentucky epidemic revealed that almost all of the survivors were completely asymptomatic (10) at the time of admission and came to the emergency room only because of the publicity associated with the early deaths. Once methanol has been found in the blood, other tests must be done to interpret the significance of the level. The serum pH and bicarbonate will indicate the extent of conversion of methanol to acidic end-products.

THERAPY

Therapy is directed towards removal of the methanol, correction of the acidosis and decreasing the rate of methanol oxidation.

1. *Removal of the Methanol:* (2, 6, 7, 8, 10, 17) Methanol can be effectively removed by peritoneal dialysis. Hemodialysis is probably more efficient but no medical center would be likely to have the equipment available to handle the epidemic form of the disease by hemodialysis. Dialysis is about 5 to 10 times as effective as forced diuresis in the removal of methanol. Peritoneal dialysis should be seriously considered even in the asymptomatic patient when the serum methanol level is above 100 mg per 100 ml. Serum methanol in excess of 100 mg per 100 ml associated with decreased serum pH and bicarbonate are an entirely different matter and dialysis is almost mandatory.
2. *Correction of Acidosis:* (3, 5, 10, 13, 14) Intravenous sodium bicarbonate is given until a normal blood pH is achieved and maintained (7, 10, 12). This is the principle therapy for those patients who have already converted the bulk of their methanol to the acidic end products and no longer have the methanol available for removal by dialysis.
3. *Decrease Conversion of Methanol:* (1, 4, 10, 11, 16) Ethyl alcohol will inhibit the oxidation of methanol in the liver by alcohol dehydrogenase and thus delay the formation of the acidic end products which are responsible for the symptoms of the poisoning. Methyl alcohol disappears from the blood at the rate of about 5 mg per 100 ml per hour. In the presence of ethyl alcohol at a level of 100 mg per 100 ml, methyl alcohol will disappear from the blood at the rate of only 2 mg per 100 ml per hour. The time gained may be used to remove the methyl alcohol by dialysis. It is important to remember that there is a loading dose of ethyl alcohol which must be given to reach the level of 100 mg per 100 ml. One common error made is to calculate the maintenance dose of alcohol and to begin the infusion with this dose. The patient burns the alcohol as fast as it is given and never at-

tains the desired level of 100 mg per 100 ml ethyl alcohol necessary to inhibit conversion of methyl alcohol.

REFERENCES

1. Agner, K., Höök, O., and von Porat, B.: The treatment of methanol poisoning with ethanol. Quart. J. Stud. Alcohol., *9:*515-522, 1949.
2. Austin, W. H., Lape, C. P., and Burnham, H. N.: Treatment of methanol intoxication by hemodialysis. New Eng. J. Med., *265:*334-336, 1961.
3. Bennett, I. L., Jr., Cary, F. H., Mitchell, G. L., Jr., and Cooper, M. N.: Acute methyl alcohol poisoning: a review based on experiences in an outbreak of 323 cases. Medicine, *32:*431-463, 1953.
4. Chew, W. B., Berger, E. H., Brines, O. A., and Capron, M. J.: Alkali treatment of methyl alcohol poisoning. JAMA,*130*:61-64, 1946.
5. Cooper, J. R., and Kimi, M. M.: Biochemical aspects of methanol poisoning. Biochem. Pharmacol., *11:*405-416, 1962.
6. Cowen, D. L.: Extracorporeal dialysis in methanol poisoning. Ann. Intern. Med., *61:*134-135, 1964.
7. Erlanson, P., Fritz, H., Hagstam, K., Liljenberg, B., Tryding, N., and Voigt, G.: Severe methanol intoxication. Acta. Med. Scand., *177:*393-408, 1965.
8. Felts, J. H., Templeton, T. B., Wolff, W. A., Meredith, J. H., and Hines, J.: Methanol poisoning treated by hemodialysis. Southern Med. J., *55:*46-47, 1962.
9. Harrop, G. A., and Benedict, E. M.: Acute methyl alcohol poisoning associated with acidosis. JAMA, *74:*25-27, 1920.
10. Kane, R. L., Talbert, W., Harlan, J. Sizemore, G., and Cataland, S.: A methanol poisoning outbreak in Kentucky. Arch. Environ. Health, *17:*119-129, 1968.
11. Kaplan, K.: Methyl alcohol poisoning. Am. J. Med. Sci. *244:*170-174, 1962.
12. Pfister, A. K., McKenzie, J. V., Dinsmore, H. P., and Edman, C. D.: Extracorporeal dialysis for methanol intoxication. JAMA, *197:*211-213, 1966.
13. Pohl, J.: Ueber die oxydation des methyl — und aethylalkohols in thierkoerper. Arch. f. exp. Path. u. Pharm., *31:*281-302, 1893.
14. Potts, A. M., and Johnson, L. V.: Studies on the visual toxicity of methanol. Am. J. Opthal. *35* (pt. 2) :107-123, 1952.
15. Röe, O.: Methanol poisoning. Acta. Med. Scand. 126 Suppl., *182:*1-253, 1946.
16. Röe, O.: The roles of alkaline salts and ethyl alcohol in the treatment of methanol poisoning. Quart. J. Stud. Alcohol, *11:*107-112, 1950.
17. Stinebaugh, B. J.,: The use of peritoneal dialysis in acute methyl alcohol poisoning. Arch. Intern. Med., *105:*613-617, 1960.
18. Van Harken, T. R., Tephly, T. R. and Mannering G. J.: Methanol metabolism in the isolated perfused rat liver. J. Pharmacol. Exp. Ther., *149:*36-42, 1965.
19. Zatman, L. J.: The effect of ethanol on the metabolism of methanol in man. Biochem. J., *40:*LXVII-LXVIII, 1946.

Chapter 32B

Measurement of Methanol in Biological Fluids

IRENE E. ROECKEL, M.D., and
WILMIER M. TALBERT, Jr., M.D.

INTRODUCTION

Methanol, because of its unusual toxic effects in man, (blindness and profound metabolic acidosis) takes a special place in the analysis for volatile poisons in biological fluids. Since wet chemical methods are technically difficult and cumbersome, a specific, rapid determination by gas chromatography is recommended.

PRINCIPLE

Gas-liquid chromatography consists of a separation column at a constant temperature. The phenomenon of flame ionization is utilized which is dependent on an optimal gas flow of a mixture of hydrogen, air, and helium. The detector response is recorded for a standard mixture of volatiles and the unknown specimen processed with an internal acetone standard added to serve as a marker and permit quantitation.

STANDARD SOLUTIONS

1. *Acetone, internal standard.* Exactly 1.5 ml of acetone is diluted to 1 liter in a volumetric flask and stored at room temperature in a polyethylene bottle with screw cap.

2. *Poly-alcohol standard.* One ml each of acetone, absolute ethyl alcohol, methanol and isopropyl alcohol are added to a 1 liter volumetric flask and diluted with distilled water. The standard is stored at room temperature in a screw cap polyethylene bottle.

3. *Individual alcohol standards.* One ml of each of the alcohols in the polyalcohol mixture are added to a 1 liter volumetric flask.

SPECIAL APPARATUS

1. Flame ionization gas chromatograph with recorder (Perkin-Elmer Model F-11).

2. Column:* 6 foot 1/8 inch column, stainless steel packed with Hallcomid M'18 and carbowax 600 on a Teflon-6 support.

3. Hamilton microsyringes, fixed needle, 10 microliter capacity (701N).

PROCEDURE

1. The helium, compressed air, hydrogen tanks are turned on in this order. The pressure regulators read for helium 40 pounds, compressed air 24 pounds, and hydrogen 24 pounds. The flow meter

*DE-111 Column for alcohols obtainable from Perkin-Elmer, Norwalk, Conn.

for helium is adjusted to give a retention time for ethyl alcohol of about 2 minutes.

2. The temperature in the column is allowed to equilibrate at 60°C (about 10 minutes). The slow warmup of the injection chamber is the limiting factor.

3. Equal volumes of serum or tissue fluid and internal acetone standard are mixed in a test tube.

4. Equal volumes of the methyl alcohol standard and internal acetone standards are mixed in a test tube.

5. About one microliter of the poly-alcohol standard is injected into the column. The syringe is immediately rinsed several times with distilled water.

6. About one microliter of the sample without internal standard is injected and if no peaks are present, no further analysis has to be done. If the specimen contains acetone and an alcohol, a new internal standard has to be prepared by adding an alcohol that is not present in the sample.

7. If methyl alcohol is present, one microliter of the serum-acetone mixture is injected.

8. Measure the retention time of standard poly-alcohol mixture to assure positive identification of unknown peaks.

9. Measure peak heights of alcohols and internal standard.

CALCULATION

$$\text{Alcohol in mg per 100 ml} = \frac{\text{unknown alcohol peak}}{\text{standard alcohol peak}} \times \frac{\text{concentration}}{\text{standard}} \times \frac{\text{standard acetone peak}}{\text{unknown acetone peak}}$$

SOURCES OF ERROR

The Hamilton syringes are so small that the needle gets easily clogged with protein from the sample unless they are properly washed.

Carry over from alcohol standard to specimen must be avoided by thoroughly washing the syringes. One μl of distilled water injected between the poly standard and the unknown specimen will, if negative, demonstrate an uncontaminated system.

DISCUSSION

A positive identification of the alcohol can usually be given within 20 minutes of obtaining the sample. Exact quantitation takes a few minutes more. The value of the system lies (1) in the rapid exclusion of ethanol as a cause of coma where low levels are demonstrated and (2) the rapid identification of methanol or isopropanol as a cause of intoxication.

REFERENCES

1. Eriksen, S. P., and Kulkarui, A. B.: Methanol in normal human breath. Science, *141*:639-640, 1963.
2. Feldstein, M., and Klendshoj, N. C.: Determination of methanol in biological fluids by microdiffusion analysis. Anal. Chem., *26*:932-933, 1954.
3. Goldbaum, L. R., Schloegel, E. L., and Dominguez, A. M.: Progress in Chemical Toxicology. Academic Press, 1963, pp 14-39.
4. Kane, R. L., Talbert, W., Harlan, J., Sizemore, G., and Cataland, S.: A. methanol poisoning outbreak in Kentucky. Arch. Environ. Health, *17:* 119-130, 1968.
5. Parker, K.D., Fontan, C. R., Yee, J.L., and Kirk, P.L.: Gas chromatographic determination of ethyl alcohol in blood for medicolegal purposes. Anal. Chem., *34*:1234-1236, 1962.

Chapter 33A

Lead Poisoning

HERBERT DERMAN, M.D.

History

The alchemist's symbol for lead was the sign of Saturn, the Roman deity who reigned in a Golden Age of happiness and virtue. In his honor, the annual feast of Saturnalia[1] was celebrated with support from wine sweetened by lead salts and stored in leaden containers. From the time of Hippocrates[2] to the 19th century, there have been clinical descriptions of saturnine intoxication more attributable to the containers than the contents. These descriptions often had colorful geographic designations such as Poitou colic, Devonshire colic, and West Indian dry-gripes. Poitou colic began as an outbreak of lead poisoning in southern France in 1572[3] as a result of the presence of lead in wine and cider presses. In 1739, Huxham[4] described Devonshire colic in England without recognizing its cause. It remained for Sir George Baker[4, 5] to observe in 1767 that colic in Devon was endemic at cider time and to identify lead in the brew derived from the vats and cider presses. When Baker used cider from neighboring Herefordshire as a negative control from vats and presses without lead, he was castigated from the pulpit as a "faithless son of Devon."[4]

Thomas Cadwalader[6, 7] described lead intoxication with painful clarity in the first American contribution to the literature in 1745. The presentation of abdominal pain, constipation, encephalopathy, and peripheral paralysis was in a volume entitled, *An Essay on the West-India Dry-Gripes* published by none other than Benjamin Franklin. Altho Cadwalader associated the illness with the drinking of rum distilled in lead vessels, he, like Huxham, failed to link the metal to the clinical picture.

In 1870, de Morveau[8] wrote of the dangers of industrial lead poisoning. Ramazzini[9] had written as early as 1700 of the occupational disease in potters who used "burnt and calcined lead for glazing . . . we scarcely see a potter that has not a leaden cadaverous complexion. They seldom have recourse to a physician, till the use of their limbs is taken from them and their viscera grown hard. . .". In a letter written about 1784,[10] the ubiquitous Ben Franklin described the sources of occupational lead poisoning among printers, plumbers, painters, glaziers, stonecutters, solderers, and rum drinkers. The first comprehensive documentation of the clinical picture of poisoning in lead workers was the classic work in 1830 of Tanquerel des

Planches,[11,12] who, in his study of 1200 cases, left little for subsequent investigators to add to our knowledge of the signs and symptoms.

Incidence and Metabolism

Lead poisoning was a formidable industrial and public health problem in the 19th century. The hazard of contaminated water and wine supplies from the use of leaden pipes and other accessories became known thru the studies of de Mussy,[13] Baker, and others. The poisoning of workers in the many industries utilizing lead was commonplace, especially in those engaged in pottery glazing, lead ore smelting, and the manufacture of lead compounds like the basic carbonate, white lead pigment. In Great Britain alone, there were 1058 reported cases of lead poisoning in 1900.[14] Despite an increasing consumption of lead during the 20th century the incidence of lead poisoning has decreased sharply, in the clinical sense at least, due to stern and careful industrial hygiene. There is, however, growing concern that a serious hazard may result from the increasing respiratory exposure to lead in urban areas of air pollution and motor vehicle exhaust.[15, 16, 17, 18] Lead can accumulate in mammalian tissues under certain levels of exposure and these levels appear to have been reached in the United States and in a few foreign countries.[15, 19] Altho experimental lead intoxication has been induced in animals with tissue concentrations similar to those of humans, no evidence of toxicity in human subjects with the same exposure has yet been found.

Meaningful statements are difficult on the incidence and potential risk of lead poisoning because of the necessity to delineate lead exposure from lead toxicity, and to interpret correctly the concept of the human body burden of lead.[15] Lead poisoning in today's world may be conveniently examined in terms of population exposure and individual exposure.

In studies extending over more than 30 years, Kehoe[20] has found measurable lead in all persons in the United States and in primitive areas, and in the environment. The "average" person in the United States ingests approximately 0.3 mg of lead daily in his food and beverages, with extremes of 0.1-0.6 mg. This same "average" adult in a city like Cincinnati inhales 30-40 μg per day, of which he absorbs not more than half. Kehoe therefore places the daily total intake of lead on the order of 0.33 mg per day. This is balanced by his findings of daily output of lead in feces and urine of approximately 0.33 mg. Schroeder and Tipton[15] suggest that Kehoe's hypothesis of a balanced absorption and excretion may hold for foreign subjects but not for Americans. Their data indicate that Americans had a greater burden of lead in their tissues than foreigners, and that in distinction from foreigners, the accumulation of lead increased with age through the fourth decade. This increase is ascribed to growing pollution of air and soils from motor vehicle exhausts. While no evidence of human toxicity was discovered in the subjects studied, they warn that the steadily increasing pollution with particular lead may lead to toxicity. Other authors discount the likelihood.[21]

Bone appears to be the major site of lead storage with 91% of the total body burden. Measurements of lead in blood or urine are considered by Schroeder and Tipton to be reflections of current exposure but unrelated to the actual body stores. To evaluate the body burden of lead they suggest its measurement in serum, erythrocytes, urine, and bone marrow. Many studies by Kehoe and coworkers[20, 22, 23] support this suggestion. Lead salts were fed daily in amounts from 0.3 to 3.0 mg to human volunteers for periods up to four years without the development of abnormal levels of lead in urine or blood despite the accumulation of up to 118 mg in the tissues. The experimental subjects showed no signs of toxicity. In general, Kehoe observes that the clinical severity of intoxication varies not so much with the total quantity of lead in the body but more with the general level of concentration in the soft tissues.[24] A high rate of absorption over a short time may produce a high soft tissue concentration with a low body burden but a severe clinical intoxication. In his human volunteer experiments with lead feeding, Kehoe made the corollary observation that the rate of excretion of lead is more dependent on the time of accumulation rather than the total quantity accumulated. This line of reasoning tends to calm the concern over the effects of the potential long term pollution from motor vehicle exhausts.

In 1960, Haeger-Aronsen[25] reported that delta-aminolevulinic acid (ALA), an intermediate metabolite in porphyrin and hemoglobin biosynthesis, is increased with exposure to lead. The steps in the biosynthesis are as follows:[26]

glycine + pyridoxal – P + succinyl – CoA
↓ ALA-synthetase
delta-aminolevulinic acid
↓ ALA-dehydrase
porphobilinogen
↓
uroporphyrinogen III
↓
coproporphyrinogen III
↓
protoporphyrin – 9
↓ Fe^{++}
heme

Lead interferes in the synthesis of hemoglobin at two levels. It inhibits ALA-dehydrase which catalyzes the coupling of two molecules of ALA to form porphobilinogen. This is attributed by Bonsignore and Cartesegna[27] to the oxidation by lead of the sulfhydryl groups needed to activate the ALA-dehydrase. The inhibition of the ALA-dehydrase accounts for the increased ALA excretion. It is surprising[28] that porphobilinogen is also increased in lead exposure since it is formed from ALA by ALA-dehydrase. Although lead inhibits the ALA-dehydrase, it is assumed that the remaining activity is still enough in the face of increased ALA to produce increased porphobilinogen excretion. Inorganic lead also interferes with the incorporation of iron into protoporphyrin-9 to form the heme molecule, thus causing increased erythrocyte protoporphyrin-9, increased serum iron, and ultimately decreased hemoglobin. The cause of the anemia in lead toxicity seems to be due to inhibition of the "incorporation enzyme" (Goldberg enzyme) rather than by inhibiton of ALA-dehydrase.[28]

Clinical Criteria for Diagnosis

The exposure of individual adults to lead is primarily an industrial problem with less common opportunities in the home or garage.

The symptomatology of lead poisoning may be divided into three forms: an alimentary form in which colicky pain as a result of bowel spasm is the primary feature; a neuromuscular form in which weakness of a muscle group precedes actual paralysis; and an encephalopathic form which manifests itself in coma, convulsions, mania, or delerium. Symptoms common to all forms are anemia, insomnia, headache, dizziness, and irritability.[29]

Industrially induced inorganic lead intoxication is not difficult to diagnose since the symptoms are well-defined and laboratory results are generally conclusive.[30] The typical pattern of intoxication generally begins several days or even a week or two before the onset of colic. The worker develops a headache frequently accompanied by generalized muscle pain. Constipation and abdominal pain develop later, with nausea and even vomiting if obstipation occurs. Diarrhea rather than constipation infrequently may set in. Loss of appetite results in loss of weight and the worker may complain of fatigue and a bad taste in his mouth. The once-claimed "lead line," caused by a lead sulfide deposit along the gingival margin of some or all the teeth, is rare. This is due to better oral hygiene in today's worker and the fact that the diagnosis of lead poisoning is made earlier, usually when the worker consults a physician because of intestinal colic.[30] It is exceptional today for a worker to appear with neuritis, tremor or wrist drop. Stippling of the retina adjacent to the optic disc has been described as an early sign in lead poisoning.[31] Recent studies indicate that the toxic effect of lead on the eyes causes lesions of the optic nerve.[32]

Organic lead intoxication occurs almost exclusively in the petroleum industry and even more specifically in the use of tetraethyl and tetramethyl lead as antiknock agents in gasoline.[33] Tetraethyl lead concentrations in air should be below 0.1 mg per m^3.[29] Massive exposure to this compound nearly always results in the encephalopathic form of intoxication.[29] The toxicity of the tetraalkyl leads is believed to be due to their conversion in the body to the corresponding trialkyl lead derivatives which have a dominant action on the central nervous system.[34]

Lead poisoning in children usually results from the oral ingestion of chips of lead-containing paint or the mouthing of plaster, wallpaper or putty.[35-38] Children who go through an extended period of time with "pica," an abnormal appetite manifesting itself by a compulsive habit of chewing inedible substances, are understandably the primary targets. Although certain lead compounds (e.g., PbS) are relatively insoluble, nevertheless toxic amounts may be dissolved in the body.[2] Ingested lead is absorbed from the gastrointestinal tract, deposited in the liver and subsequently released into the systemic circulation.[29] Small amounts of lead may be ingested over a protracted period before symptoms develop. Since the signs and symptoms of lead poisoning are frequently similar to those of other common childhood diseases, lead poisoning in children is often overlooked.[35] Acute manifestations may develop indicating involvement of the central nervous, gastrointestinal, and/or hematologic systems.[37] The almost invariable hematologic disorder in childhood plumbism is microcytic hypochromic anemia. Lead poisoning should be suspected in any young child with a microcytic hypochromic anemia which does not respond to iron therapy.[37] The gastrointestinal symptoms most commonly encountered are vague abdominal pains, constipation and recurrent vomiting. The most serious form of intoxication is encephalopathy which may present with symptoms varying from undue drowsiness to coma to grand mal. Focal or generalized convulsions with or without fever may occur. According to Smith,[37] plumbism deserves special consideration if convulsions change in a few hours from one side to the other and then become generalized. Encephalopathy has a 25% fatality rate in children; recurrent seizures and significant neurologic defects in survivors of lead encephalopathy, and mental retardation in victims of lead intoxication with or without encephalopathy, are important sequelae.[36, 37]

Laboratory Criteria for Diagnosis

"The manifestations of overt lead poisoning are well documented, but the clinical relevance of the many tests used for its diagnosis has not yet been clearly defined."[39] With the new understanding of the site of action of lead in the synthesis of heme, insight is developing to permit objective criteria to be added to the clinical acumen historically needed to distinguish lead exposure from lead toxicity.[30, 40, 41, 42] The measurement of lead in blood and urine is a finicky procedure requiring a type of care, precision and experience available only in certain reference centers. The criteria of toxicity of Kehoe[20] have been useful as a standard retrospectively, but are not conveniently useful in prospective case finding, as in industrial surveillance or epidemiologic studies.[38] His criteria are:

(1) Urine lead excretion of 0.15 mg/liter means probable absorption of a potentially dangerous quantity of lead,

(2) Whole blood lead of 0.08 mg/100 gm means probable absorption of a potentially dangerous quantity of lead,

(3) It is safe to breathe air with 0.15 mg of lead/cu.meter.

Gibson *et al.*[39] studied 100 lead workers to determine criteria for the distinction of presymptomatic exposure from frank poisoning. They demonstrated no correlation between the tests of absorption of lead (urinary and blood lead levels), and those which measure interference with tissue enzymes (hemoglobin level, urinary coproporphyrin, delta-aminolevinic acid, and porphobilinogen levels). The latter measurements reflect toxicity of lead, since they are significant effects upon hemoglobin metabolism. Their data are in substantial agreement with those of deBruin and Hoolboom[28] who studied 50 Dutch auto workers exposed to lead. Both groups found a high correlation between coproporphyrin and delta-ALA as the earliest manifestations of lead exposure. However, the groups disagree on which substance appears first in the urine. deBruin and Hoolboom's data suggest that ALA excretion increases before coproporphyrin and quote similar observations by Djuric *et al.* and Balbo *et al.*[44] Gibson *et al.*[39] mention unpublished experiments in rabbits which showed urinary coproporphyrin to be the more sensitive response to lead exposure. It rose immediately as compared with one or two weeks of continual dosage before an increased excretion of ALA occurred. Porphobilinogen was found to increase only after several weeks of continual dosage, and only with the onset of symptoms. The presence of coproporphyrinuria is less specific than ALA since it may reflect conditions other than lead exposure.[29, 36, 45] Nevertheless it is useful as a more simple laboratory procedure for following potentially exposed individuals.

Gibson *et al.*'s criteria for lead toxicity are worthy of attention. They are in essential agreement with those of DeBruin and Hoolboom.

Evidence of Toxicity[39]

Measurement	*Danger Level*
Hemoglobin	<13 g %, or falling
Urinary coproporphyrin	>80 μg/100 mg.creatinine (800 μg/liter)
Urinary ALA	>2.0 mg/100 mg.creatinine (2.0mg%)
Blood lead	>60 μg/100 g blood
Urine porphobilinogen	>0.15 mg/100 mg. creatinine (0.15 mg%)

Crepet and Chiesura[46] attempt to distinguish between the intoxication of organic and inorganic lead compounds. These workers suggest that poisoning owing to organic lead causes a significant increase in the levels of free protoporphyrin in erythrocytes while intoxication from exposure to inorganic lead salts tends to increase urinary excretion of ALA and coproporphyrin. In addition, dosage and mode of entry may affect the distribution of lead in the tissues of experimental animals and may account for some of the discrepancies in the literature.[27, 47, 43]

TREATMENT

A number of drugs have been found to be effective in the treatment of lead poisoning. Calcium di-sodium edetate ($CaNa_2$-EDTA) is recognized as the antidote.[49, 50] This compound, administered intravenously, forms a soluble lead chelate which is rapidly eliminated by the kidneys and may yield increased excretions that are 25 to 40 times the normal values.[49, 51] It should be mentioned that prolonged administration of $CaNa_2$-EDTA may produce alterations in the kidneys and liver of experimental animals.[52, 53] D-Penicillamine, administered orally in dosages of 20 to 40 mg per kg per day appears to be without serious side effects and is regarded as the agent of choice for the treatment of moderate lead intoxication.[29, 54, 55] Disodium dimercaptosuccinate has also been found to be effective as an antidote in lead poisoning.[56, 57] It has a low order of toxicity (intraperitoneal LD_{50} in mice = 3.163 g per kg) and is particularly effective in increasing urinary excretion of lead deposited in tissues.[57]

Prevention of lead poisoning in industrial atmospheres where the hazard is known to exist has been promoted to some extent by the giving of free milk to workers.[58] The ingestion of milk appears to reduce the severity of lead poisoning and favors the elimination of lead from the organism and not its deposition into bone.[59]

REFERENCES

1. Bulfinch, T.: The Age of Fable. Heritage Press, New York, 1942.
2. Brieger, H., and Rieders, F.: Chronic lead and mercury poisoning: Contemporary views on ancient occupational diseases. J. Chron. Dis., *9:* (2) 177-84, 1959.

3. Garrison, F. H.: History of medicine, 4th ed., reprinted. W. B. Saunders Co., Phila. and London. 1960, pp. 242, 271, 272, 367.
4. *Ibid.*, p. 361.
5. Editorial: J.A.M.A., *204*:541, 1968. Sir George Baker (1722-1809).
6. Garrison, F. H.: p. 376.
7. Editorial: J.A.M.A., *207*:553-554, 1969.
8. Garrison, F. H.: p. 837.
9. Ramazzini, Bernardini. DeMorbus Artificum. 1700. Compiled by Herman Goodman, M.D., 1933. Medical Lay Press, New York City.
10. Franklin, Benjamin: Letter written about 1784. Arch. Indust. Hlth., *14*:591-592, 1956.
11. Garrison, F. H.: p. 659.
12. Hunter, D.: The Diseases of Occupations. Little Brown and Co., Boston, 1955, p. 219, p. 220.
13. Garrison, F. H.: p. 781.
14. Hunter, D.: p. 220.
15. Schroeder, H. A., and Tipton, I. H.: The human body burden of lead. Arch. Environ. Hlth., *17:* (6) 965-78, 1968.
16. Goldsmith, J. R., and Hexter, A. C.: Respiratory exposure to lead: Epidemiological and experimental dose-response relationships. Science, *158*:132-4, 1967.
17. Thomas, H. V., Milmore, B. K., Heidbreder, G. A., and Kogan, B. A.: Blood levels of persons living near freeways. Arch. Environ. Hlth., *15:* (6) 695-702, 1967.
18. Kehoe, R.A.: Normal metabolism of lead. Arch. Environ. Hlth., *8*:232-235, 1964.
19. Patterson, C.C.: Contaminated and natural lead environments of man. Arch. Environ. Hlth., *11:* 334-360, 1965.
20. Kehoe, R. A.: Metabolism of lead under abnormal conditions. Arch. Environ. Hlth., *8*:235-243, 1964.
21. Haley, T. J.: Chronic lead intoxication from environmental contamination myth or fact? Arch. Environ. Hlth., *12*:781-785, 1966.
22. Kehoe, R. A., Cholak, J., Hubbard, D. M.; Bambach, K., McNary, R. R., and Story, R. V.: Experimental studies on the ingestion of lead compounds. J. Indust. Hyg., *22*:381-400, 1940.
23. Kehoe, A. A.: The Harben Lectures, 1960: The metabolism of lead in man in health and disease, Lecture II, J. Roy Inst. Public Health, *24*:101-120, 129-143, 1961.
24. Kehoe, R. A.: *Ibid.* Lecture III, *24*:177, 203, 1961.
25. Haeger-Aronsen, B.: Studies on urinary excretion of delta-aminolevulinic acid and other haem precursors in lead workers and lead-intoxicated rabbits. Scand. J. Clin. Lab. Invest., *12* (suppl. 47) :1-128, 1960.
26. Tschudy, D. P.: Porphyrin biosynthesis. In, Hemoglobin. Its Precursors and Metabolites (ed., Sunderman, F. W., and Sunderman, F. W., Jr.). J. B. Lippincott Co., Phila., 1964, pp. 159-163.
27. Bonsignore, D., and Cartasegna, C.: The erythrocyte aminolevulinic acid dehydratase in experimental lead poisoning. Lav. Umano, *18:* (12) 529-36, 1966.
28. de Bruin, A., and Hoolboom, H. Early signs of lead-exposure. A comparative study of laboratory tests. Brit. J. Indust. Med., *24*:203-212, 1967.
29. Beeson, P. B., and McDermott, W., ed.: Cecil-Loeb Textbook of Medicine. W. B. Saunders Company, Philadelphia, 1967.
30. Johnstone, R. T.: Clinical inorganic lead intoxication. Arch. Environ. Hlth., *8:* (2) 250-5, 1964.
31. Sonkin, N.: Stippling of the retina. A new physical sign in the early diagnosis of lead poisoning. New Eng. J. Med., *269*:779, 1963.
32. Unseld, D. W.: Lesions of the optic nerve from lead. Med. Welt, *9*:444-5, 1966.
33. Sanders, L. W.: Tetraethyl lead intoxication. Arch. Environ. Hlth., *8:* (2) 270-7, 1964.
34. Cremer, J. E.: Toxicology and biochemistry of alkyl lead compounds. Occp. Hlth Rev., *17:* (3) 14-19, 1965.
35. Schroeder, H. A.: Lead poisoning in children 1950 - 1964. Philadelphia Dept. Public Hlth., July 1964.
36. Davis, J. R., Abrahams, R. H., Fishbein, W. I., and Fabrega, E. A.: Urinary Delta-aminolevulinic acid (ALA) levels in lead poisoning. II. Correlation of ALA values with clinical findings in 250 children with suspected lead ingestion. Arch. Environ. Hlth, *17:* (2) 164-71, 1968.
37. Smith, H. D.: Pediatric lead poisoning. Arch. Environ. Hlth., *8:* (2) 256-61, 1964.
38. Jacobziner, H.: Lead poisoning in childhood; epidemiology, manifestations, and prevention. Clin. Ped., *5*:277-286, 1966.
39. Gibson, S.L.M., Mackenzie, J. C., and Goldberg, A.: The diagnosis of industrial lead poisoning. Brit. J. Industr. Med., *25*:40-51, 1968.
40. Collins, R. P. Difficulties in the evaluation of lead poisoning. Arch. Environ. Hlth., *14*:523-528, 1967.
41. Corrigan, C. E.: Fallacies in the diagnosis of chronic lead poisoning in industry. Manitoba Med. Rev. *47*:559-560, 1967.
42. Rathus, E. M.: The clinical diagnosis of lead poisoning. M. J. Aust., *1*:371-375, 1967.
43. Djuric, D., Novak, L., Milic, S., and Kalic-Filiporic, D.: Med. d. Lavoro., *57:161,* 1966 Quoted by de Bruin and Hoolboom.
44. Balbo, W., Gualdi, G., and Marucci, V.: Folia med. (Napoli), *48*:554, 1965. Quoted by de Bruin and Hoolboom.
45. Saita, G., Morea, L., and Croce, G.: Porphyrin

metabolism in chronic saturnism and in non-saturnine anemias and liver diseases. Med. Lavoro, *57:* (3) 167-74, 1966.

46. Crepet, M., and Chiesura, P.: Porphyrins in tetraethyl lead poisoning. Panminerva Med., *8:* (7-8) 295-301, 1966.
47. Bernthal, I., Faibus, A., Rotaru, N., Negru, T., Rebedea, I., and Mihalcea, F.: Experimental poisoning with salts of lead. Stud. Cercet. Fiziol., *10:* (1) 75-87, 1965.
48. Mole, R., and Pesaresi, C.: Amino-levulinic acid dehydrogenase (ALD) in Human and experimental lead poisoning. Folia Med., *47:* (1) 73-9, 1964.
49. Moeschlin, S.: Poisoning in general practice. Clin. Toxicol., *1:*(2) 149-60, 1968.
50. Chenoweth, M. B.: Clinical uses of metal-binding drugs. Clin. Pharmacol. Ther., *9:* (3) 365-87, 1968.
51. Castellino, N., and Aloj, C.: Effects of calcium sodium ethylenediamine-tetra-acetate on the kinetics of distribution and excretion of lead in the rat. Brit. J. Indust. Med., *22:*172-80, 1965.
52. Sroczynski, J., and Zajusz, K.: Some histochemical reactions in the preventive administration of disodium calcium versenate in experimental lead poisoning in rabbits. Arch. Immunol. Ther. Exp., *15:* (3) 428-34, 1967.
53. Reuber, M. D.: Hepatic lesions in young rats given calcium disodium edetate. Toxicol. Appl. Pharmacol., *11:*321, 1967.
54. Chisolm, Jr., J. J.: The use of chelating agents in the treatment of acute and chronic lead intoxication in childhood. J. Pediat., *73:* (1) 1-38, 1968.
55. Teisinger, J., and Srbova, J.: Effect of D-penicillamine on urinary excretion of mercury and lead. Pracov. Lek., *16:* (10) 433-5, 1964.
56. Tati, M., and Miyata, S.: Use of dimercaptosuccinate in lead poisoning. Igaku to Seibutsugaku, *73:* (1) 35-42, 1966.
57. Matsuda, Y.: Sodium dimercaptosuccinate. Gifu Daigaku Igakuba Kiyo, *15:* (3) 869-88, 1968.
58. Komura, S.: Prevention of lead poisoning in the patenting shop. Wire Prod., *42:* (6) 982-4, 1967.
59. Gontea, I., Sutescu, P., Rujinski, A., and Cocora, D.: Effect of milk on lead retention in experimental lead poisoning. Igiena, *16*: (4) 199-206, 1967.

Chapter 33B

The Dithizone Method for the Measurement of Lead in Biological Fluids

J. HENRY WILKINSON, D.Sc., Ph.D.

INTRODUCTION

Lead intoxication is a well-known industrial hazard especially in the lead-paint and battery manufacturing industries, whose workers are regularly subjected to screening tests for lead in blood or urine. Small children are liable to chew painted wooden surfaces of their toys and furniture and if a lead paint is used (though in many countries this is illegal), they are at risk of lead poisoning. It is essential therefore that methods for the determination of lead in body fluids should be available for the diagnosis of lead poisoning and for following the course of treatment.

The method described in this section is based upon the well-known reaction of dithizone with heavy metals[1, 2] which has been adapted to blood and urine by Bessman and Layne.[3]

PRINCIPLE

Lead is extracted from a basified acid digest with a chloroform solution of diphenylthiocarbazone (dithizone) with which it forms a red complex. Other metals such as copper and iron also form complexes with dithizone but interference can be eliminated by washing the chloroform extract containing the lead-dithizone complex with an ammonium hydroxide-cyanide solution. This washing process also removes excess dithizone. The red color remaining in the extract is determined colorimetrically.

REAGENTS

1. *Digestion Reagent.* Lead-free concentrated sulfuric acid (28 ml) is added to lead-free concentrated nitric acid (70 ml).

2. *Buffer Solution.*[3, 4] Dibasic ammonium citrate (118 gm) is dissolved as quickly as possible in a mixture of concentrated ammonium hydroxide solution (75 ml) and double distilled (or demineralized) water (50 ml). The solution is transferred to a borosilicate measuring cylinder and the volume adjusted to 250 ml with double distilled (or demineralized) water. After cooling to room temperature, potassium cyanide (5 gm) and sodium sulfite (2.5 gm) are added.

At this stage the buffer solution should be tested for its lead content by shaking with the dithizone solution (Reagent No. 6). The chloroform layer should retain its green color. If a red color develops it indicates heavy metal contamination, and extraction with dithizone solution should be repeated until the latter remains green.

The aqueous layer should then be transferred to a 1 liter stoppered borosilicate bottle and mixed with concentrated ammonium hydroxide solution (500 ml).

3. *Wash Reagent.* A freshly prepared solution of potassium cyanide (5 gm) in concentrated ammonium hydroxide (250 ml) and double distilled (or demineralized) water (250 ml).

4. *Phenol Red Indicator,* 0.1 percent.

5. *Perchloric Acid,* C.P. 70 percent (or 60%). Beware of spilling. Any spillage should immediately be flushed with lots of water.

6. *Dithizone Reagent.* Diphenylthiocarbazone (30 mg) is dissolved in one liter of chloroform. The solution should be kept in a brown bottle in the refrigerator.

Standard Solutions 7. *Stock Lead Standard.* Lead acetate trihydrate (36.6 mg) is dissolved in double distilled (or demineralized) water and the volume made up to one liter in a volumetric flask.

8. *Working Standard.* Ten ml of the stock standard is diluted to 100 ml with double distilled (or demineralized) water. One ml contains 2 μg of lead.

Special Apparatus 1. *Digestion-extraction tubes.* Borosilicate glass digestion tubes (25 x 200 mm) fitted with 24/40 standard taper joints and stoppers. The overall lengths of the tubes are 260 mm.

2. *Glass beads,* borosilicate or silica. They should be washed successively with glacial acetic acid, tap water, distilled water, and finally with double distilled (or demineralized) water, or alternatively with glacial acetic acid and three rinses with demineralized water.

3. *Digestion rack.*

PROCEDURE

1. For blood, digestion tubes are prepared according to the following scheme:

	Test	*Blank*	*Standard*
Oxalated blood	2 ml	—	—
Oxalated water	—	2 ml	—
Demineralized water	—	—	1 ml
Working standard	—	—	1 ml
Digestion reagent	5 ml	5 ml	5 ml
Glass beads	3 or 4	3 or 4	3 or 4

For urine, digestion tubes are prepared as follows:

	Test	*Blank*	*Standard*
Urine	10 ml	—	—
Demineralized water	—	10 ml	9 ml
Working standard	—	—	1 ml
Digestion reagent	5 ml	5 ml	5 ml
Glass beads	3 or 4	3 or 4	3 or 4

2. The contents of the tubes are digested until dense white fumes appear (1 to 1½ hours).

3. After cooling for about 5 minutes, 20 drops of perchloric acid are added.

4. Digestion is then continued until the digest has completed the following changes: yellow, colorless, yellow with frothing, and finally colorless. With blood specimens the digest may remain faintly yellow. The time required for this stage varies according to the source of heat, but in the writer's laboratory where electrically heated Kjeldahl furnaces are used, about 2 to 2½ hours are needed. Gas heated furnaces generally give quicker digestion.

5. After cooling, demineralized water (5 ml) is added to each digestion tube. The contents are mixed by swirling and 1 drop of phenol red indicator is added. Concentrated ammonium hydroxide is

then added with cooling in ice-cold water until the phenol red remains red. About 4 to 5 ml is required.

When determining lead in blood, operations 6, 7, and 8 should be carried out within a minute or two. A yellow color, believed to be due to a complex of iron cyanide and dithizone, develops in the chloroform layer on prolonged standing and the dithizone-chloroform mixture becomes incapable of extracting lead. Thus it is best to perform steps 6, 7, and 8 with not more than two tubes at a time.

No such difficulties occur with urine.

6. Buffer solution (10 ml) is added and mixed by swirling. Without delay, dithizone solution (3 ml) is added, the tube is stoppered and shaken vigorously in a horizontal direction about 20 times. Shaking on a vortex mixer for about 20 seconds is satisfactory.

If the dithizone-chloroform layer is colored red, indicating the presence of about 10 μg or more of lead in the specimen, another 3 ml of the dithizone solution should be added and shaking repeated.

7. The upper aqueous layer is removed as quickly and completely as possible without loss of the chloroform layer. Suction from a water-pump is suitable for this purpose.

8. If additional dithizone solution has not been necessary, chloroform (3 ml) is now added. The combined chloroform solution is then washed by shaking 20 times (as in 6 above) or on a vortex mixer with 10 ml wash reagent. The supernatant layer is removed by suction.

9. The chloroform layer is transferred to a colorimeter cuvette, preferably stoppered, and allowed to stand 5 to 10 minutes until clear. Clearing can be accelerated by gentle centrifugation or by placing the cuvettes in a 37° water-bath.

10. The absorbance (A) is read at 510 nm against chloroform in a suitable spectrophotometer.

11. *Calculation*

For Blood

$$\text{Lead content} = \frac{A_T - A_B}{A_S - A_B} \times 100\ \mu\text{g per 100 ml}$$

For Urine

$$\text{Lead content} = \frac{A_T - A_B}{A_S - A_B} \times 200\ \mu\text{g per liter}$$

DISCUSSION

Lead is rather a ubiquitous impurity, traces being found in foods, water supplies and chemicals of all descriptions. Though limit tests are prescribed, the amounts of lead found in laboratory reagents and in water are often sufficient to necessitate further purification before they can be used in the analysis of lead in blood and urine.

Ordinary distilled water is frequently contaminated by foaming or splashing in the still and a second distillation is needed to produce lead-free distilled water of the required quality. Alternatively demineralized water prepared by treatment with an ion-exchange resin (The Crystalab Deeminizer is an example of a suitable system).

The Bessman-Layne method described has the important advantage over earlier procedures in that all manipulations up to the final colorimetry are performed in the digestion tube. The separating funnels formerly used are no longer needed, and as quantitative transfers are eliminated an important source of inaccuracy is removed.

The authors[3] have demonstrated that the lead-dithizone color reaction obeys Beer's law at concentrations up to 10 μg per tube, and that the recovery of lead added to blood and urine is about 95%. The differences between duplicate determinations on blood averaged 7.5% while the mean of the corresponding figures for urine was 3.9%.

SOURCES OF ERROR

1. *Contamination of apparatus.* Glassware should be washed with a detergent, rinsed first with ordinary distilled water, then thoroughly with demineralized water.

2. *Contamination of water.* Double distilled or demineralized water should be used for all aqueous reagents.

3. *Other metals.* Copper and iron-dithizone complexes are removed with the wash reagent at stage 8 of the procedure. If the presence of bismuth is suspected, this can be removed at stage 5 by adding ammonium hydroxide to the digestion solution to about pH 3.4 and extracting with dithizone solution (5 ml). The chloroform layer is completely removed and discarded, after which the phenol red is added and basification continued.

4. *Losses due to sputtering during digestion.* A small beaker should be placed over the mouth of each digestion tube during stage 4.

NORMAL RANGES

Blood: 0 to 32 μg per 100 ml.
Urine: less than 80 μg per 24 hours.

RESUME OF CLINICAL INTERPRETATIONS

Values in excess of the normal ranges are indicative of excessive ingestion of lead. In some individuals, toxic symptoms may appear with blood levels in the 30 to 40 μg per 100 ml range, but others have remained symptomless with levels of about 100 μg per 100 ml.[5] The urinary output can reach 300 μg per 24 hours in acute lead poisoning, but when exposure to lead ceases, values return to normal within a few weeks.

Determination of lead in body fluids is also valuable for following the course of therapy in the treatment of lead poisoning with chelating agents such as calcium ethylenediamine-tetraacetate.[3]

REFERENCES

1. Fischer, H.: Uber den Nachweis von Schwermetallen mit Hilfe von "Dithizon". Z. Angew. Chem., *42:*1025-1027, 1929.
2. Bambach, K., and Burkey, R. E.: Microdetermination of lead by dithizone with an improved lead-bismuth separation. Indust. Eng. Chem., Anal. Ed., *14:*904-907, 1942.
3. Bessman, S. P., and Layne, E. C., Jr.: A rapid procedure for the determination of lead in blood or urine in the presence of organic chelating agents. J. Lab. Clin. Med., *45:*159-166,1955.
4. Amdur, M. O.: Rapid determination of lead in old urine samples. Arch. Indust. Hyg., *7:*277-281, 1953.
5. Tompsett, S. L., and Anderson, A. B.: Lead-Poisoning. Lead Content of Blood and of Excreta. Lancet, *1:*559-562, 1939.

Chapter 33C

Determination of Lead by Atomic Absorption Spectrophotometry

M. LUBRAN, M.D.

INTRODUCTION

Atomic absorption spectrophotometry, which combines specificity with sensitivity, has proved satisfactory for the measurement of trace quantities of metals in biological material. The theory and general applications of the technique will not be given here, — they have been adequately described in recent books and articles.[1-4] The particular application of atomic absorption to the measurement of low concentrations of lead in blood and urine described in this article has been based to a large degree on the work of Berman and co-workers[5, 6] and Hessel,[7] although many other investigators have described suitable methods. Some changes have been made, in order to make the methods more suitable for routine work; for the same reason, the description of the procedures has been simplified; in particular, the mode of use of the atomic absorption spectrophotometer has been described in some detail.

Although atomic absorption provides adequate specificity, with little interference from other metals, the very low concentration of trace elements found in biological material is often at the lower limit of detection by this technique. In general, it is necessary to concentrate the metal. A satisfactory procedure is to chelate the metal and extract it into an organic solvent. In addition to concentration, chelation and solvent extraction removes interfering anions and provides a medium of constant composition; standard and blank solutions can then be readily prepared in the same medium as the test material.

Instrumentation becomes of great importance when trace quantities are to be measured. High intensity hollow cathode lamps should be used; the spectrophotometer should have great stability (double beam instruments are satisfactory), and sensitive detectors. It is usually necessary to amplify the signal, both by scale expansion within the instrument and by an external recorder. Stability and sensitivity are improved by the use of a three slot burner (Boling burner), suitable for burning a mixture of acetylene and air. There is not much to be gained in the determination of lead by burning a mixture of nitrous oxide and acetylene. The techniques described here are based on the use of a Perkin-Elmer 303 atomic absorption spectrophotometer; however, any equivalent instrument can be used. It is necessary to employ a recorder with a fast response time, as the signal to be recorded may last only a few seconds. A molten cathode lead lamp (e.g., P-E "Intensitron") should be used.

An important part of trace element analysis is sample preparation. Most atomic absorption techniques require the element to be in solution, which is then aspirated into the flame through an atomiser. Recently, a method has been described in which the dry sample is combusted; indeed, much work is now being carried out on flameless methods of atomic absorption analysis.[8] These procedures are, so far, experimental — established techniques still require the metal be in solution.

Tissue lead can be put into solution by either dry ashing at a low temperature, or by digestion with a mixture of sulphuric and nitric acids. Complete destruction of organic matter is not essential, as the lead is liberated from organic combination before all organic matter has been destroyed. Wet digestion introduces considerable errors through the contamination of the reagents with lead — consequently, the blanks are high. Dry ashing is preferable, but is time consuming. Further, it may not be possible to recover all the lead from the vessel in which the ashing is carried out. Detailed information on the treatment of tissues can be found in the book by Sandell.[9] Whatever procedure is used, the solution obtained should be neutralised and then treated by the procedure given for measuring lead in urine. Appropriate reagent blanks should be run.

Lead in blood is found mainly in the erythrocytes where it is protein-bound; it is therefore important to use whole blood for the analysis. Heparin is the best anticoagulant; EDTA must not be used; the other anticoagulants may contain significant amounts of lead. The metal may be freed from protein combination by treatment with trichloroacetic acid, which both frees the lead and precipitates the protein; or, it may be freed by a strong detergent. Both procedures will be described. No special treatment of urine is necessary, unless it contains large amounts of protein. The trichloroacetic acid procedure should then be employed. In patients treated with EDTA, the lead in the urine is excreted as the EDTA complex. Extraction procedures using chelating agents do not give complete recovery of the lead. However, as the concentration of lead in the urine of these patients is usually high, it is satisfactory to aspirate the urine, without previous treatment, directly into the flame, using aqueous standards of lead. Errors due to the high salt content of the urine can be reduced by dilution of the urine, or by use of special devices which compensate for the flame effect.

In trace metal procedures, whether the element is measured by a color reaction or by atomic absorption spectrophotometry, particular attention must be paid to the cleanliness and nature of the glassware used. Borosilicate glass should be used. It must not be assumed, without verification, that plasticware is lead free. Glassware should be thoroughly washed with hot water, then soaked for about an hour in a hot solution of non-ionic detergent and then rinsed with deionised water. Next, the glassware is completely immersed in 50% (v/v) nitric acid for about 30 minutes, then thoroughly rinsed with deionised water, dried and wrapped, to exclude atmospheric contamination.

DETERMINATION OF LEAD IN URINE[3]

Principle

Lead is chelated with sodium diethyldithiocarbamate and the complex extracted into methylisobutyl ketone, which is aspirated into the flame. Standard solutions of lead are treated similarly.

REAGENTS

1. *Methyl Isobutylketone (4-methyl-2-pentanone).* The solvent *must* be saturated with water. The pure solvent and the water saturated solvent are aspirated at different rates into the flame for a given air flow. The solvent should be vigorously shaken with two or three times its volume of deionised water, the phases allowed to separate, and the upper phase (referred to as MIBK) stored in a tightly-stoppered bottle. It keeps indefinitely.
2. *Sodium Diethyldithiocarbamate Solution,* 1% (w/v) in deionised water. It keeps indefinitely, if stored in a dark bottle at 4 to 6°.
3. *1 N Hydrochloric acid.*
4. *1 N Sodium Hydroxide Solution.*

STANDARD SOLUTIONS

1. *Stock Lead Solution (1 mg Pb per ml).* Exactly 0.7992 gm of reagent grade lead nitrate are dissolved in deionised water to a volume of 500 ml. The solutions keep indefinitely.
2. *Working Standard Solutions* (50, 100, 200, 300 μg Pb per 100 ml). These are prepared, as required, by appropriate dilution of the stock lead solution. In order to avoid the use of large quantities of water, it is convenient to prepare an intermediate standard, containing 10 μg Pb per ml, by diluting the stock lead solution to one-hundredth of its strength. The working standard solutions do not keep well; they should be discarded at the end of the day's work.

PROCEDURE

Fifty ml of urine are pipetted into a 100-ml glass-stoppered tube, the pH adjusted to 6.5 to 7 (pH paper) with hydrochloric acid or sodium hydroxide solution, 3 ml of 1 percent sodium diethyldithiocarbamate solution are added, and the tube shaken to mix its contents. Exactly 3 ml of MIBK are then added, the tube is stoppered, and shaken vigorously for two minutes, then centrifuged to separate the phases (alternatively, a separatory funnel may be used, — in this case, complete separation of the phases may not be achieved; it will then be necessary to centrifuge the upper phase). A smaller volume of urine may be used, if the lead content is expected to exceed 3 μg per ml. The MIBK (upper) phase is transferred to a clean, narrow tube for aspiration into the flame. A reagent blank is prepared by treating 50 ml of deionised water similarly. A standard calibration curve is prepared by diluting exactly 5 ml of each working standard to about 50 ml with deionised water (carry this out in a 100-ml tube) and treating this solution in the same way as the urine samples. Details of the use of the spectrophotometer and calculation of the concentration of lead in the urine are given in the blood lead procedure.

Determination of Lead in Blood

A. WITH PRECIPITATION OF PROTEIN

Principle

Lead is freed from combination with protein by trichloroacetic acid, which also precipitates the protein. The lead is chelated with sodium diethyldithiocarbamate and extracted into MIBK.

Reagents

1. *Trichloroacetic Acid, 10% (w/v) in deionised water.*
2. *Trichloroacetic Acid, 5% (w/v) in deionised water.*
3. *2.5 N Sodium Hydroxide Solution.*
4. *Bromphenol Blue Solution,* 0.1% (w/v) in ethanol.
5. *Sodium Diethyldithiocarbamate Solution.*
6. *MIBK.*

Reagents 5 and 6 and the standard lead solutions are prepared as described in the urine lead method.

Procedure

Macro-method.[3] To 10 ml of 5 percent trichloroacetic acid in a 25-ml round-bottomed tube are added, dropwise with mechanical mixing (e.g., a Vortex mixer), 5 ml of well-mixed, heparinished, whole blood. The tube is set aside for not less than one hour, after which it is centrifuged at high speed to pack the precipitate tightly. The supernatant is decanted as completely as possible into a 50-ml stoppered tube. The precipitate is broken-up with a thin, glass rod and washed with 10 ml of 5% trichloroacetic acid. The tube is then recentrifuged and the supernatants combined. One drop of bromphenol blue solution is added to the combined supernatants, the pH of which is then adjusted to 6.5 to 7 with 2.5 N NaOH (about 1.5 ml); 1 ml of sodium diethyldithiocarbamate solution is added, followed by 3 ml of MIBK. The tube is stoppered and shaken vigorously by hand for about two minutes. A reagent blank is prepared by carrying 20 ml of 5% trichloroacetic acid through the neutralisation, chelation, and extraction procedures. A standard calibration curve is prepared by adding 5 ml of each of the respective working standard solutions to 20 ml of 5% trichloroacetic acid. The diluted standards are then treated in the same way as the reagent blank. After extraction into MIBK, the tubes are centrifuged and the supernatant MIBK transferred to clean, narrow tubes for aspiration into the flame. The volume of blood can be reduced to 2 ml, the total volume of trichloroacetic acid to 8 ml and the volume of MIBK to 1 ml. If less blood is available, the micromethod should be used.

Micro-method.[4] Exactly 0.25 ml of heparanised whole blood are washed into 1 ml of deionised water in a 10 x 75 mm tube and mixed until hemolysis is complete; then 1 ml of 100% trichloroacetic acid is added dropwise, with mechanical mixing. The tube is covered with Parafilm, and set aside for not less than one hour, during which time it is shaken at intervals of about 20 minutes. It is then centrifuged, and the supernatant decanted quantitatively into a 13 x 100 mm tube. The precipitate is broken up with a fine glass rod, and the rod, precipitate, and walls of the tube washed with 1 ml of 5% trichloroacetic acid to which has been added one drop of bromphenol blue solution. After recentrifugation, the supernatants are combined and the pH adjusted to 6.5 to 7 with 2.5 N NaOH (about 0.2 ml). Exactly 0.2 ml of 1% sodium diethyldithiocarbamate solution and 1 ml of MIBK are then added to the neutralised supernatants, the tube is sealed with a stopper covered with Saran wrap (or similar plastic insoluble in MIBK) and shaken vigorously by hand for about one minute. After centrifugation to separate the phases, the MIBK layer is transferred as completely as possible to a small, narrow tube for aspiration into the flame. It is possible, after practice, to aspirate the MIBK supernatant layer without previous transfer. Standards and the reagent blank are prepared by carrying 0.25 ml of each working standard solution and deionised water through the procedure. More conveniently, although with slightly less accuracy, 0.25 ml of standard and water can be added to 3 ml of 5% trichloroacetic acid, which is then neutralised, chelated, and extracted.

B. WITHOUT PROTEIN PRECIPITATION[5]

Principle

Whole blood is rapidly hemolysed by the addition of a detergent Triton X-100, which also liberates lead from combination with protein. The lead is chelated with ammonium pyrrolidine dithiocarbamate and extracted into methyl isobutyl ketone.

Reagents

1. *Triton X-100,* 5 percent (v/v) in deionised water.
2. *Ammonium pyrrolidine dithiocarbamate,* (ammonium 1-pyrrolidine-carbodithioate, or APDC). Two percent (w/v) in deionised water.
3. *MIBK* (methyl isobutyl ketone).
4. *Lead Stanadard Solutions.* Reagent 3 and the lead standard solutions are prepared as described in the urine lead method.

Procedure

Into each of five 16 x 130 mm tubes are pipetted 5 ml of water or working standard solutions; 5 ml of well-mixed heparinised whole blood are pipetted into a sixth tube. To each tube is added, dropwise, 1 ml of Triton X-100 solution, while the tube is rapidly agitated on a mechanical mixer (e.g., a Vortex mixer). Rapid hemolysis is essential. One ml of APDC solution is then added to each tube followed by 5 ml of MIBK. The tubes are sealed with a stopper covered with Saran wrap and shaken vigorously by hand for about one minute. They are then centrifuged to separate the phases, and the upper layer is transferred to a clean, narrow tube for aspiration into the flame. The volume of blood can be reduced to 1 ml with corresponding reductions in the volumes of the other reagents.

Method of Use of the Atomic Absorption Spectrophotometer with MIBK

Because MIBK acts as a fuel, thereby reducing the requirement for acetylene, a special technique is needed for the measurement of lead in MIBK solution. Details will be given for the Perkin-Elmer 303 instrument; similar considerations apply to other instruments.

The apparatus is adjusted as follows: hollow cathode lead lamp at 30 ma; slit — 4; scale expansion — 5; noise suppression — 2; resonance line at 2833 A; chart speed — 0.75″ per minute. The burner is lit under normal conditions and the acetylene flow reduced until the flame is almost colorless. At this stage, the aspiration of *water-saturated* MIBK is started. The flame becomes yellow. The acetylene flow is now further reduced to 3.5 to 4 on the flowmeter and the air flow adjusted until all traces of yellow have disappeared from the flame (about 7 to 8 on the flow meter). The flame may lift at the edges from the burner head during the adjustments; should this happen, the air flow should be slightly increased to prevent the flame from blowing out. After the final adjustments have been made, the burner must not be allowed to operate for more than a few seconds without MIBK being aspirated, as the very hot flame will otherwise damage the burner head.

As maximum sensitivity is required, it is worthwhile spending some time to obtain optimum flame conditions. It is convenient to aspirate a MIBK solution containing 3 μg Pb per ml in order to obtain the best flame. The percentage absorption should be noted, so that conditions can be repeated on future occasions. The instrument should not be finally adjusted until all solutions are ready for aspiration. After final adjustment, MIBK should be aspirated and a steady base line established on the recorder. The solutions should then be aspirated without delay, MIBK being aspirated between samples until the pen returns to the base line. Each sample must be aspirated until a peak appears; as the volume of solvent may be as small as 1 ml, a fast response time for the recorder is essential. Linear chart paper calibrated in percent should be used.

CALCULATION

A calibration curve can be obtained by plotting peak height against concentration of lead in the corresponding standard or blank solution. From this curve, the concentration of lead in the test solution can be obtained by interpolation. The calibration curve obtained by this method is not linear. It is better, therefore, to divide the peak height (expressed as percent absorption) by 5 (the scale expansion factor) and convert the answer to absorbance by means of the tables provided with the instrument or by the formula:

$$\text{absorbance} = 2 - \log_{10}(100 - \text{corrected percent absorption}).$$

The absorbance of the blank is subtracted from the other absorbances. A linear calibration curve passing through the origin is obtained by plotting the corrected absorbance of the standard against its concentration. From this curve, the concentration of lead in the test solutions can be obtained. This concentration is the same as the concentration of lead in the blood in the blood methods, in which equal volumes of blood and sample are used. In the urine method, the concentration obtained from the calibration curve must be divided by ten to give the concentration of lead in the urine. Appropriate factors must be used if different volumes of urine or blood are used.

DISCUSSION

The principles of the methods and the precautions to be taken to ensure reliable results have been described. The major source of error in the blood methods is incomplete extraction of the lead. Care must be taken, in the precipitation methods, to ensure a fine, granular precipitate, which must be thoroughly broken up in the re-extraction stage. The Triton X-100 method avoids these difficulties. It is the preferred method, but has not yet been adapted to very small volumes of blood. The concentration of lead in MIBK in the micromethod is one quarter of that in the macromethod. The precision of the micromethod is thus lower than that of the macromethod. As large a volume of blood as possible should be used. Sensitivity may be improved when the newer methods of introduction of the sample into the flame, and flameless methods, have been worked out. The measurement of lead in the blood and urine of patients receiving EDTA therapy presents some problems. Urine may be aspirated directly into the flame, as described previously. However, it has proved unsatisfactory to aspirate blood directly, even after hemolysis and precipitation of proteins. The lead of blood is often incompletely extracted in the presence of EDTA. The problem will not be completely extracted in the presence of EDTA. The problem will not be completely solved until solid sample techniques become practicable.

RANGE OF VALUES IN HEALTH AND DISEASE

Concentrations of lead in the blood and urine of subjects not exposed to lead are lower when measured by atomic absorption spectrophotometry than by colorimetry. Whole blood levels are less than 20 μg per 100 ml in healthy unexposed subjects; concentrations greater than 60 μg per 100 ml are abnormal and characteristic of lead poisoning; intermediate values are in keeping with exposure to lead, not necessarily with toxicity. Healthy unexposed subjects excrete less than 100 μg of lead daily in the urine; most excrete less than 40 μg a day. As lead is deposited in bones, from which it is transmitted gradually to the urine, chronic lead poisoning can coexist with apparently normal values of blood and urine lead. However, during treatment with chelating agents or parathyroid hormone, lead is mobilised and the urinary excretion increases; blood lead may not rise as dramatically, but an elevation is usually present. Repeated determinations of urinary lead excretion provide a better guide to the success of therapy than blood lead measurements. Determination of blood lead is of greater value in the diagnosis of acute lead poisoning. Very little lead is found in plasma; whole blood should always be examined.

REFERENCES

1. Robinson, J. W.: Atomic Absorption Spectroscopy. Marcel Dekker, Inc., New York, 1966.
2. Elwell, W. T., and Gidley, J. A. F.: Atomic Absorption Spectophotometry, 2nd ed. Permagon, New York, 1966.
3. Willis, J. B., The analysis of biological materials by atomic-absorption spectroscopy. Clin. Chem., *11:*251-258, 1965.
4. Kahn, H. L.: Principles and practice of atomic absorption. Trace inorganics in water. Adv. Chem. Ser., *73:*183-229, 1968.
5. Berman, E.: The determination of lead in blood and urine by atomic absorption spectrometry. Atomic absorption newsletter, *3:*111-113, 1964.
6. Berman, E., Valavanis, V., and Dubin, A.: A micromethod for determination of lead in blood. Clin. Chem., *14:*239-242, 1968.
7. Hessel, D. W.: A simple and rapid quantitative determination of lead in blood. Atomic absorption newsletter, *7:*55-56, 1968.
8. Koirtyohann, S. R.: Recent developments in atomic absorption and flame emission spectroscopy. Atomic absorption newsletter, *6:*77-84, 1967.
9. Sandell, E. B.: Colorimetric determination of traces of metals, 3rd ed. Interscience Publishers, New York, 1959, pp. 579-583.

Chapter 34A

Inorganic Arsenic Intoxication

ROBERT A. KYLE, M.D.

Arsenic has been a favorite poisoning agent for more than 2,000 years. The absence of taste or smell makes it easy to put in the victim's food or drink. Although many people believe that arsenic poisoning is uncommon now, my colleagues and I have seen a number of such patients in our practice.

Acute arsenic poisoning is characterized by burning and dryness of the oral cavity, esophagus, and stomach. Nausea, abdominal pain, protracted vomiting, and diarrhea frequently follow. Oliguria, shock, and death occur in severe cases. Occasionally, restlessness, vertigo, muscle spasm, delirium, and coma occur. Conjunctivitis and swelling of the face (particularly the eyelids) have been seen.

Chronic arsenic intoxication is manifested by malaise and fatigue. Intermittent nausea, vomiting, and diarrhea are prominent features. The patient may recognize that symptoms began shortly after eating food or drinking coffee. Hyperpigmentation is common and usually involves the skin of the face, trunk, or extremities. Occasionally, pigmentation of the buccal mucosa occurs, and this plus weakness and fatigue indicates the possibility of Addison's disease. Hyperkeratosis of the palms and soles is not uncommon. Epitheliomas may develop years later. Paresthesias and numbness, frequently in a symmetric stocking-glove distribution, and muscular weakness are common features. The peripheral neuropathy that involves both sensory and motor modalities may be so severe that the patient is unable to walk. This peripheral neuropathy is the most significant problem after ingestion of arsenic has been stopped and frequently prevents normal activity for many months. Splenomegaly of modest degree may appear. This regresses when arsenic ingestion is discontinued. Mees' lines are transverse pale bands of the fingernails or toenails and appear 4 to 6 weeks after arsenic poisoning. These lines also may be seen after the ingestion of other poisons, such as thallium or fluorides.

Anemia is moderate and basically normocytic and normochromic, although some hypochromasia may be seen. Considerable anisopoikilocytosis and increased polychromasia are present in the peripheral blood smear. Basophilic stippling is prominent and is seen in virtually all cases. Rouleau formation is minimal. My colleagues and I have seen levels of normoblasts as high as 8% and have seen myeloid immaturity in many patients. An elevated level of reticulocytes and an increased disappearance of chromium-tagged red cells indicate a hemolytic component. Disturbed production of erythrocytes, indicated by bone-marrow changes, also has a role in the anemia. Thus, the anemia is probably from a combination of increased destruction and decreased production of the red cells.

Leukopenia (Table 1) is prominent, and three of our six patients had a leukocyte level of less than 1,000/cu mm. Leukopenia most often is a result of a decrease in neutrophils although the number of lymphocytes also is decreased. Despite the pronounced neutropenia, bacterial infections are not a significant clinical problem. Frequently, eosinophilia is mentioned in arsenic poisoning, but there are few data supporting absolute increases in these cells. All six of our patients had eosinophil counts of 6% or greater, but only one patient had absolute eosinophilia. Thrombocytopenia may occur but is rarely, if ever, severe enough to produce bleeding.

TABLE 1. LABORATORY DATA IN SIX CASES OF ARSENIC INTOXICATION

Case No.	*Hemoglobin gm/100 ml*	*Leukocytes x10³*	*Neutrophils %*	*Eosinophils %*	*Platelets x10³*
1	14.8*	0.45	7	19	Decreased
2	10.0	1.4	61	7	72
3	7.9	0.70	51	6	36
4	10.5	0.75	21	21	119
5	9.1	1.6	33	13	...
6	10.7*	2.1	39	9	211

*Had received blood transfusions.

The most striking change in the bone marrow is an increase in erythropoiesis. It is predominantly normoblastic, but a few megaloblastoid forms are seen. Karyorrhexis, producing an irregular pyknotic nucleus, is a prominent feature in the polychromatic and orthochromatic normoblasts. Increased numbers of mitotic figures are seen, and occasional binucleated red-cell precursors are present. Partial "maturation arrest" of granulocytic elements is common. This may well represent increased utilization of the more mature granulocytic elements rather than an arrest in maturation. The overall cellularity of the marrow is generally normal.

The hemoglobin value and leukocyte and platelet counts usually return to normal levels in 2 or 3 weeks provided that exposure to arsenic is discontinued.

The diagnosis of arsenic poisoning is confirmed by the finding of increased amounts of arsenic in the urine, hair, or nails. The Gutzeit method is the standard procedure for the determination of arsenic. Arsenic is found in a trivalent form in the body and is oxidized to the pentavalent state by sulfuric acid and nitric acid in the Gutzeit method. Stannous chloride reduces arsenic to the trivalent form, and the trivalent atom is combined with hydrogen from the action of acid on zinc to form arsine. Arsine is trapped in mercuric bromide, which produces an orange color. The absorption is determined in a spectrophotometer and compared with known standards. Our laboratory uses a modified Gutzeit procedure with perchloric acid instead of sulfuric acid and silver diethyl dithiocarbamate in pyridine rather than mercuric bromide. We believe that this modification increases the reproducibility of the determination, with only a small loss of sensitivity.

Normal values of arsenic in a 24-hour urine specimen have been reported to range from 0.00 to a mean of 0.126 mg/liter[4-6] in patients without a known exposure to arsenic (Table 2). Thus, urine containing more than 0.2 mg/liter is abnormal and strongly suggestive of arsenic poisoning.

TABLE 2. ARSENIC CONTENT IN URINE, HAIR, AND NAILS OF SIX PATIENTS WITH ARSENIC INTOXICATION

Case No.	*In Urine mg/L*	*In Hair mg/100 gm*	*In Nails mg/100 gm*
1	1.65	1.76	2.58
2	0.68	8.5	42.0
3	0.348	4.2	9.7
4	3.46	2.7	0
5	1.7	5.0	7.0
6	3.36	7.1	0.415
Normal	Less than 0.2	Less than 0.1	Less than 0.1

Because arsenic is deposited in the hair and nails, these are excellent tissues to study when the condition is suspected. Arsenic has been found in the hair as early as 30 hours and as late as 9 years after ingestion of the poison.[7] Normal values are variable and range from 0.025 to 0.10 mg/100 gm of hair.[1-3] A reasonable normal value would be less than 0.10 mg/100 gm of hair.

The differential diagnosis of arsenic intoxication must include thallium poisoning because of the similarity of clinical symptoms. The gastrointestinal symptoms of thallium intoxication may closely resemble those from arsenic, but the onset of symptoms in thallium intoxication is delayed for 12 to 24 hours. Alopecia is much more common in thallium poisoning. The presence of hematologic abnormalities and hyperkeratosis is suggestive of arsenic poisoning rather than thallium intoxication. Lead poisoning differs clinically from arsenic intoxication by the presence of a lead line and wrist drop rather than a bilateral peripheral neuropathy with predominant sensory involvement. Increased urinary excretion of coproporphyrin is indicative of lead poisoning. The Guillain-Barré syndrome may be confused with the neuropathy of arsenic intoxication, but the gastrointestinal symptoms, hyperpigmentation, and hyperkeratoses should easily help to differentiate these entities. Cranial-nerve involvement and high protein content in the spinal fluid are more indicative of Guillain-Barré syndrome. In spite of these points, this syndrome was diagnosed initially in two of our patients with arsenic poisoning. Addison's disease may resemble arsenic intoxication superficially, but the presence of hyperkeratoses and peripheral neuropathy strongly indicates the latter. The differentiation of arsenic poisoning from intoxication by some other metal such as mercury or gold and from the neuropathies of periarteritis nodosa, alcoholism, and diabetes mellitus is usually not difficult.

In patients with arsenic poisoning, one must exclude therapeutic agents such as Fowler's solution which contains potassium arsenite, as well as rodent poisons and insecticides. The source of arsenic poisoning is infrequently discovered and may involve the efforts of the homicide department. One of our patients recalled that nausea, vomiting, abdominal pain, and diarrhea developed whenever he and his wife had guests. His wife later admitted that she put ant poison containing arsenic in his tea or coffee before any family gathering or social function because she was extremely jealous of him and did not want him talking to other people. Another of our patients did not have further symptoms after she refused to return to her husband, a pharmacist and pharmaceutical salesman, and she divorced him subsequently. Still another patient had no more gastrointestinal symptoms after divorcing his wife. This patient, a fruit farmer, had used a spray containing arsenic for his apples. The symptoms, however, did not coincide with the spraying and analysis of the apples did not show significant amounts of arsenic. The personal physician of another of our patients believed that marital discord had a part in the patient's arsenic intoxication. One of my colleagues had a patient to whom his wife brought milk shakes spiked with large amounts of arsenic. Recently, she was convicted in criminal court for attempted murder. Thus, the etiology is not always found, but the spouse is commonly suspected.

Treatment of arsenic intoxication consists of BAL (Britsh anti-Lewisite or dimercaprol) 2.5 mg/kg every 4 to 6 hours for 1 to 2 days and then twice daily for approximately 10 days. Gastric lavage and saline cathartics should be given if the poisoning is acute.

Arsenic intoxication is simple to diagnose when the symptoms are classic and the possibility is considered. However, the frequent presenting symptoms of fatigue, malaise, nausea, vomiting, and diarrhea are so nonspecific that the possibility is generally not considered until the more obvious findings of pigmentation, keratosis, and peripheral neuropathy indicate the proper diagnosis. Ordinarily, arsenic intoxication is not considered when thrombocytopenia, severe leukopenia (neutropenia), or anemia is present. Arsenic can cause these abnormalities, however, and should be considered in all cases of pancytopenia.

REFERENCES

1. Camp, W. J. R., and Gant, V. A.: Arsenic content of normal hair in Chicago area. Federation Proc., *8*:279, 1949.
2. Fordyce, J. A., Rosen, I., and Myers, C. N.: Quantitative studies in syphilis from clinical and biological point of view. II. Normal arsenic. Arch. Int. Med. (Chicago), *31*:739-757, 1923.
3. Herman, F. A.: Arsenic content of hair. Canad. M. A. J., *71*:496, 1954.
4. Pinto, S. S., and McGill, C. M.: Arsenic trioxide exposure in industry. Indust. Med., *22*:281-287, 1953.
5. Watrous, R. M., and McCaughey, M. B.: Occupational exposure to arsenic In manufacture of arsphenamine and related compounds. Indust. Med., *14*:639-646, 1945.
6. Webster, S. H.: Lead and arsenic content of urines from 46 persons with no known exposure to lead or arsenic. Public Health Rep., *56*:1953-1961, 1941.
7. Young, E. G., and Smith, R. P.: Arsenic content of hair and bone in acute and chronic arsenical poisoning: Review of two cases examined posthumously from medicolegal aspect. Brit. Med. J., *1*:251-253, 1942.

Chapter 34B

Determination of Arsenic in Urine

J. M. KAUFFMAN, M.S., and
F. WILLIAM SUNDERMAN, M.D., PH.D.

INTRODUCTION

This procedure is recommended for the determination of trace amounts of arsenic in urine. Both inorganic and organically bound arsenic are included in the determination. Recoveries of the order of 90 to 100 percent have been obtained for urine, over the range of 0.25 to 1.0 mg per liter.

PRINCIPLE

The urine sample is concentrated then digested using a magnesium oxide-magnesium nitrate slurry. The resultant ash is dissolved in 1:1 hydrochloric acid then reacted with metallic zinc and acid in a Fisher arsenic generator to liberate arsine. The arsine is freed of hydrogen sulfide and other contaminating hydrides by passage through cotton which is saturated with lead acetate solution. The arsine is absorbed in silver diethyldithiocarbamate to form a soluble red complex. The absorbance of this complex, which is proportional to concentration over a wide range, is measured spectrophotometrically at 560 mμ.

Metals or salts of metals such as cobalt, mercury, nickel, silver, palladium, copper, chromium, and molybdenum are said to interfere with the evolution of arsine. The last three do so when present in large amounts. Antimony, which forms stibine, is the only metal likely to interfere in the color development. This forms a red color with maximum absorbance at 510 mμ.

REAGENTS

1. *Absorbing Solution* (Silver Diethyldithiocarbamate-Pyridine Solution) Five gm of silver diethyldithiocarbamate are dissolved in 1 liter of pyridine. The solution is stored in an amber bottle.
2. *Acetone, reagent grade*
3. *Arsenic Standard Solution,* concentrated. Approximately 1.32 gm of primary standard arsenic trioxide is dissolved in 10 ml of 40% sodium hydroxide (w/v), diluted to 1 liter with deionized distilled water, and mixed thoroughly. Ten ml of this solution are transferred to a 100 ml volumetric flask and diluted to the mark with deionized distilled water and mixed. This is Solution "A". Ten ml of Solution "A" are transferred to a 100-ml volumetric flask, diluted to volume with deionized distilled water, and mixed thoroughly. This solution contains approximately 10 mg of arsenic per liter. The arsenic concentration is calculated as follows:

4. *Arsenic Standard Solution,* diluted Ten ml of Solution "A" (prepared for the Arsenic Standard Solution, concentrated) are transferred by pipet to a 1 liter volumetric flask, diluted to volume with deionized distilled water, and mixed thoroughly. This solution contains approximately one mg of arsenic per liter. The arsenic concentration is calculated as follows:

Arsenic, mg per liter =
Weight of Sample, gm × 0.7574

5. Ether, reagent grade
6. *Hydrochloric Acid,* Equal volumes of concentrated hydrochloric acid and deionized distilled water are mixed, adding the acid to the water.
7. *Lead Acetate Solution* Ninety gm of lead acetate are dissolved in 900 ml of deionized distilled water and mixed thoroughly.
8. *Magnesium Oxide-Magnesium Nitrate Slurry* Seventy-five gm of magnesium oxide, MgO, and 105 gm of magnesium nitrate, $Mg(NO_3)_2 \cdot 6H_2O$, are suspended in enough deionized distilled water to make 1 liter and agitated vigorously. (The suspension is allowed to stand approximately 24 hours before using, since freshly prepared slurry gives an ash which is easily disturbed by air currents.)
9. *Methanol,* reagent grade
10. *Nitric Acid:* Approximately 45 ml of concentrated nitric acid are added to 255 ml of deionized distilled water and mixed thoroughly.
11. *Potassium Iodide Solution* Exactly 135 gm of potassium iodide are dissolved in 900 ml of deionized distilled water and mixed thoroughly.
12. *Pyridine,* reagent grade
13. *Silver Diethyldithiocarbamate,* A. R.
14. *Sodium Hydroxide:* Forty gm of sodium hydroxide pellets are dissolved in 60 ml of deionized distilled water and mixed thoroughly.
15. *Stannous Chloride Solution:* Sixty gm of stannous chloride ($SnCl_2 \cdot 2H_2O$) are dissolved in 150 ml of concentrated hydrochloric acid.
16. *Starch Glycerite:* Fifty gm of starch and 1 gm of benzoic acid are triturated with 100 ml of deionized distilled water in an 800 ml beaker until a smooth mixture is produced, then 350 ml of glycerine in approximately 50 ml increments are added slowly with constant stirring. The mixture is heated on a sand bath to a temperature between 140 and 144°C, with constant but gentle stirring, until a translucent jelly-like mass results which is then strained through muslin.
17. *Zinc,* granular 20 mesh, low arsenic, reagent grade

APPARATUS

Arsine Generator (Fisher Scientific Co. No. 1-405) *

Beaker, stainless steel, 5500 ml

Crucible, Porcelain, Coors 230, size 3, 100 ml

Glass Beads, solid, 5 mm. New glass beads are boiled in a solution containing equal volumes of concentrated nitric

*The generator consists of a 125 ml Erlenmyer flask 24/40, a scrubber unit and a 12 ml absorber unit 24/40.

acid and deionized distilled water for at least ten minutes. The beads are allowed to cool and are then rinsed with deionized water and dried.

Glass Wool, Pyrex

Spectrophotometer, Beckman, Model DU

PROCEDURE

Caution: All reagents, glassware, and water used in this determination must be very low in arsenic. (A blank consisting of 25 ml of deionized distilled water is carried through all steps of the procedure.)

I. Sample Preparation

Twenty ml of sample are pipetted into a 100 ml porcelain crucible. (Note 1) The contents are evaporated to dryness on a steam hotplate. Approximately 10 ml of well-mixed magnesium oxide-magnesium nitrate slurry are added by graduated cylinder, together with enough deionized distilled water to permit thorough mixing with a glass stirring rod. The stirring rod is rinsed and the sample is dried at 100°C and ashed 2 to 4 hours at 550 to 600°C (slight carbon residue does not interfere).

The crucible is removed from the oven, covered with a watch glass, and cooled to room temperature. The residue is moistened with deionized distilled water and about 15 ml of 1:1 hydrochloric acid are added. The crucible is covered with a watch glass and allowed to stand overnight to allow the residue to dissolve. (Note 2)

The solution is quantitatively transferred to a 125-ml Erlenmeyer flask.

The sides of the crucible are rinsed with hot deionized distilled water to insure complete transfer, obtaining approximately 30 ml of solution in the Erlenmeyer flask. Five ml of concentrated hydrochloric acid are added by graduated cylinder.

II. Arsine Evolution

Safety Precaution:

The arsine evolution step must be done in a well-ventilated, explosion-proof hood since poisonous arsine and explosive hydrogen are evolved. If for any reason the arsine is not collected in the trap (e.g., discontinuation of an analysis after the acid is added to the flask), it is important that the flask be kept in a well-ventilated hood until all visible reaction in the flask ceases.

Two ml of potassium iodide solution are added to the Erlenmeyer flask, followed by 8 drops of stannous chloride solution. The flask is swirled and allowed to stand for 15 minutes. If the solution immediately appears yellow, small amounts of deionized distilled water are added while swirling the flask until the solution becomes clear.

The absorber of the arsine generator is attached to the scrubber unit and placed on a convenient stand. To each absorber are added, by pipet, 3 ml of absorbing solution.

Approximately 3 gm of zinc are added to the Erlenmeyer flask of the arsine generator and the scrubber-absorber assembly is immediately attached in such a manner that no arsine will be lost. A convenient method for accomplishing this is described in Note 3.

The evolution of arsine is allowed to continue for at least 30 minutes. If the solution becomes too dark (i.e., an absorbance of greater than 0.8 absorbance units, by visual estimation based on previous experience) as many 3 ml aliquots as necessary are added to dilute the solution to a readable absorbance. The number of aliquots of absorbing solution used are recorded (Note 4). If a colored ring appears on the absorber, the open end of the absorber is plugged with the finger, providing enough pressure to cause the solution to reach and dissolve the ring.

When the evolution of arsine is complete, the absorbance of the solution is determined by the use of a Beckman DU Spectrophotometer under the following conditions:

Source Lamp	Tungsten
Cell	10 mm glass
Slit Width	0.03 mm
Filter	In
Phototube	Out (blue)
Wave Length	560 mμ
Ref. Solution	Silver diethyldithiocarbamate-pyridine solution

After each reading the cells are rinsed with warm, deionized distilled water, acetone and ether in that order, and air-dried.

The concentration of arsenic is estimated by interpolation from a prepared calibration curve (Section IV).

III. Procedure for Cleaning Glassware

The glass wool is removed from the scrubber and the scrubber and absorber are rinsed with hot water, removing as much starch glycerite from the scrubber as possible. The absorber and scrubber are placed into a freshly prepared, hot, 15 percent nitric acid solution for at least 10 minutes (Notes 5 and 6). The apparatus is carefully removed from the nitric acid solution and rinsed with hot water. Each scrubber and absorber is dipped into methanol, then acetone and allowed to dry.

The contents of the generating flask are discarded after recovering the glass beads. The liquid contents are poured down a drain with copious amounts of water and the spent zinc is discarded in a solid waste container. The flask is washed with cleanser, rinsed well with deionized distilled water, and allowed to drain and dry.

IV. Preparation of Calibration Curve

Zero, 2.0, 4.0, 6.0, 8.0, 10.0, and 12 0 ml aliquots of diluted Arsenic Standard Solution (see Reagents Section) are pipetted into separate, clean, numbered 125-ml Erlenmeyer flasks. The neck of each flask is rinsed with 3 to 4 ml of deionized distilled water. Enough water is added to make a total volume of approximately 30 ml, then 5 ml of concentrated hydrochloric acid are added. The procedure is continued as described under Section II, "Arsine Evolution."

The concentration of the standard solution is plotted as the abscissa and the absorbance is plotted as the ordinate on rectangular coordinate graph paper. The best straight line is drawn through the points and the concentration of the unknown is estimated by interpolation.

V. Preparation of Control Standard

An arsenic control standard containing a known amount of arsenic should be run with each set of samples (Notes 7 and 8).

NOTES

1. A larger amount of sample must be used if the arsenic content is below 0.075 mg per liter. A maximum of 70 ml of sample may be added directly to the crucible and evaporated on a steam bath.

2. In order to reduce the amount of analytical time necessary, the sample may also be heated on a water bath with agitation until the ash dissolves.

3. The suggested apparatus for this technique is a small plastic cup to con-

tain the zinc, a support for a 50 mm filtering funnel (a 3 x 1½" plastic vial may be used), and a 3 ml pipet which has been shortened to a height of 4 inches from the bottom. The funnel is placed into its holder and the pipet end is inserted into the center of the funnel. The zinc is poured into the funnel. The funnel is placed in the neck of the generating flask and the pipet end is removed from the funnel allowing the zinc to drop into the generating flask. The scrubber joint is immediately attached to the neck of the flask.

4. The technique of adding additional volumes of silver diethyldithiocarbamate pyridine solution is an emergency measure to salvage the analysis when the arsenic content of the sample is higher than anticipated. This procedure may result in low values owing to the possible loss of arsine when insufficient absorbing solution is present. For most precise results the analysis should be repeated using a smaller sample.

5. Splash-proof acid goggles are worn when handling concentrated nitric acid or hot nitric acid solutions.

6. The following procedure should be followed to prevent injury in case the beaker containing 15% nitric acid should break:

The 4000-ml glass beaker containing the nitric acid should be placed in a 5500 ml stainless steel beaker which contains a ½ inch layer of sand. The steel beaker can then be placed on a hot plate.

7. The concentration of arsenic in the control samples should be representative of the arsenic levels of the samples analyzed. These may be varied from time to time as experience dictates.

8. The arsenic-free samples are obtained from persons who have had no exposure to arsenic compounds.

REFERENCES

1. Vasak, V., and Sedivec.: Colorimetric determination of arsenic. Chem. Listy, *46:*341-344, 1952.
2. Anon.: Determination of Arsenic in Air. Manual of the American Conference of Government Industrial Hygienists, 1956.
3. Powers, G. W., Jr., Martin, R. L., Piehl, F. J., and Griffin, J. M.: Arsenic in naphthas. Anal. Chem., *31:*1589-1593, 1959.
4. Albert, D. K. and Granatelli, L.: Determination of microgram quantities of arsenic and naphthas with the oxyhydrogen burner. Anal. Chem., *31:*1593-1596, 1959.
5. Liederman, D., Bowen, J. E., and Milner, O. I.: Determination of arsenic in petroleum stocks and catalysts by evolution as arsine. Anal. Chem., *31:*2052-2055, 1959.

Chapter 35A

Toxicity from Exposure to Mercury

JAMES J. HUMES, M.D.

Historically, accounts of the toxic properties of mercury can be traced to the time of Hippocrates. As early as 1700, Ramazzini reported on mercury poisoning in surgeons using mercurial unctions. Review of the literature of the past several years reveals evidence of the continuing importance of mercury as a toxic agent. Potential sources of exposure include a gamut of situations ranging from mining operations through ore processing and manufacturing of mercury filled gauges, meters and control instruments to routine laboratory operations. In addition, there are the all too frequent reports of accidental and even suicidal exposures to various compounds of mercury.

Mercury exerts its deleterious effects in biologic systems by release of the Hg^{2+} ion which serves as a protein precipitant and general cellular poison. Rodin and Crawson[9] have localized the mitochondria as the apparent site of initial damage in the renal tubular epithelial cells of experimental animals. Numerous investigators[1, 6, 7, 8, 13, 14] have studied cellular enzyme defects in experimental mercury poisoning and have reported on alterations in succinic dehydrogenase activity. These enzyme changes have been thought by some to explain the physiologic effects of mercurial diuretics.

The toxic effects of mercury in the human depend on the type of compound, the concentration and mode of absorption, and the duration of exposure. Mercury may be absorbed through the skin or mucous membranes, inhaled, ingested or injected. The clinical illness, thus produced, may be categorized as acute, sub-acute or chronic with some degree of overlap depending on the variables previously mentioned.

The initial symptoms due to acute absorption of soluble compounds of mercury such as $HgCl_2$ are related to coagulation and corrosion of mucous membranes of the portal of entry. There rapidly follows an astringent metallic taste, salivation, thirst, abdominal distress and pain. In severe cases weakness, prostration, excitement, tachycardia, albuminuria, oliguria, anuria, colitis, hepatitis, stupor, circulatory collapse and death may ensue. There may be considerable variation in the severity of involvement of different organ systems from case to case but the kidneys, liver and central nervous system are particularly susceptible.

In acute toxicity owing to inhalation, the initial symptoms may be those of a severe respiratory illness in which dyspnea and cough predominate. If the exposure has been sufficiently prolonged or to high concentrations of mercury vapor, these initial symptoms will be shortly followed by evidence of other organ system involvement as mentioned above. At this stage, these symptoms will be essentially indistinguishable from those produced by ingestion of a soluble salt of mercury.

Sub-acute or chronic toxicity may occur from exposure to both inorganic and organic compounds. The time required for clinical manifestations of toxicity to appear varies greatly again depending on the route of exposure, type of compound and concentration. Thus, some cases have been reported after exposures of only a few weeks while others have required many years to develop.

The clinical picture in cases of chronic toxicity is often dominated by evidence of involvement of the central nervous system characterized by psychic and emotional disurbances. There may be increased irritability, combativeness, defective concentration, generalized weakness, loss of memory and disturbances of sleep patterns. The central nervous system involvement is also responsible for tremors and various ocular disturbances. Stomatitis, gingivitis and excessive salivation are often prominent.

One clinical illness which apparently represents a bizarre type of toxic reaction to mercury is worthy of separate consideration. This is the condition which pediatricians now classify as acrodynia or pink disease, and which was formerly known as Feer's disease or Swift's disease. This distressing illness affects infants and young children who have been exposed to mercury in one form or another. In some regions, the condition has been related to the use of mercury containing teething powders while in others mercury containing vermifuges or accidental exposures have been incriminated.

Acrodynia is characterized by a distinct pinkish discoloration of the skin of the fingers and toes which progresses to involve the palms and soles. The face is sometimes also involved. In characteristic cases there is evidence of central nervous system involvement with marked hypotonia and the production of the picture of a typical "floppy baby." These infants have been compared to a rag doll with hypotonia so severe that when placed in a given position the child will remain immobile for protracted periods of time. More complete accounts of this complex syndrome are available in the literature but two of the additional more constant findings are intense pain in the extremities and excessive sweating with profound depletion of chlorides particularly in warm weather.

The diagnosis of mercury poisoning, as in most areas of toxicology, depends on a complete and accurate clinical history. The examiner should be aware of the wide variety of industrial processes which offer the potential for exposure. The clinical course of the illness may be more or less characteristic but the *sine qua non* for the diagnosis rests with the demonstration of mercury in the urine in acute clinical cases or in the tissues in post-mortem material. The correlation between clinical symptoms of patients with chronic mercury poisoning and urinary excretion has been inconstant in reported series. Urine levels of 6 to 16 micrograms of mercury per liter have been reported in apparently unexposed subjects.

Prevention of unnecessary exposure to potentially toxic quantities of mercury or its compounds is to be preferred over treatment. The American Conference of Governmental Industrial Hygienists has recommended that a level of 0.1mg of Hg/cu meter of air be established as the upper limit for safety in industrial exposure. Clinical laboratory directors should be ever conscious of the hazard created by careless handling of this material.

In recent years the most important contribution in the treatment of mercury poisoning has been the adoption of dimercaprol (British anti-Lewisite) as the chelating agent of choice. Other chelating agents have been used in the treatment of mercury poisoning with inconstant results.

REFERENCES

1. Barron, E. S. G., and Kalnitsky, G.: The Inhibhibition of Succinoxidase by Heavy Metals and Its Reaction with Dithiols.
2. Bilderback, J. B.: Acrodynia, In, Nelson-Textbook of Pediatrics. W. B. Saunders Co., Phil., 1964.
3. Burke, W. J., and Quagliana, J. M.: Acute inhalation mercury intoxication. J. Occupat. Med., *5:*157-160, 1963.
4. CPC from the Children's Hospital Medical Center, Boston, Mass. J. Pediatrics, *68:*480-487, 1966.
5. Forsyth, C. C.: Pink disease. Brit. Med. J., *1:* 767, Mar. 23, 1968.
6. Handley, C. A., and Lavik, P. S.: Inhibition of kidney succinic dehydrogenase system by mercurial diuretics. J. Pharacol. & Exper. Therap., *100:*115-118, 1950.
7. Mustakallio, K. K., and Telkka, A.: Histochemical localization of the mercurial inhibition of succinic dehydrogenase in rat kidney. Science, *118:*320-321, 1953.
8. Rennels, E. G., and Ruskin, A.: Histochemical changes in succinic dehydrogenase activity in rat kidney following administration of mercural diuretics. Proc. Soc. Exper. Biol. & Med., *85:*309-314, 1954.
9. Rodin, A. E., and Crawson, C. N.: Mercury nephrotoxicity in the rat. Am. J. Path., *41:*485, Oct. 1962.
10. Schneider, W. C., and Potter, V. R.: The assay of animal tissues for respiratory enzymes. II Succinic dehydrogenase and cytochrome oxidase. J. Biol. Chem., *149:*217-227, 1943.
11. Sollmann: A Manual of Phamacology. W. B. Saunders, New York.
12. Stokinger, H. E.: In, Industrial Hygiene & Toxicology, Vo. II, p. 1090. Interscience Publishers, New York, 1963.
13. Wachstein, M., and Meisel, E.: E. Influence of experimental renal damage on histochemically demonstrable succinic dehydrogenase activity in the rat. Am. J. Path. *30:*147-165, 1954.
14. Wachstein, M., and Meisel, E.: On the histochemical localization of the mercurial inhibition of succinic dehydrogenase in rat kidney. Science, *119:*100, 1954.

Chapter 35B

The Determination of Mercury in Biological Fluids

WILLIAM J. HERMANN, JR., B.S., JAMES W. BUTLER, B.S., and RALPH G. SMITH, PH.D.

INTRODUCTION

The analysis of mercury in biological fluids has always proven a difficult task due mainly to the extreme sensitivity of the metal to heat. Various methods of chemical digestion with low heat have been reviewed by Campbell and Head,[1] yet all had the intrinsic problem of possible mercury loss due to the heat and the long digestion time necessary under low heat. Consequently, more rapid and sensitive methods of analysis for mercury were considered making use of the metal's heat sensitivity. Jacobs, Goldwater, and Gilbert[2] coupled the ease of vaporization with the principle of atomic absorption in the last step of an analytical procedure in which the mercury was isolated from the digestion mixture with dithizone. The mercury was vaporized by heat from the dithizone and passed through a Mercury Vapor Meter which operates on the principle of atomic absorption. The utilization of dithizone resulted from the report by Lindstrom,[3] that various chemical interferences occurred when a urine sample was combusted and the vapor passed directly into a Mercury Vapor Meter. These interfering substances include sulfates, sulfur, and iodine. The method of Lindstrom closely parallels the theory and operation of this method; however, there are some drawbacks. These drawbacks include the previously mentioned interferences, the necessity for sample preparation steps for solid samples, and the use of a flame which gives off additional background interferences. However, the basic principle of oxidizing the sample matrix, vaporizing the mercury and determining the concentration of the vapor stream by atomic absorption at 2537 Å is similar. Monkman, *et al.*[4] used a CdS pad absorption technique and heated the pad to release the mercury into an atomic absorption apparatus. Thilliez[5] recently used a platinum trap to isolate the mercury from the sample matrix, then heated to trap to distill off the trapped mercury into an atomic absorption device.

PRINCIPLE

Since mercury is characterized as having a relatively high vapor pressure at room temperature (10^{-3} mm Hg) and reaching a vapor pressure of 1 atmosphere at 357°C, the metal may be easily vaporized from any combustible or noncombustible matrix. The metal, if present in trace amounts, can be carried as a vapor in an airstream at room temperaure and below without significant condensation. Thus, this dynamic system introduces the metal as a vapor into a rapidly moving airstream by heating the crude sample in a furnace. While the mercury vaporizes, the sample matrix is pyrolyzed. The airstream is then filtered to remove substances emitted from the sample that absorb light at 2537 Å besides mercury. Determination of the mercury concentration of the airstream follows, using the principle of atomic absorption.

REAGENTS

1. *Mercury trap solution.* Ten gm of potassium permanganate are dissolved in one liter of 20% sulfuric acid.
2. *Filter reagents:*
   a. *Magnesium Perchlorate,* anhydrous
   b. *Ascarite®* 8-20 mesh
   c. *Soda lime* 8-14 mesh

STANDARD SOLUTIONS

1. *Stock standard mercury solution* (1 mg per ml). Exactly 1.000 gm of metallic mercury is dissolved in a 20% nitric acid solution.
2. *Working standard mercury solution* (100 Ng per ml). The stock standard is diluted with distilled water and approximately 1 mg of NaCl is added to every 100 ml of solution.

SPECIAL APPARATUS

1. Beckman Model 23 Mercury Vapor Meter, fitted with a sampling tube with one quartz window at either end and an inlet and outlet on the side.
2. Dyna-Vac Pump (Universal Electric Co.) rated at 3000 rpm.
3. Pyrolyzing Furnace (see discussion for complete details on construction and operation).
4. Recorder (with integrator for greatest convenience).

PROCEDURE

The furnace is turned on and allowed to heat. Upon reaching near maximum heat, the condenser water should be started circulating and the vacuum pump turned on. This will allow the system to "clean itself" and will lengthen the life of the furnace's heating elements. Any water in the bottom of the inverted condenser or cold trap should be removed. A standard of suitable concentration is prepared from a 1 mg per ml Stock standard (see Standard Solutions section). The concentration of the working standard will vary with the estimated sample concentration. A very common working standard has the concentration of 10 Ng per 0.1 ml or 0.1 ppm. All samples and standards if in a liquid state are injected into the entrance port of the furnace in 0.1 ml volumes with syringes of suitable size to allow accuracy in measuring the 0.1 ml aliquots. Syringes are used so that the technician may pierce the top of the vacutainer or plastic bottle and allow shaking of the sample to occur while withdrawing the aliquots. Disposable syringes are recommended since a new syringe is needed for each sample.

The working standard is injected into the furnace to begin the analysis and the system is calibrated. The standard must yield repeatable results before proceeding. Next, a blank sample of the substance or matrix in which the mercury is to be found must be passed through the system to check the combustion and filter efficiency. This blank matrix should read zero or a level which is insignificant to the estimated level of mercury concentrations in the samples. The samples are then run in rapid succession in 0.1 ml aliquots for liquid samples. In the case of solid samples, an amount of known weight (approximately 0.1 gm) is introduced at the entrance port. In the case of wet or moist solid samples, such as tissue, small pieces are cut and allowed to dry. Drying will allow more rapid combustion and more uniform emission of mercury. Oxygen is fed into the open entrance port at a rate of 1 to 2 l per m to enrich the burning atmosphere. No alteration in the system need occur between running samples of different matrixes, which may be interchanged freely.

The curves formed on the recorder in response to the output of the Mercury Vapor Meter are of Gaussian shape, and the area under the curve is the measurement of mercury concentration. Different matrices have different rates of burning. Consequently, a urine curve appears sharper and more rapidly than the curve for slower burning blood.

The dry chemical filter is changed approximately every 50 samples, although its life depends on the type of sample being run. Indications to the operator that the filter needs changed are: first, a white appearance of spent Ascarite accounting for approximately ¾ of the Ascarite present; second, a broadening of the curves indicating a clogging of the filter; and, third, an excessively wet appearance. The presence of any one of these conditions merits a filter change.

The samples are usually run in duplicate to check reproducibility. The working standard, made fresh daily, is run frequently throughout the analysis to check the calibration. The blank matrices are also run periodically to check furnace and filter efficiency.

DISCUSSION

Construction and Operation of Direct Determination of Mercury Analytical System

Briefly, the system consists of a pyrolyzing furnace of sufficient volume, surface area and temperature to break down the sample matrix and vaporize the mercury and numerous other substances, some of which will interfere with mercury in an atomic absorption detector by absorbing light energy at 2537Å. Consequently, a filtering system is introduced between the furnace and the atomic absorption unit. This filtering system consists of a condenser to remove water vapor (an additional cold trap may be necessary, depending on the tap water temperature). A dry chemical filter follows the condenser, which serves to remove H_2O, CO_2, NO_2 and SO_2, and contains $MgClO_4$, Ascarite (NaOH on inert particles) and soda lime. An atomic absorption unit follows the filtering system. This laboratory has had much success using the Beckman Model 23 Mercury Vapor Meter. However, it is conceivable that other, more versatile, instruments that are more widely distributed could be adapted for this system as long as the basic principle of atomic absorption is common to all.

Furnace Construction and Operation

Temperature is the first and most critical factor in a successful furnace. This must exceed 1000°C with an air stream of at least 7 lpm flowing through it. This temperature must be maintained throughout the operational zones of the furnace. The high temperature is needed to burn organic hydrocarbons and aromatics to CO_2. No matter how long the combusted vapor remains in the furnace, if the temperature is insufficient for cracking, then none will occur and those substances capable of light energy absorption at 2537 Å, other than mercury, will be emitted from the furnace.

Time and hot surface area encountered by the combusted sample as it travels through the furnace are the next most critical factors, and are closely associated with each other. Sufficient time must be allowed for the cracking process to take place. As stated above, 7 lpm is the airflow found to be most satisfactory in allowing sufficient burning. The airflow rate has a lower limit since the vacuum pulling the sample through the furnace must exceed the rate of expansion of the water vapor and combustion gases upon hitting the hot combustion plate. The time factor may be compensated for in part by providing excessive amount of hot surface area to the vapor stream. If surface area is sufficiently large the rate of air flow has nearly unlimited possibilities, within reason, on the high side. With regard to surface area, first a combustion plate should be present at the injection port to retain large pieces of the sample until they are combusted at least to the liquid or vapor stage; second, the entire furnace should be filled with granules of sufficiently small size to give maximum surface yet little impedance to the air flow. Granules of size 5 to 10 mesh are optimal. These granules and the combustion plate should be made of quartz, ceramic, or some other material of similar properties with respect to chemical and thermal stability. Most ordinary metals (including stainless steel) have been found to be inadequate due to corrosion.

Volume is the fourth factor to consider. The present system operates with a furnace approximately four feet in length and one inch in diameter. The furnace tubing is made of ceramic but could be made of other substances which fulfill the requiremnts stated above for the surface area granules. The construction of a furnace apparatus of similar dimensions might be a three-foot horizontal section connected to a one-foot vertical section with an open end for sample introduction.

Oxygen, the fifth factor, should be introduced at the furnace's open end to provide the optimal oxidizing atmosphere, thus coming as close as possible to an instantaneous burning of the sample at the combustion plate.

With these empirical requirements in mind, one may proceed from a theoretical discussion to practical application. Unless a standardized furnace is built, each laboratory wishing to work with this method must build their own furnace. All of the preceding five factors have been stated at their optimal levels, *but* many times these levels are not practically attainable or suitable for the specific laboratory. When a furnace is constructed which closely approximates the requirements stated above, the test is for a blank sample (containing no mercury) to be passed through the furnace and other apparatus of the system without a deviation of the base line mercury level. The requirements in this case depend on the sensitivity desired. The sensitivity attained is directly related to the efficiency of the combustion apparatus. Present levels of sensitivity which are now obtained in the operating model are 10 ppb or 0.01 ppm. For most operations, this is considerably more sensitive than the minimum requirement. Any of the preceding five factors, except temperature, may be altered in furnace construction, so that one gets a furnace capable of attaining the sensitivity levels desired.

This method will analyze any substance for mercury for which a blank reading can be attained with sufficient sensitivity. One can see that the limits so far as sensitivity and substances which can be analyzed are dependent entirely on the construction of an adequate combustion apparatus and the electronic sensitivity of the detection device.

The construction of a satisfactory furnace is a difficult task, and all factors discussed previously should be studied before proceeding with a design. The design is an option to the builder. It is hoped that a furnace of less bulky dimensions can eventually be constructed.

Filtering Apparatus

The vapor stream containing the combustion products and vaporized mercury must be filtered to remove undesirable contaminants which absorb energy emitted from the mercury vapor lamp at 2537 Å These substances include CO_2, NO_2, SO_2, and H_2O. The hydrocarbons and aromatics should have been oxidized in the furnace apparatus to CO_2. Water vapor is largely removed by an inverted Friedrichs condenser. The water found in the bottom of the condenser should be checked frequently for mercury content. It should be free of mercury. The condenser is attached to the furnace outlet by a teflon tube approximately one foot in length. Following the condenser is a dry chemical filter using the following stratification. Glass wool ($\frac{1}{2}''$) is followed by anhydrous $MgClO_4$ (1″) to remove any last traces of H_2O vapor which pass the condenser. A mixture of soda lime to ascarite (1:1, 6″) removes CO_2, NO_2, and SO_2 when slightly moist. The moisture is provided by the initial reactions with CO_2 and the NaOH of the ascarite. This moisture produced in the CO_2 filtering reaction must then be removed by another layer of anhydrous $MgClO_4$ (½″) and finally glass wool (½″) to maintain the contents of the filter (dimensions for a ½″ I.D. glass tube). The purified air stream is then ready to be read for mercury concentration. Recovery data and rerunning of water trapped in the condenser reveal that insignificant amounts of mercury may condense in the condensing and filtering apparatus.

Mercury Vapor Detection

The principle for detection of the concentration of the mercury in the air stream is provided by atomic absorption. The vapor stream passes through a sample tube fitted with quartz windows at each end. A beam of light of 2537 Å is passed through the length of the sample tube. The operating system uses a Beckman Mercury Vapor Meter Model 23 as the atomic absorption unit. However, a system was recently set up using a Perkin-Elmer 303 atomic absorption unit with the flame atomizer removed and a sample tube inserted in the light path. The electronic signal generated is then fed to a suitable recorder and the *total area* under the curve measured. A planimeter can be used to trace around the curves or an integrator may be used on the recorder.

Precision of Replicate Analyses of Urine Mercury

The precision of 50 replicate analyses of a single urine specimen was 0.116 mg per 1 ± 0.008 mg per 1. This concentration is the approximate level of mercury one would expect to find in a worker with chronic exposure to low concentrations in the air.

Precision of Replicate Analyses of Blood Mercury

The precision of 30 replicate analyses of a single blood specimen was 14.0 μg per 100 ml ± 1.7 μg per 100 ml. This concentration is the approximate level of mercury one would expect to find in a worker with chronic exposure to low mercury concentrations.

Application of the System

The great bulk of the analyses done with this method has been on blood, urine and tissue. Other types of samples could conceivably be analyzed as long as one could obtain a zero response from the sample's matrix which would contain no mercury or a level of response insignificant to the concentrations expected in the samples. Food products, cloth, and ores are among the possibilities. Cloth has been analyzed successfully on one occasion. The extremely small amounts of sample needed for analysis removes some of the limitations of other methods.

Sensitivity of the System

The level of sensitivity thus far obtained is 0.01 ppm for blood, urine, and tissue. At this level, the operator may maintain a high degree of confidence. The sensitivity is a function of the efficiency of the furnace in pyrolyzing the sample matrix. The filter device is not a limiting factor at this sensitivity level. It is the belief of the authors that a more sensitive system could be developed by producing a better furnace apparatus, i.e., of higher temperature and greater combustion surface area.

Recovery of Mercury Added to Urine

Varying amounts of mercury were added to urine samples. The following recoveries were obtained:

Hg Added (mg per liter)	*Recovery (mg per liter)*
.23	.21
.05	.05
.09	.11
.06	.05
.13	.15
.03	.03
.17	.17
.01	.01

These mercury concentrations span the range of values most frequently found in urine of exposed persons.

Recovery of Mercury Added to Blood

Hg Added (μg per 100 ml)	*Recovery (μg per 100 ml)*
1.1	1.7
4.8	5.1
7.0	7.1
27.0	31.7
9.1	11.0
15.0	19.5
Blank	Blank
20.0	24.2
2.0	1.2

These mercury concentrations span the range most frequently observed in blood of exposed persons. An adequate method for adding mercury to tissue samples has not been developed and consequently recovery data for tissue is not available. However, confidence that tissue and other materials difficult to spike may be analyzed stems from three facts. First, the running of a blank sample of the matrix and obtaining zero response and comparing this to an exposed sample, the only difference being the mercury itself. Second, the recovery data on blood and urine gives a high degree of confidence in the system's capability to pass a sample through without mercury loss. Third, the diversity in the matrices of blood and urine and the close similarity of tissue and blood with respect to chemical composition leads to the opinion that the system will treat the tissue samples no differently than the blood and urine once the sample passes through the furnace.

SOURCES OF ERROR

The major source of error comes in the injection technique. As stated previously, in this method a disposable syringe is recommended for introduction of the sample into the furnace. However, the smallest disposable syringe available is 0.5 ml in graduations of 0.1 ml. The technician must exercise extreme care to inject exactly 0.1 ml each time, since a single drop could mean a 10 percent error. Although this sounds a bit crude, experiments with 0.1 ml automatic pipettes with disposable tips have proved to have many disadvantages. All of the recovery data and replication studies were done with the 0.5 ml syringes.

Another source of error is the stability of the Mercury Vapor Meter. It is suggested that the meter be allowed to equilibrate for at least one hour before an analysis. A third source of error is introduced if the air stream's velocity is not sufficient to overcome the expansion of the sample when it first falls on the combustion plate in which case some mercury will be lost from the injection port. Thus, care should always be exercised in checking the system for undue resistance to the air stream. This problem usually arises from a wet filter. A heavily acidified solution cannot be analyzed by this method since large amounts of acid condensing in the water traps will dissolve mercury out of the air stream. Outside of these mechanical factors, there is not a great chance of error. In this method no reagents or glassware are needed, which could be contaminated, and there is no transferring of solutions between containers.

APPLICATIONS OF THE SYSTEM TO CLINICAL MEDICINE

Speed in diagnosis is highly essential in any case of disorders due to toxic agents. This method provides an extremely rapid diagnosis of mercury poisoning. A single sample can easily be analyzed from crude sample to result in one minute after instrument warm-up and calibration. The principle and operation of the system do not require a high degree of chemical knowledge to use it. In the field of industrial medicine, where constant monitoring of worker's blood and urine is necessary (especially in the chlorine industry), this system provides a rapid and simple method for accurate monitoring. Sample size requirements of the system is another advantage. Since the metabolism and physical state of an individual having severe acute mercury intoxication are greatly diminished, the taking of a 50 ml urine sample or large blood sample may be extremely difficult and hazardous (this is especially true in the case of children who so often are the patients). This method has been employed to analyze over 150 samples from one hospital alone (Children's Hospital, Detroit, Michigan). In two cases, the symptoms were extremely severe. The rapidity of analysis allowed the doctors to monitor the mercury levels and consequently assisted in regulating the treatment with dimercaprol (BAL).

REFERENCES

1. Campbell, E. E., and Head, B. M.: The determination of mercury in urine. Am. Ind. Hyg. Assoc. Quart., *16*:275-279, 1955.

2. Jacobs, M. B., Goldwater, L. J., and Gilbert, H.: Ultramicrodetermination of mercury in blood. Am. Ind. Hyg. Assoc. Quart., *22*:276-279, 1961.
3. Lindstrom, O.: Rapid microdetermination of mercury by spectrophotometric flame combustion. Anal. Chem., *31*:461, 1959.
4. Monkman, J. L., Maffett, P. A., and Doherty, T. F.: The determination of mercury in air samples and biological materials. Am. Ind. Hyg. Assoc. Quart., *17*:418-420, 1956.
5. Thilliez, G.: Determination precise et rapide par absorption atomique de traces de mercure dans l'air et dans les milieux biologiques. Chimie Analytique, *50*:226-232, May 1968.

Chapter 36

Nickel Poisoning

F. WILLIAM SUNDERMAN, M.D., PH.D.

It is only within the past three or four decades that the hazards of exposure to nickel and nickel compounds have come to be recognized. In 1943, during World War II, it became apparent that exposure to nickel and certain of its compounds was a serious health hazard and a handicap to the furtherance of research work in atomic energy. As a consequence, studies were initiated to provide safeguards for the handling of nickel compounds during the war and these studies have continued until the present time. Obviously, an enormous amount of data has been collected which can only be epitomized in this chapter.

The increasing industrial use of nickel in recent years has focused attention upon the varied clinical syndromes that may be encountered after exposure to nickel. These syndromes range from nickel dermatitis, pulmonary eosinophilia (i.e., Loeffler's syndrome), acute and subacute pneumonitis with adrenal cortical insufficiency, and pulmonary cancer. The factors that determine the clinical response depend upon the nature of the nickel compound, its molecular state and reactivity, the dosage, the speed and method of exposure, and the sensitivity and resistance of the host.

Values pertaining to the toxicity of nickel are given in Table I. It will be seen that solutions of colloidal nickel or nickel salts have a high degree of toxicity when given either intravenously or subcutaneously. On the other hand, the ingestion of nickel or nickel salts has a relatively low degree of toxicity. It will be seen that dogs are able to tolerate doses of metallic nickel and nickel compounds as high as 3 grams per kilogram body weight. It should also be mentioned that in so far as has been ascertained up to the present time the ingestion of milligram quantities of nickel

TABLE I: TOXICITY OF NICKEL AND ITS COMPOUNDS

Nickel	
Colloidal (Intravenous — Dogs)	LD = 10 to 20 mg/kg[1]
Powdered (Actual Oral — Dogs)	Tolerated: 1 to 3 gm/kg[2]
Nickel Salts (Cl, NO_3, SO_4, O)	
Intravenous — Dogs	LD = 10 to 20 mg/kg[1]
Subcutaneous — Rabbits	LD = 1.3 gm/kg[8]
Acute Oral—Rats	LD_{50} = 2.0 gm/kg[4]
Chronic Oral — Cats	Tolerated: 25 mg/kg/day for 200 days[5]
Nickel Carbonyl — $Ni(CO)_4$	LD_{50} = 0.067 mg/L for 30 min.[6]
Mice	LD_{50} = 0.24 mg/L for 30 min.[6]
Rats	1:10,000 soln of $NiCl_2$ may
Nickel Skin Sensitivity	evoke dermal sensitivity.[7]

contained in food and also derived from food cooked in stainless steel utensils is without detectable deleterious effects on the health of people.

The most commonly observed toxic reaction to nickel and nickel compounds is nickel dermatitis and skin sensitivity. The increasing prevalence of nickel dermatitis and sensitivity has been emphasized by many investigators. It has been estimated that 5% of all cases of eczema are caused by contact with nickel or nickel compounds.[8] The dermatitis arises from direct contact of the skin with metals containing nickel, such as costume jewelry, garter buckles, watches, metal straps, spectacle frames, pins, hair clips, sissors and coins.[8, 9] Although most of the investigators have directed attention to the dermatologic manifestations of nickel sensitivity, nevertheless, it is noteworthy that other allergic phenomena, such as pulmonary eosinophilia (i.e., Loeffler's syndrome) may also be encountered.[10, 11]

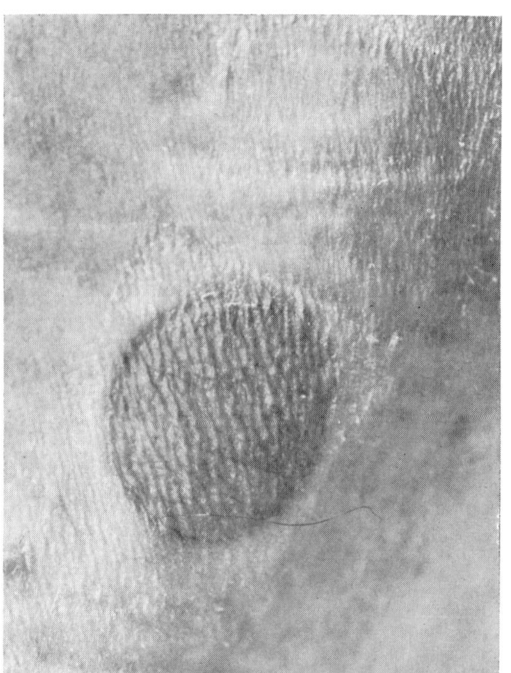

Figure 1. Response to patch testing with five-cent coin.

The type of skin reaction that may be encountered in persons hypersensitive to nickel is illustrated in the photograph (Fig. 1).[10] The patient, who was patch-tested, was a chemical engineer who had been exposed to low concentrations of nickel carbonyl for several months during the installation of a chemical plant. On one occasion, he was exposed to a relatively high concentration of nickel carbonyl for a few minutes. After this high single exposure the patient developed severe paroxysmal asthmatic attacks and pulmonary eosinophilia (Loeffler's syndrome). Eventually, he became so hypersensitive to nickel that the skin reaction shown on the photograph developed within two hours after the application of a five-cent coin (75% copper and 25% nickel).

The most toxic of all of the compounds of nickel that are encountered in industrial operations is nickel carbonyl and its vapors. It will be seen in Table I that the LD_{50} values for a 30-minute exposure to nickel carbonyl for mice and rats are 0.067 and 0.24 mg per liter, corresponding to 10 and 35 parts per million, respectively.[6] For the purposes of this presentation, emphasis will be placed upon the toxicity of inhaled nickel carbonyl.

NICKEL CARBONYL

Whenever finely divided nickel or its compounds come in contact with carbon monoxide, nickel carbonyl is formed. Nickel carbonyl is widely used commercially and is one of the most toxic gases encountered in industrial operations. The American Conference of Governmental Industrial Hygienists has placed the threshold limit value for a working day at 1 part per billion (by comparison, hydrogen cyanide was placed at ten parts per million — a 10,000 times greater concentration).[12] The gas ($Ni(CO)_4$) is unstable under atmospheric conditions and if inhaled, nickel is presumed to be deposited in highly active form on the respiratory mucosa when the gas comes into contact with it. The high volatility of nickel carbonyl creates a special hazard of exposure by inhalation during handling.

Walter Reppe, a German chemist, made a major contribution in the field of chemistry when he discovered the Oxo and related reactions with nickel carbonyl as a catalyst. As a result of his work, nickel carbonyl has been introduced into many of the large chemical industrial processes. In addition to the separation of nickel from its ores, one of the important recent uses is as an intermediate in the synthesis of acrylic esters for the production of plastics (plexiglas). It is also employed in nickel-plating operations and as a medium for depositing thin layers of metallic nickel in electronic circuits and magnetic tapes. Nickel is magnetic and a highly purified sample of metallic nickel may be deposited on tapes by means of nickel carbonyl. It is also now being used for casting operations and in making dies for machine parts. It is used in the preparation of organic syntheses, sometimes at extremely high pressures. It should also be mentioned that nickel carbonyl may be formed inadvertently whenever carbon monoxide comes into contact with any active form of nickel. In the latter case, the hazards of exposure are increased because the presence of nickel carbonyl may not be easily recognized. Nickel carbonyl lacks any strong or penetrating odor to warn of its presence.

It is suspected that nickel carbonyl poisoning may not be too uncommon an occurrence, and that poisoning from it often goes unrecognized. Furthermore, severe symptoms may develop insidiously hours or even days after exposure. In a tragic accident reported from our laboratories a number of years ago,[13] approximately 100 men were accidentally exposed to nickel carbonyl in an oil refinery of which 31 required hospitalization and 3 eventually died. It is noteworthy that in this accident, nickel carbonyl was not recognized as the offending agent until 4 days after exposure.

The acute symptoms which follow exposure to nickel carbonyl are of two types — immediate and delayed (Table II).[14] Even in exposure sufficiently severe to cause death, the initial symptoms are usually mild and not specific, disappearing quickly upon removal of the subject to uncontaminated air. On the other hand, the delayed symptoms which may appear from 12 to 36 hours after the initial symptoms (at times they merge immediately from the initial symptoms) are apt to be severe and usually indicate a grave prognosis.

Within the past twelve years, an opportunity has been afforded of studying over 200 workers who suffered from acute nickel carbonyl poisoning.[13, 14, 15] The initial symptoms in these patients usually include frontal headache, vertigo, nausea, vomiting and sometimes sternal and epigastric pain. In those patients who develop delayed reactions, constrictive pain in the chest is usually the first symptom. This is followed by cough, hypernoea, cyanosis, occasionally gastrointestinal symptoms and a pro-

TABLE II: SYMPTOMS IN ACUTE NICKEL CARBONYL POISONING

Immediate	*Delayed*
Mild, non-specific Symptoms disappear when subject is removed to uncontaminated air Frontal headache, vertigo, sweating, nausea, vomiting and sternal pain	Symptoms appear 12 to 36 hours after exposure Constrictive pains in chest, cough, dyspnea, profound weakness Temp. 101°; Tachycardia WBC — 12,000 per cmm Death — 4th to 14th day

found weakness (adrenal exhaustion). These patients become so weak that they may have difficulty turning in bed. The temperature in these patients seldom goes above 101°F and leukocytosis above 12,000 per cmm is infrequent. The pulse rate is usually increased but not in proportion to the increased respiratory rate. Physical signs compatible with pneumonitis or bronchopneumonia are elicited in the chest. Excepting for the pronounced weakness and hypernoea, the physical findings and symptoms resemble those of a viral or influenzal pneumonia. Terminally, the patients frequently become delirious. In the fatal cases death occurs between the 4th and 11th days after exposure.

NICKEL METABOLISM

Early studies on nickel metabolism were undertaken by means of balance studies on dogs.[16] The results of the nickel balance measurements are portrayed in Figures 2 and 3. The nickel content of food and excretion of nickel in the stools and urine were measured for eight 3-day metabolic periods in four dogs. It will be seen that under normal conditions approximately 90% of the ingested nickel is excreted in the stool and only 10% in the urine. When balance studies were made on dogs exposed to nickel carbonyl, it was observed that during the first three days after exposure more than twice as much nickel was excreted in the urine as in the feces. This observation that there is a sharp increase in the nickel excretion in the urine immediately after exposure to nickel carbonyl proved to be of major practical value and led to the development of procedures for detecting exposure in workers to minimal amounts of nickel carbonyl in concentrations which are too low to produce acute symptoms.

NICKEL IN URINE

The mean concentration of nickel in the urine of 107 normal subjects was found to be 2.0 mcgm per 100 ml with a standard deviation of ± 1.1 (Table III). Our nickel analyses are made on urine specimens collected over an 8-hour working period. The standard deviation using this method of collection is obviously greater owing to the greater variations in volume than would be obtained if the results were expressed in terms of daily excretion. These data have led to the conclusion, however, that only one specimen in 50 selected from a normal population will be found to exceed a value of 5.3 mcgm per 100 ml of urine. This value has therefore been selected as the upper limit of normal. In ten years, 18,-

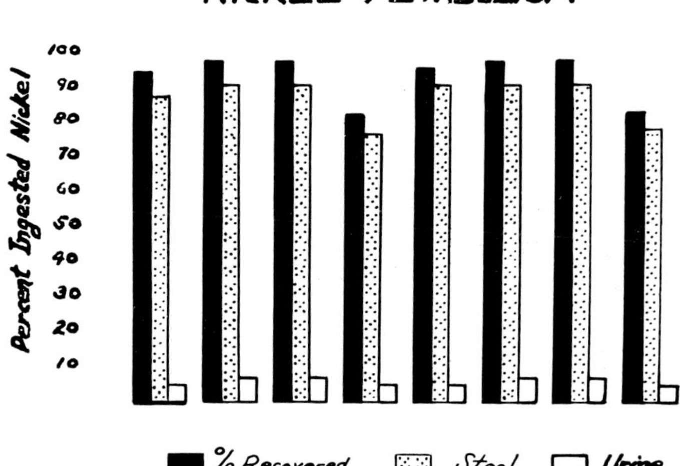

Figure 2.

815 routine analyses were undertaken on urine specimens collected over 8-hour periods. All of these specimens had a nickel concentration below 6 mcgm per 100 ml of urine. Measurements of nickel concentration in urine have proved to be more satisfactory than estimations of total nickel excretion because of the difficulty of obtaining from industrial workers reliable estimations of the volume of urine excreted within stipulated periods of time. Furthermore, the time-saving factor has proved important in critical cases.

PATHOLOGIC CHANGES OBSERVED IN ANIMALS FOLLOWING ACUTE EXPOSURE TO $Ni(CO)_4$

The most striking gross changes observed at necropsy in experimental animals after acute exposure to nickel carbonyl are found in the lungs.[17] The lungs of animals that die soon after exposure show a severe degree of congestion and pulmonary edema whereas the lungs of animals that survive for one to five days after exposure usually show extensive pneumonitis.

TABLE III: NICKEL IN URINE (Normal Population)

		mcgm
Excretion per day		15 to 50
Mean concentration	(per 100)	2.2 ± 1.1
18,815 Routine analyses	(per 100)	< 6.0
One analysis in fifty	(per 100)	> 5.3

An autopsy was obtained on a worker who died following the accidental acute exposure. This man had been a strong, healthy, muscular, well-nourished man, 29 years of age and a pipe-fitter by occupation. He died 13 days after exposure to nickel carbonyl.

The main pathologic changes were found in the lungs which contained many consolidated areas of fibroblasts and only a relatively small amount of aerating tissue (Fig. 4). In many places the pulmonary parenchyma was found to be practically consolidated with fibroblasts (Fig. 5).

This amazingly rapid infiltration of fibroblasts in pulmonary tissues within two weeks after exposure was also observed by Baader in two cases.[18]

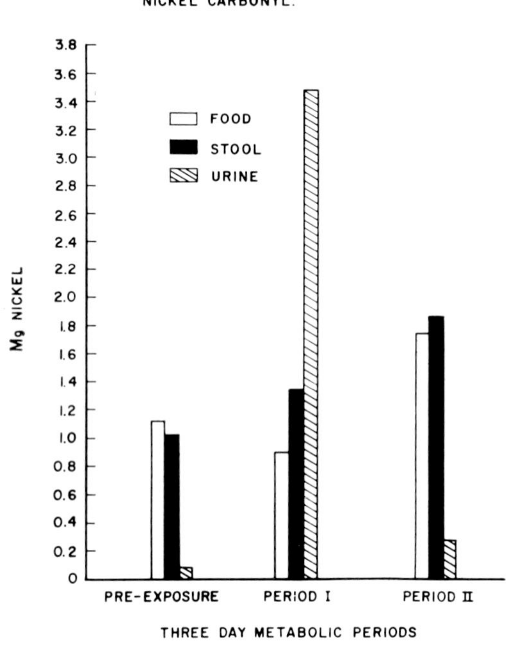

Figure 3.

NICKEL AS A CARCINOGEN

Nickel and nickel carbonyl have been under suspicion as carcinogens for human beings for several decades. An historical resumé of some of the published studies on the relation of nickel to cancer is presented in Table IV.

A number of investigations from our laboratory have established the fact that pulmonary cancer may be induced in rats exposed to a single heavy concentration of nickel carbonyl as well as in rats exposed to repeated inhalations of sublethal concentrations for a period of a year.[17, 31, 37, 42] It is noteworthy that cancers were not observed in the animals until two or more years after the initial exposure. It might be emphasized that the induction of pulmonary cancer in a laboratory rat is a severe challenge since spontaneous pulmonary neoplasms occur only rarely in this animal.

Since inhalation of minute amounts of nickel was found to be carcinogenic in experimental animals, nickel was investigated and evaluated as a possible carcinogenic agent in smoking tobaccos.[32] Nickel is a ubiquitous element present in trace amounts in practically all soils and plants. It has been shown to be present in tobacco in concentrations of 2 mcgm per gm.

Nickel has a great affinity for carbon monoxide. In the burning of tobacco, carbon monoxide is formed in amounts estimated to be from 2 to 6.6% of the smoke. Nickel or nickel compounds in a finely divided state will unite with carbon monoxide to form nickel carbonyl, even at environmental temperatures; however, maximal concentrations at normal pressure are obtained at 45 to 50°C which is within the range of the temperature of the combustion gases from burning cigarettes. In a burning cigarette, all of the reactants and the reaction conditions are present which are known to lead to the formation of nickel carbonyl. In view of these facts, it would appear obvious that tobacco smoke provides a ready means for transporting an active form of nickel into the respiratory system.

It will be seen in Table V that the average amount of nickel in the mainstream smoke of a single cigarette is 0.37 mcgm. The carcinogenic dose for rats chronically exposed to nickel carbonyl for a period of a year is 1930 mcgm. This amount is contained in the inhaled mainstream smoke from 260 packs of cigarettes.

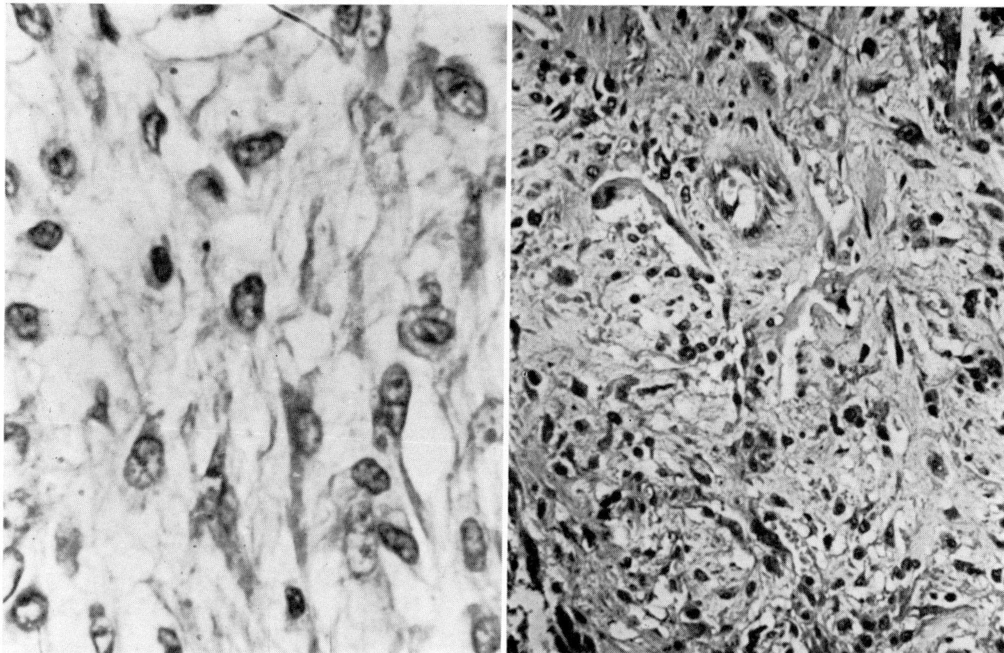

Figure 4. Figure 5.

TREATMENT OF $Ni(CO)_4$ POISONING

For the treatment of acute nickel carbonyl poisoning, sodium diethyldithiocarbamate trihydrate (Dithiocarb) has proved to be dramatically effective.[43, 44]

The metal-binding property of the dialkyldithiocarbamates was first reported by Delepine in 1908.[45, 46] However, it was not until 21 years later that this property found application in analytical chemistry. Callan and Henderson in 1929[47] first applied the metal-binding property of dithiocarb to a colorimetric method, which is now a classical method for the determination of trace amounts of copper.

Recognition of the metal-binding and biologic properties as well as the low toxicity of the dithiocarbamates has formed the foundation for studies on the mobilization of nickel and copper in acute nickel carbonyl poisoning[44] and has ultimately brought to light the therapeutic effectiveness of Dithiocarb.[48]

SUMMARY

A resumé of nickel poisoning has been presented. A number of clinical syndromes may be encountered after exposure to nickel. These syndromes range from nickel dermatitis, pulmonary eosinophilia, acute and subacute pneumonitis with adrenal cortical insufficiency and pulmonary cancer. Special emphasis has been placed on the toxicity of exposure to nickel carbonyl.

Experimental studies indicate that inhaled gaseous nickel is carcinogenic to the lungs of rats, a species generally con-

TABIE IV: HISTORICAL RESUMÉ OF NICKEL AS A CARCINOGEN

1931-1932	*Report of the Chief Inspector of Factories,* Great Britain, for 1931 listed several cases of nasal cancer which had occurred among workers in a nickel refinery at Clydach, South Wales.[19]
1933	*Stephens* suggested that nickel was one of the agents responsible for industrial epitheliomato.[20]
1937	*Baader* announced a high incidence of pulmonary cancer in nickel workers.[18]
1944	*Campbell* suggested that incidence of lung cancer in mice was increased after exposure to "nickel dust."[21]
1949	*Ministry of Pensions,* Great Britain, officially designated cancer of respiratory tract in nickel workers as an industrial disease.[22,23]
1950	*Loken* reported 5 cases of lung cancer in nickel workers in Norway.[24]
1952	*Barnett* reported 82 cases of lung cancer in nickel workers in Norway.[25]
1957	*Sunderman et al.* demonstrated extensive squamous metaplasia of the bronchial epithelium in rats exposed to nickel carbonyl. Surviving rats were observed for pulmonary carcionogenesis.[26]
1958	*Morgan* reported 131 cases of lung cancer and 61 of nasal cancer in Welsh nickel workers.[27]
1958	*Doll* reported 35.5 percent of all deaths among nickel workers in Glamorganshire to be due to cancer of the respiratory tract.[28]
1958	*Williams* reported a pathologic study of 5 cases of lung cancer in Welsh nickel workers.[29]
1958	*Hueper* found metaplastic and anaplastic changes in lungs of rats and guinea pigs exposed to nickel dust.[30]
1959	*Sunderman et al.* induced pulmonary cancer in rats by inhalations of nickel carbonyl.[31]
1961	*Sunderman and Sunderman, Jr.,* implicated nickel as a pulmonary carcinogen in tobacco smoke.[32]
1962	*Passey* tabulated 144 deaths from lung cancer in nickel workers. Average age at death, 57.6 years; average years in nickel refineries, 27 years; average time between first exposure and death, 30 years.[33]
1963	*Sunderman and Sunderman, Jr.,* observed that after chronic exposure of rats to nickel carbonyl, microsomal and supernatant fractions of lungs and liver as well as nuclear and mitochondrial fractions of the lung contained increased amounts of nickel.[34]
1964	*Sunderman, Jr.* found increased concentration of nickel in high molecular weight RNA from lung and liver after inhalation of nickel carbonyl by rats.[35]
1964	*Heath and Daniel* observed that powdered metallic nickel injected intramuscularly into rats produced tumors of striated muscle origen.[36]
1965	*Sunderman and Donnelly* found six of 89 rats exposed to nickel carbonyl and living for two or more years after the initial exposure developed pulmonary carcinomas with metastases. These lesions included squamos cell carcinoma, adenocarcinoma and anaplastic carcinoma.[37]
1967	*Tatarskaya* reported an increase in the incidence of cancer of the nose and sinuses among industrial nickel workers in Russia.[38]
1967	*Hackett and Sunderman, Jr.,* observed that the administration of nickel carbonyl parenterally induced the same type of lesions in the lungs of rats as those observed in animals exposed to the inhalation of nickel carbonyl.[39]
1968	*Hackett and Sunderman, Jr.,* reported their observations of the ultrastructure of the lungs of animals exposed to nickel carbonyl.[40]
1968	*Sunderman, Jr. and Selin* showed by means of radioactive nickel carbonyl, $^{63}Ni(CO)_4$, that the lung is a major route for the excretion of nickel carbonyl.[41]

TABLE V: NICKEL IN TOBACCO

	Micrograms of Nickel Inhaled
Average amount of nickel in mainstream smoke of a single cigarette	0.37
Carcinogenic dose for rats. One year of chronic exposures (30 minutes — 3 times weekly)	1930 (equivalent to 260 packs of cigarettes)

sidered to be peculiarly resistant to pulmonary cancer. The lesions included the common types of pulmonary cancer — squamous cell carcinoma, adenocarcinoma and anaplastic carcinoma. All of the pulmonary lesions were found between 24 and 27 months after the initial exposure to nickel carbonyl.

The amount of nickel capable of inducing lung cancer in the rat is comparable to the amount of nickel inhaled by persons smoking less than 15 cigarettes per day for a period of a year.

REFERENCES

1. Caujolle, J., and Canal, G.: Toxicology of nickel. J. pharm. chim., *29:*391-409, 1939.
2. Mastromatteo, E.: Nickel: A review of its occupational health aspects. J. Occup. Med.,*9:*127-36, 1967.
3. Caso, B.: Folio Medica, *24:*1625, 1932. Cited in Scudier, U., and Tinazzi, V.: Experimental research in nickel poisoning and its treament with $Na_2CaEDTA$. Med. Lavoro, *47:*161-6, 1956.
4. Mellon Institute of Industrial Research: University of Pittsburgh Special Report, 1951.
5. Lehman, K.B.: Hygienic studies on nickel. Arch. f. Hyg., *68:*421-65, 1908-1909.
6. Kincaid, J. F., Strong, J. S., and Sunderman, F. W.: Nickel poisoning. I. Experimental study of the effects of acute and subacute exposure to nickel carbonyl. Arch. Ind. Hyg. Occup. Med. *8:*48-60, 1953.
7. Gaul, L. E.:Incidence of sensitivity to cromium, nickel, gold, silver and copper compared to reactions to their aqueous salts including cobalt sulfate. Ann. Allergy, *12:*429-44, 1954.
8. O'Driscoll, B. J.: Allergy to nickel: A common cause of eczema. J. Irish Med. Assn, *56:*162-3, 1965.
9. Fisher, A. A., and Shapiro, A.: Allergic eczematous contact dermatitis due to metallic nickel. JAMA, *161:*717 21, 1956.
10. Sunderman, F. W., and Sunderman, F. W., Jr.: Loeffer's syndrome associated with nickel sensitivity. Arch. Intern. Med., *107:*405-8, 1961.
11. Arvidsson, H., and Bogg, A.: Transitory pulmonary infiltration: Loffer's syndrome; in acute generalized dermatitis. Acta dermat.-venereol., *39:*30-4, 1959.
12. American Conference of Governmental Industrial Hygienists. Threshold Limit Values for 1968.
13. Sunderman, F. W., and Kincaid, J. F.: Nickel poisoning. II. Studies on patients suffering from acute exposure to vapors of nickel carbonyl. JAMA, *155:*889-94, 1954.
14. Kincaid, J. F., Stanley, E. L. Beckworth, C. H., and Sunderman, F. W.: Nickel poisoning. III. Procedures for detection, prevention, and treatment of nickel carbonyl exposure including a method for the determination of nickel in biological materials. Am. J. Clin. Path., *26:*107-19, 1956.
15. Unpublished studies.
16. Tedeschi, R. E., and Sunderman, F. W.: Nickel poisoning. V. The metabolism of nickel under normal conditions and after exposure to nickel carbonyl. Arch. Ind. Health, *16:*486-8, 1957.
17. Sunderman, F. W., Range, C. L., Sunderman, F. W., Jr., Donnelly, A. J. and Lucyszyn, G. W.: Nickel Poisoning. XII. Metabolic and pathologic changes in acute pneumonitis from nickel carbonyl. Am. J. Clin. Path., *36:*477-91, 1961.
18. Baader, E. W.: In, Berufskrebs-neure Ergebnisse auf dem Gebiefc der Krebskrankheiten, Adam, C and Auler, D., eds., pp. 116-7. S. Hirzel Verlag, Leipzig, c. 1937.
19. Annual Report of H. M. Chief Inspector of Factories, 1931. His Majesty's Stationery Office, London, 1932. Cited in Heath, J. C., and Daniel, M. R.: The production of malignant tumors by nickel in the rat. Brit. J. Cancer, *18:*261-4, 1964.
20. Stephens, G. A.: Med. Press, *187:*194, 216 and 283, 1933. Cited in Heath, J. C., and Daniel, M. R.: The production of malignant tumors by nickel in the rat. Brit. J. Cancer, *18:*261-4, 1964.
21. Campbell, J. A.: Lung tumors in mice and man. Brit. Med. J., *1:*179-83, 1943.
22. Doll, R.: Cancer of the lung and nose in nickel workers. Brit. J. Ind. Med., *15:*217-23, 1958.
23. Goldblatt, W. M.: Occupational carcinogenesis. Brit. M. Bull., *14:*136-41, 1958.
24. Lóken, A. C.: Lung cancer in nickel workers. Tiddskr. norske laegefore, *70:*376-8, 1950.
25. Barnett, G. P.: Annual Report of the Chief Inspector of Factories for the Year 1948, p. 158. Her Majesty's Stationery Office, London, 1949.
26. Sunderman, F. W., Kincaid, J. F., Donnelly, A. J., and West, B.: Nickel Poisoning. IV. Chronic exposure of rats to nickel carbonyl: A report after one year of observation. Arch. Ind. Health, *16:*480-5, 1957.
27. Morgan, J. G.: Some observations of the incidence of respiratory cancer in nickel workers. Brit. J. Ind. Med., *15:*224-34, 1958.
28. Doll, R.: In Carcinoma of the Lung, Bignall, J. R., ed. pp. 45-59. E. & S. Livingstone, Ltd., Edinburgh and London, c. 1958.
29. Williams, W. J.: The pathology of the lungs in five nickel workers. Brit. J. Ind. Med., *15:* 235-42, 1958.
30. Hueper, W. C.: Experimental studies in metal carcinogenesis. IX. Pulmonary lesions in guinea pigs and rats exposed to prolonged inhalation of powdered metallic nickel. Arch. Path., *65:* 600-7, 1958.
31. Sunderman, F.W., Donnelly, A. J., West, B., and Kincaid, J. F.: Nickel Poisoning. IX. Carcinogenesis in rats exposed to nickel carbonyl. Arch. Ind. Health, *20:*36-41, 1959.
32. Sunderman, F. W., and Sunderman, F. W., Jr.: Nickel poisoning. XI. Implication of nickel as

a pulmonary carcinogen in tobacco smoke. Am. J. Clin. Path., *35:*203-9, 1961.

33. Passey, R. D.: Some problems of lung cancer. Lancet, *2:*107-12, 1962.
34. Sunderman, F. W., Jr., and Sunderman, F. W.: Studies of nickel carcinogenesis: The subcellular partition of nickel in lung and liver following inhalation of nickel carbonyl. Am. J. Clin. Path., *40:*563-75,1963.
35. Sunderman, F. W., Jr.: Studies of nickel carcinogenesis: Fractionations of nickel in ultracentrifugal supernatants of lung and liver by Dextran Gal chromatography. Am. J. Clin. Path., *42:*228-36, 1964.
36. Heath, J. C., and Daniel, M.R.: The production of malignant tumours by nickel in the rat. Brit. J. Cancer, *18:*261-4, 1964.
37. Sunderman, F. W., and Donnelly, A. J.: Studies of nickel carcinogenesis: Metastasizing pulmonary tumors in rats induced by the inhalation of nickel carbonyl. Am. J. Path., *46:*1027-41, 1965.
38. Tatarskaya, A. A.: Cancer of the respiratory tract in nickel workers. Vop. Onkol., *13:*58-60, 1967.
39. Hackett, R. L., and Sunderman, F. W., Jr.: Acute pathological reactions to administration of nickel carbonyl. Arch. Environ. Health, *14:* 604-13, 1967.
40. Hackett, R. L., and Sunderman, F. W., Jr.: Pulmonary alveolar reaction to nickel carbonyl. Arch. Environ. Health, *16:*349-62, 1968.
41. Sunderman, F. W., Jr., and Selin, C. E.: The metabolism of nickel-63 carbonyl. Toxicol. Appl. Pharmacol. *12:*207-18, 1968.
42. Sunderman, F. W.: In, Lung Tumors in Animals. Proceedings of the 3rd Quadrennial International Conference on Cancer. Perugia, Italy, 1965, pp. 551-64.
43. Sunderman, F. W., and Sunderman, F. W., Jr.: Nickel poisoning. VIII. Dithiocarb: A new therapeutic agent for persons exposed to nickel carbonyl. Am. J. Med. Sci., *236:*26-31, 1958.
44. Sunderman, F. W.: The mobilization of copper and nickel by sodium diethyldithiocarbamate. J. New Drugs, *4:*154-61, 1964.
45. Delépine, M. M.: Composés sulfurés et azotes derivés de sulfure de carbone. XII. Thiosulfocarbamates métalliques. Bull. Soc. Chim. Paris, *3:*643-52, 1908.
46. ——————: Proprietés des thisosulfocarbamates métalliques. Comptes Rendus Acad. Sci., *146:*981-5, 1908.
47. Callan, T., and Henderson, J. A. R.: A new reagent for the colorimetric determination of minute amounts of copper. Analyst, *54:*650-3, 1929.
48. Sunderman, F. W., Paynter, O. E., and George, R. B.: The effects of the protracted administration of the chelating agent, sodium diethyldithiocarbamate (Dithiocarb). Am. J. Med. Sci. *254:*24-33, 1967.

PART IV

CLINICOPATHOLOGIC CONSIDERATIONS

Chapter 37

Use of Dialysis in the Treatment of Poisoning

ERVIN A. GOMBOS, M.D.

Both hemodialysis and peritoneal dialysis have proved to be valuable in a variety of types of poisoning and excessive ingestion of drugs. It is however by no means the only recourse to the physician. Poisons have been removed by the use of other methods such as chelation, forced diuresis (using osmotic loading with mannitol, urea or soluretic agents) or by gastric or pulmonary lavage.

KINETICS OF DIALYSIS

The artificial kidney represents a system consisting of 2 compartments separated by a membrane. One compartment contains blood which is flowing by virtue of being pumped by an artificial pump assist or the action of myocardial contraction itself. The other side of the membrane contains the bath fluid, usually refered to as dialysate, also flowing. Substances which are to be removed from the blood enter into the circulation from both the intravascular and extravascular compartments. At the outset of dialysis, when the concentration of the substances to be removed is the greatest, the transfer into the bath is also the greatest. As soon as the dialysate bath fluid contains the substance, the transfer across the membrane occurs in both directions. In order to maintain a high rate of transfer throughout the dialytic period and thus maximize the efficiency of the procedure, most up-to-date equipment utilizes a single pass of dialysate through the dialyzing device rather than the older re-circulating tank systems. The rate of diffusion of a particular substance affected by the permeability of the membrane, is also influenced by the rate of ultrafiltration and by osmotic pressure gradients. All these factors independently and in concert affect the rate of removal of the toxic substances and thus exert influence on the rate of clinical recovery.

One of the means of assessing the effect of dialysis on the rate of diffusion of a particular substance is by measuring dialysance. Wolf *et al.* (32) define dialysance in a hemodialyzer as the rate of shift of a substance between blood and dialysate bath per unit of blood-dialysate concentration gradient. It is comparable to the clearance concept of the natural kidney where the rate of blood flow from which a substance is completely removed is expressed in ml/min.

The rationale in the use of dialysis in removal of toxic substances is dependent on several factors:

a. The dialyzed substance must have

a reasonable rate of diffusion through the dialytic membrane

b. Diffusible poisons must be present in plasma water in significant quantities. There should be a dynamic equilibrium with whatever part is protein bound in blood and distributed and bound in the tissues.

c. The intoxication is directly related to the blood concentrations and the duration of exposure to the poison.

d. The amount of poison dialyzed must significantly add to the amount disposed of by normal physiological mechanisms.

Tables I and II indicate some of the currently known dialysable poisons.

TABLE I: DIALYSABLE POISONS*

Barbiturates	*Sedatives*	*Analgesics*
Barbital	Glutethemide	Acetylsalicylic Acid
Phenobarbial	Diphenylhydantoin	Methylsalicylate
Amobarbital	Primidone	Acetophenetidin
Pentobarbital	Meprobamate	Dextropropoxyphene
Butabarbital	Ethchlorvynol	
Secobarbital	Methypyrlon	
Cyclobarbital	Pargyline	
	Heroin	
	Paraldehyde	
	Chloral Hydrate	
Alcohols	*Halides*	*Metals*
Ethanol	Bromide	Strontium
Methanol	Chloride	Calcium
Isopropanol	Iodine	Iron
Ethylene Glycol	Fluoride	Lead
		Mercury
		Arsenic
		Sodium
		Potassium
		Magnesium

*This list is incomplete. Other compounds in whom the kinetics of dialysis are unknown have been omitted.

TABLE II: DIALYSABLE POISONS*

Antibiotics	*Endogenous metabolic products*	*Other substances*
Streptomycin	Ammonia	Digoxin
Kanamycin	Bilirubin	Dextroamphetamine
Neomycin	Uric Acid	Carbon Tetrachloride
Vancomycin	Lactic Acid	Ergotamine
Penicillin	Pyruvic Acid	Cyclophosphamide
Ampicillin		5-Fluorouracil
Sulfonamides		Methotrexate
Cephalin		
Cepheloridine		
Chloramphenicol		
Tetracycline		
Nitrofurantoin		
Polymyxin		
Isoniazid		
Cycloserine		
Colistin		

*This list is incomplete. Other compounds in whom the kinetics of dialysis are unknown have been omitted.

It is clear from experience that dialysance of substances vary and that although improvement usually follows dialysis, the degree of this change is unpredictable. The support of the laboratory in the process of the assessment of the poisoning and subsequent management is invaluable. An important aspect of information that must be sought from the laboratory, especially in situations where poisoning led to a comatose state, is the nature and concentration of the agent. Ideally, the physician responsible for the management of the patient could profit most from the laboratory before deciding on the mode of management. The knowledge of the nature of the intoxication and its degree may greatly affect the decision for aggressive therapy. Since dialysis is a life saving measure and usually requires prompt intervention, it is equally clear that it is impossible in most instances to wait for the laboratory to indicate the nature of the poisoning. Thus, in the majority of instances, careful assessment of the circumstances may give clues as to the nature of the intoxication. (3, 10).

BARBITURATES (11, 12, 28)

There has been a significant decrease in the mortality from barbiturate intoxication by the use of forced diuresis and maintenance of circulation. In addition, alkalinisation of the urine increases excretion phenobarbitol but not of short acting barbiturates.

Still, with severe intoxications, dialysis is needed to speed up recovery. Depending on the specific drug, hemodialysis removes barbiturates 10 to 30 times faster than diuresis. Maximal dialysance ranges from 65 ml/min for *secobarbital* to 100 ml/min for *phenobarbital*. Protein binding and sequestration in body fat limits removal of short acting barbiturates. Dialysis is usually indicated on clinical grounds, and should be considered after ingestion of more than 3.0 gm of short or 5.0 gm of long acting barbiturates. Blood levels above 3.5 mg% (short acting) and 8.0 mg% (long acting) are indications for dialysis.

GLUTETHIMIDE (3, 14, 19, 24)

Intoxication with *glutethimide* (Doriden) is usually severe. Dialysance values may be 70-90 ml/min but clinical results with dialysis are discouraging. Dialysis shortens coma, blood levels decline and dialysate may contain 30-200 times the amount removed by urinary excretion. Removal of glutethimide is hampered by protein binding and low circulating blood levels. This is due to a 10-15 fold concentration in body fat. Because of high mortality and slow removal by simpler means, dialysis is recommended for prolonged coma, severe intoxications, blood levels above 3.0 mg% or after ingestion of more than 10 gm or 0.15 gm/Kg.

OTHER SEDATIVES AND TRANQUILIZERS (1, 17, 27)

Hemodialysis has been reported as useful in intoxications with *diphenylhydantoin* (Dilantin®), *primidone* (Mysoline®) or *meprobamate*. Dialysis should be considered after ingestion of more than 10 gm of *ethchlorvynol* (Placidyl®) or when blood levels are above 7.0 mg%. Hemodialysis produces clinical improvement also in poisoning with *methypyrlon* (Noludar®), *heroin*, *paraldehyde* and *chloral hydrate*.

Phenothiazines are not dialyzable.

ANALGESICS (5, 8, 26)

Acetylsalicylic acid is rapidly removed

by dialysis. Dialysance is 100 ml/min and rates equal 3 to 5 times those lost by diuresis. Dialysis is indicated after ingestion of more than 0.5 gm/kg or with a blood level above 70 mg%. *Methyl salicylate* and *acetophenetidin* (Phenacetin®) have been dialyzed out with good clinical results. Intoxication with *propoxyphene* (Darvon) may be severe with Nalomorphine as the specific antidote. Clinical response to dialysis is only fair due to small quantity in circulating blood.

HALIDES (22)

Dialysis of *bromide* is rapid and clinical improvement is dramatic. Dialysance may exceed 200 ml/min and serum half life is reduced from over 100 hours with no therapy to one hour with dialysis. Dialysis may be indicated with blood levels above 20 mEq/L.

Radioiodide is dialysable *in vitro,* but removal at low plasma concentrations is limited by protein binding. Organic *iodide* can be removed by dialysis.

Fluoride is dialysable in vitro from plasma but in fluoride poisoning, the course is usually too rapid to achieve clinical benefit in spite of some clinical improvement.

ALCOHOLS (7, 20)

Clinically, *ethanol* intoxication responds to dialysis which is rarely needed because of the rapid metabolism and excretion of this alcohol. Dialysis is indicated for *methanol* intoxication to relieve coma and prevent blindness. Dialysance is about 100 ml/min. The toxic metabolite formic acid is also rapidly cleared. Indications for dialysis are a definite history of ingestion, a blood level above 100 mg% severe acidosis or visual impairment.

METALS (4, 18, 23, 31, 32)

Calcium is freely dialyzable (150 ml/min) but clinical results in hypercalcemia have been variable. This is attributed to rapid mobilisation of bone calcium.

Magnesium is also dialysable and at rates comparable to calcium (100 ml/min).

Iron is dialysable and a significant increase in removal was reported by combined chelation and with diethylenetriaminopentaacetic acid (DTPA) and hemodialysis.

The dialyzance of BAL – *mercury* complex is 5 ml/min. Dialysance of *lead* versenate is 31 ml/min but clinical results are poor. Dialyzability of *arsenic* has been reported.

Sodium and *potassium* are freely dialyzable and their dialyzance can reach 250-350 ml/min.

ANTIBIOTICS (2, 6, 9, 15, 16, 21, 25, 29, 30)

In patients with renal failure impaired excretion of antibiotics may lead to toxic manifestations.

Streptomycin induced ototoxicity has been reported improved and blood levels significantly decreased. Persistence of *Kanamycin* in the blood may cause ototoxicity and nephrotoxicity. Dialysis effectively lowers blood levels. *Neomycin* may also accumulate and cause ototoxicity and nephrotoxicity. Dialysis significantly reduced blood levels. *Vancomycin* retention produces nephrotoxicity. It is poorly dialyzable partly due to protein binding.

In renal failure, *penicillin* persists in blood. Neuromuscular toxicity and hypersensitivity reactions may be indications for dialysis which effectively reduces penicillin levels in the blood. *Oxa-*

cillin and *methicillin* are also accumulated in renal failure. They are dialyzed only slowly, partly due to protein binding. *Ampicillin* is also retained in renal failure and is dialyzable. *Cephalothin* and *Cephaloridine* are only slowly removed by dialysis. *Sulphonamides* are also dialyzable. *Polymyxin B* and *Colistin* can produce neurotoxicity. They are only slowly dialyzable. *Isoniazid* is dialyzable.

REMARK

This review is by necessity sketchy and incomplete. The interested reader is advised to peruse the annual reviews on the subject in the Transactions of the American Society for Artificial Internal Organs.

BIBLIOGRAPHY

1. Avram, M. M. and McGinn, J. T.: Extracorporporeal hemodialysis in phenothiazine overdosage. J.A.M.A., *197:*142, 1966.
2. Bulger, R. J., Lindholm, D. D., Murray, J. S., and Kirby, W. W. M.: Effect of uremia on methicillin and oxacillin blood levels. J.A.M.A., *187:*319, 1964.
3. Chandler, B. F., Meroney, W. H. Czarnecki, S. W., Herman, R. H., Cheitlin, M. D., Goldbaum, L. R., and Herndon, E. G.: Artificial hemodialysis in management og glutethimide intoxication. J.A.M.A., *170:*914, 1959.
4. Covey, T. J.: Ferrous sulphate poisoning: A review, case summaries and therapeutic regimen. J. Pediat., *64:*218, 1964.
5. Doolan, P. D., Walsh, W. P., Kyle, L. H., and Wishinsky, H.: Acetyl salicylic acid intoxication, A proposed method of treatment. J.A.M.A., *146:*105, 1951.
6. Edwards, K. D. G., and Whyte, H. M.: Streptomycin poisoning in renal failure. An indication for treatment with an artificial kidney. Brit. Med. J., *1:*753, 1959.
7. Erlanson, P., Fritz. H., Hagstam, K. E., Liljenberg, B., Tryding, H., and Voigt, G.: Bevere methanol intoxication. Acta Med. Scan., *177:* 393, 1965.
8. Fennely, J. J., and Lasker, N.: Acute renal failure following acetophenetidine ingestion. J. Med. Soc. New Jersey, *61:*115, 1964.
9. Gombos, E. A., Katz, S., Fedorko, J., Allnoch, H., and Lee, T. H.: Dialysis properties of newer antimicrobial agents. Antimicrobial Agents Chemother., *4:*373, 1964.
10. Hagstam, K. E., and Lindholm, T.: Treatment of exogenous poisoning with special regard to the need for artificial kidney in severe complicated cases. Acta Med. Scan., *175:*507, 1964.
11. Hagstam, K. E., Larsson, L. E., and Thysell, H.: Experimental studies on charcoal perfusion in uremia including histopathologic findings. Acta Med. Scan., *180:*593, 1966.
12. Henderson, L. W., and Merrill, J. P.: Treatment of barbiturate intoxication. With a report of recent experience at Peter Bent Brigham Hospital. Ann. Int. Med., *64:*876, 1966.
13. Jorgensenm, H. E., and Wieth, J. O.: Dialysable poisons, Hemodialysis in the treatment of acute poisoning. Lancet, *1:*81, 1963.
14. Kier, L. C., Whitehead, R. W., and White, W. C.: Blood and urine levels in glutethimide (Doriden) intoxication. J.A.M.A., *166:*1861, 1958.
15. Kunin, C. M., Problems of antimicrobial drug therapy in renal failure. Proc. 3rd Int. Congr. Nephrol. *3:*193, 1966.
16. Lindholm, D. D., and Murray, J. S.: Persistence of vancomycin in the blood during renal failure and its treatment by hemodialysis. New England J. Med., *274:*1047, 1966.
17. Loeser, W. D., Fisher, C. J., and Boulis, G.: Forty-three dialyses in a community hospital, J.A.M.A., *192:*809, 1965.
18. Maher, J. F., and Schreiner, G. E.: The dialysis of mercury and mercury-BAL complex. Clin. Res., *7:*298, 1959.
19. Maher, J. F., Schreiner, G. E., and Westervelt, F. B.: Acute glutethimide intoxication. I. Clinical experience (22 patients) compared to acute barbiturate intoxication (62 patients) . Amer. J. Med., *33:*70, 1962.
20. Marc-Aurele, J., and Schreiner, G. E.: The dialysance of ethano- and methanol: A proposed method for the treatment of massive intoxication by ethyl or methyl alcohol. J. Clin. Invest., *39:*892, 1960.
21. Mackay, D. N., and Kaye, D.: Serum concentration of colistin in patients with normal and impaired renal function. New England J. Med., *270:*394, 1964.
22. Merrill, J. P., and Weller, J. M.: Treatment of bromism with the artificial kidney. Ann. Int. Med., *37:*186, 1952.
23. Mehbod, H.: Treatment of lead intoxication. Combined use of peritoneal dialysis and edetate calcium disodium. J.A.M.A., *201:*972, 1967.
24. Parsons, F. M.: The use of the artificial kidney in salicylate poisoning. Salicylates, an International Symposium, Empire Rheumatism Coun-

cil, Ed., Dixon, A. St. J., Martin, B. K., Smith, M. J. H., and Wodd, P. H. N. Boston, Little Brown and Co., 1963, p. 281.

25. Ruedy, J.: Effects of peritoneal dialysis on physiolgical disposition of oxacillin, ampicillin and tetracycline in patients with renal disease. Canad. M. A. J., *94*:257, 1966.
26. Schreiner, G. E., Berman, L. B., Griffin, J., and Feys, J.: Specific therapy for salicylism. New England J. Med., *253*:213, 1955.
27. Schultz, J. C., Crouder, D. G., and Medart, W. S.: Excretion studies in ethchlorvynol (Pacidyl) intoxication. Arch. Int. Med., *117*:409, 1966.
28. Setter, J. G., Maher, J. F., and Schreiner, G. E.: Barbiturate intoxication. Evaluation of therapy including dialysis in a large series selectively referred because of severity. Arch. Int. Med., *117*:224, 1966.
29. Sitprija, V., and Holmes, J. H.: Isoniazid intoxication. Amer. Rev. Resp. Dis., *90*:1174, 1965.
30. Skimming, L. H., Knies, P. T., Anthony, M. A., and Melaragno, E. S.: Hemolytic anemia caused by sulfamethoxpyidazine. Report of a case successfully treated with hemodialysis. Ohio Med. J., *57*:280, 1961.
31. Smith, H. D., King, L. R., and Margolin, E. G.: Treatment of lead encephalopathy: the combined use of EDTA and hemodialysis. Amer. J. Dis. Child., *109*,332, 1965.
32. Wolf, A. V., Remp, D. G., Kiley, J. E., and Currie, G. D.: Artificial kidney function: kinetics of hemodialysis. J. Clin. Invest., *30*:1062, 1951.

Chapter 38

Clinicopathological Considerations of Acute Toxic Nephropathy

ROBERT C. MUEHRCKE, M.D.

Etiolgy and Pathogenesis

The kidney with its rich blood supply and superior excretory function is particularly vulnerable to the adverse effects of chemicals, biological products and drugs (1, 2). Although the kidney comprises 0.4% of the total body weight, it requires a high oxygen consumption. To achieve this requirement the kidneys receive approximately 20 to 25% of the heart output. When compared to other organs, the relatively small kidney mass have the greatest surface area of endothelial cells. Moreover, the kidneys are second to the liver in the most complex metabolic function of any organ. Finally, the kidneys have an extremely vascular renal medullae with its rete mirabile that functions in the final dilution and concentration of the urine. This complex mechanism results in hypertonicity of the renal interstitium with concentration of nephrotoxic chemicals and drugs.

Nephrotoxic chemicals, plants, venoms, and drugs have exerted these adverse effects of the kidney through any one, or a combination of several pathopharmacological mechanisms. The most common mechanism is the direct action of the nephrotoxic substance as a protoplasmic poison (3). As the nephrotoxic agent passes through the glomerular filter, it is present in an amount proportionate to the filtered plasma water. The nephrotoxic substance is foreign to the kidney and has no specific renal tubular transport process as it moves down the nephron it is progressively concentrated within the tubular lumen. The concentrated nephrotoxic agent is of such sufficient quantity that it directly damages the tubular epithelial cells. Moreover, other nephrotoxic substances are reabsorbed and may increase in their concentration to reach toxic levels within the medullary interstitium by the osmotic concentration of fluids. When sufficient quantity is accumulated, the kidney interstitium is damaged. An excellent example of this latter effect is chronic phenacetin nephritis (4).

Some nephrotoxic substances penetrate the cell to interact with cellular constituents and, subsequently poisons the cell. One example of this mechanism is the nephrotoxic effects of Mercuhydrin. It reacts with enzyme systems of the sulfhydryl groups within the mitochondria. Other nephrotoxins couple with enzymes to inactivate them. Some nephrotoxins affect enzymes within the mitochondria (Kreb cycle) while other toxins affect cytoplasmic enzymes (Glycolytic cycle). This functional interference may result in a biochemical dysfunction. When the tissue is studied by light or electron microscopy, no apparent tubular morphological abnormalities are noted. Other protoplasmic toxins when concentrated may coagulate protein and result in either severe tubular necrosis or diffuse bilateral renal cortical necrosis.

Other nephrotoxic agents produce their adverse effects through a pathopharmacological mechanism of hypersensitivity. The sulfonamides are the best example of such a model. The morphological site involved is usually the large endothelial surface of the glomerular capillaries, arterioles, arteries and renal interstitium. The interstitial hypersensitivity reaction was reported over 75 years ago by Councilman (5). It is known as Councilman's interstitial nephritis and is characterized by interstitial infiltrates of plasma cells, small lymphocytes and eosinophils. Examples of this hypersensitivity reactions are drugs such as; phenindione, nitrofurantoin, Dilantin, methicilin, penicillin and Mercuhydrin.

In general, substances toxic to the kidney include chemicals, plant poisons, venoms, and drugs in any physical state; liquids, solids and gases, biological products such as bee, spider, and snake venom; plant toxins (mushrooms); horse serum (vaccines); and drugs given by the oral or parenteral route.

A. CHEMICALS

The more common nephrotoxins producing acute renal failure are heavy metals, organic solvents, glycols, aniline, insecticides, arsine, cresol and a miscellaneous group of chemicals Table I. They usually act directly on the tubular cells to disrupt their metabolic and morphological integrity.

TABLE I: COMMON CHEMICALS AND DRUGS THAT INDUCE OLIGURIC RENAL FAILURE

Amphotericin B	Mercuhydrin
Aniline	Mercury compounds
Aristolochic acid	Methicillin
Arsenic	Naphthalene (mothballs)
Arsine gas (AsH_3)	Neomycin
Bacitracin	Nitrofurantoin
Bismuth	Orabilex
Camphor	Oxalates
Carbon tetrachloride	Para-aminosalicylic acid
Chlordane	Paradichlorobenzene
Chloroform	Parathione
Chlorothiazide	Penicillin
Colistin	Pentachlorophenol
Copper compounds	Phenacetin
Creosote	Phenindione
Dilantin	Phenol
Essential (volatile) oils	Phenylbutazone
Ethylene dichloride	Phosphorus, yellow
Ethylene glycol	Polymyxin B
Ferrous sulfate	Propylthiouracil
Formaldehyde (formalin)	Quinine sulfate
	Resorcinol
Gold salts	Salicylates
Guaiacol	Sodium acetrizoate
Horse serum	Sulfonamides
Hydralazine	Tetrachloroethane
Iodides	Thiourea
Kanamycin	Thymol

1. MERCURY COMPOUNDS

The inorganic salt-bichloride of mercury (mercuric chloride) is also known as corrosive sublimate. Mercury compounds were used in mediaeval times to poison one's enemies. Today, mercuric chloride is usually ingested accidentally, in suicidal attempts (6) or followed its use as an abortive agent. The dose required to induce renal failure is difficult to assess. In most reports, the patients with acute renal failure had ingested 2 or 3 tablets (0.5 gm tablets). When more than four tablets were taken acute oliguric renal failure was fatal. Renal lesions developed within three hours after ingestion.

Schreiner and Maher (2, 7) described 11 patients with mercuric chloride-induced acute oliguric renal failure. Five patients who survived were treated within 48 hours after ingesting mercuric chloride using hemodialysis and BAL inffusion. Six patients were treated after uremia occurred and only three survived. BAL appears to enhance the removal of mercuric ions by 7 to 11% using hemodialysis.

The clinical symptom of inorganic mercury poisoning begins with a lingering bitter and metallic taste in the mouth. The patient experiences a sensation of throat constriction, suffocation, substernal burning, gastritis, abdominal pain, and, finally nausea and vomiting. Persistent vomiting leads to retching of blood. On examination, ulceration may be noted in the palate. The patient goes into circulatory failure; the pulse becomes weak and rapid. Syncope and shock is followed by a scanty urinary output. Finally, a fatal anuria develops. Jaundice occurs in approximately 35% of the patients.

The most striking morphological abnormalities occur in the proximal convoluted tubules. Less striking abnormalities are found in the ascending limbs, distal convoluted tubules and collecting tubules. The proximal tubule are dilated and appear lined by flat epithelial cells. Patchy calcification may occur in severely damaged tubules. Interstitial edema is noted early and should oliguria be prolonged interstitial fibrosis ensues.

2. Carbon Tetrachloride

Carbon tetrachloride ($C\,Cl_4$) is widely used as an industrial solvent, as a household cleaning agents, as a constituent in certain types of fire extinguishers, in some hair lotions, as an antihelminthic agent and as a vermifuge. It is a volatile, heavier than air liquid which accounts for the high incidence of exposure in poorly ventilated areas. Carbon tetrachloride is toxic in concentration above 100 p.p.m. It is absorbed through the lungs, the skin, and the gut. It is found concentrated in fatty tissue such as the brain and bone marrow.

Carbon tetrachloride is soluble in ethanol. Therefore, the drinking of alcoholic beverages and the simultaneous exposure to carbon tetrachloride tend to enhance carbon tetrachloride absorption and subsequent toxicity. *In vitro,* carbon tetrachloride is oxidized to phosgene and later can condense with ethyl alcohol to form ethyl chloroformate. The later is an extremely nephrotoxic substance. In the absence of ethyl alcohol, phosgene condenses with ammonia to form urea (4).

Carbon tetrachloride appears to be more dangerous in obese or in under nourished individuals. In France, carbon tetrachloride was the commonest agent producing acute renal failure. An excellent description of the clinical features can be found in Hamburger's textbook on nephrology (8). The clinical features of acute poisoning is extremely variable. Males are more afflicted by a ratio of 14:1 over females. Inhalation is the most frequent route of exposure. Toxicity due to ingestion carries a grave prognosis. Initially, the patient has surface or superficial irritation to the exposed skin and mucus membranes. Later, the patient has headaches, nausea, vomiting, abdominal pain, mental confusion, leading to convulsion and coma. Although liver damage is a very striking feature of carbon tetrachloride toxicity, acute renal failure is the most frequent cause of death.

The onset of oliguria is prolonged and may be 7 to 10 days after exposure (Fig. 1). Some patients may have forgotten their exposure to this solvent. Absolute

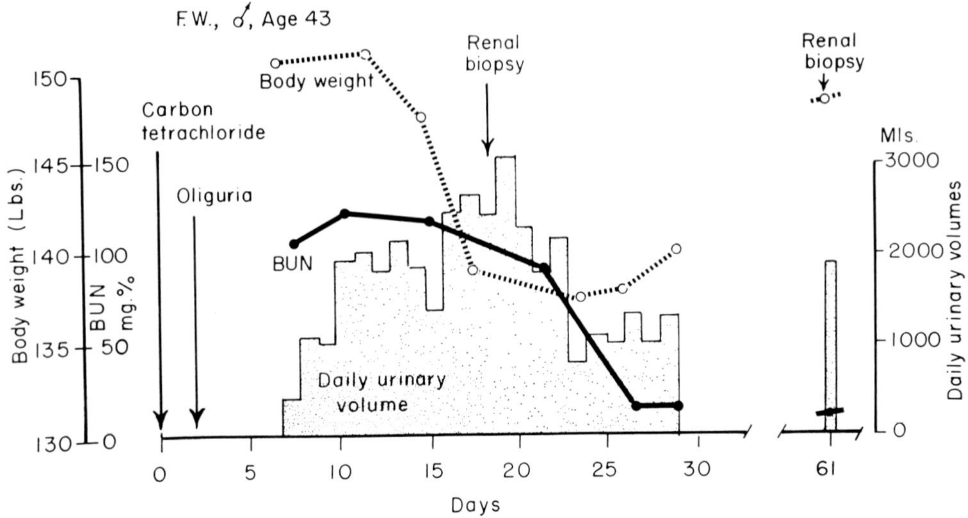

Figure 1. Clinical course of patient with acute renal failure due to carbon tetrachloride. A 43-year-old laborer used carbon tetrachloride to clean neck ties. Two days later he had oliguria and was admitted to hospital. Conservative measures were used to treat him. This included fluid restriction and high carbohydrate diet.
On the seventh day after exposure to CCl_4, he entered the diuretic phase and gradually recovered. A renal biopsy study was done on the eighteenth day. Tubular regeneration and interstitial edema were noted. On the twenty-sixth day, the blood urea nitrogen was stabilized. A repeat biopsy was done during the recovery period. Diffuse interstitial fibrosis was noted.

anuria may last from one day to several weeks. One patient had carbon tetrachloride-induced oliguria for 67 days (5) . In the author's experience, patients with acute renal failure due to carbon tetrachloride were usually "do-it-yourselfers." They usually worked indoors, e.g., in a poorly ventilated basement during the winter months. They usually drank several cans of beer or a few mixed alcoholic drinks while they worked on refinishing furniture, cleaning outboard motors, or cleaning clothes — usually neckties.

Morphological abnormalities occurred in the cortical convolutions and Henle's loops (Fig. 2). Tubular necrosis was most prominent in the out-most cortical portion. Acute tubular necrosis may be severe with tubular coagulation and degranulation.

3. Tetrachloroethylene

Tetrachloroethylene is a colorless liquid with an ethereal odor. It is soluble in 1:10,000 in water and mixable with organic solvents. Tetrachloroethylene has replaced carbon tetrachloride in the treatment of hookworm infestation. It is placed in soft gelatin capsules as either 0.2, 1.0 or 2.5 ml. Tetrachloroethylene produces inebriation, giddiness and liver damage. It is less nephrotoxic than carbon tetrachloride and has produced acute oliguric renal failure due to acute tubular necrosis.

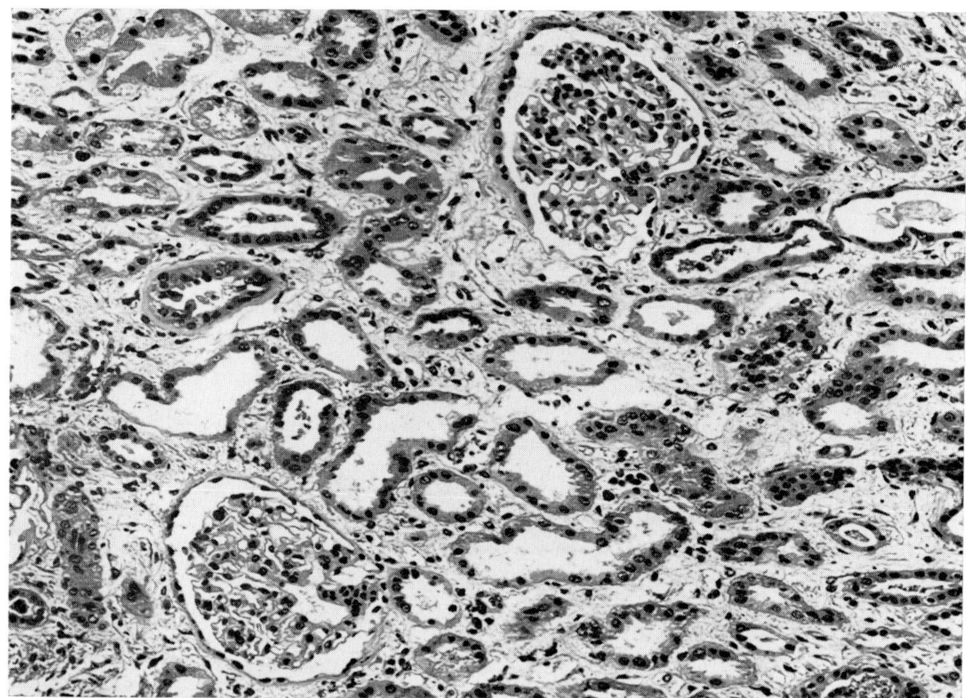

Figure 2. Carbon tetrachloride induced tubular necrosis. This microphotograph is the renal biopsy taken from the patient described in Figure 1. Renal biopsy study revealed acute tubular necrosis with tubular regeneration associated with interstitial edema. (H & E X375)

4. Glycol Toxicity

Glycols are found in automobile antifreeze, in solvents for plastics, in paints; especially lacquers, textiles, cosmetics and flavoring extracts. Allen (9) has classified the toxic glycols. The more important nephrotoxic glycols are ethylene glycol and diethylene glycol. Ethylene glycol dinitrite, a yellow liquid used in the explosive industry, produces symptoms resembling those of nitroglycerol toxicity. Methemoglobinuria and acute tubular necrosis are the prominent renal features. Propylene glycol produces hemoglobinuria and prolonged oliguria without crystals in the tubular lumen. Ethylene dichloride may produce shock, pulmonary edema and tubular necrosis.

5. Aniline

Acute poisoning due to pure aniline is rare (10). However, it does occur in industrial workers and children exposed to inks, colored wax crayons and shoe polishes. Diapers freshly stamped with aniline marking ink have resulted in fatal methemoglobinuria and acute renal failure in infants (11).

Aniline poisoning has been caused by the percutaneous absorption of aniline from freshly dyed shoes or blankets. Aniline and its derivative produces hemolysis, methemoglobinuria, shock, cyanosis, anoxia and acute renal failure. In patients with sublethal poisoning, the clinical manifestations are cyanosis, dyspnea, headache, dizziness and blurring of mental functions. If the aniline poisoning is severe, the manifestations are shock, cyanosis, coma, anemia, and finally a fatal anuria.

The diagnosis is made on finding methemoglobinuria. This is detected as a well defined absorption band at the 630 wave length and immediately disappears after the addition of a few drops of 5% KCN solution. Diazo-reacting compounds can be found in the blood, urine and hemodialysate. Comparisons of the diazo-reacting compounds in blood, urine, and dialysate are used to obtain an optimal clinical end point for dialysis.

Treatment is to remove aniline from the patient by gastric lavage, purges and hemodialysis. This permits the reducing enzyme system of the erythrocyte to rapidly reconvert methemoglobin to hemoglobin. Intravenously injected methylene blue in dosage of 1.0 to 2.0 mgm per kilogram of body weight should be given over a period of several minutes. This dose very rapidly reconverts methemoglobin to hemoglobin. It may be necessary to repeat methylene blue injections at hourly intervals. The blood pressure should be supported by giving whole blood transfusions, vasopressive agents and hemodialysis. Dialysis should be maintained for longer and repeated periods than usually used in treating acute renal failure. This will remove toxic derivative mobilized as a lipid soluble material from body tissues. Acute tubular necrosis is the common morphological burn found in aniline poisoning.

6. Insecticides

The two main groups of nephrotoxic insecticides are the chlorinated hydrocarbons (chlorathane) (9) and the organo-phosphates (parathion) (10). Acute tubular necrosis is the common morphological finding in patients with acute oliguric renal failure.

7. Hexol

Hexol is a mixture of a steam distilled pine oil derivative. (70%) and neutral soap (30%). The pine oil derivative is a mixture of terpine alcoholic predominantly terpineol with 5% to 10% each of terpene, borneol and terpene ethers. Hexol is used in the United States as a household disinfectant.

The common toxic effects of pine oil distillates are local irritation on the skin or burning pain in the mouth. They produce central nervous system excitation and, later depression. Hexol produces headaches, giddiness, ataxia, stupor and death in respiratory failure due to central nervous system depression (11).

The pine oil distillates have produced dysuria, hematuria, proteinuria and glycosuria. In general renal damage is transient and completely reversible.

8. Arsine

Arsine (AsH_3) induced renal failure usually occurs as an occupational hazard. When anuria occurs the prognosis is grave (12). Arsine is inhaled and readily combines with the hemoglobin within the erythrocyte to form an arsine-oxyhemoglobin complex. This is initially oxydized to AsH_2-hemoglobin. As the oxidation process continues, an arsenic-hemoglobin bound product occurs. Intravascular hemolysis occurs and results in methemoglobinuria and massive hemoglobinuria. Hemoglobin and erythrocyte casts fill the tubular lumen. A number of simultaneous conditions occur. The ischemia due to anemia, the presence of hemoglobin, methemoglobin and erythrocyte casts and the direct tissue anoxia of arsine on the respiratory enzymes of the nephron all either singly, or in combination, produce acute tubular necrosis.

9. Cresol

Cresol shares the generalized nephrotoxicity of carbolic acid, naphtol, guaiacol, creosote and other phenols. Lysol® (Cresol) has been taken for suicide purposes or in excessive concentrated solutions via vaginal douches to induce abortion. Cresol is lethal in a dose of 50 to 100 ml. It produces mucus membrane necrosis without the patient aware of the toxic effect. The clinical features are nausea, vomiting, dizziness, ataxia, abdominal pain and shock. Severe intravascular hemolysis occurs followed by hemoglobinuria, proteinuria, hematuria, acute cystitis and acute oliguria due to acute tubular necrosis. The penetrating smell of cresol makes the diagnosis easier. The mucus membrane of the mouth and tongue may be burned and appear a dull, white with phenol and darker brown with cresol. The patient may require dialysis.

10. Potassium Bromate

Accidental poisoning with potassium bromate occurs in infants and children. Potassium bromate was primary chemical constituent of the neutralizing solution used after "Toni Permanent Wave" or "Coldwave." Dunsky (13) reported a 17-month-old infant with fatal acute oliguric renal failure following ingestion of the neutralizing solution. At autopsy, the patient had generalized edema and acute tubular necrosis. Warren and Gross (14) reported a 2-year-old infant who accidentally was fed "Toni Neutralizer." After 38 days of anuria and oliguria, the child gradually recovered.

11. Chlorate Compounds

Sodium and potassium chlorate is used in the manufacture of matches, explosives, toothpaste, synthetic pigments and as weed killers. Potassium chlorate is used as an oxidizing agent in lozenges and gargles.

Should the patient develop acute renal failure, the onset stage varies from three to fifteen hours. The clinical features are fever, hypotension, jaundice, abdominal pain, nausea, vomiting, diarrhea, extreme fatigue, nervousness and headache. The skin and mucus membranes are deeply cyanosed with a brownish-gray color. The patient has massive hemolysis with hemoglobinuria. Acute tubular necrosis is the common morphological lesion.

A clinical test can make the diagnosis of chlorate poisoning. Ten grams of kidney is minced in 16 ml of warm distilled water and an equal volume of acetone is added. The mixture is centrifuged, the acetone is evaporated and the mixture filtered. The aqueous filtrate is decolorized by a few drops of a dilute solution of indigo sulfate followed by a few drops of sulfurous acid. Silver nitrate is added followed by sulfurous acid. Silver chloride forms a white precipitate and is used for a quantitative estimate of the chlorates.

12. Miscellaneous Chemicals

Acute oliguric renal failure has followed exposure to a wide variety of "common chemicals." Listed in Table II are these common chemicals. Some of the listed chemicals have produced acute renal failure in a rare patient. These include arsenic, phenols, formalin, pyrogallal, tartaric acid, phosphorous and sodium tetrathionate.

B. BIOLOGICAL PRODUCTS

Acute renal failure can result from biological products due to acute reactions such as anaphylactic allergic reactions or from delayed reactions due to horse serum, vaccines, plant toxins as found in mushrooms, and venom of snakes, bees and spiders.

TABLE II: COMMON CHEMICALS WHICH INDUCE ACUTE TOXIC NEPHROPATHY

Chemical	MLD (Approximately per 70 kg)
Aniline	10 gm
Arsine Gas (AsH_3)	MAC 30 ppm
Camphor	2 gm
Carbon Tetrachloride	4 ml (MAC 25 ppm)
Chlordane	8 gm
Chloroform	25 ml
Copper Comopunds	15 gm
Creosote	10 gm
Essential (Volatice) Oils	1 gm
Ethylene Dichloride	MAC 100 ppm
Ethylene Glycol	100 ml
Formaldehyde (Formulin)	30 ml
Gualacol	2 gm
Mercury Compounds	MAC 0.1 mg/M^3 1 gm
Naphthalene (Moth Balls)	5 gm
Oxalates	5 gm
Paradichlorophenol	1 gm
Pentachlorophenol	1 gm
Phenol	10 gm
Phosphorus, yellow	0.05 gm (MAC 1 gm/H^3)
Resorcinol	2 gm
Tetrachloroethane	MAC 5 ppm
Thymol	2 gm

MAC = Maximum Allowable Concentration

1. ANAPHYLACTIC ALLERGIC REACTIONS

Acute oliguric renal failure has resulted from anaphylactic shock due to horse serum, and venom of snakes, spiders or bees. They produced sudden and prolonged hypotensive states resulting in acute tubular necrosis.

2. HORSE SERUM-INDUCED FATAL GLOMERULONEPHRITIS

In 1962, LaPava and colleagues (15) reported 3 patients who had malignant tumors and were treated with horse anti-human-cancer serum. All developed a fatal acute renal failure. At autopsy, a proliferative glomerulonephritis with epithelial crescents was present. The kidney was studied using electron microscopy. Epithelial humps on the glomerular lamina densa were found. They were similar to humps of antigen antibody complex seen in poststreptococcal glomeulonephritis (16), dextran-induced glomerulonephritis (16) and in patients with renal disease due to syphilis. The use of large dosages of adrenocortical steroids has been most beneficial in resolving these lesions of drug-induced diseases.

A horse serum-induced disease was first observed by Rackemann, Longcope and Peters (17). They noted water retention, decreased urinary output and retention of chloride. They were the first to point out that the mechanisms of horse serum-induced renal failure was on an immunological basis. Later, the specific immunological reaction was found to be due to soluble antigen-antibody complexes in the presence of excessive antigen.

3. PERTUSSIS VACCINE

Acute oliguric renal failure due to pertussis vaccine is rare (19). Fatal renal failure has followed 8 injections of pertussis vaccine over a six week period. One week after the eighth injection the patient developed fever, arthralgia, adenopathy and progressive renal failure. On the eighth day he was comatosed, had mild hypertension and his blood urea nitrogen was 201 mg per 100 ml. A diffuse healing vasculitis was found involving the medium and small arteries, arterioles and veins. The pathological findings in the kidney were multiple infarction in the cortex and medulla. There were numerous anti-mortem thrombi and extensive papillary necrosis.

4. TYPHOID VACCINE

Four patients given typhoid vaccine intravenously for 2 to 3 days died in shock and acute oliguric renal failure. One patient died in acute renal failure four days after receiving the vaccine. Another patient (20) developed the "hepatorenal syndrome." The third patient died 6 hours following the vaccine. Acute tubular necrosis and acute necrosis of the liver was noted.

The fourth patient, a 7-month-old boy with hereditary agammaglubolinuria developed complete anuria following one injection of typhoid vaccine. At autopsy, acute renal cortical necrosis was found. In addition, there was diffuse thrombosis of the glomerular capillaries. This patient may have had an increased susceptibility to the typhoid vaccine in view of an inadequate or "under developed" reticuloendothelial system.

5. Plant Poisons

The toxins of Amanita phalloides produce a characteristic clinicopathological course. Initially, gastrointestinal toxicity occurs followed by other conditions that are fatal to the patient. These dread complications are acute oliguric renal failure, (21, 22) hepatitis, acute yellow atrophy, myocardial injury, central nervous system disease, and hypoplastic anemia. The exact mode of action of mycetous toxins is not known. However, Wieland and Wieland (19) suggested a mechanism for mycetous toxins as an inhibitor of mitochondrial oxidative phosphoryl action with consequent interference with specific enzymes necessary for cellular metabolism.

Prolonged anuria may result from the mycetous toxins of Amanita phalloides. Acute tubular necrosis is the common morphological lesion and involves both proximal and distal convoluted tubules. The glomeruli are usually not affected.

C. SNAKE, SPIDER AND WAX BEE VENOM

Acute oliguric renal failure induced by venom of snakes, spiders and wax bees have been reported from Lima, Peru, by Piazza and co-workers (20) and from Sao Paulo, Brazil by Silva and colleagues (21). Acute intravascular hemolysis was common in all afflicted patients and probably resulted on an immunohemolytic basis.

1. Snakes

Of the snake species in the United States, approximately 10% are venomous. Snake bites inflicted by the pit viper, Crotalus terrificus (rattlesnake) and Brohtrups zararaca species usually produce local pain and swelling. The greater the area of edema and erythema around the fang marks the greater the venomation. Severe venomation occurs twelve or more inches of surrounding edema and erythema within the first 12 hours of the snake bite. The Ancistrodon contortrix mokeson (copperhead), the Ancistrodon piscivorus (water moccasin) and the Micruroides (coral snake) are other important venomous snakes. Their venom usually contains a variety of enzymes, cytolysins and neurotoxins which produce a variety of neurological disturbances, circulatory collapse, shock and acute renal failure. Other clinical features are dizziness, severe headaches, visual impairments, paralysis of neck muscles, respiratory depression and urinary findings of myoglobin, proteinuria and hematuria.

Snake venom-induced oliguria occurs in a small percentage of those patients suffering a greater degree of renal damage. When acute renal failure develops acute tubular necrosis is the common renal lesion found. One patient with a fatal bite by a Brothrups species developed bilateral renal cortical necrosis with an associated afibrinogenemia.

A bite of the Echiscarinatus (sand viper) near Lake Rudolph in Kenya produced bilateral renal cortical necrosis. The bite of the Atracepaspis Microlapidata (small African snake) can result in severe tubular necrosis with complete anuria.

2. Spider Bites

The Loxosceles reclusus and Loxosceles laeta (tarantula) spiders live in homes, outdoor privies and also in gardens. They seldom bite man. When the spider does the injected "poison" produces a local necrotic and angry cutaneous lesion usually in buttocks and genitalia. Some bites have caused extensive tissue sloughing at the site of the bite. In others, the lesion had healed locally in several weeks, leaving a healed scar. The spider's poison, a "toxalbumin" usually affects the nerve endings. Should it reach the systemic circulation a marked hemolysis occurs (25). This is followed by anemia, jaundice and acute oliguric renal failure. The Loxosceles laeta spider produces a prolonged anuria that is usually fatal.

In addition to present accepted methods of treating acute renal failure, use of anti-loxoscele serum is most helpful in neutralizing the spider antigen. The bite of the Amanrobius ferox results in severe intravascular hemolysis with production of a dark urine as seen in black water fever. Methemoglobinuria and hemoglobinuria occurs. Antivenom and intravenous injections of calcium gluconate has been helpful. The Latrodectus mactans (common black widow spider) predominately produces a neurotoxin. The patient experiences pain in the kidney area similar to renal colic. In addition, the patient has severe dehydration and oliguria.

3. Wax Bee

Immunohemolytic anemia and subsequently acute oliguric renal failure has followed the bite of hundreds of wax bees Appis mellificus. The skin becomes edematous, red, painful and itches. The clinical course and renal lesions of acute renal failure are not as severe as produced by snake or by spider venom.

4. Portuguese Man-of-War Stings

The sea nettle (Portuguese Man-of-War) produces a sharp sting at the site of its tentacle strike. The venom injected into the skin has resulted in local swelling, local secondary infection and angioneurotic edema. Hypersensitivity reactions include anaphylactic shock, urticaria and eosinophilia. Patients have had gastroenteritis with severe abdominal pain and generalized muscle cramps and spasms.

Acute oliguric renal failure and less severe renal disease has followed sea nettle stings. These usually occur to the unsuspecting tourist who swims or bathes in ocean waters. Adrenocortical steroids have suppressed the hypersensitivity reaction and produced recovery.

D. DRUGS

Drug-induced acute oliguric renal failure is a by-product of man's ever increasing exposure to a vast array of noxious chemicals and drugs resulting from industrial and medical progress. In the author's experience, approximately 20 to 25 percent of all patients with acute oliguria have renal failure induced by chemicals or drugs (17, 26).

In general, the nephrotoxicity mechanism is the most common and is dose related; in general, excessively large doses of drugs are used. Some drugs can produce acute oliguric renal failure when used in either the usual dosages or in very small amounts. These include methicillin, penicillin, phenylbutazone, sulfonamide, Dilantin, phenindione and Mercuhydrin. This mechanism of acute renal failure is one based on hypersensitivity.

Some drugs such as tetracyclines may produce prerenal azotemia on a metabolic mechanism such as their anti-anabolic action (22) on (23) the proximal tubules. This is reflected by proteinuria, aminoaciduria, phosphaturia, hypokalemia, a low plasma urate and acidosis. Tetracycline may undergo spontaneous degradation during storage especially under warm and moist conditions. Anhydro tetracycline and epianhydrotetracycline are the nephrotoxic degradation products that produce the Fanconi syndrome.

The author will review nephrotoxic drugs on a therapeutic classification and emphasis will be placed on the morphological site of drug-tissue interaction.

Drugs interact at specific morphological sites within the kidney to produce acute renal failure. On a structural basis, drugs interact at all four major components; the vessels, the glomeruli, the tubules and the interstitium. Arteritis has resulted from arsenic, bismuth, Dilantin, gold salts, horse serum, iodides, penicillin, propylthiouracil, chorothiazides and sulfonamides. Glomerulonephritis has followed hydralazine, Orabilex, phenylbutazone and sulfonamides.

Acute tubular necrosis has followed a large variety of drugs. These include amphotericin B, aristolochic acid, bacitracin, Colistin, ferrous sulfate, kanamycin, Mercuhydrin, neomycin, Orabilex, paraaminosalicylic acid, penicillin, phenylbutazone, quinine sulfate, salicylates and sodium acetrizoate (Urokon).

Acute interstitial nephritis and subsequent acute renal failure has followed treatment with Mercuhydrin (24), methicillin (25), nitrofurantoin (30), penicillin, phenacetin, phenindione (26), Polymyxin B (27), sulfonamides (28), Dilantin (29) and phenylbutazone.

1. Radiological Contrast Medium

The essential ingredient in all absorbable radiological contrast media is iodine. Individuals sensitive to iodine in any form may have mild to severe hypersensitivity reactions to contrast media. When inorganic iodine was used such as sodium iodide in a concentration of 80 to 100%, numerous hypersensitivity reactions occurred including acute renal failure. Although contrast media containing organic iodides are safer than inorganic iodides, they have been implicated in a steady flow of sporadic reports of severe nephro-toxicity.

Physicians depend on the use of radiological contrast media for diagnosis of biliary diseases, vascular diseases, diseases of the kidneys and diseases of the genitourinary tract. These agents are usually taken by mouth to evaluate the biliary tract, by intravenous injection to evaluate the arterial circulation and the kidneys, and by retrograde injections into the renal pelvis to evaluate the upper genito urinary tract.

a. *Cholecystographic Medium*

Iodine is the essential component of all contrast media used in roentgenography. Because of individual sensitivity to iodine, a significant number of allergic reactions occur. This was especially noted following the introduction of 100% sodium iodide in 1929. The use of organic iodide preparation has reduced the number of hypersensitivity reactions, however, sporadic reports have occurred due to nephrotoxicity of the cholecystographic medium. When the patient has delayed excretion of the contrast material due to biliary disease, an increased load of a potentially nephrotoxic agent is presented to the kidney.

The oral contrast medium iopanoic acid (Telepaque) (30) and bunamiodyl (Orabilex) (31, 36, 37) have resulted in acute renal failure. The use of bunamiodyl in a double oral dose was more prone to induce acute renal failure. This may be explained on a basis that bunamiodyl has an iodine content of 57% and is more completely absorbed from the gut than other cholecystographic material. Due to a local alteration of pH within the nephron an enhancing dissociation to inorganic iodine occurs. Physiochemically, the cholecystographic media are similar to the sulfonamides in that both groups of compounds are weak acids and their solubility increases directly with increases in pH.

This may explain the crystalluria of bunamiodyl and deposits of birefringent green-brown crystals can be found at the base of the tubular epithelial cells. The nephrotoxicity is further enhanced by the relatively dehydrated state of the patient prior to the roentgenographic procedure. The inorganic iodine may produce a hypersensitive mechanism in inducing acute oliguric renal failure.

Over the past five years, 26 patients were reported to have developed acute renal failure following Orabilex.® Most of these patients were given a double dose. The nephrotoxic lesion of acute tubular necrosis was the common morphological lesion reported. Although mild glomerular lesions were reported severe hypersensitivity glomerulonephritis was rare. Bunamiodyl has been withdrawn from the drug market by the United States Food and Drug Administration because of its nephrotoxicity. Acute renal failure induced by other cholecystographic material is rare.

b. *Aortography*

Nephrotoxicity was the most significant complication in 13,207 patients (32) following abdominal aortograms. Twelve patients of this group died in acute oliguric renal failure and 27 patients had reversible nephrotoxicity. Fatal acute renal failure following translumbar aortography has appeared in numerous reports. Proteinuria, cylindruria, pyuria, hematuria and progressive azotemia and impaired renal function persisted for months should one recover from acute oliguric renal failure.

Crawford and co-workers (33) reported 31 patients with aortographic nephrotoxicity. Twenty percent died in acute oliguric renal failure. Schreiner and Maher (2) reported three deaths out of 9 patients with renal injury in a series of 300 aortograms. The morphological lesions involved the glomeruli and tubules with acute damage associated with interstitial hemorrhage.

c. *Pyelographic Medium*

Retrograde and intravenous pyelogram are implicated in reports of nephrotoxicity but not to the frequency of cholecytograms.

1. Retrograde Pyelography

The first described report of reversible acute oliguric renal failure following retrograde pyelography was by Morten (34), in 1923. The patient developed oliguria following a bilateral retrograde pyelography utilizing sodium bromide as a contrast medium. In 1939, Quinby and Austen (35) described four patients who developed a reversible acute oliguric renal failure following within 24 hours of a retrograde and intravenous pyelogram using sodium iodohippurate and sodium methiodal. In addition to the risk of hypersensitivity reactions, retrograde pyelography carries a principal risk of infection.

In 1945, papillary necrosis following bilateral retrograde pyelography was reported by Eskelund. He used 10 ml of 25% sodium iodohippurate. The papillary necrosis probably resulted from local irritation caused by the "hypotonic solution" of sodium iodohippurate. It is also possible that the contrast media entered the papillary ductules with subsequent obstruction due to epithelial necrosis.

Sirota and Narins (36) attributed oliguria and rapidly progressive azotemia following retrograde pyelography to edematous obstruction of the ureteral orifices. In three patients, they found bullous edema of both ureteral orifices on cystoscopy. They attributed the edema to idiosyncratic reactions from an unusual sensitivity of the bladder and ureteral mucosa to trauma and to either the formaldehyde used in sterilization of the catheters or the pyelographic contrast media.

Grieve and Lowe (37) attributed anuria due to interstitial edema following severe pyelotubular backflow. In the author's experience, renal interstitial edema has accompanied acute anuria in two patients following use of Retrografin. Both required peritoneal dialysis before recovery.

Epstein and co-workers (38) reported a patient who developed anuria following retrograde pyelography using 30 ml of a 50% solution of Retrografin. Repeat ureteral catheterization failed to exclude parenchymal renal disease. Their patient did not undergo a spontaneous diuresis as expected. In that patient, it was very likely that the nephrotoxic antibiotic (neomycin) may have recirculated and produced intrinsic renal disease on a hypersensitivity basis.

2. Intravenous Pyelography

Intravenous urography results in fewer complications than does arteriography. This can be explained on the use of a less concentrated contrast material and the admixture of the media with blood. Pendergrass and co-workers (39, 40) reported 31 patients who died out of 3,-800,000 patients who had intravenous pyelograms. Twenty-five deaths occurred immediately after the intravenous injection of the contrast media. The patients usually died in anaphylactic shock, cardiac arrest or symptoms of drug sensitivity. Three patients died as a result of acute oliguric renal failure.

Perillie and Conn (41) focused attention on the potential danger of intravenous pyelography in patients with multiple myeloma. Acute oliguric renal failure occurred in five patients with plasma cell myeloma following intravenous pyelography. Dehydration appears to predispose patients with multiple myeloma to acute oliguric renal failure. The pathogenesis of pyelogram-induced oliguric renal failure in patients with multiple myeloma is related to precipitations of concentrated urinary proteins and contrast media within tubular lumen. The sudden blockage of a large percentage of the renal tubules may result in sudden suppression of urine flow. The combination of Bence-Jones protein in a concentrated urine and dehydration induced by purgatives leads to protein precipitation within the lumen of the nephron. The author suggests all efforts should be made to exclude multiple myeloma before pyelography is done. Once the diagnosis of multiple myeloma is made, the patient should be adequately hydrated before intravenous pyelography is done.

2. Antibiotics and Chemotherapeutic Agents

Antibiotics and chemotherapeutic agents have become indispensable in the treatment of urinary tract infection as well as in the treatment of systemic and local infections. As these agents become more extensively used, their adverse side effects and nephrotoxicity becomes more apparent. In the presence of underlying renal disease, it may be difficult to recognize nephrotoxicity of a specific antibiotic. Moreover, when antibiotics are used in combination with other antibiotics or with chemotherapeutic agents, their exact nephrotoxic effect may be impossible to determine as well as the specific agent to blame for the adverse reaction. The author has not observed nephrotoxicity due to chloramphenicol nor erythromycin.

a. *Sulfonamides*

Damage to the kidney is the most serious and frequent complications of sulfonamide treatment. Sulfonamides were the first effective chemotherapeutic agents to have nephrotoxic properties. The incidence of renal abnormalities varies considerably and depends in a great part on the solubility of sulfonamides. Acute oliguric renal failure has been induced by sulfonamides due to parenchymal lesions as well as due to an obstructive uropathy caused by sulfonamide crystallization of the unchanged drug or of its acetyl derivative within the renal pelvis (Fig. 3). The prevention

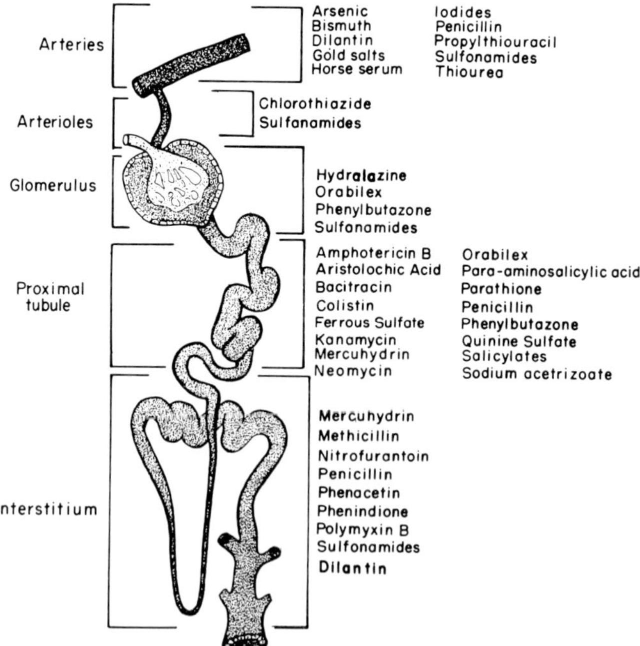

Figure 3. Morphological sites of drug induced renal failure. This figure illustrates the specific morphological sites where drugs interact to produce renal damage and subsequent acute renal failure. Some drugs such as phenylbutazone produce lesions at multiple sites.

of sulfonamide obstructive uropathy is the preferential use of a more soluble sulfonamide, adequate hydration and alkalinization of the urine with sodium bicarbonate. Obstructive uropathy due to the low solubility of sulfonamides is more frequently observed than are the parenchymal lesion of tubular necrosis, focal granulomatous interstitial lesions, diffuse interstitial nephritis, hypersensitivity glomerulonephritis and acute hypersensitivity arteritis (48).

Several hundred patients with renal failure due to sulfonamide crystallization have been reported. The most frequent sulfonamides implicated were sulfapyridine, sulfathiazole and sulfadiazine. The solubility of sulfonamides depends on a number of factors which include the drug concentrations, state of dehydration, the urinary pH and the renal function. Sulfadiazine is the most dangerous. Sulfadimidine and sulfisoxazole form more soluble crystals and are less hazardous. The finding of sulfonamide crystals in the urine leads the physician to suspect a diagnosis of acute sulfonamide crystallization within the renal pelvis. Treatment is to do a retrograde catherterization of the ureters with lavaging the renal pelvis with warm alkalinized solution (10% NaH CO_3).

Acute tubular necrosis can occur with and without sulfonamide crystallization. The tubular lumen are plugged with amorphous debris containing erythrocytes, leucocytes, hemoglobin casts and crystals. When sulfonamides induce a hypersensitivity renal lesion, one of three sites are involved. In some hypersensitivity reactions, the intrarenal arteries were involved with an angiitis or a polyarteritis nodosa. In a second type of hypersensitivity reaction the glomeruli were involved with a hypersensitivity glomerulonephritis. The third site for sulfonamide induced hypersensitivity reaction was the renal interstitium. Acute interstitial nephritis was the more common interstitial lesion and was similar to a Councilman acute interstitial nephritis. A focal interstitial granulomatous interstitial nephritis was a less common interstitial lesion.

b. *Polymyxin B*

The polymyxin B and E are a closely related cyclic polypeptides. Polymyxin B is an antibiotic composed of amino acids and a fatty acid. Polymyxin B is antibacterially more active than polymyxin E and can be used intravenously. Nephrotoxicity of polymyxin is dose related. Following administration of polymyxin B, proteinuria, epithelial cells and casts appear in the urine and azotemia develops. In the presence of normal renal function, the nephrotoxicity is negligible at 2 mg per kg per day.

Beirne and colleagues (27) reported a 44-year old male who developed an acute oliguric renal failure due to acute interstitial nephritis. Polymyxin B sulfate seemed the most capable of several antecedent agents. The patient had an eosinophilia of 25% but no dermatological lesion. On withdrawal of polymyxin B, the patient gradually recovered. A Councilman type of acute interstitial nephritis was found on renal biopsy study.

c. *Colistin Methanesulfonate*

Colistin differs from polymyxin B only by the absence of a single amino acid and is known to be identical with polymyxin E (42). Because of this close structural relationship colistin shares some of the nephrotoxic proportion of polymyxin B.

Toxicity studies in animals have demonstrated that colistin produces impaired renal function and renal lesions. Partial to complete necrosis of the proximal tubules was found on histological examination. In man, the effect of intramuscular colistin on renal function is unpredictable. Healthy individuals and patients ill with chronic pyelonephritis and other forms of renal disease (33, 34) have received the drug without significant changes in urinalysis or blood urea nitrogen. In other patients with azotemia, further elevation of blood urea nitrogen has occurred.

The author (45) has reported acute oliguric renal failure in four patients following treatment with colistin administered intramuscularly. Three patients were given dosages greater than 5 mg/kg/day and died in uremia. The lesion of acute tubular necrosis were found in the kidney (Fig. 4). A fourth patient developed oliguria after a dosage of 5 mg/kg/day but recovered and survived. Randall (46) reported a patient with acute oliguria due to acute tubular necrosis following nine days of intramuscular Colistimethate (6.3 mg/kg/day). Recovery followed four weeks of hemodialysis.

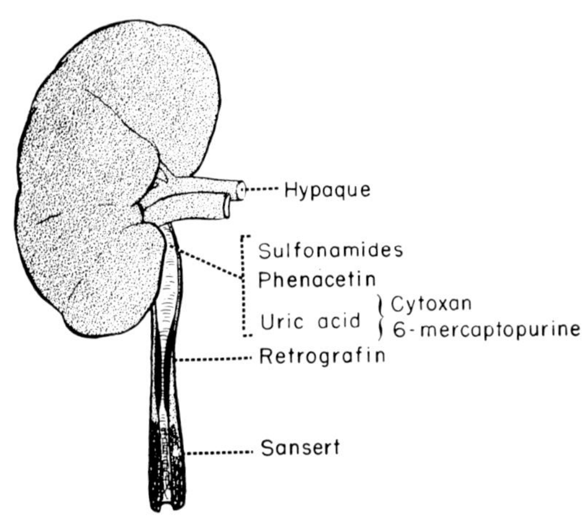

Figure 4. Drug induced acute renal failure. This figure illustrates the gross anatomical sites where various drugs induce acute renal failure. Sansert causes periureteral fibrosis and subsequent ureteral obstruction. Retrografin induces ureteral obstruction by producing edema of the ureters. Sulfonamides and uric acid may obstruct urinary flow by crystallization within the renal pelvis. Phenacetin induces renal papillary necrosis and the slough-off papillae produces obstructive uropathy.

Although the mechanism of colistin nephrotoxicity is unknown, it may be related to the ability of the drug to disrupt the integrity of certain cell membranes (47), probably by acting as a cationic detergent which destroys the cellular osmotic barrier, combines with polyphosphates thus allowing leakage of substances essential to cell function (55).

d. *Streptomycin*

Streptomycin, vancomycin, kanamycin and neomycin have several features in common. They are relatively strong organic bases which cross cell membranes very slowly. Therefore, they are poorly absorbed from the gut. They are almost entirely distributed in the extracellular fluid and mainly excreted in the urine. In addition, all four antibiotics have ototoxicity. The nephrotoxicity is increased in patients with a reduction of glomerular filtration rate. Should these antibiotics be used in combination, their nephrotoxicity is greatly increased.

In individuals with normal renal function, approximately 70% of parenterally injected streptomycin is excreted unchanged in the urine within 24 hours. In patients with renal insufficiency, less than 2% of an injected dose of streptomycin is excreted in the urine. Vestibular damage due to streptomycin is frequent in patients with severe renal failure. Dialysis has been useful in the removal of streptomycin in the treatment of neurotoxicity and nephrotoxicity.

During the course of treatment with streptomycin, occasionally proteinuria and cylinduria may occur. McDermott (48) reported a patient with acute oliguric renal failure due to acute tubular necrosis following a dosage schedule of 4 gm of streptomycin daily.

e. *Kanamycin*

The nephrotoxicity of kanamycin has been described in numerous reports whenever the clinical application of kanamycon was mentioned. Kanamycin nephrotoxicity was neither related to dose level nor to duration of treatment but occurred more frequently in elderly patients. Kanamycin nephrotoxicity occurred in doses over 200 mgm per kilo per day and was evident clinically by mild proteinuria, nitrogen retention, microscopic hematuria and fine granular casts in the urinary sediment. In approximately 10% of patients on treatment with kanamycin, there was azotemia. Severe tubular necrosis was reported by Kleeman and Maxwell (49) and Schrienner and Maher (2).

Ototoxicity was the most serious toxic effect of kanamycin. It was more likely to occur in patients with renal insufficiency or dehydration. When kanamycin was given to patients ill with anuria or oliguria, or a diabetic patient with nephropathy, it was imperative to reduce the dose by careful calculation of the dose and giving kanamycin in "spread out" doses. A recommended kanamycin dosage of 0.5 gms can be given every three or four days. Approximately 29 to 63% of the injected dose of kanamycin was removed by effective peritoneal dialysis. In an anuric patient, approximately 30% of kanamycin can be removed by hemodialysis in an eight-hour period.

However, during peritoneal dialysis, kanamycin, 25 mgm daily can be given with safety. The morphological site of nephrotoxic damage was the level of its proximal tubules. When acute oliguric renal failure occurred, it was the result of acute tubular necrosis. On stopping kanamycin, diuresis followed within five days and renal function usually returned to normal within two months.

f. *Bacitracin*

The use of Bacitracin is limited to topical application and local infiltration. Transitory urinary abnormalities of proteinuria, cylinduria, azotemia and occasional oliguria were noted in nearly all reported patients. Bacitracin is very nephrotoxic and produces both proximal and distal tubular necrosis.

Genkins, Uhr and Bryer (50) reported a 57-year-old housewife with prior normal renal function. She developed a fatal acute oliguric renal failure following five divided doses of 50,000 units daily of bacitracin. On the third day of bacitracin treatment, she developed proteinuria, oliguria and azotemia. She died on the tenth day after intramuscular bacitracin treatment. Acute tubular necrosis was found on autopsy.

g. *Neomycin*

Neomycin is primarily a topical antibiotic and is used for its local antibacterial action within the lumen of the gut. It is extremely nephrotoxic and damages the eighth cranial nerve. Although the drug is poorly absorbed, it crosses the peritoneal cavity much more readily.

Emmerson and Pryse-Davis found neomycin very nephrotoxic and caused severe proximal tubular necrosis. Randall (46) reported four patients with adverse effects of neomycin due to total injections of 4, 6, 8, and 72 gm of neomycin. Patients developed deafness. One patient developed acute oliguric renal failure and one subsequently had permanent renal insufficiency. Hemodialysis and peritoneal dialysis removed large amounts of neomycin and mannitol prevented acute renal failure in two patients. Hemodialysis rapidly reduced serum neomycin concentration in two patients while mannitol diuresis removed significant amounts in another. Peritoneal dialysis was the less effective of all methods.

h. *Penicillin*

Penicillin induces acute oliguria through a hypersensitivity mechanism. Dehydration was a possible contributing factor in two infants with abnormal renal function. When acute oliguria occurs, it is usually associated with dermatological lesions and eosinophilia.

Randall (46) reported acute oliguric renal failure due to hypersensitivity manifestations of ampicillin, oxacillin, oral penicillin and intramuscular penicillin G. Two patients died. One was a 24-year-old student who received oral penicillin; he developed clinical features of the hemolytic uremic syndrome. At autopsy, he was found to have necrotizing arteriolitis. The other patient had a marked acute interstitial nephritis characterized by interstitial cellular infiltrates of plasma cells.

i. *Methicillin*

Methicillin (Staphicillin) does not differ in its sensitizing potential from other penicillins (51). The hypersensitivity clinical features of methicillin are dermatological lesions, nephropathy and eosinophilia. During the past few years, methicillin-induced nephropathy has been reported by several individuals (59). The clinical manifestations of renal disease were proteinuria, hematuria, dysuria and azotemia with and without oliguria. Nephropathy usually appeared between 7 to 21 days on treatment and, in most instances, subsided within 24 to 48 hours after cessation of treatment with methicillin.

Patients with methicillin-induced nephropathy have additional manifestations of hypersensitivity. The most common was an eosinophilia. In some patients thrombocytopenia was observed. Hypersensitivity dermatological lesions were noted; they included hemorrhagic-bulla, urticaria, maculopapular lesions, purpura with petechiae, and exfoliative dermatitis. None of these reported patients with methicillin-induced nephropathy had a renal biopsy study. In general, knowledge is insufficient as to the overall morphological renal changes. The complete reversibility of methicillin-induced nephropathy together with other allergic manifestations suggest that a hypersensitivity mechanism occurs.

Histological abnormalities of the kidney include an acute interstitial nephritis with or without tubular damage. This interstitial nephritis is characterized by cellular infiltrates of eosinophils, plasma cells and small lymphocytes (Figs. 5 and 6). Adrenocortical steroids has been effective in resolving this drug induced lesion.

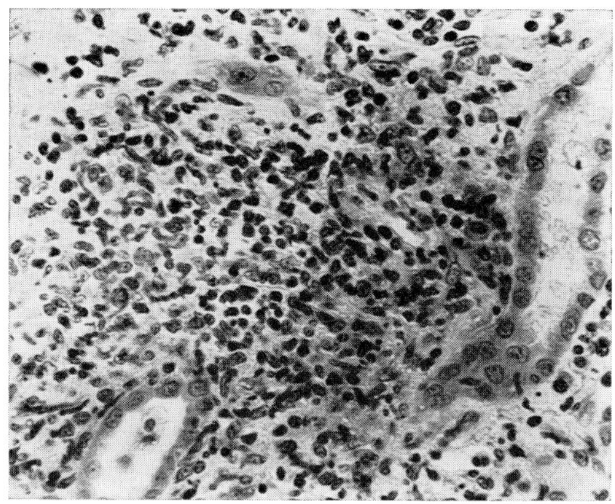

Figure 5. Acute interstitial nephritis. Acute renal failure followed Methicillin therapy. An acute interstitial nephritis was found. A portion of tubules is shown above and to the right and also below and to the left. Over a wide area, there is accumulation of large number of cellular infiltrates possibly polymorphonucleocytes, plasma cells, eosinophils and lymphocytes. Slight interstitial fibrosis is seen. (H & E X650)

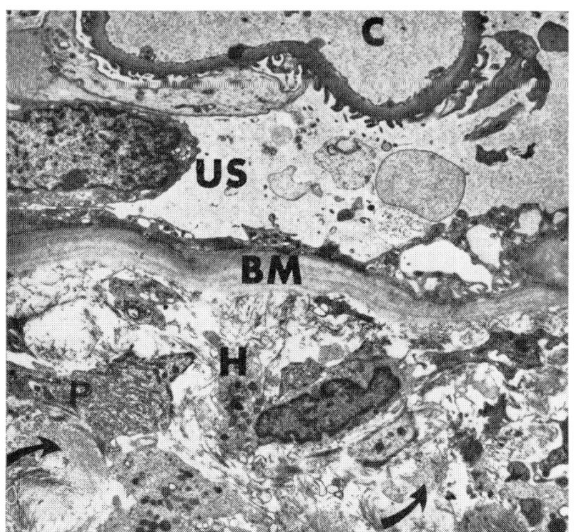

Figure 6. Electron micrograph of acute interstitial nephritis. This electromicrograph illustrates acute interstitial nephritis in a periglomerular area. A normal glomerular capillary loop (C) is seen above. Normal epithelial foot processes are seen projecting into the urinary space (US). Proteinaceous material is seen both within the glomerular capillary lumen and the urinary space. Bowman's membrane (BM) is laminated and thickened. The interstitium is edematous and contains numerous bundles of collagen fibers (**arrows**). A portion of a plasma cell (P) is seen at the left. A histocyte (H) is in the center. (Uranyl acetate and lead citrate X3,500.)

j. *Tetracycline*

Tetracycline, a so-called "broad spectrum antibiotic," is produced by several streptomycin species. When storage degeneration occurs to the tetracyclines, they may produce proximal tubular damage. Chemical deterioration is more likely to occur if the drug is improperly stored under moist or warm conditions. Anhydrotetracycline and epianhydrotetracycline are the nephrotoxic products. The formation of these products is accumulated by temperature elevation, high humidity and reduced pH. They were especially likely to occur when citric acid was added to tertacycline. However, tetracycline preparations containing lactose are less likely to degenerate into nephrotoxic products.

Aged, outdated or degenerated tetracycline produces a reversible Fanconi syndrome, (52, 53) associated with polyuria, proteinuria, renal glycosuria, phosphaturia, aminoaciduria, acidosis, hypokalemia and a low plasma urate. In most patients with tetracycline-induced Fanconi syndrome, the condition is a slowly reversible once the drug is discontinued.

Acute non-oliguric renal failure has been reported by Solomon, Galloway and Patterson (54). They gave tetracycline, two grams daily, and observed an increase in blood urea nitrogen from 63 mgm to levels of 161 mgm per 100 ml. Tetracycline toxicity is also directly related to existing renal insufficiency. Large doses of oxytetracycline has produced azotemia (63). Prerenal azotemia may be induced by a negative nitrogen balance producing anorexia, nausea, vomiting and death.

k. *Para-Aminosalicylic Acid*

Renal involvement due to Para-aminosalicylic acid (PAS) was uncommon and was usually confined to patients who had hepatitis. Inasmuch as PAS is an organic acid, it requires a fixed cation to accompany its excretion. Therefore, hypokalemia can occur as well as an acidosis in children.

Owen (55) reported a 31-year-old Irshman with pulmonary tuberculosis on treatment with calcium PAS for 83 days without mishap. After 35 days of sodium PAS treatment, he developed fever, a pink vesicular rash, massive proteinuria and acute oliguria without hepatitis. The blood urea reached 245 mg per 100 ml and spontaneously fell to normal. The patient made a rapid and complete recovery from acute renal failure.

1. Cephaloridine

Adverse reactions of cephaloridine occurred in 35% of 76 patients (56). In general, they were minor reactions and included allergic phenomena, phlebitis at infusion sites, transient leukopenia and gastrointestinal symptoms. More serious reactions include acute renal failure, Coombs' positive hemolytic anemia, superinfections and anaphylaxis. For example, cephaloridine produced anaphylaxis in a nurse who prepared an injection of the drug.

Renal damage due to cephaloridine appears to be on a nephrotoxic mechanism. The drug had been localized by autoradiographic studies to the renomedullary interstitium and proximal tubular cells. Cephaloridine is accumulative and dose related. In large doses, it produces a severe nephropathy; while in low doses it has produced proteinuria, hematuria and cylindruria. On discontinuing the drug urinary abnormalities disappeared.

The author would predict that cephaloridine will also produce an acute oliguric renal failure due to a (hypersensitivity) interstitial nephritis.

3. Diuretic Agents

In the majority of instances, the kidney responds favorably to diuretic agents with a prompt diuresis. However, the kidney also becomes the target organ to untoward effects of diuretic agents. It is not unlikely that acute oliguric renal failure developed in patients following treatment with Mercuhydrin, the thiazides and aristolochic acid.

a. *Mercurial Diuretic Agent*

The primary action of the mercurial diuretic agents is their ability to inhibit sulphydryl-containing enzyme systems which normally supply energy for sodium reabsorption. Most organic mercurials are rapidly excreted by active renal tubular secretion bound with cysteine. Mercurial diuretic agents usually produce acute oliguric renal failure due to acute tubular necrosis. Schreiner and Maher (2) believe that organic mercurials are slowly converted to inorganic mercury secondary to abnormal renal retention by the kidneys.

Mercuhydrin-induced acute oliguric renal failure has developed as the result of acute tubular necrosis. This is probably due to a nephrotoxicity mechanism. In a rare patient, acute oliguric renal failure exfoliative dermatitis, fever and eosinophilia has followed several injections of Mercuhydrin (Fig. 7.) Adrenocortical steroids were used to reverse this condition. This hypersensitivity reaction produces an acute interstitial nephritis (Fig.

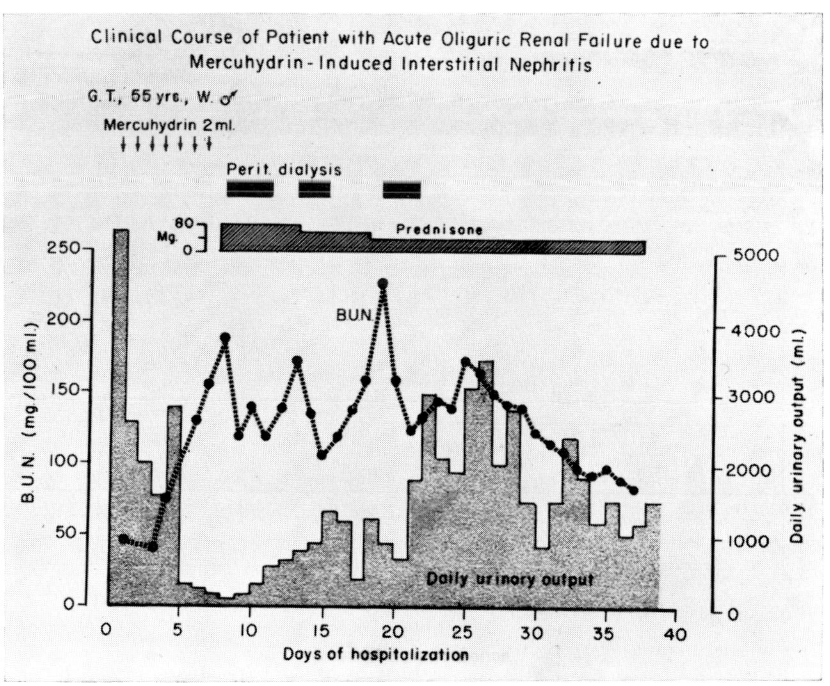

Figure 7. Clinical course of patient with mercuhydrin-induced acute renal failure. A 55-year-old truck driver received Mercuhydrin 2 ml daily for seven days. On the fifth day, he had an exfoliative dermatitis, eosinophilia, and oliguria. An acute interstitial nephritis was found on study of his kidney (Fig. 8). Peritoneal dialysis and Prednisone were used to treat the renal lesions and dermatitis.

8). In a rare report, nephritis developed following Mercuhydrin treatment. The morphological lesion was tubular degeneration associated wtih interstitial nephritis.

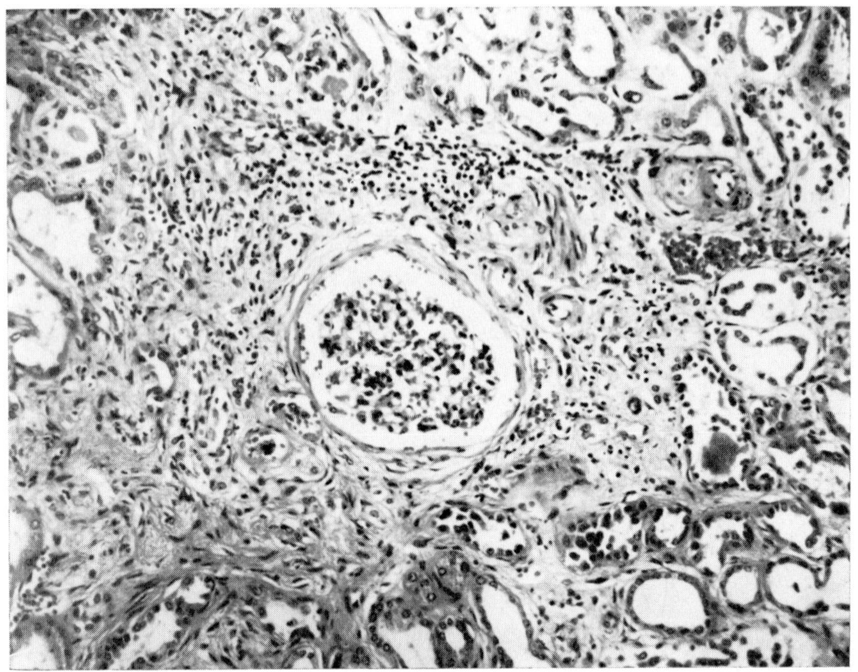

Figure 8. Mercuhydrin-induced acute interstitial nephritis. An acute interstitial nephritis was found. The interstitium was edematous and contained numerous plasma cells, eosinophils and lymphocytes. (H & E X320)

b. *Thiazide Diuretic Agents*

The untoward effects of the thiazide diuretic agents on the kidney are potassium deficiency, aggravation of pre-existing diabetes mellitus, aggravation of gout and blood dyscrasias. The latter include leukopenia, thrombocytopenic purpura and aplastic anemia.

Chlorothiazide and hydrochlorothiazide have produced acute oliguric renal failure on two specific mechanisms. The first is due to acute renal parenchymal damage due to one of three lesions: 1) Acute renal necrotizing angitis, 2) glomerulonephritis with interstitial nephritis and, 3) acute tubular necrosis.

Kjellbo and co-workers (57) observed a patient with acute necrotizing angiitis simultaneously in the skin and kidney. Their patient was a 62-year-old mildly hypertensive woman who developed fever, right kidney pain, gross hematuria, proteinuria and azotemia. Renal biopsy study revealed interstitial granulomatous inflammatory nodules enclosing necrotic arteriols. The glomeruli appeared normal. The granulomas were composed of lymphocytes, histiocytes, plasma cells and neutrophilic leukocytes. Fatal glomerulonephritis with interstitial nephritis has complicated "allergic purpura" due to chlorothiazide. Abry and Cavusoglu (58) reported a patient with fatal acute oliguric renal failure due to acute tubular necrosis following chlorothiazide treatment. Others have observed co-existing

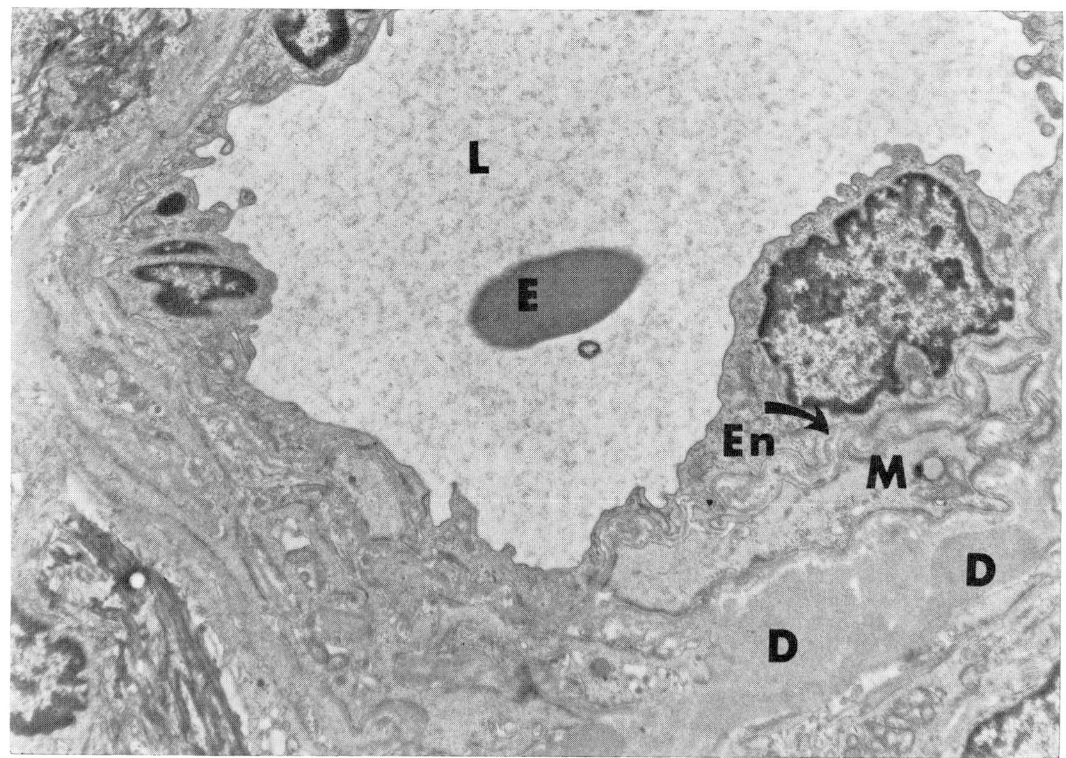

Figure 9. Necrotizing angiitis. A 53-year-old laborer developed a necrotizing angiitis following treatment with erythromycin. He had hypertension, azotemia, gross hematuria and impaired renal function. Light microscopic examination revealed necrotizing angiitis. By electron microscopic study, "so-called electron denser deposits" (D) were noted within the arterial wall. The arterial lumen (C) contains proteinaceous material and a portion of an erythrocyte (E). Endothelial cells (En) line the lamina elastica (arrow). A smooth muscle cell (M) is noted. (X8,000.)

thrombocytopenic purpura and acute oliguric renal failure following thiazide treatment.

The second mechanism of acute oliguric renal failure is the more common. Thiazides have induced acute oliguric renal failure in patients with mild impaired renal function by a gradual and chronic reduction in the effective circulating blood volume associated with severe hyponatremia. Treatment consists of fluid and sodium chloride replacement. The physician must take great care so not to error in the direction by excessively expanding the blood volume and precipitate the primary illness, e.g., congestive heart failure.

c. *Aristolochic Acid*

Aristolochic acid was used experimentally as a diuretic agent as well as an anticancer drug. It has produced renal damage in horses, rabbits, rats and mice. Aristolochic acid can abolish the anti-diuretic effect of vasopressin in rabbits and, therefore, was thought to have diuretic properties. Peters and Hedwall (59) intensively studied the effects of aristolochic acid toxicity in rats. They found that a single injection of 30 mg/kg of the drug induced reversible renal failure associated with a decrease in glomerular filtration rate and a urea nitrogen and creatinine increase. A maximum polyuria occurred on the eighth day. Their data reveals a decrease in the permeability of the collecting ducts and proximal tubules to urea.

The author has observed two entirely opposite effects of aristolochic acid; in one patient it produced a tremendous diuresis and the other patient resulted in a severe acute tubular necrosis with fatal acute oliguric renal failure.

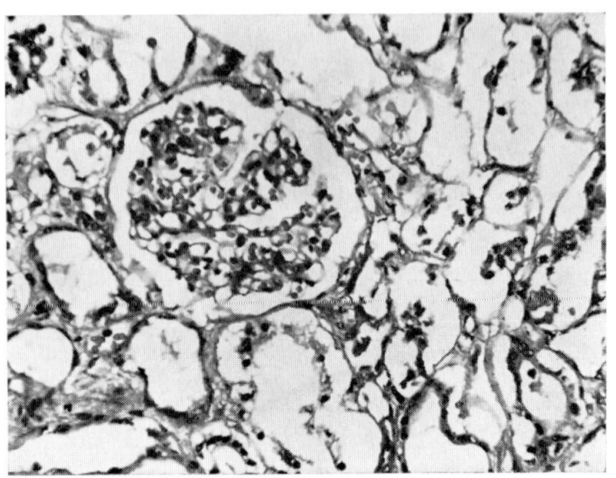

Figure 10. Aristolochic acid induced acute tubular necrosis. Acute renal failure followed intravenous injection of aristolochic acid. Severe acute tubular necrosis was found. In many areas, the tubular epithelial cells were destroyed down to the tubular basement membrane. The glomeruli appeared normal. (H & E X360)

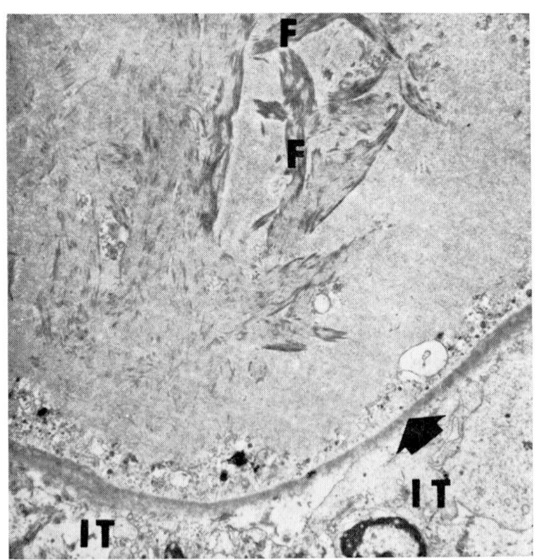

Figure 11. Acute tubular necrosis. Electron microscopic study of patient described in Figure 10. Coagulated necrosis of tubular epithelium was found containing fibrinoid material (F). The tubular basement membrane is indicated by an arrow. The interstitial tissue (IT) was edematous and contained loose collagen fibers. (X4,100)

4. Anticoagulants

Bishydroxycoumarin (Dicumarol) and Phenindione (Hedulin) have been implicated in inducing acute oliguric renal failure.

a. *Bishydroxycoumarin*

Bishydroxycoumarin in the therapeutic range has produced nausea, vomiting and diarrhea. Excessive doses cause bleeding. In general, painless gross hematuria is the first evidence of toxicity. This bleeding may arise from the kidney and, in some patients, it is followed by renal pain, ureteral colic and gross hematuria. Ureteral obstruction has followed blood clots within the ureters.

In one patient (60), retroperitoneal hematoma has dissected down around the urinary bladder to produce an external ureteral obstruction and acute oliguria.

b. *Phenindione*

Phenindione is known as phenylindanedione (P.I.D.), Danilone,® Hedulin® and Eridone.® It was used as a "short acting" anticoagulant as it is rapidly absorbed from the gut and rapidly excreted by the kidney. Proteinuria is commonly observed during the first day of phenindione treatment. Heavy proteinuria has occurred to result in the nephrotic syndrome (31).

Six patients with severe and significant renal damage due to phenindione were reported (61). Four patients developed acute oliguric renal failure; one had the nephrotic syndrome and the sixth had a heavy proteinuria. The other clinical features were fever, skin rash, jaundice and eosinophilia.

The histological renal abnormalities in patients with oliguria was an acute diffuse interstitial nephritis characterized by interstitial infiltrates of plasma cells, eosinophils and small lymphocytes. In addition, there was intersititial fibrosis and intimal fibrosis of the interlobular artery. The glomeruli were usually normal. Adrenocortical steroids were beneficial in reversing the acute interstitial nephritis due to phenindione hypersensitivity.

5. Calcium Versenate

Calcium versenate is a synthetic water soluble polyaminoacid (calcium disodium ethylenediamine tetracetic acid). It is an organic chelating agent used in the treatment of heavy-metal poisonings.

In 1957, Vogt and Cottier (62) reported a 38-year-old man with chronic lead poisoning. Their patient was treated with calcium versenate, 600 mg per kilo of body weight, daily for four days (tenfold the average dose). Acute tubular "necrotizing nephrosis" (necrosis) was found with dilated proximal tubular epithelial cells.

In 1957, Moeschlin (63) described two patients treated for lead intoxications with calcium versenate. Both died in uremia due to acute oliguric renal failure. At autopsy, acute tubular necrosis was found.

In 1958, Weinig and Schward (64) described acute renal failure associated with a bleeding tendency in a 59-year-old factory worker who received 3 grams of calcium versenate. Acute tubular necrosis with dilated proximal tubules were found at autopsy.

In 1960, Renher and Bradley (65) reported a 1-year-old girl who had lead intoxication. The child was treated with calcium versenate in a dose of 1 gm (125 mg per kilo of body weight) daily, subcutaneously for three days. She developed acute oliguric renal failure twelve days after the first injection. She died four days later. Acute tubular necrosis with dilated proximal tubules were found.

The author again emphasized the important need to use caution when one exceeds recommended dosages of any medication (calcium versenate of 75 mg/kilo/of body weight). Moreover, the physician should carefully screen the patient for kidney disease before administering calcium versenate.

6. Dextran

Low molecular weight dextran (Dextran-60 Gentran) has a molecular weight of 40,000. It passes through the glomerular membrane. It is used in clinical medicine as a short term flow-improver in small blood vessels and as a "plasma volume expander." The high urinary concentration of dextran creates a urine of high viscosity. An increase in blood clotting time has occurred in a substantial number of individuals receiving dextran. Adverse reactions due to dextran are hypersensitivity in origin and include urticaria, angioneurotic edema, bronchospasm and severe anaphylatic shock. Hypersensitivity glomerulonephritis due to an arthus phenomenon and acute oliguric renal failure are two renal conditions induced by dextran.

a. *Hypersensitivity Mechanism*

Dextran is a potent antigen with a molecular weight similar to many antigens. It may be given by injection without any reaction. However, subsequent injections of dextran such as iron-dextran can precipitate an immunological reaction leading to acute renal failure (16).

Iron-dextran, U.S.P. injected intramuscularly is a stable complex of ferric hydroxide and dextran in 019% sodium chloride solution. Dextran is known as a potent antigen. In man, the injection

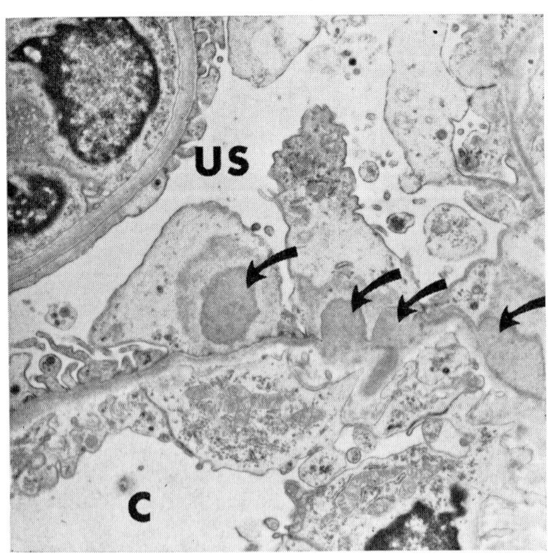

Figure 12. Dextran induced proliferative glomerulonephritis. A 40-year-old woman was given iron dextran as treatment for an iron deficient anemia due to hemorrhage from a peptic ulcer. Several days later, she was given dextran intravenously. Fever, hematuria, proteinuria and azotemia followed. A renal biopsy study revealed an acute proliferative glomerulonephritis. Numerous epithelial humps (arrows) were noted on electron microscopy. The glomerular capillary lumen (C) was patent. Proteinaceous material was noted in the urinary space (US). (X6,200)

of such small amounts as 1 mg can lead to the development of precipitins and cutaneous erythema and wheal reactions (74). Dextran is a polysacchride with a molecular weight similar to many antigens.

The morphological renal lesions of humps on the epithelial side of the glomerular basement membrane support a soluble antigen-antibody complex in an excess antigen reaction. The clinical improvement following adrenocortical steroids supports the immunological aspects of this reaction (17).

b. *Tubular Obstructive Mechanism*

Acute oliguric renal failure induced by low molecular weight dextran has produced two distinct renal lesions. The first was observed by Morgan and colleagues (66) in three hydrated patients with acute oliguria following dextran infusion. They did renal biopsy studies on each patient and found grossly swollen tubular cells crammed with a foamy material. The distended cells completely occluded the tubular lumen. Special stains revealed large quantities of dextran within the tubules but none in the tubular lumen.

The second lesion occurred in dehydrated patients given dextran infusion. Acute oliguric renal failure was associated with finding dextran casts obstructing the tubular lumen. Once within the tubular lumen, the dextran becomes concentrated and a highly viscous urine is formed. This results from the proximal tubular reabsorption of electrolytes and water. The highly concentrated viscous dextran urine forms tubular casts which resulted in urine flow obstruction and subsequent acute oliguric renal failure. Mannitol infusions as a 20% solution have been effective in initiating a diuresis.

7. Ferrous Sulfate

The ingestion of large doses of ferrous sulfate by children quite frequently produces iron poisoning. The mortality rate in a large series of children with "iron poisoning" was approximately 50% (76). Acute oliguric renal failure occurred as a result of acute tubular necrosis. This renal lesion may be related to gastrointestinal tract damage.

8. Aminopyrine

Aminopyrine is used clinically as analgesic and antipyretic. Aminopyrine is rapidly and virtually completely absorbed from the gut and is demethylated in the liver.

The toxic effect of aminopyrine is a severe, and often fatal, agranulocytosis. It can cause herpes labialis and angioneurotic edema in hypersensitive individuals. Eknoyan and Matson (67) reported a 37-year-old woman who developed acute oliguric renal failure. Al though their patient did manifest renal damage following a brief course of amphotericin B, a marked decrease in renal function occurred coincident with aminopyrine administration. Recovery occurred after stopping aminopyrine. There was a dramatic decrease in renal function coincident with a second course of aminopyrine. The patient died in uremia. Unfortunately, no autopsy was done.

9. Phenylbutazone

Phenylbutazone (Butazolidin) is a congener of aminopyrine and can induce damage to the skin, lungs, heart, liver, bone marrow, adrenal glands and gut. Phenylbutazone has produced both acute non-oliguric renal failure and acute oliguric renal failure.

Phenylbutazone-induced acute oliguric renal failure results by three distinct morphological lesions. These include acute tubular necrosis, acute interstitial nephritis and thrombotic thrombocytopenic purpura (78). Lipsett and Goldman (68) reported a patient with reversible acute oliguric renal failure following phenylbutazone. A renal biopsy study done on the fifth day of oliguria revealed acute tubular necrosis. Herrmann, Hopfeld and Berning (69) reported a patient with fatal acute oliguric renal failure due to phenylbutazone. At autopsy, an acute interstitial nephritis was found. Dunea and the author reported a 44-year-old housewife who was treated with phenylbutazone, 600 mg daily for three days followed by acute anuria and jaundice (78). She remained anuria until her death thirty-one days after ingesting phenylbutazone. A renal biopsy study, during the third week of her illness, revealed thrombotic thrombocytopenic purpura associated with a hemolytic anemia.

10. Bismuth Compounds

Bismuth compounds have induced nephrotoxicity through repeated intramuscular injections, rectal suppositories, accidental ingestion and idiosyncrases to heavy metals. The proximal renal tubules are the most sensitive target organs to injury.

The toxicity of bismuth compounds is directly related to the rapidity of absorption. Approximately 90% of the absorbed dose of a soluble bismuth salt is excreted by the kidneys. Bismuth tends to concentrate in renal tissue to amounts five fold that in the liver. Therefore, damage occurs to the kidney. Proximal tubular necrosis with intranuclear inclusion bodies are frequently observed in bismuth nephropathy. In addition to kidney damage, these compounds have produced damage to the gut, the liver and the central nervous system. Acute oliguric renal failure was the chief cause of death in patients poisoned with bismuth.

Robinson and Wong (70) consider bismuth compounds as the second most common cause of nephrotoxicity in children. In 1932, Beerman (71) reviewed the literature and found 22 patients with fatal bismuth toxicity. Barnett (72) described 4 patients and Weinstein (73) added 11 children with fatal poisoning due to bismuth containing suppositories. Dowd (74) had 3 patients who died due to bismuth toxicity, two had acute renal failure. McClendon (75) reported two children who received a single injection of bismuth thioglycollate (Thio-bismol) for Vincent's stomatitis. Both recovered from prolonged acute oliguria. In 1946, Boyette (76) reported a child who died in acute oliguric renal failure thirteen days after injection of bismuth. Although the child had an excellent diuresis, he suddenly died. At autopsy widespread tubular regeneration was found.

Chamberlain and Franks (77) reported a 9-year-old school girl with acute oliguric renal failure following an intramuscular injection of 3 gr of bismuth thioglycollate. She was treated with BAL and recovered. The efficacy of BAL treatment was questioned by the authors. In general, bismuth thioglycollate has produced death in approximately 50% of all patients with bismuth toxicity. Bismuth tartrate had produced the nephrotic syndrome in a patient with rhumatoid arthritis (89). Gzerninsici and Ginn (90) found ingestion of 1.5 gm of bismuth compounds produced the Fanconi syndrome with reversible renal insufficiency.

Summary

Acute toxic nephropathy is the by-product of man's ever-changing environment and of medical progress. Toxic nephropathy can result from a large variety of chemicals, in any physical state, drugs, and biological substances, such as plant toxins and venoms of snakes, wax bees and spiders.

The prompt recognition of the clinical features of acute toxic nephropathy will lead to immediate and effective therapy. In some situations, the nephrotoxic substance must be removed from the body by use of dialysis or exchange transfusion; or its effects must be neutralized, such as by anti-venom, adrenal corticosteroids or such agents as B.A.L.

Nephrotoxic agents damage the kidney through several pathopharmocological mechanisms either singly or in combination. The toxic substances may interact with cellular constituents to damage a specific kidney site in one individual and an entirely different cellular site in another individual.

Through the combined efforts of physicians and clinical pathologists working as a team, can we begin to understand acute toxic nephropathy. The cellular mechanisms and enzyme systems involved in toxic nephropathy are far from understood.

REFERENCES

1. Bull, G. M., Joekes, A. M., and Lowe, K. G.: Acute renal failure due to poisons and drugs. Lancet, *1*:134, 1958.
2. Schreiner, G. E., and Maher, J. F.: Toxic nephropathy. Amer. J. Med., *38*:409, 1965.
3. Oliver, J., MacDowell, M., and Tracy, A.: The pathogenenes is of acute renal failure associated with traumatic and toxic injury. Renal ischemia, nephrotoxic damage, and the ischemic episode. J. Clin. Invest., *30*:1307, 1951.
4. Zollinger, H. U.: Relationship of renal toxicity of drugs to pyelonephritis. In, Biology of Phelonephritis, 1st ed. Boston, Little, Brown & Co., 1960.
5. Councilman, W. T.: Acute interstitial nepritis. J. Exp. Med., *3*:339, 1898.
6. Bouchard, C. J.: Lecons sur les auto-intoxications dans les maladies. Recueillies et publiees par P. Le Gendre, vol. 1. Paris, Savy, 1887, p. 138.
7. Maher, J. F., and Schreiner, G. E.: Clinical Aspects and Pathology of Toxic Nephropathy, vol. 2. Proc.-3rd int. Congr. Neprol. Washington, 1966, pp 276-290.
8. Hamburger, J., Richet, G., Crosnier, J., Funck-Brentano, J. L., Antoine, B., Ducrot, H., Mery, J. P., and DeMontera, H., Nephrology. Philadelphia, W. B. Sanders Co., 1968.
9. Allen, A. C.: The Kidney. Medical and Surgical Diseases. vol. 1. New York, Grune and Stratton, 1951, p. 583.
10. Hamilton, A.: Hygienic control of the anilin dye industry in Europe. U. S. Month. Labor Rev., *9*:167, 1919.
11. Graubarth, J., Bloom, C. J., Coleman, F. C., and Solomon, H. N.: Dye poisoning in nursery; review of 17 cases. JAMA, *128*:1155, 1945.
12. Muehrcke, R.C., and Pirani, C. L.: Arsine-induced anuria. a correlative clinc-pathological study with electron microscopic observations. Ann. Int. Med., *68*:853, 1968.
13. Dunsky, I.: Potassium bromate poisoning. Amer. J. Dis. Child., *74*:730, 1947.
14. Warren, S. A., and Gross, W. V., Jr.: Clinical recorvery from prolonged anuria in an infant two (2) months of age. Pediatrics, *5*:954, 1950.
15. De LaPava, S., Nigogosyan, G., and Pickren, J. W.: Fatal glomerulonephritis after receiving horse anti-human-cancer serum. Arch. Int. Med., *109*:67, 1962.
16. Thiele, K. G., Muehrcke, R. C., and Berning, H.: Nierenerkrankungen durch medipamente. Deutsche, Med. Wschr., *36*:1632, 1967.
17. Rackermann, F. M., Longscope, W. T., and Peters, J. P.: The excretion of chlorides and water and the renal function in serum disease. Arch. Int. Med., *18*:496, 1916.
18. Bishop, W. B., Carlton, R.F., and Sanders, L. L.: Diffuse vasculitis and death after hyperimmunization with pertussis vaccine. New Eng. J. Med., *274*:616, 1966.
19. Wieland, T., and Wieland, O.: Chemistry and toxicology of toxins of Amanita Phalloides. Pharmacol Rev., *11*:87, 1959.
20. Piazza, A., Chaname, W., Cauti, D., and Maya, L.: Acute renal failure due to spider bite

(Loxosceles Laeta). International Congress of Nephrology, Sept. 25-30, Washington, D. C., 1966.

21. Silva, H. B., Brito, T., Lima, P. R., Penaa, D. O., Almedia, S. S., and Mattar, E.: Acute anuric renal insufficiency (ARI) due to snake, waxbee and spider bites. Clinical and pathological observations in 8 cases. Int. Congress of Nephrology, Sept. 25-30, Washington, D. C., 1966.
22. Faloon, W. W., Downs, J. J., Duggan, K., and Prior, J. T.: Nitrogen and electrolyte metabolism and hepatic function and histology in patients receiving tetracycline. Amer. J. Med. Sci., *233:*653, 1957.
23. Gabuzda, G. J., Gocke, T. M., Jackson, G. G., Grisby, M. E., Love, B. D., and Finland, M.: Some effects of antibiotics on nutrition in man, including studies of the bacterial flora of the feces. Arch. Int. Med., *101:*476, 1958.
24. Muehrcke, R. C.: Intersitial Nephritis. Chicago Med., *71:*211, 1968.
25. Muehrcke, R. C., Pirani, C. L., and Kark, R. M.: Interstitial nephritis: a clinicopathological and renal biopsy study. Ann. Int. Med., *66:* 1052, 1967.
26. Angervall, L., Lehmann, L., and Lincoln, K.: On the effect of phenacetin and NAPA (N-acetyl-p-aminophenol) on the development of bacterial interstitial nephritis in the rat. Acta. Path. & Microbiol. Scand., supp., *154:*61, 1962.
27. Beirne, G. J., Hansing, C. E., Octaviano, G. N., and Burns, R. O.: Acute renal failure caused by hypersensitivity to polymyxin B sulfate. JAMA, *202:*62, 1967.
28. French, A. J.: Hypersensitivity in pathogenesis of histopathologic changes associated with sulfonamide chemotherapy. Amer. J. Path., *22:* 697, 1946.
29. Heptinstall, R. H.: Pathology of the Kidney. Boston, Little Brown and Co., 1966, p. 45.
30. Fink, H. E., Jr., Roenigk, W. R., and Wilson, G. P.: An experimental investigation of the nephrotoxic effects of oral cholecystographic agents. Amer. J. Med. Sci., *247:*201, 1964.
31. Rennie, I. D. B.: Acute renal changes after oral cholecystography. Lancet, *2:*645, 1964.
32. McAfee, J. G.: A survey of complications of abdominal aortography. Radiology, *62:*825, 1957.
33. Crawford, E. S., Beall, A. C., Moyer, J. H., and DeBakey, M. E.: Complications of aortography. Surg. Gynec. & Obstet., *104:*129, 1957.
34. Morton, H. D.: Temporary suppression of urine following double pyelography. J. Urol., *10:*261, 1923.
35. Quinby, W. C., and Austin, G., Jr.: Suppression of urine complication of pyelography. New Eng. J. Med., *221:*814, 1939.
36. Sirota, J. H., and Narins, L.: Acute urinary suppression after ureteral catheterization. New Eng. J. Med., *257:*1111, 1957.
37. Grieve, J., and Lowe, K. G.: Anuria following retrograde pyelography. Brit. J. Urol., *27:*63, 1955.
38. Epstein, E., Shelp, W. D., and Weinstein, A. B.: Acute Renal Failure following retrograde pyelography. Invest. Urol., *2:*355, 1965.
39. Pendergrass, E. P., Chamberlain, G. W., Godfrey, W. E., and Burdick, E. D.: Survey of deaths in unfavorable sequalae following administration of contrast media. Amer. J. Roentgenol., *48:*741, 1942.
40. Pendergrass, E. P., Hodes, P. J., Tondreau, R. E., Powell, C. C., and Burdick, E. D.: Further consideration of deaths and unfavorable sequalae following the administration of contrast media in urography in the United States. Amer. J. Roentgenol., *74:*262, 1955.
41. Perilie, P. E., and Conn, H.O.: Acute renal failure after intravenous pyelography in plasma cell myeloma. JAMA, *167:*2186, 1958.
42. Jawetz, E.: Laboratory and clinical observations on polymyxin B and E. Amer. J. Med., *10:*111, 1951.
43. Holmes, K. K.: Toxicity of colistin and polymyxin B. New Eng. J. Med., *271:*633, 1964.
44. Petersdorf, R. G., and Plorde, J. J.: Colistin, a reappraisal. JAMA, *183:*123, 1963.
45. Erlanson, P., and Lundgren, A.: Ototoxic side effects following treatment with antibiotics. Connection with dosage and renal function. Acta. Med., *176:*147, 1964.
46. Randall, R. E., Jr.: Renal failure following antibiotic. Ann. Int. Med., *66:*1056, 1957.
47. Feingold, D. S.: Antimicrobial chemotherapeutic agents: the nature of their action and selective toxicity. New Eng. J. Med., *269:*900, 1963.
48. McDermott, W.: Toxicity of streptomycin. Amer. J. Med., *2:*491, 1957.
49. Kleeman, C. R., and Maxwell, M. H.: The Nephrotoxicity of Antibiotics; A Review. In, Biology of Pyelonephritis. Edited by Quinn, E. L. & Kass, E. H. Boston, Little, Brown & Co., 1960.
50. Genkins, G., Uhr, J. W., and Bryer, M. S.: Bacitracin nephropathy; report of a case of acute renal failure and death. JAMA, *155:*894, 1954.
51. Bulger, R. J., Lindholm, D. D., Murray, J. S., and Kirby, W. M. M.: Effect of uremia on methicillin and oxacillin blood levels. JAMA, *187:* no. 5, 1964.
52. Frimpter, G. W., Timpanelli, A. E., Eisenmenger, W. J., Stein, H. S., and Ehrlich, L. I.: Reversible "Fanconi syndrome" caused by degraded tetacycline. JAMA, *184:*111, 1963.
53. Shils, M. E.: Renal disease and the metabolic

effects of tetracycline. Ann. Int. Med., *58:*389, 1963.

54. Solomon, M., Galloway, N. C., and Patterson, R.: The kidney and tetracycline toxicity. Missouri Med., *62:*283, 1965.
55. Owen, D.: Renal failure due to para-aminosalicylic acid. Brit. Med. J., *2:*483, 1958.
56. Atkinson, R. M., Caisey, J. D., Currie, J. P., Middleton, T. R., Pratt, D. A. H., Sharpe, H. M., and Tomich, E. G.: Subacute toxicity of cephaloridine to various species. Toxicology and applied Pharmacology, *8:*407, 1966.
57. Kjellbo, H., Stakeberg, H., and Mellgren, J.: Possibly thiazide-induced renal necrotizing vasculitis. Lancet, *1:*1034, 1965.
58. Abry, J., and Cavusoglu, M.: Fatal tubular recrosis during chlorothizide administration. New York State J. Med., *60:*1638, 1960.
59. Peters, G., and Hedwall, P. R.: Aristolochic acid intoxication: a new type of impairment of urinary concentrating ability. Arch. Int. Pharmacondyn, *145:*334, 1963.
60. Kaden, W. S., and Friedman, E. A.: Obstructive uropathy complicating anticoagulant therapy. New Eng. J. Med., *265:*283, 1961.
61. Baker, S. B. de C., and Williams, R. T.: Acute interstitial nephritis due to drug sensitivity. Brit. Med. J., *1:*1655, 1963.
62. Vogt, W., and Cottier, H.: Nekrotisierende nephrose nach behandlung einer subakutchronischen bleivergiftung mit versenat in hohen Dosen. Schweiz med. Wchnschr., *87:*665, 1957.
63. Moeschlin, S.: Zur klinik und therapie der bleivergiftung mit bericht uber eine todliche toxische nephrose durch CaEDTA (Calciumversenat). Schweiz Med. Wchnschr., *87:*1091, 1957.
64. Weinig, E., and Schwerd, W.: Nil nocere. Gefahren bei der behandlung der bleiintoxikation mit calciumversenat ("Mosatil Komplexon"). Munchen. Med. Wchnschr., *100:*1788, 1958.
65. Reuber, M. D., and Bradley, J. E.: Acute versenate nephrosis occurring as a result of treatment for lead intoxication. JAMA, *174:*BFC, 1960.
66. Morgan, I. O., Little, J. M., and Evans, W. A.: Renal failure associated with low molecular weight dextran infusion. Brit. Med. J., *2:*737, 1966.
67. Eknoyan, G., and Matson, J. L.: Acute renal failure caused by aminopyrine. JAMA, *190:*934, 1964.
68. Lipsett, M. B., and Goldman, R.: Phenylbutazone toxicity; report of a case of acute renal failure. Ann. Int. Med., *41:*1075, 1954.
69. Herrmann, W. P., Hopfeld, G., and Berning H.: Uber niereentzundungen nach Irgapyrin — behandlung (Nephritis after Irgapyrin therapy) Klin. Med., *154:*302, 1956.
70. Robinson, G. C., and Wong, L. C.: Acute tubular necrosis in infancy and childhood. J. Dis. Child., *95:*417, 1958.
71. Beerman, H.: Fatalities due to bismuth in treatment of syphilis. Arch Derm. Syph., *26:*797, 1932.
72. Barnett, R. N.: Reactions to Bismuth Compound. JAMA, *135:*28, 1947.
73. Weinstein, I.: Fatalities associated with analbis suppositories. JAMA, *133:*962, 1947.
74. Dowds, J. H.: Poisoning by sodium bismuth tartrate injections. Lancet, *2:*1039, 1936.
75. McClendon, S. J.: Toxic effects with anuria from single injection of bismuth preparation: report of 2 cases. Amer. J. Dis. Child., *61:*339, 1941.
76. Boyette, D. D.: Bismuth nephrosis with anuria in an infant. J. Pediat., *28:*493, 1946.
77. Chamberlain, III, J. L., and Franks, R. C.: Nephropathy resulting from bismuth. Southern Med. J., *56:509,* 1963.
78. Czerwinski, A. W. and Ginn, H. E.: Bismuth nephrotoxicity. Amer. J. Med., *37:*969, 1964.

Chapter 39

Clinicopathological Correlations in Chronic Toxic Nephropathies

M. FORLAND, M.D. and B. H. SPARGO, M.D.

The occurrence of a specific nephropathy from chronic exposure to a potential toxin has long been recognized and studied. A clinical appreciation of the significance of such lesions was first applied to problems related to industrial exposure and has been of particular importance in the heavy metal industries. In a number of areas throughout the world, the likelihood that chronic toxic exposure is responsible for an unusually high regional incidence of renal disease has more recently attracted attention. The high incidence of chronic nephritis in Queensland, Australia has been attributed to excess lead exposure, a chronic interstitial nephritis with papillary necrosis first recognized among the factory workers of Switzerland has been associated with analgesic abuse, and investigations are underway to define the causes of the endemic nephritis in Southeastern Europe, which has been termed Balkan Nephropathy.

I. LEAD

The clinical observation of proteinuria and postmortem finding of granular contracted kidneys in lead industry workers dates back to observations of Olivier in 1863 (61). An early renal tubular lesion followed by the development of an interstitial nephritis was described by Oliver in England before the turn of the century (60), and Dickinson, his American contemporary, described granular kidneys in 26 of 42 workers in the lead trade who died from disease or accident (25). He noted, "the constancy with which permanent albuminuria and granular degeneration are produced by the saturnine occupations is one of the most definite facts in pathology."

This association was placed in broader perspective by a group of observations related to the high incidence of chronic nephritis in young people in the Australian state of Queensland. Epidemiologic data in the '20's revealed a death rate from renal disease more than three times as great as in neighboring states (59). Studies appeared to rule out an infectious etiology and in seeking a toxic source the extraordinary incidence of plumbism in the children of Queensland was apparent. Houses in this semi-tropical area were built with broad, covered verandas bordered by railings and coated with white paint of high lead carbonate content. Youngsters usually played on these areas and were exposed to the dry, flaking paint through habits of nail-biting, finger-sucking, and the licking of rain drops. In 1922, legislation was passed in the state limiting the concentration of lead in paint and by the early '30's the problem of plumbism markedly lessened.

In a series of publications, Henderson emphasized the significance of the association between lead exposure and chronic nephropathy (42-45). In tracing 352 of 401 Queensland children diagnosed as having lead poisoning between 1915 and 1935, he found 165 had died. Chronic nephritis or vascular disease was the cause of death in 108 (65%) (42). The interval was six to thirty-five years after the diagnosis of plumbism. The lead content of bone from patients dying of chronic renal disease in Queensland was then anlyzed and found to be significantly higher than those with a similar diagnosis from Sydney (45). In addition, those whose renal insufficiency was of unknown etiology had higher bone lead concentration than those with known chronic glomerulonephritis or chronic pyelonephritis.

Emmerson (26) studied the effect of a standardized infusion of calcium disodium edetate (EDTA) upon the urinary excretion of lead. He found it elevated in 22 Queensland patients with varying degrees of renal insufficiency associated with childhood lead poisoning, in comparison to a group of normal controls and others with renal disease attributable to differing causes. The author also reemphasized the high incidence of gouty arthritis in patients with chronic lead nephropathy.

American industrial hygienists have tended to minimize the significance of lead exposure in the development of chronic renal insufficiency, perhaps because of the early introduction of industrial precautions in this country. Tepper (75) traced 139 of 165 cases of childhood plumbism in Massachusetts for a 20-year follow-up. He found only one dead of chronic renal disease of unknown etiology. Renal function was screened in 42 without finding convincing evidence of impairment. The striking difference in these reported experiences may be related to the more acute type of exposure seen in Massachusetts, where many of the patients presented with lead encephalopathy. In contrast, the Australian group often had a peripheral neuropathy, suggesting the renal lesion may correlate with a more chronic exposure and consequently higher total body accumulation.

In a recent report from Alabama, Morgan *et al.* (57) have described 13 patients with known chronic lead poisoning and renal failure without apparent cause. Lead exposure was excessive in all and generally related to the use of illegal alcohol of high lead concentration due to processing and additives. A clinical picture of anemia, normal or decreased renal size and function, without characteristic urinary findings or infection, and a protracted course with frequent hypertension and proven gout in six of the 13 was reported. The pathological findings in 11 were similar to Case 1.

Case 1.
O.L.
U.C. 910657-6

A 47-year-old Negro lead smelting worker was seen in the outpatient clinic for evaluation of anemia. The patient had been employed in the lead industry for seven years and was asymptomatic but for recent fatty food intolerance relieved by antacids. Physical examination was unremarkable but for slight epigastric tenderness. Hemoglobin was 9.8 gm per 100 ml; hematocrit, 30%; red blood cells, 3,220,000 per cubic mm; stool benzidine was 1+. The initial diagnostic impression was iron deficiency anemia secondary to gastrointestinal bleeding and arrangements were made for hospitalization.

Prior to admission, the patient was seen in the emergency room with an exacerbation of abdominal pain, nausea and vomiting. Abdominal examination now included decreased bowel sounds, epigastric guarding and rebound tenderness. X-ray suggested a distended loop of midline small bowel. Lead poisoning was considered, but an abdominal exploration was performed with a suspicion of acute appendicitis. A mild serositis was the only finding.

In the post-operative period laboratory studies included: blood lead, 284 mcg per 100 ml (normal, <20 mcg); 24 hr urinary lead excretion, 1800 mcg; (normal, <120 mcg); urinary coproporphyins III, strongly positive; delta amino-levulinic acid, 56.8 mg per 24 hours (normal, 2-4 mg); urinary porphobilinogen, 3 mg per 24 hrs; serum uric acid, 8.05 mg per 100 ml; BUN, 50-56 mg per 100 ml; repeat urinalyses showed only occasional granular casts. Serum iron, iron-binding capacity and urinary aminoacids were normal. A renal biopsy was performed (Fig. 1-5).

The post-operative course was uneventful. A diagnosis of lead poisoning was considered established and the patient was discharged from the hospital for out-patient follow-up in regard to further renal function studies and EDTA therapy, however, he failed to return. BUN at the time of discharge was 39 mg per 100 ml.

The presence of intranuclear acid-fast inclusion bodies in the liver and tubular epithelium of the kidneys in cases of lead poisoning was first reported in 1936 by Blackman (11) who also succeeded in reproducing them in experimental animals (Fig. 1). Landing and Nakai (51) observed them in sloughed renal tubular epithelial cells in the hematoxylin and eosin stained urinary sediment of children with acute lead poisoning. These lesions have been studied with the electron microscope and their development observed to be independent of the nucleolus with early changes occurring in the mitochondria as well as within the nucleus (2) (Figs. 2-5). Similar observations have been made by Richter *et al.* (68), who found the fibrils and amorphous material in the lead inclusion bodies were composed of protein other than histone and the fibrils neither contained nucleic acid nor were related to the nucleoli or nucleolar products. Inclusions with similar renal localization have been observed in patients treated with bismuth and their persistence for periods up to 31 years following treatment has been reported (5). They differ from those of lead by their spherical symmetry, fine punctate granularity and intracytoplasmic, as well as intranuclear site (6).

As might be postulated from the tubular localization of the early morphologic changes, renal functional changes also indicate predominantly tubular dysfunction. Historically renal glycosuria was an early observation (56, 36). A generalized aminoaciduria with normal plasma amino-acids has been observed, in conjunction with a proportionate renal glycosuria (79). These findings were confirmed by Chisholm (19) who noted hypophosphatemia as well in nine

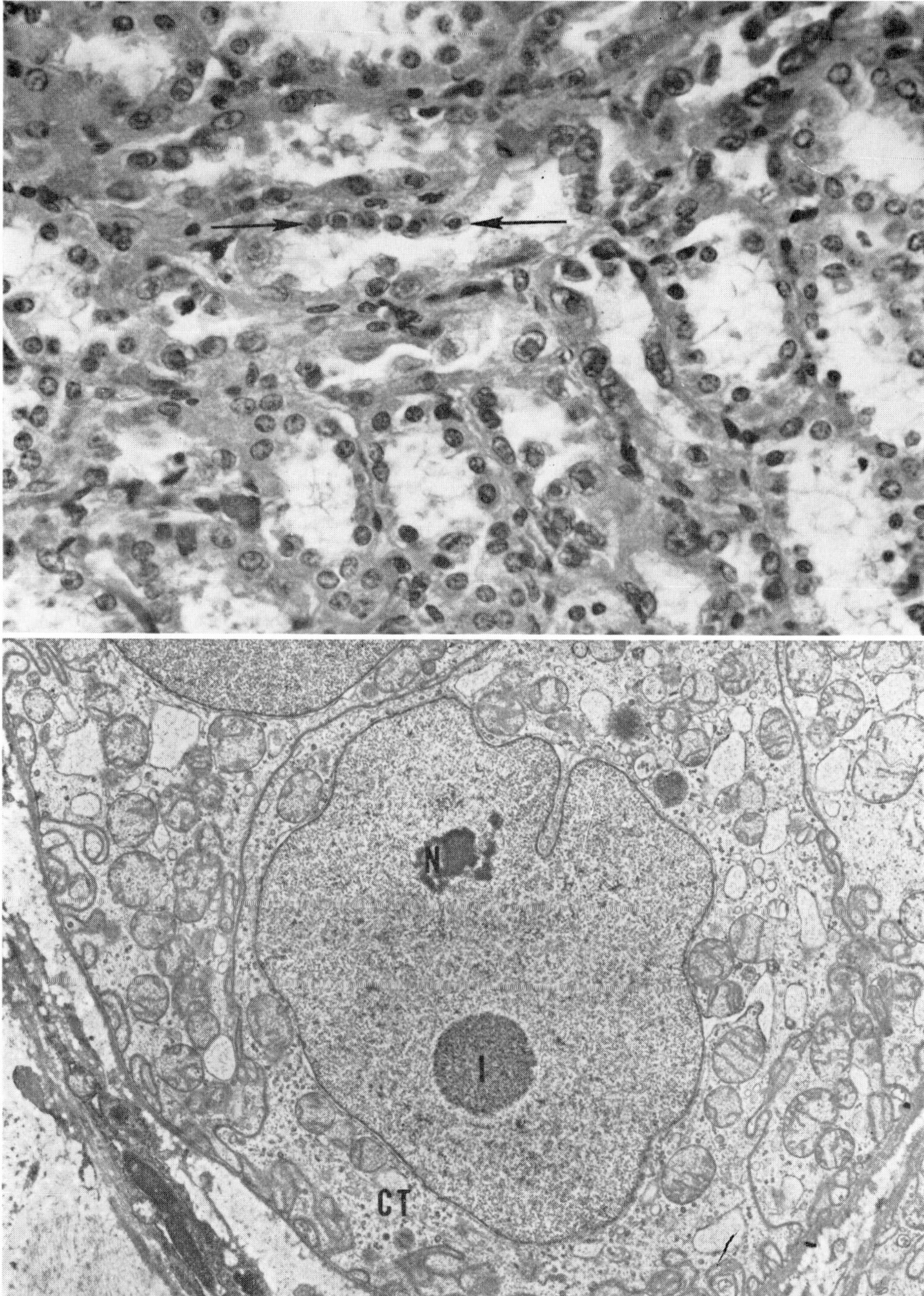

Figure 1. Lead nephropathy. Renal biopsy from case 1 reveals numerous nuclear inclusions (6 between arrows). The inclusions are acid fast and are shown to be numerous especially in the first portion of the collecting tubule. Occasional bizarre nuclei and abnormal mitoses are found, but there is little evidence of tubular necrosis. H & E, fixed in Zenker's, Mag. 350 X

Figure 2. Lead nephropathy. Ultrastructurally the nuclear inclusions are easily distinguished from the nuclelous. The inclusions have a spherical shape with irregular punctate densities that are osmophilic. Enzymatic studies have been interpreted as indicating that these structures are neither RNA nor DNA. The cytoplasm of the collecting tubule cells is only moderately altered with some increased vacuolization, dilatation of the cisternae of the endoplasmic reticulum and mitochondrial enspherulation. Uranyl acetate and lead hydroxide stain. Mag. 11,000 X

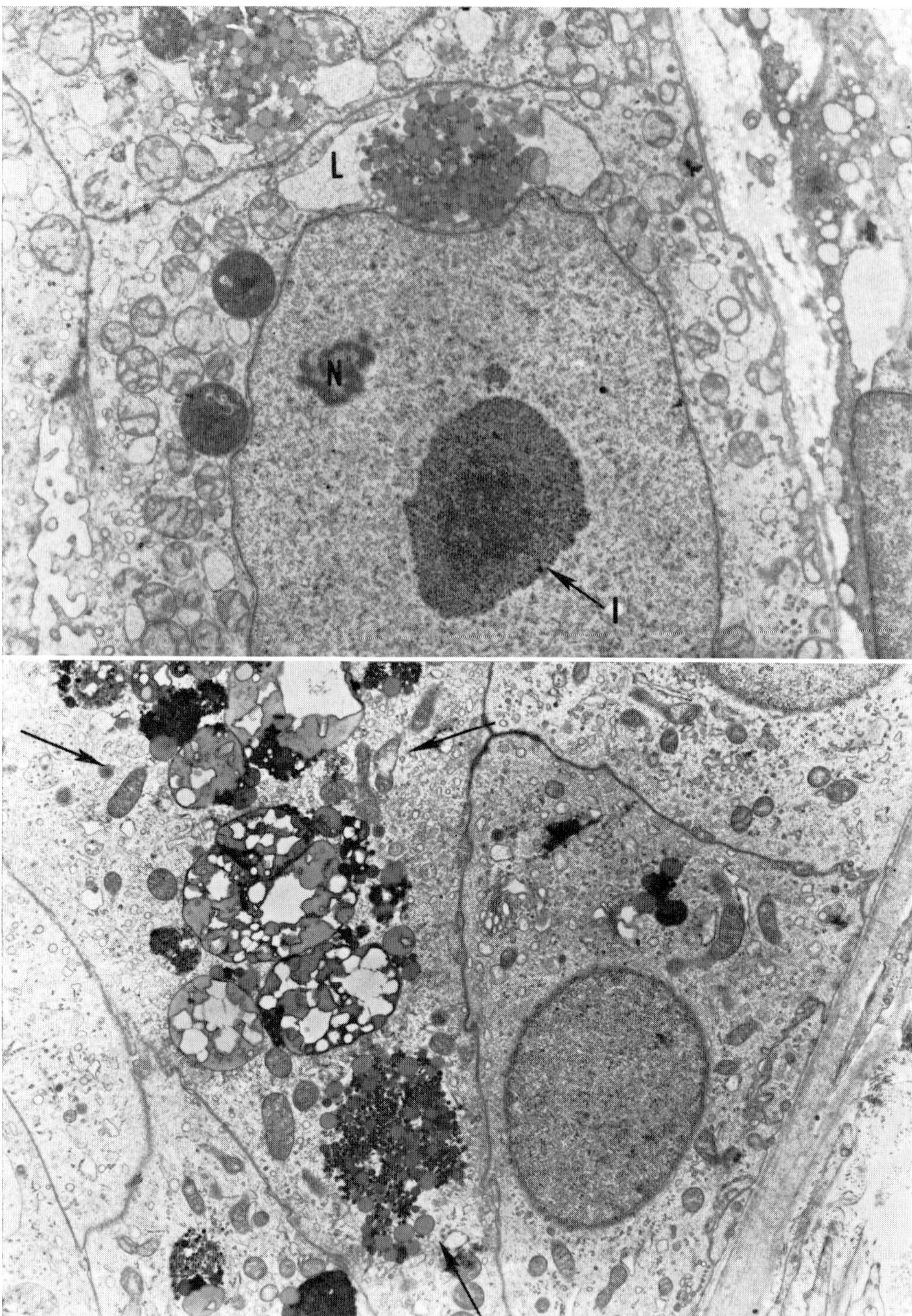

Figure 3. Lead nephropathy. Some collecting tubule cells with larger nuclear inclusions have large collections of lipochrome pigment in more than the usual amounts. Although the origin of this lipo-pigment is not known, it seems probable that lipo-chrome results from destruction of cytoplasmic components in cytosomes. Its formation is stimulated by mild cellular injury and it is especially conspicuous with lead nephropathy. The nuclear inclusion has a central osmophilic zone surrounded by a slightly fibrillar lighter zone. Mag. 14, 1000 X

Figure 4. Lead nephropathy. Occasional cells contain a large collection of polymorphic bodies with areas of light material and dense granules. These do not contain ferruginous material and are interpreted as lipochrome or "wear-and-tear" pigments. A large collection is shown in one cell between the arrows. Mag. 11,000 X

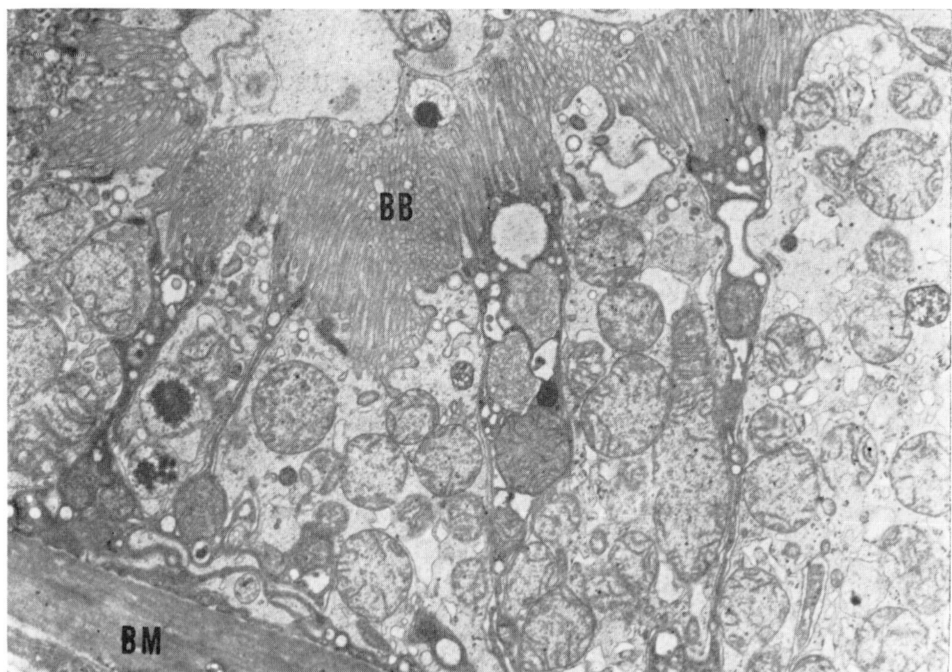

Figure 5. Lead nephropathy. A proximal tubule has some simplification of the cytoplasm with a decrease in particulates partially masked by the prominent enspherulated mitochondria. Cristae lysis is shown with conspicuous loss of the transverse cristae pattern characteristic of these usually elongated cigar-shaped mitochondria. In addition, there is a decrease in the height of these columnar proximal tubule cells and loss of some of the basilar membrane infolding. Mag. 11,000 X

of 23 children with acute lead intoxication. The occurrence of a coincident fructosuria and citraturia set this apart from other childhood Fanconi-type syndromes and suggested a less localized tubular cellular injury. The functional changes cleared with treatment or amelioration of the intoxication. With the development of aminoaciduria in the lead-intoxicated rat, mitochondrial swelling, as well as intranuclear inclusions, have been emphasized (37). This swelling, accompanied by shortening and margination of the cristae, has suggested an impairment in energy metabolism in the proximal tubule. Upon isolation of such mitochondria, a decreased rate of respiration and partial uncoupling of oxidative phosphorylation were found which were partially reversible by the addition of EDTA. Consequently, a divalent cation was suggested as possibly responsible for the metabolic defect (38).

II. ANALGESIC ABUSE

A toxic nephropathy with perhaps wider implications was suggested by Spühler and Zollinger during an investigation of interstitial nephritis (73). They noted a considerable increase in the incidence of this postmorten finding after 1950, particularly in the absence of diabetes mellitus or urinary tract infection. They first suggested a causal relationship between chronic interstitial nephritis and analgesic or sulphonamide ingestion.

Additional observations soon appeared in the European literature. Patients admitted to a county and municipal hospital in Denmark were questioned in regard to phenacetin consumption and a strongly positive correlation was found between the total amount of phenacetin consumed and impaired renal concentrating ability (52). The incidence of reduced renal function increased with total dosage and duration of ingestion; 17 of 21 patients whose total consumption exceeded seven kilograms had both impaired concentrating ability and reduced glomerular filtration rates. Although urinary tract infections were frequent, they were regarded as secondary. Nordenfelt and Ringertz (58) reported 30 deaths from renal insufficiency in patients whose total consumption of phenacetin was at least 10 kilograms over a 10 to 20 year period. The majority were factory workers who took the drug to increase their working ability. Microscopic examination done in 23 of the cases showed a similar picture of chronic interstitial nephritis with tubular damage and papillary necrosis or necrobiosis (Figs. 6, 7). Pyelonephritis was seen in approximately a third of the cases and was again considered secondary.

The occurrence of this clinical picture in the United States was evident from a questionnaire distributed to nephrologists and reported by Schreiner in 1962 (72). Case reports soon appeared in the American literature (66, 67). Questions, however, were also forthcoming concerning the precise etiologic significance of phenacetin in this clinical picture (35). Were the analgesics actually taken because of symptoms of underlying renal disease and consequently of secondary importance? Since the drug was almost invariably taken in combination with caffeine and/or an antiinflammatory agent such as aspirin, could one of the latter drugs be responsible? Why was there no consistent model of a phenacetin lesion in experimental animals? At the same time, conjecture concerning a mechanism for the pathogenesis of the lesion was also offered. Was the lesion mainly the result of a bacterial infection with a high incidence of papillary necrosis? Did the drug predispose to infection by primary injury and/or inhibition of the kidney's resistance to infection? Could methemoglobin and accelerated red blood cell destruction be playing a role? Was analgesic abuse a distinct entity with several causes acting singly or in combination to result in renal insufficiency?

Partial answers to some of these questions are becoming available. At least three investigators have reported the production of tubular and papillary lesions in experimental animals by the administration of phenacetin alone (1, 21,-30). Abrahams (1) reported the most severe papillary lesions occurred when phenacetin was given along with aspirin and caffeine. Prospective autopsy studies continue to affirm an association between phenacetin and renal papillary necrosis. In a study of 507 post-mortems, 40 of 42 cases with severe papillary damage independent of obstruction, diabetes mellitus or amyloidosis were correlated with the regular ingestion of phenacetin-containing analgesics (15). Sixteen patients who consumed analgesics without phenacetin showed no papillary changes. In those who ingested greater than four kilograms, 73% showed papillary degeneration and 37% died from pyelonephritis with papillary necrosis. Earlier papillary lesions correlated with smaller total doses of phenacetin.

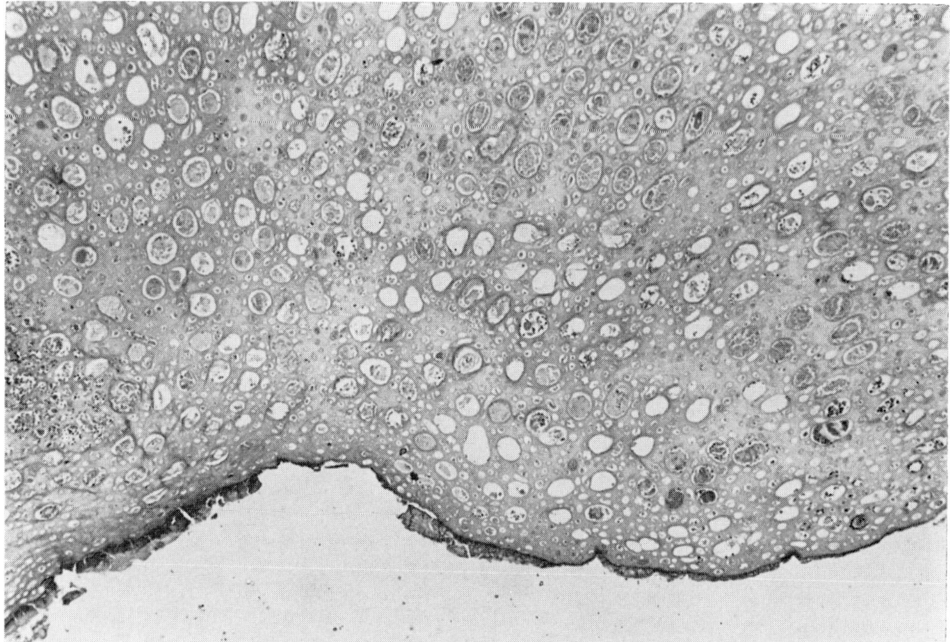

Figure 6. Papillary necrosis complicating longstanding analgesic abuse has as the primary lesion the conspicuous coagulation necrosis of the papilla with an area of superficial erosion. Along the left margin, minimal inflammatory exudate is shown. Casts are prominent despite the loss of the collecting tubule epithelium. H & E, Mag. 10 X (Slide by Dr. Conrad Pirani).

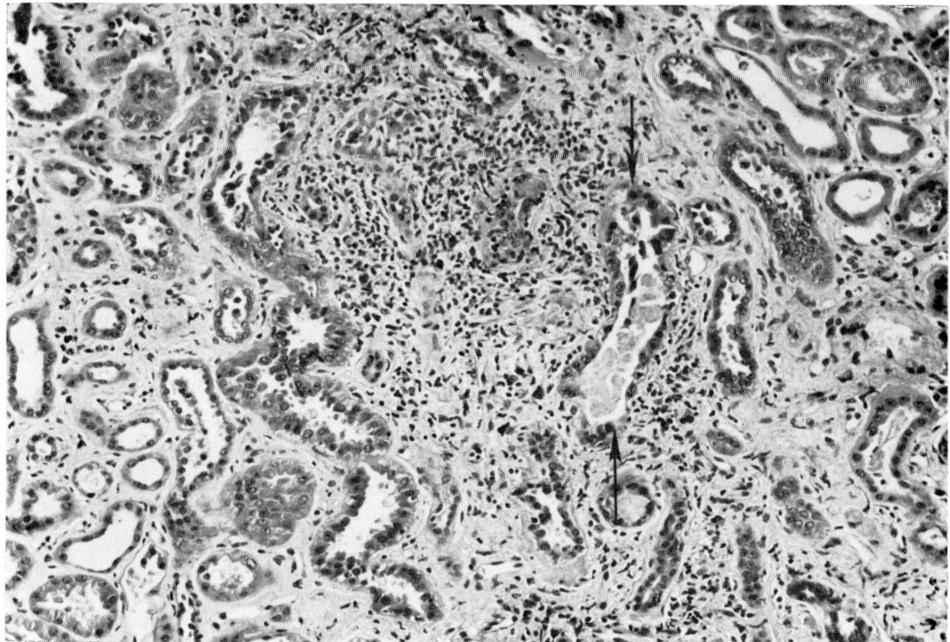

Figure 7. Analgesic abuse with marked chronic interstitial fibrosis. The tubular loss with prominent interstitial tissue is associated with only sparse focal collections of lymphocytic infiltrate. The glomeruli are relatively well preserved and there is no periglomerular fibrosis. Brown pigment of the tubules is common although not shown at this magnification. H & E, Mag 10 X (Slide by Dr. Conrad Pirani).

Three independent studies (69, 50,-14) have recently emphasized the primacy of renal papillary necrosis following long-term, high-dosage use of phenacetin. The cortical changes characterized as chronic interstitial nephritis appear secondary to parenchymal atrophy and fibrosis subsequent to the medullary lesion, particularly when infection is superimposed on the comprised kidney.

Vivaldi (76) found no increased incidence of an experimental ascending E. coli renal infection in rats fed phenacetin or N-acetyl-p-aminophenol for six to 12 months. However, animals fed aspirin had significantly more infections than others.

III. BALKAN NEPHROPATHY

Extensive investigations have been conducted concerning another localized occurrence of renal disease thought likely to be of toxic etiology (82). The Balkan Nephropathy has been described in limited areas of three countries in southeast Europe—Bulgaria, Rumania and Yugoslavia. These regions border on one another and are all situated in the basin of the Danube River. The high incidence of endemic chronic nephritis in some villages was described almost simultaneously but independently from the three countries approximately ten years ago. There are suggestions, however, that the problem may have been present as early as the post-World War I years.

The disease appears to occur in villages, rather than towns and particularly those in hilly zones, toward the bottom of valleys eroded by small rivers (10). The incidence of renal disease may be as high as five to 12% of the population in affected villages and often appears to have a strong familial incidence. Diagnosis is rare in children and greatest in the 30 to 60 age group with a somewhat higher incidence and earlier appearance in women.

The onset is usually insidious with headache, lassitude and anorexia and the findings include slight proteinuria, progressive azotemia, a normochromic anemia and renal atrophy. Sallow, copper-colored skin with xanthochromia of the palms and soles is a frequent feature. Edema, or other features of the nephrotic syndrome are not seen and hypertension is rare. In the Rumanian series, death occurred within two years after the first symptoms in 56% (10).

The pathologic picture is one of early tubular dystrophy and necrotic change leading to a progressive sclerosis with eventual secondary hyalinization of glomeruli, tubular atrophy and diffuse fibrosis, all more marked in the outer cortical zone (64). In Bulgaria, a 35% incidence of associated tumors of the urogenital tract, without metastatic dissemination, has been reported (64). This concurrent finding has not been observed in Rumania. Schourup has suggested the lesion is a primary tubular degeneration resembling that produced experimentally in phenacetin treated rats (71).

Functional changes include early impairment in concentrating ability and para-aminohippurate (PAH) secretory capacity and renal blood flow, with a later fall in glomerular filtration rate (64). The pattern of proteinuria observed in Yugoslavia has been characterized as tubular (40), with relatively small amounts of albumin and increased quantities of low molecular weight proteins of beta and gamma electrophoretic mobility. This is the pattern reported with renal damage in the proximal tubule (16). It has been observed in children as young as three years and seasonal variation in its occurrence has also been reported (40). Studies of the proteinuria in Rumania have indicated a mixed pattern, with a more prominent albumin fraction, possibly because their patients studied had more advanced disease (12).

The etiology of this nephropathy remains unexplained. In a Serbian village where 37 persons in 12 families had died of chronic nephritis and 23 of 44 living persons had evidence of renal disease, an exposure to flour heavily contaminated with lead during the milling process has been incriminated (13, 14). This has not been the finding in other areas. Investigations of trace elements in water and soil and studies of local flora and fauna have not been revealing. Evidence of viral or bacteriologic infection has not been substantiated. In both Yugoslavia (33) and Rumania (10), the affected villages are situated at a lower level than those free of the disease and a tentative hypothesis suggesting the water supply as the carrier of the potential toxin necessitates further study.

IV. HYPERCALCEMIA

The fact that chronic toxic nephropathy is not limited to remote areas of the world and must be considered in the differential diagnosis of many clinical renal problems can be appreciated from Case II:

CASE II.
L.R.H.
U.C. 746708

A 58-year-old white male was hospitalized for investigation of dull, aching upper abdominal pain of six month's duration, unrelated to meals or position. Episodic nausea and vomiting, malaise, easy fatigability, and marked obstipation had been noted during a similar period and was accompanied by a 25-pound weight loss.

Approximately eight years earlier the patient had developed low back pain diagnosed by his family physician as arthritis and was started on vitamin D in a dosage of 150,000 units daily. This was continued for approximately four years and then cut to 100,000 units daily, which he took until the time of hospitalization.

Physical examination was normal but the patient was thin and appeared chronically ill.

Pertinent laboratory findings included a hemoglobin of 11.9 gms per 100 ml; hematocrit, 35%; repeated urinalyses showed only a trace of albumin and 3-4 WBC's per high power field. BUN, 51 mg per 100 ml; urea clearance, 11 ml/min with a flow of 2.3 ml/min; serum calcium, 11.9 to 12.6 mg per 100 ml; albumin, 4.0; globulins, 2.8. Gastrointestinal x-rays were unremarkable and an intravenous pyelogram showed nephrocalcinosis. Urinary calcium excretion was greater than 300 mg per 24 hours on a 200 mg diet. A renal biopsy was performed (Fig. 8).

The patient was admitted to the hospital with a suspicion of a gastric carcinoma and it was only after the finding of a persistent hypercalcemia and hypercalciuria that vitamin D intake was acknowledged and a diagnosis of hypervitaminosis D confirmed. Dietary vitamin D and calcium intake were restricted and hydration encouraged. The patient was followed in clinic and serum calcium returned to normal by a three-month follow-up visit. BUN gradually

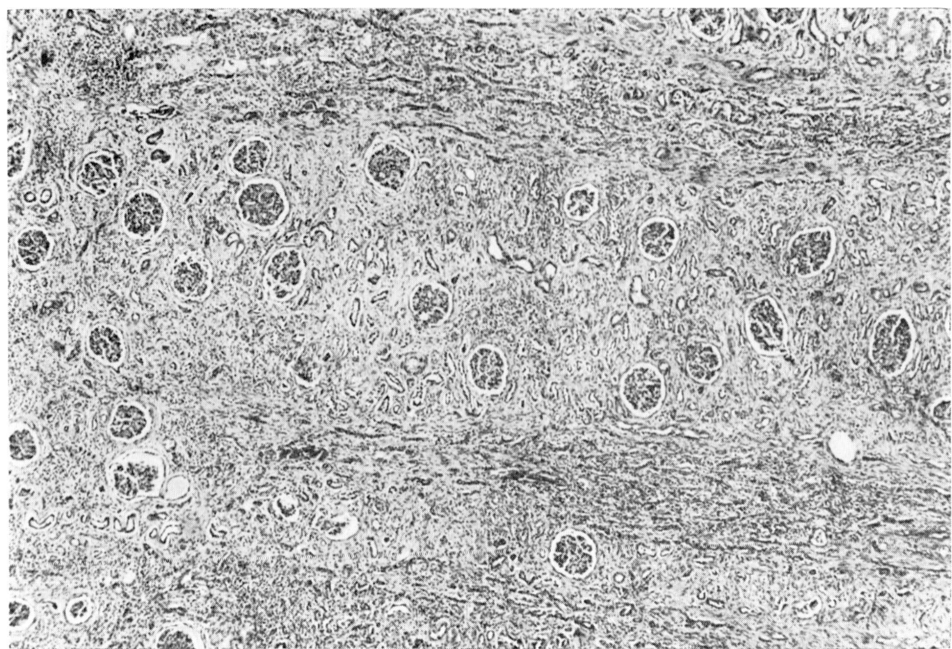

Figure 8. Hypercalcemic nephropathy. Case 2. Large calcified casts (**between arrows**) are partially fragmented during sectioning. There is tubular cell proliferation in areas of the larger casts. Many tubules are lost and it is not clear whether this is primary because of chronic obstruction or the specific early effect of the excess calcium on the mitochondria. Large areas of interstitium are well collagenized and focally infiltrated by mononuclear cells. Ultrastructurally evidence of tubular basement membrane and interstitial calcification is frequently shown in these areas. H & E, Mag. 100 X.

fell and at a nine month evaluation his urea clearance was 52 ml per min with a BUN of 14 mg per 100 ml. The patient's gastrointestinal symptoms cleared and he gradually regained weight.

Hypercalcemia even of transient nature produces structural changes in the kidney. Carone *et al.* (17) localized patchy areas of tubular epithelial degeneration, calcification and necrosis following parathyroid hormone administration to dogs for one day. The ascending limb of Henle, distal convolution and collecting system were primarily involved. Electron microscopy has revealed early mitochondrial changes with hypercalcemia from parathyroid hormone (18) or vitamin D (70), subsequently followed by calcification in the same areas. Changes with calcium gluconate were most striking in the basement membrane in portions of the proximal tubule and consisted of electron-opaque deposits thought to be calcium carbonate (18). The occurrence of intratubular casts at these sites leads to obstruction of the nephron and proximal tubular dilatation and localized interstitial reaction (Fig. 8). The persistence of hypercalcemia with increasing numbers and progression of these lesions results in significant impairment in renal function. Clinically, infection and hypertension are frequent late complications (27).

The early functional consequence of hypercalcemia is an impairment in renal concentrating ability due to an apparent defect in the tubular reabsorption of water. Carone *et al.* (17) have demonstrated this in the dog after only 24 hours of hypercalcemia induced by parathyroid hormone. Several investigators have confirmed its occurrence in patients with hypercalcemia, hypercalciuria, or both, due to a variety of causes. (34, 83). Structural damage to the tubular system interfering with the operation of the countercurrent mechanism for urinary concentration provides a possible explanation, however, the impairment is often present when the lesion is spotty or not well established. An alternate explanation for this diminution in water reabsorption can be found in the demonstration of inhibition in antidiuretic hormone (ADH) effect on water transport by calcium across a wide variety of membranes. Bentley (8) first demonstrated this in the toad urinary bladder and it has been observed in necturus kidney slices (78), and the distal tubule of the intact rat (53). A number of studies have suggested calcium does not influence ADH effect on sodium transport (9, 62). Others have found a decrease in sodium transport (22, 42) and inhibition of sodium-potassium activated adenosine triphosphatase by calcium has been suggested as a possible mechanism (28).

In addition to a defect in water reabsorption, impairment in urinary acidification has been observed to follow long-standing hypercalcemia. Fourman has observed this in four patients with hyperparathyroidism, with improvement observed two months after surgery (31). Ferris *et al.* (29) reported the development of a clinical picture of renal tubular acidosis in a patient with hypoparathyroidism who had several episodes of vitamin D intoxication. Potassium wasting was also observed in this patient and the occurrence of unexplained hypokalemia in case reports with hypercalcemia was commented upon. Heinemann reported a reversible defect in renal ammonium excretion in patients with hypercalcemia and suggested this might play a role in the impaired handling of an acid load (41).

V. OTHER HEAVY METALS

A number of other heavy metals have been implicated in the development of renal impairment following chronic exposure. Friberg (32) has studied a group of Swedish cadmium workers and reported 80% of 40 men with more than eight years exposure had proteinuria. This protein failed to precipitate with boiling or picric acid and ultra centrifugal and electrophoretic studies (63) revealed the low molecular weight globulins characteristic of renal tubular proteinuria (16). Kazantzis *et al.* (48) confirmed this finding in six cadmium pigment workers with 25 or more years of exposure. Additional findings in these patients suggestive of impaired renal tubular function included renal glycosuria, abnormal aminoaciduria, impaired concentrating ability and acid excretion, hypercalciuria and a hyperchloremic acidosis. Three of four men employed in the factory 12 to 14 years also had greater than normal excretion of a tubular pattern of proteins.

Prolonged exposure to mercury has been associated with the development of proteinuria which may be independent of other symptoms of mercury poisoning (49). Protein loss may be sufficient to produce a clinical picture of the nephrotic syndrome. The absence of renal findings among colleagues of nephrotic mercury workers, despite similar urinary excretory levels of mercury, has suggested this may represent an idiosyncratic reaction. Renal biopsy findings from nephrotic patients have varied; relatively normal appearing glomeruli have been reported, as well as a sub-epithelial deposit observed on electron microscopy of the glomerular capillary wall, suggesting a membranous nephropathy (55). Becker *et al.*, reviewed five patients with mercury associated nephrotic syndrome and found the membranous lesions were associated with the topical application of ammoniated mercury preparations, whereas the two occurrences following chlormerodrin and exposure to mercurial paint additives had more prominent tubular degenerative changes (7), which are characteristic of the experimental mercury lesion (39). The association between prolonged use of organic mercurial diuretics and the nephrotic syndrome has been frequently reported, but critical assessment of its frequency is made difficult by its independent occurrence with congestive heart failure (13).

While uranium is excreted primarily by the kidney, it is poorly absorbed following inhalation or ingestion, limiting its toxic potential for man. Studies on its intravenous effects in man (54) have demonstrated changes primarily in renal tubular function, comparable to its acute toxicity in animal studies in which lesions are localized to the distal portion of the proximal convoluted tubule (74). Aminoaciduria has been reported in workers with long-standing uranium exposure (20).

The renal effects of both acute and chronic copper poisoning have been difficult to dissociate from the associated hemolytic anemia which results in hemoglobinuria and occasionaly shock (47). However, the effects of renal copper deposition have been studied in patients with Wilson's disease (hepatolenticular degeneration) who are believed to have a genetically determined impairment in the synthesis of ceruloplasmin, the copper-binding protein. Increased copper absorption leads to tissue deposition and high renal copper concentration have been reported (81). Tubular epithelial degenerative changes have been observed to correlate with the localization of intracytoplasmic copper granules. These lesions resemble the proximal convoluted tubular changes seen in chronically copper-poisoned rats (77, 80). Renal aminoaciduria has been a frequent observation in these patients, and quantitatively parallels the level of urinary copper excretion (3). Other indications of tubular functional compromise reported have included decreased tubular secretory capacity for PAH, glycosuria, increased uricosuria, and phosphaturia, impaired urinary acidification ability and hypercalciuria associated with bony changes (4). In advanced stages of the disease, impaired glomerular filtration and renal blood flow have been reported (4).

Basic to the management of the toxic nephropathies is cessation of the damaging exposure, whether this be the hazard of an industrial setting and overzealous therapeutic effort, or insidious environmental factor. The therapeutic use of chelating agents, as we have discussed elsewhere (65), has increased the efficacy of the treatment of heavy metal poisoning by the chelator's ability to bind the potential toxin and permit its more rapid excretion in a relatively safe form. Since the urinary tract is frequently the primary excretory route, precautions are necessary in adjusting the dosage when renal function is impaired.

REFERENCES

1. Abrahams, C., Rubenstein, A. H., Levin, N. M., and Wonderlich, V.: Experimentally induced analgesic nephritis in rats. Arch. Path., *78:*222-230, 1964.
2. Angevine, J. M., Kappas, A., DeGowin, R. L., and Spargo, B. T.: Renal tubular nuclear inclusions of lead poisoning. Arch. Path., *73:*486-494, 1962.
3. Bearn, A. G., and Kunkel, H. G.: Abnormalities of copper metabolism in Wilson's Disease and their relationship to the aminoaciduria. J. Clin. Invest., *33:*400-409, 1954.
4. Bearn, A. G., Yu, T. F., and Gutman, A. B.: Renal function in Wilson's Disease. J. Clin. Invest., *36:*1107-1114, 1957.
5. Beaver, D. L., and Burr, R. E.: Bismuth inclusions in the human kidney. Arch. Path., *76:* 89-94, 1963.
6. Beaver, D. L., and Burr, R. E.: Electron microscopy of bismuth inclusions. Amer. J. Path., *42:* 609-617, 1963.
7. Becker, C. G., Becker, E. L., Maher, J. F., and Schreiner, G. E.: Nephrotic syndrome after contact with mercury. Arch. Int. Med., *110:* 178-186, 1962.
8. Bentley, P. J.: The effects of ionic changes on water transfer across the isolated urinary bladder of the toad Bufo marinus. J. Endocrin., *18:*327-333, 1959.
9. Bentley, P. J., The effects of vasopressin on the short-circuit current across the wall of the isolated bladder of the toad, Bufo marinus. J. Endocrin., *21:*161-170, 1960.
10. Biberi Moroeanu, S.: Epidemiological observations on the endemic nephropathy in Rumania. In Wolstenholme, G. E. W. and Knight, J. (eds): The Balkan Nephropathy (Ciba Foundation Study Group No. 30). Boston, Little, Brown and Company, 1967, pp. 4-13.
11. Blackman, S. S., Jr.: Intranuclear inclusion bodies in the kidney and liver caused by lead poisoning. Bull. Johns Hopkins Hosp., *58:*384-404, 1936.
12. Bruckner, I., Stoica, G., and Serban, M.: Studies on urinary proteins in endemic nephropathy In Wolstenholme, G. E. W. and Knight, J. (eds): The Balkan Nephropathy (Ciba Foundation Study Group No. 30), Boston, Little, Brown and Company, 1967, pp. 84-99.
13. Burack, W.R., Pryce, J., and Goodwin, J. F.: Reversible nephrotic syndrome associated with congestive heart failure. Circulation, *18:*562-571, 1958.
14. Burry, A. F.: The evolution of analgesic nephropathy. Nephron, *5:*185-201, 1968.
15. Burry, A. F., DeJersey, P., and Weedon, D.: Phenacetin and renal papillary necrosis. Results of a prospective autopsy investigation. Med. J. Austr., *53:*873-879, 1966.
16. Butler, E. A., Flynn, F. V., Harris, H., and Robson, E. B.: A study of urine proteins by two-dimensional electrophoresis with special reference to the proteinuria of renal tubular disorders. Clin. Chim. Acta, *7:*34-41, 1962.
17. Carone, F. A., Epstein, F. H., Beck, D., and Levitin, H.: Effects upon kidney of transient hypercalcemia induced by parathyroid extract. Am. J. Path., *36:*77-103, 1960.
18. Caulfield, J. B., and Schrag, P. E.: Electron microscopic study of renal calcification. Am J. Path., *44:*365-381, 1964.
19. Chisholm, J. D., Jr.: Aminoaciduria in lead intoxication. J. Pediat., *60:*1-17, 1955.
20. Clarkson, T. W., and Kench, J. E.: Urinary excretion of amino acids by men absorbing heavy metals. Biochem. J., *62:*361-372, 1956.
21. Clausen, E.: Histological changes in rabbit kidneys induced by phenacetin and acetylsalicylic acid. Lancet, *2:*123-124, 1964.
22. Curran, P. F., Herrera, F. C., and Flanigan, W. J.: The effects of calcium and antidiuretic hormone on sodium transport across frog skin. 2. Sites and mechanism of action. J. Gen. Physiol., *46:*1011-1027, 1963.
23. Danilovic, V.: Chronic nephritis due to the ingestion of lead-contaminated flour. Brit. M. J., *1:*27-28, 1958.
24. Danilović, V., and Stojimirović, B.: Endemic nephropathy in Kolubara, Serbia. In Wolstenholme, G. E. W. and Knight, J. (eds): The Balkan Nephropathy, (Ciba Foundation Study Group No. 30). Boston, Little, Brown and Company, pp. 44-50.
25. Dickinson, J. A.: A Treatise on Albuminuria, ed. 2. New York, William Wood & Company, 1881.
26. Emmerson, B. T.: Chronic Lead Nephropathy: The diagnostic use of calcium EDTA and the association with gout. Australas. Ann. Med., *12:* 310-324, 1963.
27. Epstein, F. H.: Calcium and the kidney. J. Chron. Dis., *11:*255-277, 1960.
28. Epstein, F. H. and Whittam, R.: Mode of inhibition by calcium of cellmembrane adenosinetriphosphatase activity. Biochem. J., *99:*232-238, 1966.
29. Ferris, T., Kashgarian, M., Levitin, H., Brandt, I., and Epstein, F. H.: Renal tubular acidosis and renal potassium wasting acquired as result of hypercalcemic nephropathy. New Eng. J. Med., *265:*924-928, 1961.
30. Fordham, C. C., III, Huffines, W. D., and Welt, L. G.: Phenacetin-induced renal disease in rats. Ann. Int. Med., *62:*738-743, 1965.
31. Fourman, P., McConkey, B., and Smith, J. W. G.: Defects of water reabsorption and of hy-

drogen-ion excretion by renal tubular in hyperparathyroidism. Lancet, *1:*619-622, 1960.

32. Friberg, L.: Chronic cadmium poisoning. Arch. Indutr. Hlth., *20:*401-407, 1959.
33. Gason, J.: Endemic nephropathy in Bosnia. In Wolstenholme, G. E. W. and Knight, J. (eds): The Balkan Nephropathy (Ciba Foundation Study Group No. 30). Boston, Little, Brown and Company, 1967, pp. 51-71.
34. Gill, J. R., Jr., and Bartter, F. C.: On impairment of renal concentrating ability in prolonged hypercalcemia and hypercalciuria in man. J. Clin. Invest., *40:*716-722, 1961.
35. Gilman, A.: Analgesic nephropathy: a pharmacological analysis. Am. J. Med., *36:*167-173, 1964.
36. Goettsch, E., and Mason, H. H.: Glycosuria in lead poisoning. Amer. J. Dis. Child., *59:*119-128, 1940.
37. Goyer, R. A.: The renal tubular in lead poisoning: I. Mitochondrial swelling and aminoaciduria. Lab. Invest., *19:*71-77, 1968.
38. Goyer, R. A., Frall, A., and Kimball, J. P.: The renal tubule in lead poisoning. II *In vitro* studies of mitochondrial structure and function. Lab. Invest., *19:*78-83, 1968.
39. Gritzka, T. L., and Trump, B. F.: Renal tubular lesions caused by mercuric chloride. Am. J. Path., *52:*1225-1277, 1968.
40. Hall, P. W., Gaon, J., Griggs, R. C., Piscator, M., Popović, N., Vasilović, M., and Zimonjić, B.: The use of electrophoretic analysis of urinary protein excretion to identify early involvement in endemic (Balkan) nephropathy. In Wolstenholme, G. E. W. and Knight, J. (eds.): The Balkan Nephropathy (Ciba Foundation Study Group No. 30). Boston, Little, Brown and Company, 1967, pp. 72-83.
41. Heinemann, H. O.: Reversible defect in renal ammonium excretion in patients with hypercalcemia. Metabolism, *12:*792-803, 1963.
42. Henderson, D. A.: A follow-up of cases of plumbism in children. Australas. Ann. Med., *3:*219-224, 1954.
43. Henderson, D. A.: Chronic nephritis in Queensland. Australas. Ann. Med., *4:*163-177, 1955.
44. Henderson, D. A.: The aetiology of chronic nephritis in Queensland. Med. J. Aust., *45:*377-386, 1958.
45. Henderson, D. A., and Inglis, J. A.: The lead content of bone in chronic Bright's disease. Australas. Ann. Med., *6:*145-154, 1957.
46. Herrera, F. C., and Curran, P. F.: The effect of calcium and antidiuretic hormone on sodium transport across frog skin. I. Examination of interrelationships between calcium and hormone. J. Gen. Physiol., *46:*999-1010, 1963.
47. Holtzman, N. A., Elliott, D. A., and Heller, R. H.: Copper intoxication: report of a case with observations on ceruloplasmin. New Eng. J. Med., *275:*347-352, 1966.
48. Kazantzis, G., Flynn, F. V., Spowage, J. S., and Trott, D. G.: Renal tubular malfunction and pulmonary emphysema in cadmium pigment workers. Quart. J. Med., *32:*165-192, 1963.
49. Kazantzis, G., Schiller, K. F. R., Asscher, A. W., and Drew, R. G.: Albuminuria and the nephrotic syndrome following exposure to mercury and its compounds. Quart. J. Med., *31:*403-418, 1962.
50. Kincaid-Smith, P.: Pathogenesis of the renal lesion associated with the abuse of analgesics. Lancet, *1:*859-862, 1967.
51. Landing, B. H., and Nakai, H.: Histochemical properties of renal leadinclusions and their demonstration in the urinary sediment. Amer. J. Clin. Path., *31:*499-503, 1959.
52. Larsen, K., and Møller, C. E.: A renal lesion caused by abuse of phenacetin. Acta Med. Scandinav., *164:*53-71, 1959.
53. Lassiter, W. E., Frick, A., Ruamrich, G., and Ullrich, K. J.: Influence of ionic calcium on water permeability of proximal and distal tubules in rat kidney. Pfluger's Arch. f. d. ges. Physiol., *285:*90-95, 1965.
54. Luessenhop, A. J., Gallimore, J. C., Sweet, W. H,. Struxness, E. G., and Robinson, J.: The toxicity in man of hexavalent uranium following intravenous administration. Amer. J. Roentgenol., *79:*83-100, 1958.
55. Mandema, E., Arends, A., Van Zeijst, J., Vermeer, G., Van Der Hem, G. K., and Van Der Slikke, L. B.: Mercury and the kidney. Lancet, *1:*266, 1963.
56. McKhann, C. F.: Lead poisoning in children. Am. J. Dis. Child., *32:*386-392, 1926.
57. Morgan, J. M., Hartley, M. W., and Miller, R. E.: Nephropathy in chronic lead poisoning. Arch. Int. Med., *118:*17-29, 1966.
58. Nordenfelt, O., and Ringertz, N.: Phenacetin takers dead with renal failure. Acta Med. Scand., *170:*385-402, 1961.
59. Nye, L. J. J.: Chronic Nephritis and Lead Poisoning. Sydney, Angus & Robertson, Limited, 1933.
60. Oliver, T.: Goulstonian Lectures on Lead Poisoning in its Acute and Chronic Manifestations. Brit. M. J., *1:*688-691, 1891.
61. Ollivier, A.: De l'albuminurie saturine. Arch. Gen. de med., *2:*530-546, 1863.
62. Petersen, M. J., and Edelman, I. S.: Calcium inhibition of action of vasopressin on urinary bladder of toad. J. Clin. Invest., *43:*583-594, 1964.
63. Piscator, M.: Proteinuria in chronic cadmium poisoning. I. An electrophoretic and chemical

study of urinary and serum proteins from workers with chronic cadmium poisoning. Arch. Environm. Hlth., *4:*607-621, 1962.

64. Puchlev, A.: Endemic nephropathy in Bulgaria. In Wolstenholme, G. E. W. and Knight, J. (eds): The Balkan Nephropathy (Ciba Foundation Study Group No. 30). Boston, Little, Brown and Company, 1967, pp. 28-39.
65. Pullman, T. N., Lavender, A. R., and Forland, M.: Synthetic chelating agents in clinical medicine. Ann. Rev. Med., *14:*175-194, 1963.
66. Rapoport, A., White, L. W., and Ranking, G. N.: Renal damage associated with chronic phenacetin overdosage. Ann. Int. Med., *57:*970-982, 1962.
67. Reynolds, T. B., and Edmondson, H. A.: Chronic renal disease and heavy abuse of analgesics. J.A.M.A., *184:*435-444, 1963.
68. Richter, G. W., Kress, Y., and Cornwall, C. C.: Another look at lead inclusion bodies. Am. J. Path., *53:*189-217, 1968.
69. Sanerkin, N. G.: Chronic phenacetin nephropathy (with particular reference to the relationship between renal papillary necrosis and 'chronic interstitial nephritis'). Brit. J. Urol., *38:*361-370, 1966.
70. Scarpelli, D. G., Tremblay, G., and Pearse, A. G. E.: Comparative cytochemical and cytologic study of vitamin D induced nephrocalcinosis. Am. J. Path., *36:*331-353, 1960.
71. Schourup, K.: Structural changes in endemic nephropathy. In Wolstenholme, G. E. W. and Knight, J. (eds): The Balkan Nephropathy (Ciba Foundation Study Group No. 30). Boston, Little, Brown and Company, 1967, p. 100.
72. Schreiner, G. E.: The nephrotoxicity of analgesic abuse. Ann. Int. Med., *57:*1047-1052, 1962.
73. Spühler, O., and Zollinger, H. U.: Die chronisch interstitielle nephritis. z. Klin. Med., *151:*1-50, 1953.
74. Stone, R. S., Bencosme, S.A., Latta, H., and Madden, S. C.: Renal tubular fine structure studied during reaction to acute urainium injury. Arch. Path., *71:*160-174, 1961.
75. Tepper, L. B.: Renal function subsequent to childhood plumbism. Arch. Environ. Hlth., *7:*76-85, 1963.
76. Vivaldi, E.: Effect of chronic administration of analgesics on resistance to experimental infection of the urinary tract in rats. Nephron, *5:* 202-209, 1968.
77. Vogel, F. S.: Nephrotoxic properties of copper under experimental conditions in mice. Am. J. Path., *36:*699-711, 1960.
78. Whittembury, G., Sugino, N., and Solomon, A. K.: Effect of antidiuretic hormone and calcium on the equivalent pore radius of kidney slices from Necturus. Nature, *187:*699-701, 1960.
79. Wilson, V. K., Thomason, M. L., and Dent, C. E:. Amino-aciduria in lead poisoning: a case in childhood. Lancet, *2:*66-68, 1953.
80. Wolff, S. M.: Copper deposition in the rat. Arch Path., *69:*217-223, 1960.
81. Wolff, S. M.: Renal lesions in Wilson's Disease. Lancet, *1:*843-845, 1964.
82. Wolstenholme, G. E. W., and Knight, J. (eds): The Balkan Nephropathy (Ciba Foundation Study Group No. 30). Boston, Little, Brown and Company, 1967.
83. Zeffren, J. L., and Heineman, H. O.: Reversible defect in renal concentrating mechanism in patients with hypercalcemia. Am. J. Med., *33:* 54-63, 1962.

Chapter 40

Drug Induced Morphologic Changes in the Liver

PETER B. HERDSON, M.B., PH.D.

Recent investigations into fine structural alterations produced in liver parenchymal cells by drugs such as phenobarbital have thrown additional light on the mechanism whereby such compounds are detoxified. They also have drawn attention to some basic biological phenomena, in particular the subjects of membrane synthesis and substrate-induced enzyme synthesis. In the present chapter, some of these current concepts will be reviewed using as a basis for discussion the biological and morphological changes which occur in the liver following such drug administration. These changes are now known to be predictable and dose-related. Also in this chapter, some of the much more extensive morphological alterations will be considered, including necrosis, inflammation, marked fat accumulation and cholestasis, which can be produced by a variety of other drugs.

The fine structure of normal rat liver parenchymal cells is well known (7, 12,-24) (Fig. 1). Briefly, the hepatocyte has one or two nuclei with prominent nucleoli. The surrounding cell membrane shows regional modifications to form bile canaliculi between adjacent cells, and to form microvilli which project into the space of Disse on the sinusoidal surface. Within the cytoplasm, rough endoplasmic reticulum is seen to consist of parallel arrays of paired membranes with attached ribosomes, while smooth endoplasmic reticulum consists of multiple interrelated smooth-walled vesicles. The rough and smooth endoplasmic reticulum together are the main components of the microsomal fraction used in biochemical investigations (1, 23). Recently, it has become possible to separate these two components as individual microsomal fractions (6, 26). Golgi apparatus is present in the hepotocyte and consists of a collection of round or flattened smooth-walled vesicles of varying sizes. Mitochondria are prominent, and microbodies with their distinctive nucleoids are seen. Characteristic glycogen particles are present in variable amounts, together with occasional fat droplets, and pericanalicular dense bodies (lysosomes).

A good deal is known about the functions of many of these organelles. Thus, all the RNA and the vast majority of the DNA produced in the cell is made in the nucleus, with the nucleolus playing a vital role in nucleic acid metabolism and protein synthesis. The mitochondria are the site of oxidative phosphorylation. Most of the protein synthesis occurring in the cell takes place in close relation to polyribosomes, which in hepatocytes are for the most part attached to the rough endoplasmic reticulum. Protein is produced both for export from the cell, and for the cell's intrinsic requirements, which include enzymes and membranes. Smooth endoplasmic reticulum is involved with cholesterol and carbohydrate metabolism, and with detoxification of a variety of endogenous and exogenous compounds. The Golgi apparatus is concerned primarily with the packaging of material for export by the cell. The chief function of lysosomes in hepatocytes is probably in the breakdown of effete organelles into their component parts, which then can be re-utilized by the cell.

The administration of phenobarbital to young rats at a daily dose of 100 mg per kg produces liver enlargement and hepatic fine structural changes (2, 11). These changes are the same irrespective of whether equivalent doses of phenobarbital are given by intraperitoneal injection, by gavage, or by incorporation of the drug into the diet. After 10 days of such medication, the livers are approximately 1.5 times as heavy as those of controls. Histologically, the parenchymal cells are of normal size but show an increased number of mitoses compared with controls. This finding, together with the fact that the fat, protein, glycogen, and water content of these livers is the same as controls, indicates that the increase in liver size induced by phenobarbital is due to hepatic parenchymal cell hyperplasia.

By light microscopy, histologic changes are apparent after about two days' medication with phenobarbital. In each lobule, there is a decrease in the size of the peripheral zone of cells containing large glycogen lakes, together with an increased number of fat globules in central cells. These changes become somewhat more pronounced as medication is continued, but even after treatment for three weeks there is always a small peripheral zone of cells with apparently normal glycogen lakes. After about a week of medication, a few hepatocytes contain characteristic eosinophilic inclusions in their cytoplasm, up to 6μ in diameter.

Electron microscopy reveals striking fine structural abnormalities in the hepatocytes of rats treated with phenobarbital (2, 11,26) (Fig. 2). After treatment for 24 hours, central cells in all lobules show an increased amount of smooth endoplasmic reticulum. Some mitochondria in these cells show dense, irregularly shaped zones within their matrix, which appear to displace the cristae. These characteristic changes of an increased amount of smooth endoplasmic reticulum together with mitochondrial abnormalities become more pronounced and affect cells further from the center of the lobule as treatment is prolonged, reaching a maximum at about 10 days. In addition, by 10 days, there are more microbodies and fewer mitochondria per unit area (2). This observation raises the possibility of a relationship between mitochondria and microbodies, but we have no additional information to add to this longstanding contentious point (28).

An increased number of lipid droplets are seen in central hepatocytes following treatment with phenobarbital for two or more days. By 10 days, a few of the cells in which there is marked proliferation of smooth endoplasmic reticulum also contain typical "myelin figures" (Fig. 3). Some of these are up to 6μ in diameter, and as noted above, can be seen by light microscopy as eosinophilic cytoplasmic inclusions. Their fine structure is interesting, in that they consist of multiple lamellae of concentric paired membranes, with up to 80 paired membranes in any one whorl. Within the core of the whorl, there are various inclusions such as mitochondria, smooth endoplasmic reticulum, glycogen particles and lipid. The concentric paired membranes are for the most part

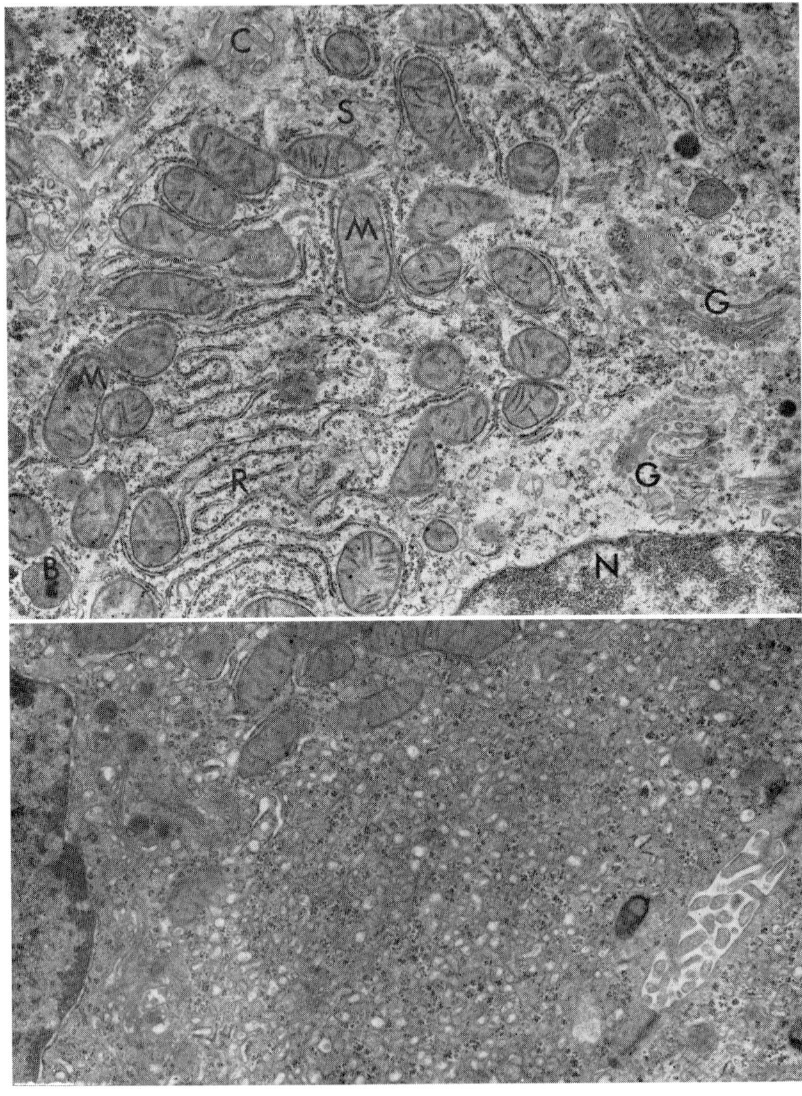

Figure 1. Control. Portion of an hepatocyte from control rat liver. N, nucleus. R, rough endoplasmic reticulum. S, smooth endoplasmic reticulum. G, Golgi apparatus. M. mitochondria. B, microbody. C, bile canaliculus. X 16,000.

Figure 2. Phenobarbital. Portions of two hepatocytes from rat liver following medication with phenobarbital, 100 mg/kg/day, for 2 days. There is a great increase in the amount of smooth endoplasmic reticulum. Note that the bile canaliculus appears normal, with no evidence of cholestasis. X 16,000.

smooth, though peripheral laminations are frequently seen to be in continuity with cisternae of rough endoplasmic reticulum.

Similar proliferation of smooth endoplasmic reticulum occurs in the livers of a variety of other animals following treatment with phenobarbital (17, 25).

Another drug which causes somewhat similar alterations in rat liver is the anticonvulsant thiohydantoin compound, Bax 422Z, which is 3-allyl-5-isobutyl-2-

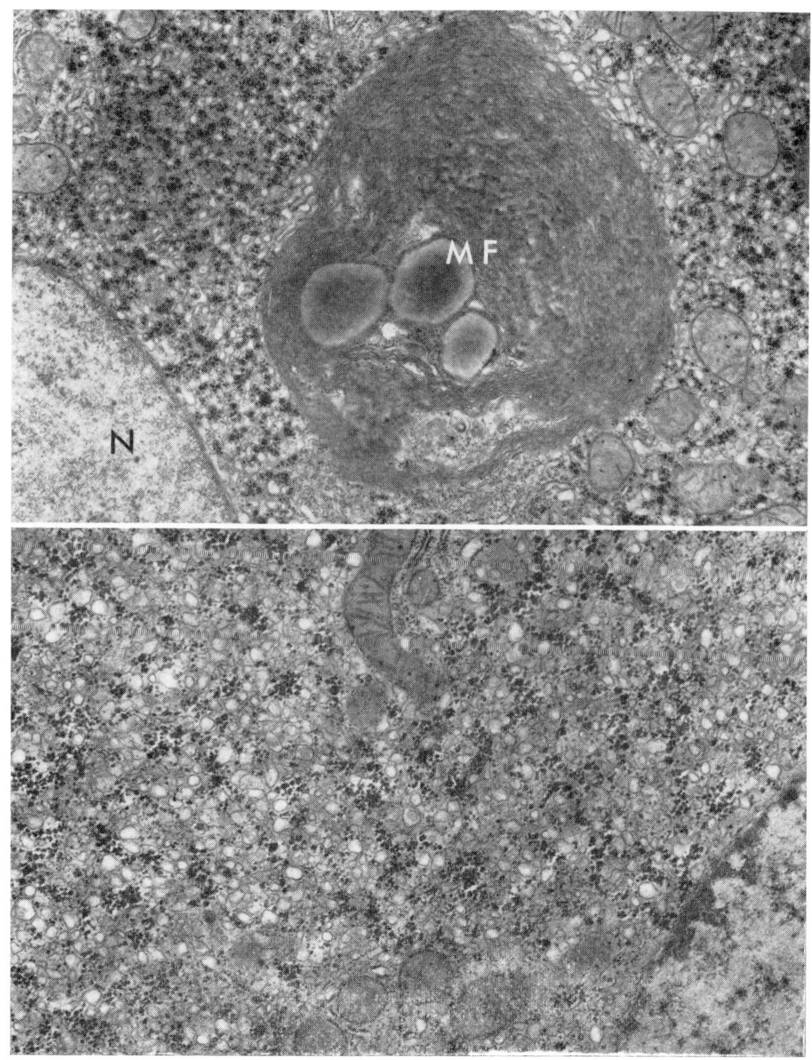

Figure 3. Phenobarbital. Part of an hepatocyte from rat liver following medication with phenobarbital, 100 mg/kg/day, for 10 days. A "myelin figure" is shown, amidst proliferated smooth endoplasmic reticulum. N, nucleus. MF, myelin figure. X 14,000.

Figure 4. 3-allyl-5-isobutyl-2-thiohydantoin (Bax 422Z). Part of an hepatocyte from rat liver following medication with high doses of Bax 422Z, 0.5%w/w in diet, for 5 days. There is a great increase in the amount of smooth endoplasmic reticulum, of similar appearance to that seen with pharmacological doses of phenobarbital. X 25,000.

thiohydantoin (9, 10). When administered to rats by incorporation into the diet at the high concentration of 0.5% w/w, this compound causes greater liver enlargement than phenobarbital, with the livers being twice normal weight after medication for 14 days. In this case, however, the individual hepatocytes have an average diameter of 46μ, twice that of controls, and there is a complete lack of mitotic activity. Taken with the findings that glycogen, protein, fat and water contents are normal in these medicated livers, the observations show that in this instance, the hepatomegaly is due to hypertrophy of individual cells, rather than to hyperplasia as is the case with phenobarbital (10).

The histological and fine structural cytoplasmic changes induced in hepatocytes by Bax 422Z are basically of the same type as those seen following phenobarbital administration (10). In particular, there is a striking increase in the amount of smooth endoplasmic reticulum (Fig. 4), seen first after medication for two days in central cells, which then involves more cells nearer the periphery of the lobule as treatment is continued. This and the other fine structural changes reach a maximum after 14 days' treatment, and even after 28 days there is a zone of apparently normal hepatocytes at the periphery of the lobule. Many more "myelin figures" are seen in livers from rats treated with Bax 422Z than with phenobarbital (Figs. 5 and 7). In addition, more autophagic vacuoles are present following medication with Bax 422Z for five days or longer (Fig. 6). These findings suggest that the hepatocytes are being more severely stressed by this dose of Bax 422Z than by the doses of phenobarbital which we have used. It should be noted, however, that even after 18 months of continuous medication with these high doses of Bax 422Z, there is no evidence of hepatic necrosis, biliary proliferation, hyperplasia or malignancy.

The fact that the histological and fine structural changes induced by phenobarbital and Bax 422Z show localization within hepatic lobules, involving central cells at first, and then cells further from central veins, is a reflection of parenchymal cell heterogeneity within hepatic lobules, and is additional evidence of regionalization of cell function within the lobule (20).

Now, it is important to point out that the proliferation of smooth endoplasmic reticulum which occurs following medication with relatively non-toxic drugs such as phenobarbital or Bax 422Z is also seen following the administration of a wide variety of compounds known to be toxic to the liver, including dichlorodiphenyltrichloroethane (22), ethionine (14, 30), dimethylaminoazobenzene derivatives (18, 24), N-2-fluorenyldiacetamide (19), and α-naphthylisothiocyanate (29). However, in addition these toxic and in some cases carcinogenic substances cause disruptive changes in hepatocytes, including swelling of the rough endoplasmic cisternae, severe mitochondrial disorganization, and frank necrosis in some cases.

The significance of the occasional "myelin figures" seen in a few liver cells following phenobarbital administration, and more commonly with Bax 422Z, is not clear. The possibility that they have some functional role in detoxication of noxious substances cannot be ruled out (10). These myelin figures have been shown to contain relatively non-specific nucleoside phosphatases (13). However, similar myeloid whorls produced in liver cells following the administration of triparanol do not show evidence of such enzyme activity (16). The fact that myelin figures do not develop until medication has been continued for seven to ten days, during which time there has been marked proliferation of smooth endoplasmic reticulum going on continuously, suggests that they may well represent foci of degenerating membranes (2). If this is so, they are a particular form of focal cytoplasmic degradation

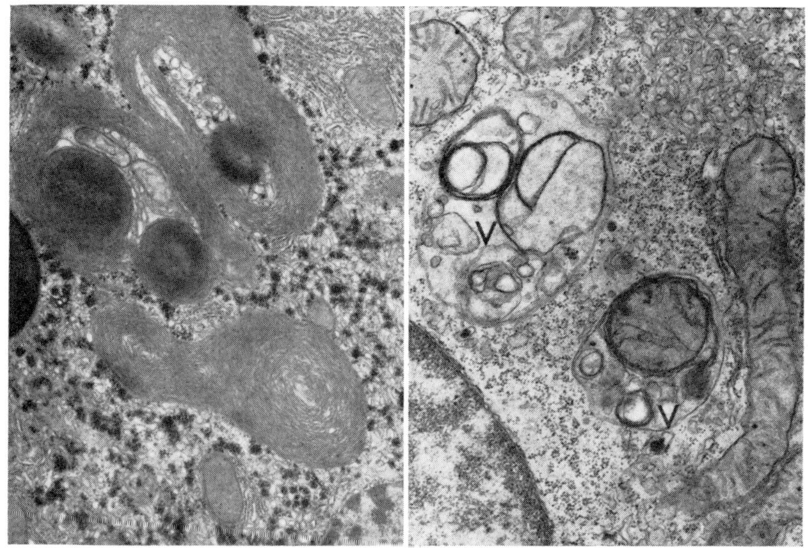

Figure 5. Bax 422Z. Portion of an hepatocyte from rat liver following high doses of Bax 422Z for 7 days. Complex myelin figure formation is seen. X 12,000.

Figure 6. Bax 422Z. Portion of an hepatocyte from rat liver following high doses of Bax 422Z for 5 days. Autophagic vacuoles (V) are prominent. X 17,000.

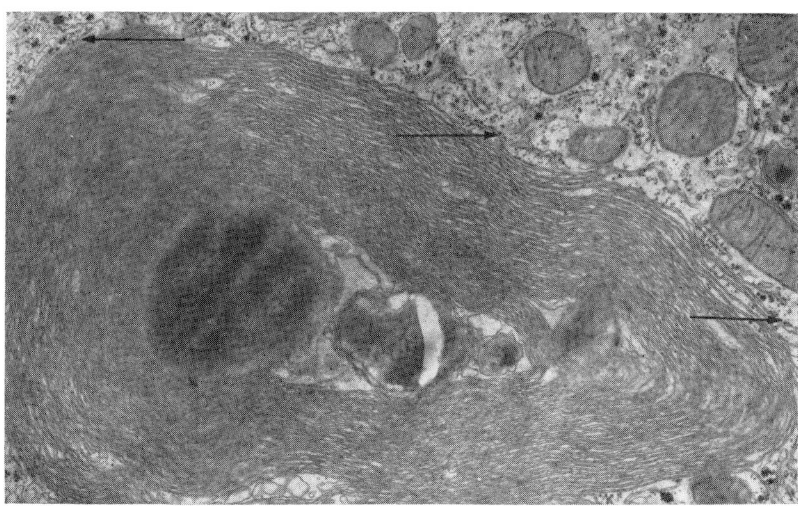

Figure 7. Bax 422Z. A myelin figure, showing the concentric array of parallel smooth membranes, and points of continuity with rough endoplasmic reticulum at the periphery (**arrows**). X 13,000.

(15), of which autophagic vacuoles are another.

It has been shown by several workers that the administration of a variety of drugs to many species of animals including rats, mice, guinea pigs, dogs, rabbits, cats and to man induces an increased tolerance to the action not only of the particular drug administered, but also to a whole group of different compounds which share the property of being hydroxylated by liver microsomal enzymes in the presence of reduced triphosphopyridine nucleotide (TPNH) (3, 21). One way in which such an increased tolerance can be demonstrated is by measurement of the "hexobarbital sleeping time." Rats given a standard dose of hexobarbital by intra-peritoneal injection loose their righting reflex for a particular time, and this sleeping time has been found to give a good measure of the activity of the drug-metabolizing enzyme system of the liver (8). Following treatment with phenobarbital or other barbiturates, and a number of other unrelated compounds, rats become resistant to the hexobarbital, as shown by much shorter sleeping times. An interesting sidelight to this matter is the finding that sleeping times are significantly decreased when rats are kept in rooms which have been sprayed with insecticides such as chlordane (8). Other experiments have shown that the chronic administration of drugs such as phenylbutazone, tolbutamide, diphenhydramine and hexobarbital to dogs causes substantial depression of the respective plasma levels of these compounds, reflecting increased activity of drug-metabolizing enzymes (3).

Two particular microsomal enzyme systems known to be involved in such drug-hydroxylating reactions are TPNH-cytochrome c reductase and carbon monoxide (CO) binding pigment. Recently these enzymes have been shown to be present specifically in the smooth microsomal liver fraction, and to exhibit increased activity following *in vivo* medication with phenobarbital (21). Clearly, there are many other enzymes involved in drug metabolizing reactions (4), and a great deal of work in this area is going on at present.

Both the proliferation of smooth endoplasmic reticulum and the associated increase in hydroxylating enzymes induced by phenobarbital decreases markedly about three days after stopping medication (27). Moreover, the induction of these changes can be prevented by administration of either actinomycin D which inhibits DNA-dependent RNA synthesis, or puromycin which inhibits protein synthesis (5, 21). These changes induced by drugs such as phenobarbital involve the synthesis of a multienzyme system, and it is believed that the proliferating membranes of the smooth endoplasmic reticulum, together with the enzymes involved, are both produced by the rough endoplasmic reticulum.

REFERENCES

1. Bernhard, W., Gautier, A., and Rouiller, C.: Le notion de "microsomes" et le problème de la basophilie cytoplasmique. Étude critique et experimentelle. Arch. Anat. Micro. Morph. Exp., *43*:236-275, 1954.
2. Burger, P. C., and Herdson, P. B.: Phenobarbital-induced fine structural changes in rat liver. Amer. J. Path., *48*:793-809, 1966.
3. Burns, J. J.: Implications of enzyme induction for drug therapy. Amer. J. Med., *37*:327-331, 1964.
4. Burns, J. J., Conney, A. H., and Koster, R.: Stimulatory effect of chronic drug administration on drug-metabolizing enzymes in liver microsomes. Ann. N. Y. Acad. Sci., *104*:881-893, 1963.
5. Conney, A. H., and Gilman, A. G.: Puromycin

inhibition of enzyme induction by 3-methylcholanthrene and phenobarbital. J. Biol. Chem., *238:*3682-3685, 1963.

6. Ernster, L., Siekevitz, P., and Palade, G. E.: Enzyme-structure relationships in the endoplasmic reticulum of rat liver. A morphological and biochemical study. J. Cell. Biol., *15:*541-562, 1962.
7. Fawcett, D. W.: Observations on the cytology and electron microscopy of hepatic cells. J. Nat. Cancer Inst., *15* (suppl.) : 1475-1502, 1955.
8. Fouts, J. R.: Factors influencing the metabolism of drugs in liver microsomes. Ann. N.Y. Acad. Sci., *104:*875-880, 1963.
9. Gesler, R. M., Lints, C. E., and Swinyard, E. Q.: Pharmacology of some substituted 2-thiohydantoins with particular reference to anticonvulsant properties. Toxic. Appl. Pharmacol., *3:* 107-121, 1961.
10. Herdson, P. B., Garvin, P. J., and Jennings, R. B., Reversible biological and fine structural changes produced in rat liver by a thiohydantoin compound. Lab. Invest., *13:*1014-1031, 1964.
11. Herdson, P. B., Garvin, P. J., and Jennings, R. B.: Fine structural changes in rat liver induced by phenobarbital. Lab. Invest., *13:*1032-1037, 1964.
12. Herdson, P. B., Garvin, P. J., and Jennings, R. B.: Fine structural changes produced in rat liver by partial starvation. Amer. J. Path., *45:* 157-181, 1964.
13. Herdson, P. B., and Kaltenbach, J. P.: Electron microscope studies on enzyme activity and the isolation of thiohydantoin-induced myelin figures in rat liver. J. Cell Biol., *25:*485-493, 1965.
14. Herman, L., Eber, L., and Fitzgerald, P. J.: Liver cell degeneration with ethionine administration. In Breese, S. S., Jr. (ed.) : Proceedings of the Fifth International Congress for Electron Microscopy. New York, Academic Press, Inc., 1962, Vol. 2, p. VV-6.
15. Hruban, Z., Spargo, B., Swift, H., Wissler, R. W., and Kleinfeld, R. G.: Focal cytoplasmic degradation. Amer. J. Path., *42:*657-683, 1963.
16. Hruban, Z., Swift, H., and Slesers, A.: Effect of triparanol and diethanolamine on the fine structure of hepatocytes and pancreatic acinar cells. Lab. Invest., *14:*1652-1672, 1965.
17. Jones, A. L., and Fawcett, D. W.: Hypertrophy of the agranular endoplasmic reticulum in hamster liver induced by phenobarbital (with a review on the functions of this organelle in liver). J. Histochem. Cytochem., *14:*215-232, 1966.
18. Lafontaine, J. G., and Allard, C.: A light and electron microscope study of the morphological changes induced in rat liver cells by the azo dye 2-Me-DAB. J. Cell Biol., *22:*143-172, 1964.
19. Mikata, A., and Luse, S. A.: Ultrastructural changes in the rat liver produced by N-2-fluorenyldiacetamide. Amer. J. Path., *44:*455-479, 1964.
20. Novikoff, A. B.: Cell heterogeneity within the hepatic lobule of the rat (staining reactions). J. Histochem. Cytochem., *7:*240-244, 1959.
21. Orrenius, S., Ericsson, J. L. E., and Ernster, L.: Phenobarbital-induced synthesis of the microsomal drug-metabolizing enzyme system and its relationship to the proliferation of endoplasmic membranes. A morphological and biochemical study. J. Cell Biol., *25:*627-639, 1965.
22. Ortega, P.: Light and electron microscopy of dichlorodiphenyltrichloroethane (DDT) poisoning in the rat liver. Lab. Invest., *15:*657-679, 1966.
23. Palade, G. E., and Siekevitz, P.: Liver microsomes. An integrated morphological and biochemical study. J. Biophys. Biochem. Cytol., *2:*171-200, 1956.
24. Porter, K. R., and Bruni, C.: An electron microscope study of the early effects of 3'-Me-DAB on rat liver cells. Cancer Res., *19:*997-1009, 1959.
25. Remmer, H., and Merker, H. J.: Drug-induced changes in the liver endoplasmic reticulum: association with drug-metabolizing enzymes. Science, *142:*1657-1658, 1963.
26. Remmer, H., and Merker, H. J.: Morphological changes in the endoplasmic reticulum of the liver cells with enzyme induction after pretreatment with several drugs. In "Drugs and Enzymes," Proceedings of the Second International Pharmacological Meeting. Oxford, Pergamon Press, 1965, 299-307.
27. Remmer, H., and Merker, H. J.: Effect of drugs on the formation of smooth endoplasmic reticulum and drug-metabolizing enzymes. Ann. N. Y. Acad. Sci., *123:*79-97, 1965.
28. Rouiller, C., and Bernhard, W.: "Microbodies" and the problem of mitochondrial regeneration in liver cells. J. Biophys. Biochem. Cytol., *2:*355-360, 1956.
29. Steiner, J. W., and Baglio, C. M.: Electron microscopy of the cytoplasm of parenchymal liver cells in α-naphthylisothiocyanate-induced cirrhosis. Lab. Invest., *12:*765-790, 1963.
30. Wood, R. L.: The fine structure of hepatic cells in chronic ethionine poisoning and during recovery. Amer. J. Path., *46:*307-330, 1965.

Chapter 41

Hepatic Manifestations of Toxic and Therapeutic Agents

GEOFFREY KENT, M.D., PH.D. and EMILIO ORFEI, M.D.

Toxic and therapeutic agents may produce a variety of hepatic injuries which range from mild biochemical changes to submassive and massive necrosis (1, 2). The injuries may be classified according to postulated mechanisms (3, 4), pharmacologic properties of injurious agents or the type of injury produced. Since their pathogenesis is not well understood, they will be discussed here on the basis of morphologic manifestations.

The histologic features encountered are readily separated into well defined groups. Toxic agents produce zonal hepatocellular injuries, while therapeutic agents give rise to cholestasis without hepatocellular damage (5) or to cellular injuries resembling viral hepatitis (Table 1).

TABLE I — REACTIONS PRODUCED BY TOXIC AND THERAPEUTIC AGENTS

Agent	*Type of Reaction*
Toxic	Zonal hepatocellular injury (toxic hepatitis)
Therapeutic	Cholestasis without hepatocellular injury
	Viral hepatitis-like hepatocellular injury

Toxic Injury

Under this heading are included injuries resulting mainly from accidental exposure to potent cellular toxins, such as carbon tetrachloride, phosphorus, ferrous sulphate and tannic acid (Table II). The injuries have been designated toxic hepatitis (1); they are dose related, appear after a short latent period, and can be reproduced in laboratory animals. The most characteristic morphologic features are a zonal distribution of the hepatocellular damage, prominence of fatty change and paucity of inflammatory cells (1, 6). Depending on the agent involved, the zonal changes may be centrolobular or periportal in distribution. In the case of carbon tetrachloride, the centrolobular cells undergo necrosis, or fatty and hydropic change, while midzonal and periportal cells are not altered (Fig. 1). Peripor-

TABLE II — AGENTS CAUSING TOXIC HEPATITIS

carbon tetrachloride
orthodichlorobenzene
chloroform
mushroom toxin
pesticides
phosphorus
ferrous sulphate
tannic acid
mercaptopurine

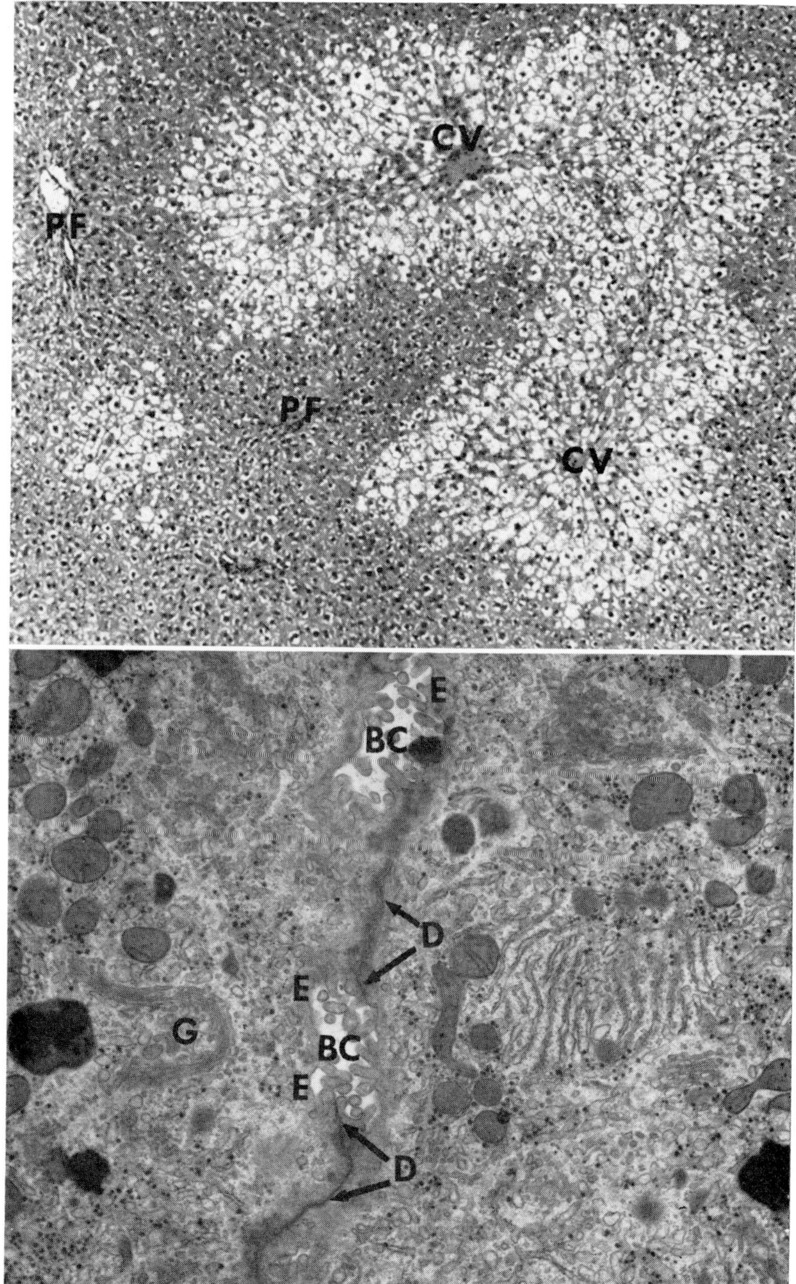

Figure 1. Carbon tetrachloride injury (rat). The injury is strictly zonal. Note hydropic and fatty changes about central veins (CV). The parenchyma about the portal fields (PF) is unaffected. X 100.

Figure 2. Bile secretory apparatus (biopsy human liver) showing Golgi apparatus (G), ectoplasm (E), desmosomes (D) and bile canaliculi (BC) almost filled with microvilli. X 12,000.

tal zonal necrosis is characteristically seen in injuries produced by phosphorus or ferrous sulphate.

Although in most cases of toxic hepatitis exposure to injurious agents is accidental, the lesion may also be observed following administration of cytotoxic agents, such as mercaptopurine (1, 7).

Injury by Therapeutic Agents

In the large majority of cases, injuries due to drugs are unpredictable and occur on the basis of individual susceptibility. They may be separated into two major morphologic variants—cholestatic and hepatitic reactions (Table III), the former being by far the most common. The two variants correlate well with clinical and biochemical findings on the one hand and with certain types of drugs on the other. However, there are numerous exceptions, and a sharp dividing line between cholestatic and hepatocellular changes cannot be drawn. Two other histologic variants (Table III), fine droplet steatosis and granulomatous disease, occur much less frequently; they are, however, distinctive enough to warrant separate listing.

TABLE III — HISTOLOGIC VARIANTS IN DRUG INDUCED HEPATIC DISEASE

Major variants
Cholestatic reaction
A. Cholestasis, uncomplicated
B. Cholestasis with inflammatory cell reaction
Viral hepatitis-like reaction
Rare variants
Fine droplet steatosis
Granulomatous reaction

CHOLESTATIC REACTIONS

According to the presence or absence of an inflammatory reaction in the liver, intrahepatic cholestasis due to drug injuries may be divided into two forms—pure or uncomplicated cholestasis and cholestasis associated with an inflammatory reaction (1, 2). The two forms of cholestasis appear to have different mechanisms.

UNCOMPLICATED CHOLESTASIS

This morphologic variant has also been named "pure" or "steroid-type" cholestasis (2). Bile stasis is the only change discernible by light microscopy. Thus, the hepatocytes appear normal, and the portal tracts contain only few, if any inflammatory cells. Bile pigment is seen mainly in dilated bile canaliculi and in hepatocytes and is most pronounced in centrolobular zones. Electron microscopy reveals alterations in the area of the bile secretory apparatus (8). The latter consists of bile canaliculi, desmosomes, ectoplasm and the Golgi apparatus (Fig. 2). Also part of the bile secretory apparatus, in a wider sense, is the smooth endoplasmic reticulum. In cholestasis, the ectoplasm is widened, the bile canaliculi are dilated and the microvilli are ballooned (Fig. 3) or attenuated (Fig. 4). Electron dense material, presumably bile constituents, are found in bile canaliculi and in liver cells (Fig. 5). The described changes, however, are not specific and are also seen in extrahepatic obstruction; they are thus probably the result rather than the cause of cholestasis.

The agents causing uncomplicated cholestasis are C 17 alkyl-substituted compounds of testosterone, such as methyl testosterone, norethandrolone (Nilevar), and methandrostenolone (Table IV). Its pathogenesis will be discussed under a separate heading.

Table IV – Therapeutic Agents and Injuries Produced

Uncomplicated Cholestasis	methyl testosterone methandrostenolone	norethandrolone norethindrone
Cholestasis with Inflammatory Reaction	chlorpromazine tolbutamide urethane chlorpropamide phenyl butazone carbasone aminosalicylic acid	mepazine methimazol isoniazid arsphenamide thiouracil erythromycin estolate sulfa drugs
Hepatitic Reaction	pheniprazine isocarboxazid pyrazinamide phenurone trimethadione halothane aminosalicylic acid	iproniazid metahexamide zoxazolamine dilantin isonicotinic acid methoxyflurane sulfa drugs

Cholestasis with Inflammatory Cell Reaction

This variant of cholestasis is characterized by the presence of a significant inflammatory reaction. Features suggesting hypersensitivity are often conspicuous, and the condition has been named sensitivity-type cholestasis (2). Prominent among the agents causing this disturbance are sulfonylurea derivatives such as phenothiazines, oral antidiabetics and thiazide diuretics (Table IV). Histologically, one sees centrolobular bile stasis and a prominent cellular infiltrate in sinusoids and portal fields (Fig. 6). The cells involved are lymphocytes and histiocytes and to a lesser degree segmented leukocytes and eosinophils. The heptatocytes show some variation in size and staining properties, but the changes are not severe and are readily distinguished from those in the following group. The predominance of a mononuclear cell infiltrate and presence of eosinophils are helpful features in differentiating this injury from extrahepatic cholestasis.

HEPATITIC REACTIONS

The hepatitic reaction is characterized by a conspicuous hepatocellular injury which resembles viral rather than toxic hepatitis (1). Complications due to drugs in this group occur much less frequently than in the previous group. However, when they do occur, they often manifest severe hepatocellular damage which may proceed to massive necrosis and lead to death in hepatic coma. The best known examples of drugs belonging to this group are mono-amino oxidase inhibitors and muscle relaxants. Other agents in this group are halothane, methoxyflurane and sulfa drugs (Table IV). Histologically, the milder lesions reveal individual cell or spotty necrosis, focal necrosis and Councilman bodies (Fig. 7). Associated with these features are a mononuclear cell infiltrate in sinusoids and portal fields and a strong mesenchymal reaction. The more severe lesions of submassive and massive necrosis are seen almost exclusively in autopsy specimens. In these instances, one notes a disappearance of liver cells

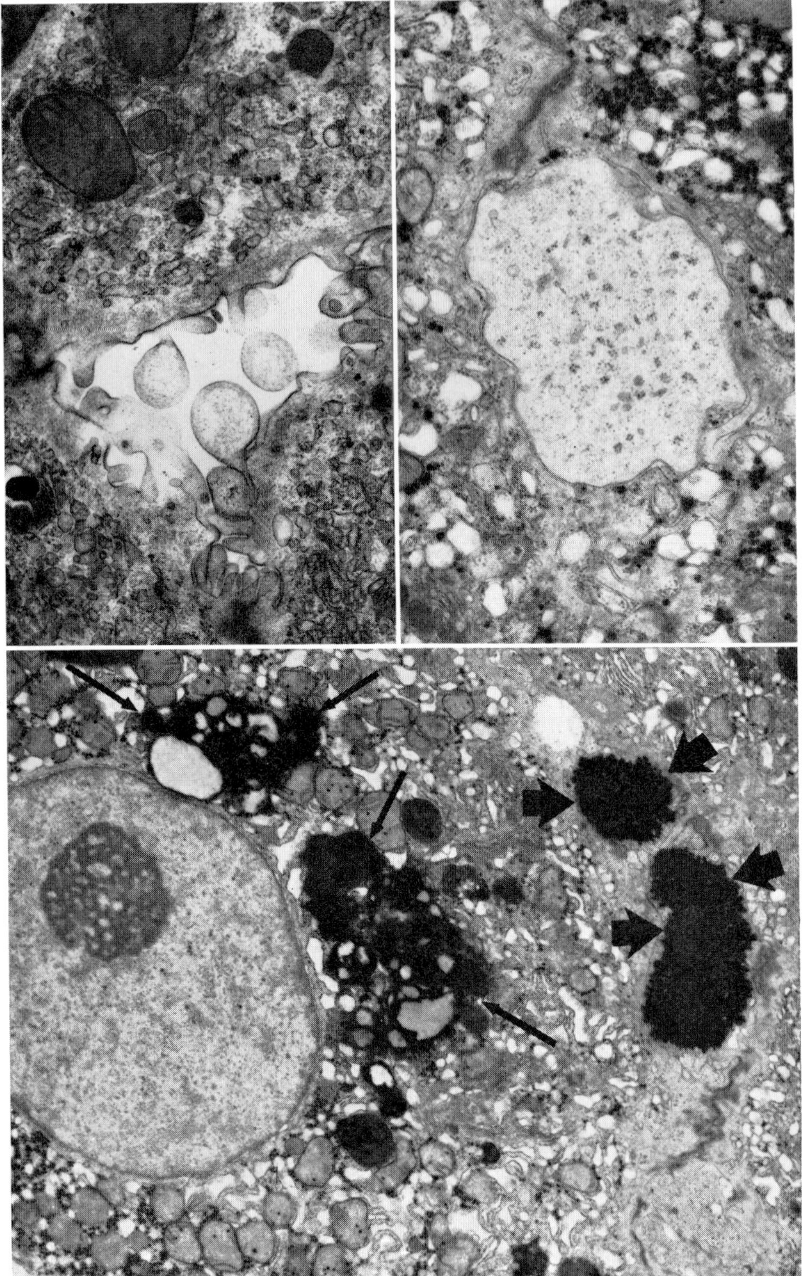

Figure 3. Bile canaliculus in cholestasis (liver biopsy). There is slight dilatation of the bile canaliculus and balooning of microvilli. X 19,000.

Figure 4. Bile canaliculus in cholestasis (liver biopsy). Note dilatation of bile canaliculus and attenuation of microvilli. X 18,000.

Figure 5. Cholestasis (liver biopsy). Electron dense material is present in bile canaliculi (short heavy arrows). Similar material associated with lipid is seen within the cytoplasm (**large slender arrows**). X 4,500.

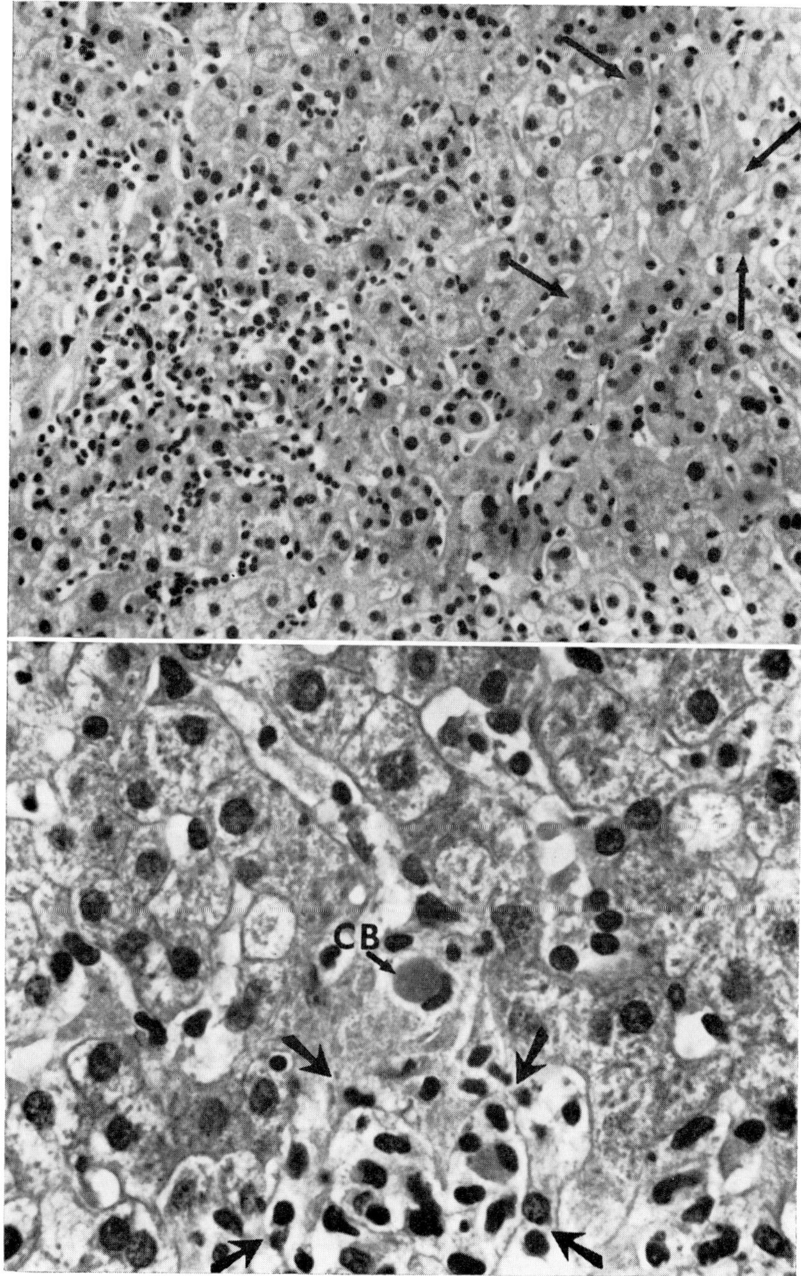

Figure 6. Cholestasis in chlorpromazine jaundice (liver biopsy). There is a heavy cellular infiltrate in portal fields and centrolobular bile stasis (arrows). The liver cells show little alteration. A sinusoidal infiltrate is also evident, but is less conspicuous. X 200.

Figure 7. Iproniazid hepatitis (liver biopsy). The histologic picture is that of viral hepatitis. Note Councilman body (CB) and area of focal necrosis (**arrows**), a mononuclear cell infiltrate and variations in size and staining—properties of cells. X 400.

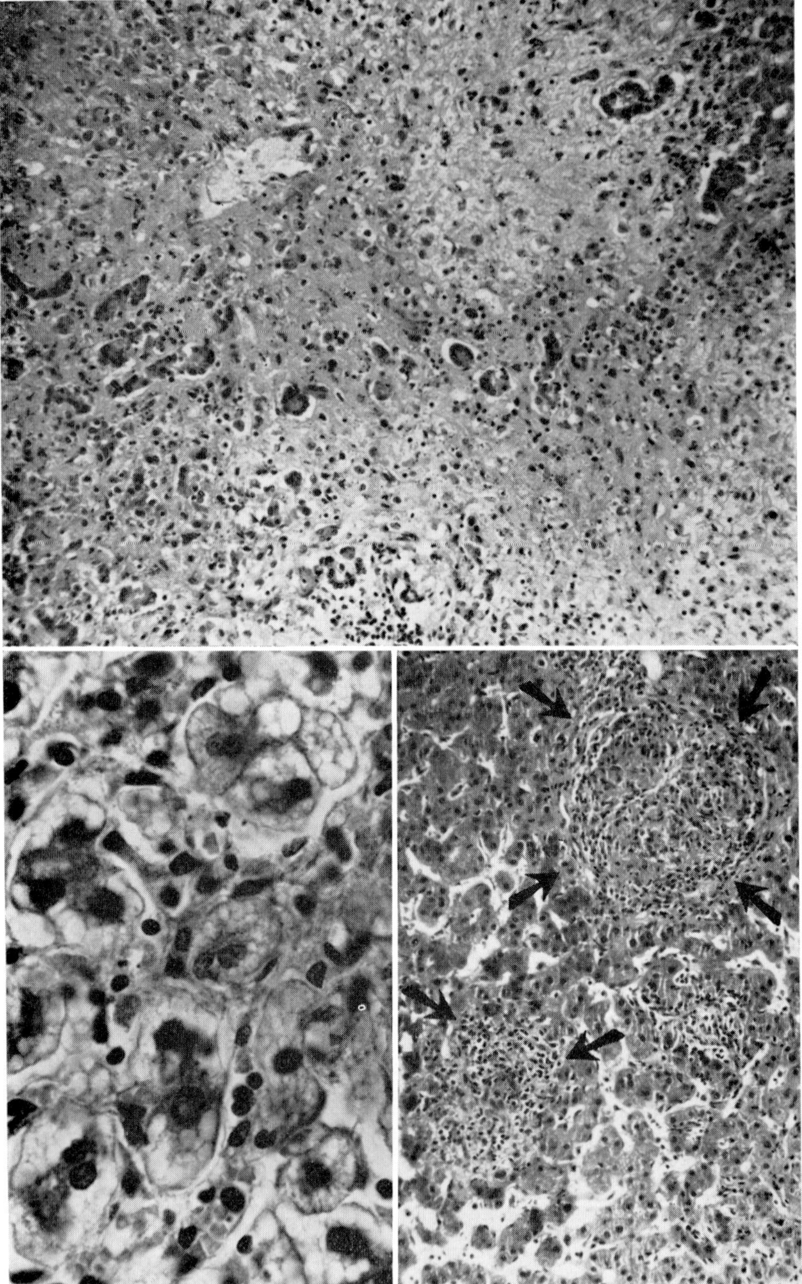

Figure 8. Massive necrosis in halothane hepatitis (autopsy). Most of the liver cells have disappeared. There is a moderate cellular infiltrate. Duct-like structures are conspicuous in periportal areas. X 100.

Figure 9. Tetracycline injury (liver biopsy). The liver cells contain fine fat droplets and the nucleus remains centrally placed. X 200.

Figure 10. Granulomatous hepatitis following sulfa drug therapy (liver biopsy). The inflammatory cell foci resemble epithelioid cell tubercles as seen in tuberculosis or sarcoidosis. X 100.

and increased number of bile ducts and ductules about portal fields (Fig. 8). Residual islands of parenchyma often show coagulation necrosis characterized by loss of nuclei and fusion of cytoplasm.

RARE MORPHOLOGIC VARIANTS

Fine Droplet Steatosis

A prime example of a serious, though rare, toxic drug reaction involving the liver is that following the intravenous administration of large doses of tetracycline. The lesion is particularly prone to occur in pregnant women and resembles the often fatal fatty liver of pregnancy (9, 10). The histological picture is characteristic, showing a fine droplet fatty change without displacement of the nucleus (Fig. 9). Although hepatocellular necrosis is not a feature, the patients are desperately sick and survival is uncommon.

Granuloma Formation

By contrast with fine droplet steatosis which appears to be a toxic reaction, granuloma formation occurs on an immunologic basis. The reaction has been observed following the use of sulfonylurea derivatives, phenyl butazone, sulfa drugs, penicillin and halothane (1,11, 12). The granulomata consist of epithelioid cell tubercles (Fig. 10) which may or may not contain Langhans type giant cells. They are located predominantly about portal fields. According to recent reports, such granulomata may have a short life span and tend to disappear rapidly which may account for the small number of reported cases.

Mechanisms

The nature of the injuries leading to the cholestatic and hepatitic reactions is still poorly understood. In the case of uncomplicated or "steroid"-type cholestasis, current knowledge favors the hepatocyte as the target organ. Morphologically, the injury appears restricted to the area of the bile secretory apparatus. Although the exact mechanism is not known, the drug is believed to interfere with the secretion of biliary constituents which are required to maintain bile flow. Of these, bile acids are the prime suspects. Patients receiving these drugs consistently show some alteration of the bile secretory apparatus (1) and impaired excretion of exogenous dyes. Similar findings have been observed in laboratory animals (13-16). The observed changes are dose dependent and hence are expressions of toxicity. The appearance of cholestasis and jaundice, on the other hand, is more unpredictable, and may depend upon some added factor.

Jaundice has also been observed following the use of oral contraceptive agents and may have a similar pathogenesis. Its incidence is exceedingly low, and a proportion of cases occurs in women who give a history of cholestatic jaundice of pregnancy (9). The reported cases, furthermore, are prevalent in certain geographic regions suggesting a genetic susceptibility.

By contrast with the "steroid"-type cholestasis in which evidence for an immune reaction is lacking, the cholestasis with an inflammatory component and the viral-like hepatitic reaction may often be suspected to be the result of an immune injury. Foremost examples are the injuries produced by chlorpromazine, para-aminosalicylic acid, sulfa drugs and halothane. Patients with these reactions often show abundant eosinophils in biopsy specimens and systemic manifestations of hypersensitivity, such as fever, skin rash, arthralgia and eosinophilia. They may display granulomas in biopsy specimens or recurrence of hepatic dysfunction upon re-exposure to small doses of the drug. The latter may be associated with the shortening of the latent period. Although the role of halothane as a cause of liver injury has been questioned for some time, recent information strongly suggests that this agent can have hepatotoxic effects (17-19), and that the injury is the result of a hypersensitivity reaction. In support of the last suggestion are the appearance of systemic manifestations, of granulomas in the liver (12, 20) and of an increased incidence and shortened latent period following a second exposure.

Whether or not hypersensitivity reactions, when in evidence, are the only underlying mechanism, is not certain. Some of the drugs in this category have such a high incidence of hepatic dysfunction that a role other than sensitivity must be suspected. The enzyme inducing property of the drug may be one such factor which may account for mild degrees of hepatic dysfunction and lead to overt jaundice in the presence of a hypersensitivity reaction.

REFERENCES

1. Popper, H., Rubin, E., Gardiol, D., Schaffner, F., and Paronetto, F.: Drug-induced liver disease. Arch. Intern. Med., *115:*128-136, 1965.
2. Sherlock, S.: Diseases of the Liver and Biliary System. Philadelphia, F. A. Davis Co., 1968.
3. Zimmerman, H.: Toxic hepatopathy. Am. J. Gastroent., *49:*39-56, 1968.
4. Schmid, M.: Hepatotoxische Reaktionen durch Medikamente. Helvetica Medica Acta Suppl., *47:*15-23, 1967.
5. Schaffner, F.: Diagnosis of drug-induced hepatic damage. J.A.M.A., *191:*466-469, 1965.
6. Kent, G., Volini, F. I., Minick, O. T., Orfei, E., and de la Huerga, J.: Effect of iron loading upon the formation of collagen in the hepatic injury induced by carbon tetrachloride. Am. J. Path., *45:*129-155, 1964.
7. Shorey, J., Schenker, S., Suki, W. N., and Combes, B.: Hepatotoxicity of mercaptopurine. Arch. Intern. Med., *122:*54-58, 1968.
8. Popper, H.: Cholestasis. Ann. Rev. Med., *19:* 39-56, 1968.
9. Sherlock, S.: Jaundice in pregnancy. Brit. Med. Bull., *24:*39-43, 1968.
10. Norman, T., Schultz, J., and Hoke, R.: Fatal liver disease following the administration of tetracycline. So. Med. J., *57:*1038-1042, 1964.
11. Espiritu, C., Kim, T., and Levine, R.: Granulomatous hepatitis associated with sulfadimethoxine hypersensitivity. J.A.M.A., *202:*985-988, 1967.
12. Rodriguez, M., Paronetto, F., Schaffner, F., and Popper, H.: Antimitochondrial antibodies in jaundice following drug administration. J.A.M.A., *208:*148-150, 1969.
13. Schaffner, R., and Kniffen, J. C.: Electron microscopy as related to hepatotoxicity. Ann. N. Y. Acad. Sci., *104:847,* 1963.
14. Heaney, R. B., and Whedon, G. D.: Impairment of hepatic bromsulphalein clearance by two 17-substituted testosterones. J. Lab. Clin. Med., *52:*169, 1958.
15. Carmichael, R. H., Wilson C., and Martz, B. L. Effect of anabolic steroids on liver function tests in rabbits. Prox. Soc. Exp. Biol. Med., *113:* 1006, 1963.
16. Arias, I. M., *et al.:* Effect of 17-ethyl-19 nortestosterone and icterogenin on hepatic metabolism of bilirubin in normal and Gunn rats. J. Clin. Invest., *40:*1023, 1961.
17. Trey, C., Lipworth, L., Chalmers, T. C., Davidson, C. S., Gottlieb, L. S., Popper, H., and Saunders, S. J.: Fulminant hepatic failure. New Eng. J. Med., *279:*798-801, 1968.
18. Klatskin, G., and Kimberg, D. V.: Recurrent hepatitis attributable to halothane sensitization in an anesthetist. New Eng. J. Med., *280:* 515-522, 1969.
19. Combes, B.: Halothane-induced liver damage — an entity. Editorial, New. Eng. J. Med., *280:* 558-559, 1969.
20. Dordal, E., and Glagov, S.: Granulomatous hepatitis due to halothane anesthesia. (In preparation.)

Chapter 42

The Pneumoconioses: Clinical Considerations

JOHN E. KASIK, M.D., PH.D.

Pneumoconiosis has been defined ". . . as a diagnosable disease produced by the inhalation of dust, dust being understood to be particulate matter in the solid phase, excluding living organisms.[33] From a clinical point of view, the pneumoconioses represent a rather heterogenous group of diseases, having in common that they all primarily effect the lung and are due to the inhalation of dust. These disorders are not all of equal severity, and in some instances, inhalation of the dust results in only an asymptomatic change in the chest x-ray. Even when a patient is exposed to a potentially hazardous dust, it may have variable effects. While in a technical sense, for example, a patient may have proven silicosis, the effects of this disease in terms of his respiratory reserve and general well being may be nil and his prognosis may be excellent. As a further complication, it is well known that the occurrence of chronic obstructive pulmonary disease has been increasing. This disorder may complicate the problem of determining the etiology of the respiratory disability in a person who has been exposed to dust, who is a heavy smoker, and also lives in a region of high air pollution. In general, the symptoms of many of the pneumoconioses are similar to those of chronic bronchitis and emphysema, and both of these conditions may be the consequence of or associated with one of the pneumoconioses.

Thus, the diagnostic problem of the clinician encountering one of the pneumoconioses can be difficult, especially in patients with borderline findings or equivocal histories of exposure. The classical approach to diagnostic problems, that of obtaining a biopsy, is not always feasible in this situation, since a lung biopsy can be hazardous, especially in a dyspneic patient with small respiratory reserve. Unfortunately, other diagnostic procedures are not always helpful because they are nonspecific.

Therefore, the purpose of this paper is to outline the clinical findings in pneumoconiosis, as available to the clinician, who is evaluating patients with a history of exposure to certain particulate matter. The effects of some of the more common dusts associated with pneumoconiosis are presented in Table 1.

SILICOSIS

In 1556, Agricola, writing about the problems of mining, stated:

TABLE I — SOME COMMON PNEUMOCONIOSES

Disease	*Cause*	*Industrial Sources*	*Effect*
Stannosis	Tin oxide	Mining	Radiological change only
Baritosis	Barium sulphate	Smelting	Radiological change only
Siderosis	Iron Oxide	Welding	Radiological change only
Silicosis	Silica	Mining, pottery, grinding,etc.	Simple silicosis and massive fibrosis, Tb.
Diatomaceous Earth Pneumoconiosis	Diatomaceous earth (Kieselguhr)	Manufacturing, Mining	Simple pneumoconiosis, Massive fibrosis, Tb
Coal-workers' pneumoconiosis	Coal dust	Mining, coal trimming	Simple and massive fibrosis, Tb.
Asbestosis	Asbestos	Manufacture, lagging, etc.	Pulmonary fibrosis, pleural plaques, carcinoma and mesothelioma
Berylliosis	Beryllium compounds	Beryllium alloys, etc.	Beryllium granulomas, diffuse interstitial fibrosis, pneumothorax

Adapted from McKerrow.[43]

"The mines are very dry and the constant dust enters the blood and lungs producing the difficulty of breathing which the Greeks call asthma. When the dust is corrosive, it ulcerates the lungs and produces consumption; hence it is in the Carpathian Mountains there are women who have married seven husbands all of whom this dreadful disease has brought to an early grave."[27]

This four-hundred-year-old quotation still is an accurate description of the clinical features of silicosis.

When symptomatic, the silicotic will complain of dyspnea of variable severity, a dry cough, and fatigue.[33] Later in the course of his disease, in addition to increasingly severe dyspnea, the patient will note anorexia, weight loss, weakness, and still later the signs of cor pulmonale. In general, the symptoms of silicosis are insidious and frequently may be out of proportion to the findings of chest x-ray.

Physical findings, where present, are indistinguishable from those of chronic obstructive pulmonary disease. Diminished breath sounds, reduced chest movement, wheezes, rhonchi, crepitation, and altered chest resonance are commonly encountered, at least in the advanced silicotic.[33, 27] Clubbing is rare, but evidence of weight loss with preservation or even hypertrophy of the accessory muscles of respiration is common. When cor pulmonale has developed, the classical findings of congestive heart failure can be observed.

X-RAY

The chest x-ray has been found to be the most important diagnostic tool in silicosis. While the chest film is not diagnostic by itself, it is characteristic enough, when associated with an adequate history of exposure to silica dust, to make the diagnosis reasonably certain, especially when evidence for other diseases is lacking.[26]

X-ray changes are related to the course of the disease. Early silicosis presents on chest x-ray as numerous small discrete nodules ranging in size from just visible to several millimeters in diameter. The lesions are generalized, though occasionally they are found in one area more than in others.[26, 49] Hilar enlargement is common, and calcification of the peripheral nodules and the hilar nodes are seen (Figs. 1, 2).

As the disease progresses, there is a tendency for the nodular masses to become confluent with the development of large conglomerate masses which appear as dense radio-opaque shadows on x-ray. Cavitation may be seen in conglomerate silicosis, with or without active pulmonary tuberculosis, the latter secondary to aseptic necrosis because of a compromised blood supply. With the conglomerate form of silicosis, cystic areas and blebs form, and secondary emphysematous changes may occur, especially in the bases (Fig. 3). Pleural thickening may be seen, though this is less prominent than with asbestosis.

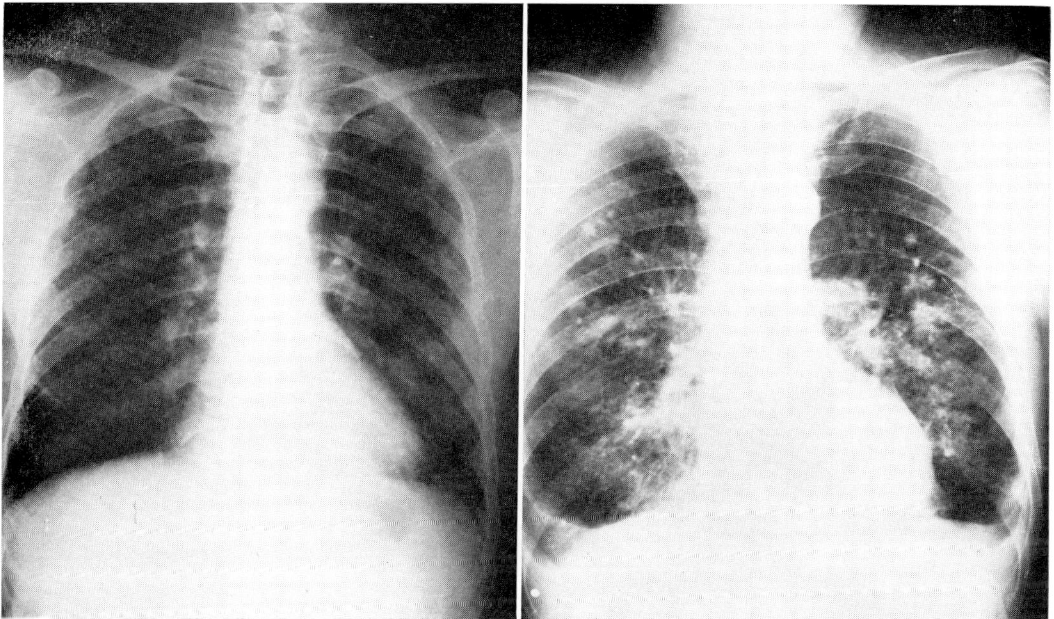

Figure 1. Nodular silicosis in a 61-year-old male with a history of foundry work.

Figure 2. Confluent silicosis with multiple calcified nodules in a 51-year-old former steel worker and miner.

Pulmonary Function

Pulmonary function changes found in silicotics are the reflection of several changes which can occur simultaneously and have opposite effects. The primary effect of silica in the lung is an intense fibrotic reaction which results in a diminished vital capacity and total lung volume, a variable effect on the residual volume, and the residual volume-total lung capacity ratio.[5,33,61] Maximum breathing capacity may be reduced, but flow rates, as expressed as timed vital capacity and maximum mid-expiratory flow rates, tend to be preserved.[54] Pulmonary compliance has been reported to be reduced as well as the diffusing capacity.[62,6] When silicosis is accompanied by secondary emphysematous changes in the lung, reductions in flow rates, as reflected in such tests as the timed vital capacity, become common.[13] Changes in blood gases are seen in far advanced silicosis and hypoxia, and hypercapnia are noted as well as the associated development of cor pulmonale, with signs, and

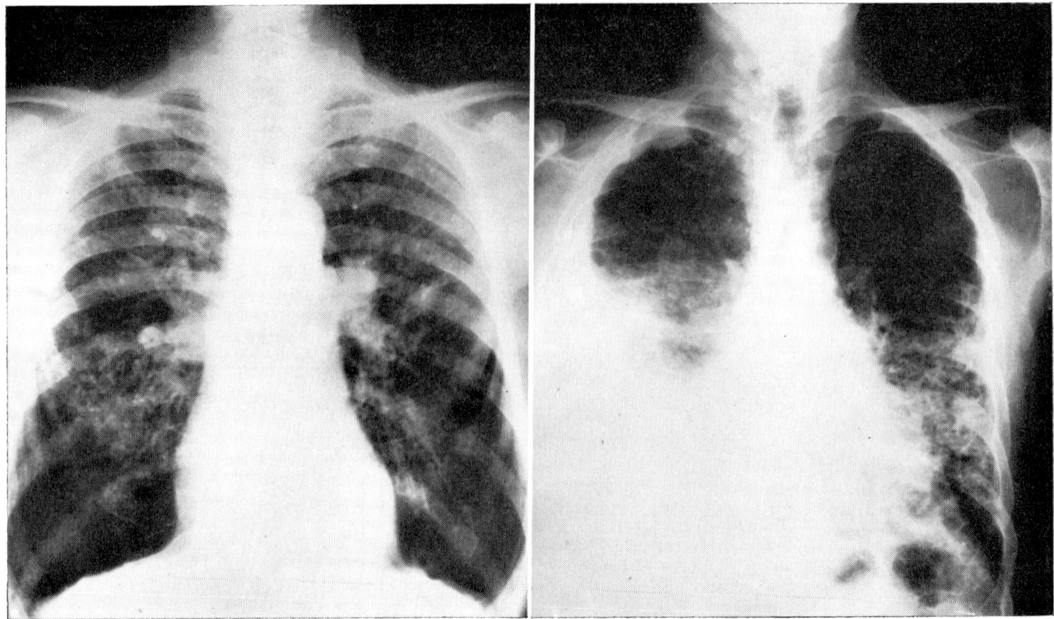

Figures 3. Silicotuberculosis with confluent peripheral masses in a 61-year-old refractory brick worker. Note emphysematous changes in the bases.

Figure 4. Asbestosis in a 51-year-old insulation worker. Note the diffuse lesions in the basilar portion of the lung, the right thickened pleural and the effusion. Subsequently, diagnosis of bronchiogenic carcinoma was made.

ECG findings compatible with that condition.[5]

It should be stated that, while pulmonary function tests are important in evaluating silicosis, they are not diagnostic of this or any other pneumoconiosis alone.

Infection

Pulmonary tuberculosis has been repeatedly demonstrated to be the frequent companion of chronic exposure to silicon dioxide.[33, 27] The clinical interrelationship of these two disorders is so close as to be at times inseperable. It is known that silicotic lungs are less resistant to tubercle bacilli than normal lungs,[23] and the presence of silicotic changes in the lung results in a smoldering, indolent infection which tends to be chronic. Expectoration of large numbers of acid-fast bacilli is infrequent in silicosis, especially when compared with the extent of the infection, and this in turn makes the diagnosis of active pulmonary tuberculosis in silicotics difficult.[46, 48]

The presence of tuberculosis also has been believed to have an unfavorable effect on the course of the disease beyond the one of a simple, superimposed infection. It has been shown experimentally that non-living products of tubercle bacilli cause an inflammatory response in silicotic lungs which accelerate the disease, causing an intense fibrotic reaction with the appearance of the conglomerate form of the diease.[24] These findings, correlated with observations on the effect of known tuberculosis in human silicosis[46] have led to the statement that the appearance of conglomerate lesions in silicosis denotes, or at least strongly suggests, superimposed active pulmonary tuberculosis.[13]

Rather surprisingly, silicosis has not been shown, either clinically or experimentally, to have an unfavorable effect on other bacterial infections. Clinical studies in silicotics have failed to associate the disease with an increased incidence of pneumonia,[4] and animal work using pneumococcal infections in mice have indicated an increased resistance.[59] These observations are rather surprising in the light of the clinical findings in patients suffering chronic obstructive pulmonary disease (e.g., emphysema or chronic obstructive bronchitis). These patients frequently have an associated, perhaps even pre-existing, chronic bronchitis and have frequent episodes of acute purulent bronchitis. Perhaps the explanation of this difference lies in the fact that while chronic obstructive pulmonary disease and silicosis have many similarities in clinical symptoms and signs, the two diseases are fundamentally different and silicosis does not predispose to bronchitis.

DIATOMACEOUS EARTH PNEUMOCONIOSIS

This form of pneumoconiosis has been recognized since 1932.[36] It is the result of inhalation of the silicious cell walls of algae deposited as sediments which are mined for various industrial purposes. The material is an amorphous silica which is sometimes treated by heating to form crystalline silica.[51] While the activity of the amorphous form as a fibrogenic material has been disputed,[51, 53, 1, 2] it appears to be clear that the crystalline material is a more serious hazard.[15]

The clinical disorder that results from the inhalation of diatomaceous earth is in many ways similar to, and in a few others different from, the features of classical silicosis. Like silicosis, the primary clinical symptoms of the disease are dyspnea, cough, easy fatigue, weight loss and anorexia. It has been stated that the physical findings are similar to silicosis and that like silicosis, clubbing of fingers is rare. In general, the clinical course of the disease appears to be more rapid than silicosis.[51]

X-RAY

The x-ray appearance of diatomacous earth penumoconiosis is different from silicosis in that the early lesion tends to be less nodular and to have a finer, more reticulated or linear pattern.[50] Where nodules occur, they are less well defined and have a less distinct outline than the silicotic nodule. In general, the early x-ray appearance of this disorder has been said to more closely resemble the pattern of fibrosis observed with berylliosis, or asbestosis.[3] Like silicosis, the pulmonary lesions of diatomaceous earth pneumoconiosis coalesce in advanced stages with dense fibrotic masses tending to appear in the upper third of the lung.[51, 50] Bleb formation and secondary emphysematous changes, especially in the bases, have been noted in the advanced stages of the disorder. Occasionally, a pneumothorax has been observed.

INFECTION

Complicating infections have been reported to occur with diatomaceous earth pneumoconioses. While not all authors agree,[51] most reports indicate an increased incidence of tuberculosis.[51, 15, 3] Similar to silicotuberculosis, an unusual clinical appearance of the infection occurs in this pneumoconiosis with slow progression, intense fibrosis and relatively infrequent expectoration of mycobacteria. Other infections have been reported in patients with this disease, both bacterial and fungal, and there is some evidence that all forms of bacterial infections of the lung are more common in this disorder.

Pulmonary functions, in general, are similar to those reported with silicosis though emphysematous changes with increased air trapping appears to be more prominent, especially in patients with coalescent lesions.[45]

COAL WORKERS PNEUMOCONIOSIS (ANTHRACOSIS, BITUMINOSIS)

Chronic inhalation of coal dust as a primary cause of pulmonary disease has been the subject of some controversy. The coincident exposure of most coal workers to silica has led some authors to conclude that silica and not coal dust is the primary malfactor.[7] This is in the face of the well recognized occurrence of pulmonary disease among coal trimmers. These men load coal on ships and are exposed to large amounts of coal dust only and yet frequently develop progressive pulmonary disease.[19]

The clinical manifestations of coal workers pneumoconiosis are similar in many respects to classical silicosis. The disorder can occur as a simple pneumoconiosis with a diffuse fibrotic pattern on chest x-ray or as progressive confluent fibrosis with large perihilar masses. The symptoms of coal workers pneumoconiosis are the classical ones of all pneumoconiosis: dyspnea and cough. The sputum frequently contains large amounts of black coal dust (melanoptysis).[43] Changes in breath sounds, expiratory wheezes, rhonchi, and hyperthrophy of the accessary muscles of respiration are commonly found on physical examination. Where the disease has been accompanied by secondary emphysema, a hyperinflated chest, low diaphragms and diminished breath sounds, especially at the bases, may be found. In general, the findings on physical examination are nonspecific[7] and similar to silicosis.

Pulmonary Function

Like silicosis, coal workers pneumoconiosis does not produce typical changes on pulmonary function testing. In the non-conglomerate form of the disease, pulmonary function tests, including diffusing capacity, may be normal.[34, 10] In the conglomerate form of this disorder, changes in pulmonary function become measurable. Loss of lung volume, as measured by vital capacity and total lung capacity without changes in the residual volume, are noted, at least in the moderately severe forms of the disease. Maldistribution of inspired gas may be noted with disturbances of the ventilation-perfusion ratios and in more severe forms of the disease, mild arterial desaturation, especially on exercise, can be found.[18] Maximum voluntary ventilation has been found to be reduced, but air-flow resistance tends to be less than in patients with emphysema, especially during quiet respiration. Lung compliance is decreased.

In general, the findings noted can be correlated with the pathological picture in coal workers pneumoconiosis of the massive replacement of normal lung with a large space occupying mass of fibrous tissue.[5] In some instances, emphysematous changes may also occur, leading to other ventilatory defects with increasing airways resistance, arterial oxygen desaturation, CO_2 retention, and ultimately cor pulmonale.

X-ray

Changes in the pulmonary roentgenogram in coal workers pneumoconiosis are not diagnostic and, in general, are similar in appearance to those encountered in silicosis.

The high incidence of the simultaneous exposure of coal miners to silica is another factor which should be considered when evaluating chest films from coal workers. Some authors have stated that the simple, non-conglomerate form of coal workers pneumoconiosis tends to be less nodular than the comparable stage of silicosis with a more reticulated pattern.[20, 39] Coal workers pneumoconiosis, like silicosis, can develop into the conglomerate form, the so-called massive progressive fibrosis of coal workers. This radiological diagnosis is the result of coalescence of masses of dense fibrotic tissue into large radiopaque lesions. Occasionally the masses may interfere with the local blood supply, and non-tuberculous cavitation occurs.[44]

Infection

Like silicosis, coal workers pneumoconiosis has been found to be frequently complicated by tuberculosis, which tends to be indolent.[14, 16] Some authors feel that the progressive massive fibrosis of coal workers pneumoconiosis is the result of secondary tuberculous infection,[16] a situation reminiscent of similar theories about the confluent lesions of silicosis.

Caplan's Syndrome

A specific problem reported in coal workers seemingly related to pneumoconiosis has been called Caplan's Syndrome. First reported in 1953,[10] the syndrome consisted of pulmonary nodules and rheumatoid arthritis in coal miners. The x-ray appearance of the lesions has been reported to be diffusely scattered, small, round, well-defined nodules resembling metastatic carcinoma.[48] It has been stated that cavitation of the lesions is not uncommon.[11]

The lesions develop rapidly and may precede, be preceded by, or coincide with the onset of rheumatoid arthritis. The disorder is not unique with coal workers, however, but has been reported in a variety of dusty occupations including silica exposure.[12] It has been shown that patients with the syndrome frequently have positive latex fixation and sheep cell agglutination tests,[12] sometimes without symptoms of arthritis.

The immunological implications of Caplan's syndrome are intriguing and, as a result, considerable attention has been paid to this disorder as a possible explanation for progressive massive fibrosis in the lung.[41] It has been postulated that dust, especially silica, initiates a hyperimmune reaction in the lung[47] and that this continuing process results in fibrosis of the lung and symptoms and signs of rhumatoid arthritis.

ASBESTOSIS

Asbestosis is the name applied to the fibrous silicates of magnesium and iron widely used in industry as insulation, fire proofing, brake linings, building materials and electrical insulation. Inhalation of significant amounts of the fiber can result in a form of pneumoconiosis, asbestosis, which has potentially serious clinical implications.

The findings in asbestosis (clinical,

radiological and to a lesser extent pulmonary function testing) are different from those found in silicosis and contrary to the other pneumoconioses; the disorder has certain oncological implications. These differences are related to the difference in the pulmonary pathology of silicosis and asbestosis. In pure active asbestosis, the fibers produce an intensive intra-alveolar fibrotic reaction with deposition of collagen tissue.[22] This active, proliferating, pneumonitis with desquamation of the alveolar cells and thickening of the alveolar walls results in subsequent reduction or obliteration of the air spaces. Edematous changes in alveolar walls are noted. Changes in the alveolar capillaries are also found with both obliteration of the capillaries and, in other regions, abnormal proliferation of small vessels. This is in contrast to silicosis, where the pulmonary intersitium is primarily affected, especially the lymphoid tissue, the perivascular lymph spaces and the regional lymph nodes, at least in the nonconfluent disease.[22] While the alveoli are affected in silicosis, this is less when compared to compatible stages of asbestosis. Plural reaction with thickening and even calcification is more common in asbestosis, especially of the basilar regions, and is much more intense than in silicosis.

Clinical Findings

The symptomatology of asbestosis is the universal ones of all the pneumoconioses of cough, dyspnea, easy fatigue and debilitation, usually of insidious onset. The cough may be severe and protracted. Physical findings are mainly in the chest with distant breath sounds, basilar rales and crepitations. Clubbing of the fingers and toes, with or without cyanosis,[48, 31] may be found.

As an ancillary finding, occasionally asbestosis corns (small, horney, wart-like, papules) are noted in the hands of asbestosis workers. These are caused by the reaction of the skin to asbestos fibers which have penetrated the epidermis during handling of the material.

Pulmonary Function

Pulmonary function changes are related to the pathology of asbestosis. The pleural thickening and intra-alveolar changes which occur in asbestosis are reflected in a diminished vital capacity and total lung capacity, but there is a tendency to preserve the residual volume, timed vital capacity, maximum mid-expiratory volume and maximum voluntary ventilation, at least when there are no associated emphysematous changes.[60, 31] Prominent among the changes in pulmonary function in asbestosis is the diminished diffusing capacity, a finding that is frequently much out of proportion to the other pulmonary functions and which may antecede symptoms and be present with a normal chest x-ray.[60, 5] While a low diffusing capacity may be found in all pneumoconioses, it tends to be proportionally much more severe in asbestosis than silicosis and this may be of diagnostic significance. These findings are compatible with the pathology of asbestosis and its relative prediliction for the alveoli and the damaging effects on small blood vessles that occur with this disease. Lung compliance may be reduced, and there is an increase in the effort of breathing.[35]

X-ray

As could be inferred from the pathology of the disease, asbestosis results in a chest x-ray that is different from silicosis. The pulmonary lesions of asbestosis are diffuse, fine and tend to be homogeneous to the extent that the term "ground glass appearance" has been widely used to describe this appearance (Fig. 4). The lesions produced are predominately in the lower third of the lung rather than general, and the disease frequently produces pleural thickening, unilaterally or bilaterally. Calcification of the thickened pleura has been occasionally observed. The cardiac border is obscured and diaphragmatic movements are limited.[48,51,31]

Asbestosis Bodies

Inhalation of asbestos fibers can result in the appearance of a club shaped artifact in biopsy specimens of the lung and in the sputa (Fig 5). These bodies measure about 3 x 70μ and can have a variety of appearances. Asbestos bodies are the result of a layering of protein material around asbestos fibers as they lie in pulmonary tissue. This coating first appears as globules strung out along the asbestos needle. They eventually coalesce and continue to enlarge at the ends taking about two months to form. Following this, the body appears to age with darkening and splitting of the protein envelope, followed by disappearance of the body leaving behind scattered granules in a ghost-like shape.[8, 27]

Asbestos bodies are found in specimens of lung from patients with asbestosis and in normal individuals with or without a history of industrial exposure.[27] In addition, the bodies become less numerous in individuals who have chronic asbestosis with considerable pulmonary disease if the exposure to asbestos fibers has ceased for a sufficient

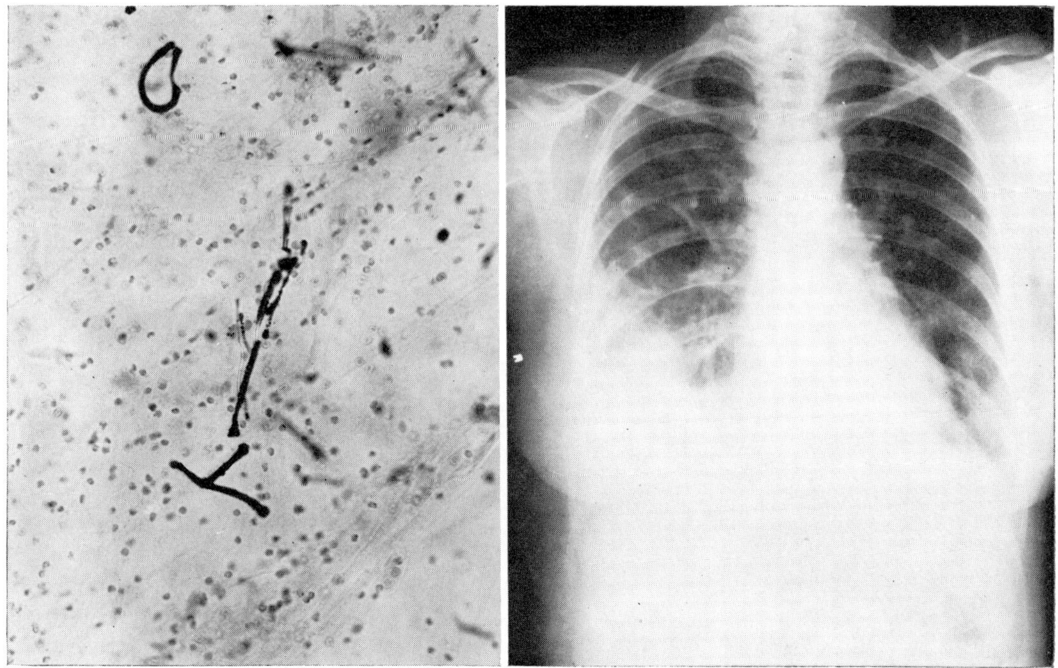

Figure 5. Asbestos body observed in a sputum cytology specimen obtained from a man with a history of 30 years employment as an insulation worker (Prussian blue stain).

Figure 6. Chronic berylliosis in a 33-year-old female with a history of industrial contact with beryllium.

period of time. Thus, the presence or absence of asbestos bodies in sputa or lung tissue must be considered in light of the history and other pertinent findings and are not, by themselves, diagnostic of asbestosis.

Asbestosis and Carcinoma

In spite of the delayed recognition of the association,[51] asbestos inhalation is associated with an increased incidence of bronchiogenic carcinoma and mesothelioma of the pleura and peritoneum.[27, 40, 37, 9] It has been reported, for example, in one study that the case rate for carcinoma of the lung is four times as great for males and ten times as great for females who had asbestosis as in the general population. In addition, there are at least suggestions that intraabdominal tumors are more common in asbestosis.[25]

Mesothelioma of the pleura and peritoneum are a special problem related to asbestos. It has been shown that a large percentage of patients with the mesotheliomas of the pleural surface have a history of exposure to asbestos.[17] The history of exposure was frequently neither severe nor prolonged, sometimes non-occupational or only through contacts with family members who were employed in jobs with asbestos exposure. In addition, there are suggestions that airborn dust in the vicinity of asbestos factories may be sufficient to induce the disease.[40] Recently, there has been increasing attention in this regard to the asbestos-containing dust produced by brake linings, floor tile and building materials which may be of considerable public health importance.

Clinically, mesotheliomas of the pleura or peritoneum are rare tumors, difficult to diagnose and almost universally fatal. The diagnosis is best established by pleural tap with examination of the cytology of the fluid and a pleural biopsy preferably with the Cope needle. Frequently, multiple taps are needed to make the diagnosis, and the appearance of a bloody pleural effusion in an individual with a history of asbestos contact, even of a minor nature, requires a careful and deligent evaluation.

TALC

Talc, hydrated magnesium silicate, is a relatively rare cause of pneumoconiosis. The disorder has a close resemblance to asbestosis: clinically, pathologically and radiologically.[28] Pulmonary function changes are similar to asbestosis.[32] No carcinogenic properties have been ascribed to talc, as yet.

BERYLLIOSIS

Beryllium is an element which has been associated with many of the spectacular accomplishments of the 20th century. It has been used in atomic research, as a moderator in nuclear reactors, in the aircraft industry, and a ceramic prepared from it has been used as heat shielding in missle nose cones. In the past, beryllium salts were a part of the phospher of fluorescent lights and it is still used in this way as in certain types of ocilloscopes. Alloys of the metal with copper are important because their special properties of hardness, resistance to corrosion, non-sparking and elastic properties.

Berylliosis, the disease produced by exposure to certain salts of the element, is not, strictly speaking, a pneumoconiosis. It is a systemic disorder, not limited to the lung, which can occur from the inhalation of fumes or vapors containing the element as well as from its dust.

Beryllium causes a multi-organ clinical disorder which superficially resembles Boeck's sarcoid to the extent that early cases of berylliosis were called "Salem sarcoid".[55] Like sarcoid, exposure of individuals to the beryllium containing dust can result in a large variety of symptoms.

Beryllium dermatitis and conjunctivitis have been described.[58] This disorder appears to be the result of the sensitization of exposed parts of the body to the element with the appearance of lesions in the skin folowing a latent period of about two weeks after exposure. In subsequent eruptions, the latent period is shortened, and the amounts of material required to produce a reaction is decreased. In the skin, the disorder is a puritic, erythematous, papular eruption, occasionally with vesicle formation. The conjunctivitis may or may not accompany the dermatitis and is sometimes associated with periorbital edema.[55]

Nasopharyngitis and trachiobronchitis may also be observed in individuals exposed to suitable beryllium compounds. These disorders have symptoms similar to an acute upper respiratory infection except that epistaxis is more common,[56] and fever is rare.

Beryllium salts can cause other dermatological problems. Ulcers of the skin and persistent granulomas have been reported.[55] Beryllium granulomas are the result of implantation of small amounts of beryllium containing material into the skin. Before 1948, this was most commonly seen with skin lacerations from fluorescent light tubes but since the use of beryllium containing salts as a phospher in these lights has been discontinued, the problem is less frequently encountered. Microscopically, these granulomas are similar to the noncaseating granuloma of sarcoid with giant cells and epithelioid cells in a dense fibrous stroma.[21] Ulceration of the lesions can occur with secondary infection and drainage.

Systemic Berylliosis

Systemic berylliosis can be divided into two types: acute and chronic. The acute form may be seen either as a fulminant disorder shortly following an exposure to large amounts of toxic beryllium compounds or as a more insidious disorder secondary to repeated exposures to lesser concentrations. The acute form of the disease most frequently begins as a dry cough which is progressive and may be accompanied by hemoptysis. Dyspnea occurs early and may be progressive and very severe. Clinically, the disorder resembles a widespread pneumonia or acute pulmonary edema with rales and rhonchi with an elevated pulse rate. If the disease is severe enough, cyanosis of the lips and hands can be observed.[55] Fever is sometimes present but tends to be low-grade.

Chest x-ray is normal early in the disease, but within weeks a diffuse hazy infiltrate appears which is generalized. Later, nodules of various size may be found that tend to persist.[58] The x-ray changes will usually clear with steroid treatment or spontaneously over a period of months, though respiratory symptoms may persist after the chest film has returned to normal. Occasionally, the x-ray changes will persist and develop into the chronic form of the disorder. Abnormal laboratory findings, as reflected in cell counts, sedimentation rates and liver chemistries, are usually absent.

Chronic Berylliosis

The disorder commonly called chronic berylliosis is the form of the beryllium disease which is most familiar to physicians. It differs from the acute form of berylliosis in that it frequently occurs many years after termination of exposure to the element, is progressive and systemic.[55]

Symptoms of the disorder are varied, though respiratory complaints predominate. Dyspnea, easy fatigue, chest tightness, orthopnea and cough are common. The cough is non-productive, frequently severe and sometimes associated with chest pain.[30] Blood in the sputum may be seen but is rare.[55] Systemic symptoms of weakness, lethargy, anorexia and weight loss are noted, and occasionally body temperature is mildly elevated.

Physical findings of rales, rhonchi and altered breath sounds are common on chest examination. Clubbing of the fingers and toes, cyanosis and the signs of cor pulmonale may be seen especially late in the course of the disease. A small percent of patients with berylliosis will have hepato-splenomegaly and skin nodules may occasionally be found.

A spectacular and serious complication of chronic berylliosis is a spontaneous pneumothorax. This problem occurs in about 15% of patients wtih chronic berylliosis, and when it occurs in an individual it tends to be recurrent. Pneumothorax may occur at any stage of the disease and can be seen in patients who have a history of beryllium exposure but with only minimal x-ray findings.[53]

Laboratory Findings

The blood picture is compatible with severe pulmonary disease, with secondary polycythemia the predominant feature. As would be expected, the sedimentation rate is elevated, but the white blood count is usually normal. Liver function tests are usually normal, but the bromsulphalein excretion may be delayed. A fairly consistent finding in chronic berylliosis, occasionally noted in the acute form of the disease, has been the reversal of the albumin-globulin ratio with an elevated serum globulin. Serum electrophoresis has demonstrated that the elevation is mainly in gamma-globulin fraction.[56] Like sarcoid, beryllium disease has been shown to be sometimes associated with an elevated serum calcium and abnormally high calcium levels in the urine. Calcium phosphate renal stones also occur. Renal function is otherwise not affected.[55]

Beryllium Assay

Beryllium analysis has been recommended as an aid to diagnosis. Spectrographic assay appears to be the most satisfactory method for detecting beryllium in biological material.[29] The method has been used with lung tissue and with urine as a diagnostic tool in suspected cases of berylliosis and as a monitoring device in possible exposure. Tissue levels of the element, as contained in lung specimens obtained either on biopsy or at autopsy, appear to correlate fairly well with a history of exposure, but no correlation can be made between the severity of the disease and beryllium tissue levels. This latter finding is not surprising, however, in light of the role that hypersensitivity appears to play in beryllium disease with wide differences in the response of different individuals to the same level of exposure.

The levels of urinary beryllium in chronic beryllium disease or suspected disease does not appear to be a reliable aid in the diagnosis of the disease. Lieben and co-workers,[38] for example, have reported that in ten cases of berylliosis and seven suspects one individual had a positive test, but all the others had no detectable beryllium in the urine. In addition, false positives were encountered in normal controls who lived in areas with a high beryllium content in the drinking water.

Pulmonary Function

In general, the pulmonary function of patients with chronic beryllium disease are similar to patients with comparable sarcoid. The usual findings early in the disease are that of a "small lung" with a decreased vital capacity, total lung capacity and residual volume. Tests measuring gas distribution (nitrogen wash-out) and airway resistance are usually unimpaired. Early in the disease, a marked decline in the diffusing capacity, the so-called alveolar-capillary block, is frequently seen.[5]

In the more chronic forms of berylliosis, secondary emphysema frequently occurs. With this change, changes in dead space, airway obstruction and maldistribution of inspired gas can be seen which are comparable to the changes noted with nonspecific chronic obstructive pulmonary disease.

The changes in pulmonary function noted with berylliosis are compatible with and reflect the pathology of the disorder. The production of large numbers of small granulomas acting as a large space occupying mass together with cellular infiltration of the alveolar walls interfering with capillary perfusion and trans-membrane gas transfer, especially of oxygen, account for the findings on pulmonary function.

X-ray Appearance

The chest x-ray in chronic berylliosis may proceed or be preceded by changes in pulmonary function and symptoms. The first evidence noted on chest film is a diffuse haziness which progresses into a diffuse fine nodulation. The nodules may appear to coalesce into larger rounded densities which are softer and less well demarcated than those of the other pneumoconiosis. Emphysematous blebs and bullae may be noted, and spontaneous pneumothorax, sometimes asymptomatic, is seen. Hilar lymphadinopathy is frequent, and linear densities may be noted. In general, the chest film resembles that of sarcoid or of the so-called Hamman-Rich syndrome, among other conditions,[56] and is not diagnostic in itself (Fig. 6).

Other Diagnostic Tests

Because of the clinical similarities in the two disorders, it has been suggested[57] that a Kveim test be used in conjunction with the beryllium patch test[42] as a method of differentiating the two diseases. The Kveim test has been noted to be negative in beryllium disease, and a negative test in a patient with compatible chest lesions would increase the suspicion of berylliosis. Thus must be interrupted, however, in the light that occasionally patients with clinically typical sarcoid have negative Kveim tests and rarely a false positive foreign body reaction can be elicited with the test. Finally, the status of the beryllium patch test as a diagnostic tool has been doubtful and controversial.[55] It has also been reported that application of the patch test may adversely influence the course of chronic beryllium disease.[52]

OTHER PNEUMOCONIOSES

Other mineral dusts that have been associated with at least changes on chest x-ray are numerous. Three that deserve at least passing mention are iron, tin and barium.

Inhalation of these compounds can cause changes on chest x-ray which at times are marked. Other than causing confusion with other pneumoconioses, the deposition of these substances in the lung appears to have little effect on respiratory function, and while occasionally the individuals involved may have symptoms such as cough or even mild dyspnea, the association between symptoms, the x-ray and the material, besides its effects as a nonspecific irritant dust, are doubtful.[48, 27, 8]

BIBLIOGRAPHY

1. Abrams, H. K.: Diatomaceous earth pneumoconiosis. Amer. J. of Public Health, *44¹*:592-599,1954.
2. Abrams, H. K.: Letters to the editor. Arch. Environ. Health, *22*:542, 1965.
3. Arch. Environ. Health; Editorial comment, *11:* 619, 1965.
4. Baetjer, A. M., and Vintinner, F. J.: The effect of silica and feldspar dusts on susceptibility to labor pneumonia. J. Indust. Hyg. and Toxicol., *26:*101-108, 1944.
5. Bates, D. V., and Christie, R. V.: Respiratory Function in Disease. Philadelphia, W. B. Saunders, 1964, pp. 382-391.
6. Battigelli, M. C.: Functional lesions in pneumoconiosis. Arch. Environ. Health, *15:*629-637, 1967.
7. Braun, D. C.: Coal. In The Pneumoconiosis, ed. by Lanza, A. J. New York, Grune and Stratton, p. 103, 1963.
8. Browne, R. C.: The Chemistry and Therapy of Industrial Pulmonary Diseases. Springfield, Thomas, 1966, p. 37.
9. Buchanan, W. D.: Asbestosis and primary intrathoracic neoplasms. Ann. N.Y. Acadm. Sci., *132:*507-517, 1965.
10. Caplan, A.: Certain unusual radiological appearance in the chest of coal miners suffering from Rhumatoid arthritis. Thorax, *8:*29-37, 1953.
11. Caplan, A.: Rhumatoid Disease and Pneumoconiosis. In Industrial Pulmonary Disease, ed. by King. E. J., and Fletcher, C. M. Boston, Little, Brown, and Company, 1960, p. 232.
12. Caplan, A., Payne, R. B., and Withey, J. L.: A broader concept of Caplan's syndrome related to rhumatic factors. Thorax, *17:*205, 1962.
13. Chatiyidakis, C. B.: Silicosis in South African white gold miners: A comparative study of the disease in different stages. Med. Proc., *9:*383, 1963.
14. Cochrane, A. L.: Tuberculosis and coal workers pneumoconiosis. Brit. J. Tuberc., *48:*274-279, 1954.
15. Dutra, F. R.: Diatomaceous earth pneumoconiosis. Arch. Environ. Health, *11:*613-619, 1966.
16. Fletcher, C. M.: Epidemological studies of coal miners pneumoconiosis in Great Britain. Arch. Indust. Health, *11:*29-40, 1955.
17. Fowler, P. B. S.: Exposure to asbestos and mesothalioma of the pleura. Brit. Med. J., 211-213, July 25th, 1964.
18. Gilson, J. C., and Hugh-Jones, P.: Lung function in Coal workers Pneumoconiosis. M.R.C. Sp. Report, Ser. No. 290, London H.M.S.O., 1955.
19. Gough, J.: Pneumoconiosis in coal trimmers. J. Path. & Bact., *51:*277-285, 1940.
20. Gough, J., James, W. R. L., and Wentworth, J. E.: Comparison of the radiological and pathological changes in coal workers pneumoconiosis. J. Fac. Radiol., *1:*28, 1949.
21. Grier, R. S., Nash, P., and Freiman, D. G.: Skin lesions and persons exposed to beryllium compound. J. Ind. Hyg. Toxicol., *30:*228, 1948.
22. Gross, P.: Pathology of asbestosis. In The Pneumoconiosis, ed. by Lanza, A. J. New York, Grune & Stratton, 1963, p. 34.
23. Gross, P., Westrick, M. L., and McNerney, J. M.: Experimental tuberculopneumoconiosis. AMA Arch. Indust. Health, *19:*320-334, 1959.
24. Gross, P., Westrick, M., and McNerney, J. M.: Experimental tuberculosilicosis. Am. Rev. Resp. Dis., *83:*510-527, 1961.
25. Hammond, E. C., Selikoff, I. J., and Chung, J.: Neoplasia among insulation workers in the U.S. with special reference to intra-abdominal neoplasms. Ann. N.Y. Acad. Sci., *132:*519-525, 1965.
26. Hodges, P. C.: Silicosis. Postgrad. Med., *28:* A75-A79, 1960.
27. Holt, P. F.: Pneumoconiosis. London, Edward Arnold, Publ., 1957.
28. Hunt, A. C.: Massive pulmonary fibrosis from the inhalation of talc. Thorax., *11:*287, 1956.
29. Keenan, R. G.: New analytical techniques for industrial hygiene. Arch. Indust. Health, *21:* 261-267, 1960.
30. Kline, E. M., and Moir, T. W.: Long-term experience with beryllium disease. Arch. Indust. Health, *19:*204, 1959.
31. Kleinfeld, M., Messite, J., and Shapiro, J.: Clinical, radiological and physiological findings in asbestosis. Arch. Int. Med., *117:*813-819, 1966.
32. Kleinfeld, M., Messite, J., Shapiro, J. Kooyman,

Y., and Swencicki, R.: Lung function in talc workers. Arch Environ. Health, *9*:559-566, 1964.

33. Lanza, A. J.: Silicosis. In, The Pneumoconiosis, ed. by A. J. Lanza. New York, Grune & Stratton, 1963, p. 1-12.
34. Leathart, G. L.: The mechanical properties of the lung in pneumoconiosis of coal miners. Brit. J. of Ind. Med., *16*:153, 1959.
35. Leathart, G. L.: Clinical bronchiographic, radiological and physiological observations in 10 cases of asbestosis. Brit. J. Ind. Med., *17*:213, 1960.
36. Legge, R. T., and Rosencrantz, E.: Observations and studies with diatomaceous silica. Amer. J. Public Health, *22*:1055-1060, 1932.
37. Lieben, J.: Malignancies in asbestos workers. Arch. Environ. Health, *13*:619-621, 1966.
38. Lieben, J., Dattoli, J. A., and Vought, V.: The significance of beryllium concentration in urine. Arch. Environ. Health, *12*:331-334, 1966.
39. Lieben, J., Pendergross, E. P., and Brieger, H. B.: The course of pneumoconiosis in coal miners. Arch. Environ. Health, *10*:786-789, 1965.
40. Lieben, J., and Pistawka, H.: Mesothelioma and asbestos exposure. Arch. Environ. Health, *14*:559-598, 1967.
41. Lindars, D. C., and Davies, D.: Rheumatoid Pneumoconiosis. Thorax, *22*:525-532, 1967.
42. McCord, C. P.: Beryllium as a sensitizing agent. Ind. Med. & Surg., *20*:336, 1951.
43. McKerrow, C. B.: Respiratory disease as an industrial hazard. The Practitioner, *195*:774-784, 1965.
44. Morrow, C. S., and Armen, R. N.: Nontuberculous pulmonary cavitation in anthrosilicosis. Ann. Int. Med., *45*:598-613, 1956.
45. Motley, H. L., Smart, R. H., and Valero, A.: Pulmonary function studies in diatomaceous earth workers. AMA Arch. Indust. Health, *13*: 265-274, 1956.
46. O'Neill, R. P., and Robin, E. D.: Relations of pneumoconiosis and pulmonary tuberculosis. Arch. Environ. Health, *8*:873-881, 1964.
47. Pernis, B.: Immunohistochemical observations in the human silicotic nodule. Med. & Lavaro., *54*:354-358, 1963.
48. Rubin, E. H., and Rubin, M.: Thoracic Diseases. Philadelphia, W. B. Saunders Company, 1961.
49. Schinz, H. R., Baensch, W. E., Friedl, E., and Uehlinger, E. (Eds.): Roentgen-Diagnostics. New York, Grune & Stratton, (1st Am. Ed.) 1953.
50. Smart, R. H., and Anderson, W. M.: Pneumoconiosis due to diatomaceous earth. Clinical and x-ray aspects. Ind. Med. & Surg., *21*:509, 1952.
51. Smith, K. W.: Diatomaceous earth pneumoconiosis. In, The Pneumoconiosis, ed. by A. J. Lanza. New York, Grune & Stratton, 1963, p. 26.
52. Sneddon, I. B.: Berylliosis: A case report. Brit. Med. J., *1*:1448-1450, 1955.
53. Spain, D. M.: Letters to the editor. Arch. Environ. Health, *12*:542, 1966.
54. Teculescu, D. B., Stanescu, D. C., and Pilat, L.: Pulmonary mechanics in silicosis. Arch. Environ. Health, *14*:461-468, 1967.
55. Tepper, L. B., Hardy, H. and Chamberlin, R. I.: Toxicity of Beryllium Compounds. New York, Elsvier, 1961.
56. VanOrdstrand, H. S.: Berylliosis. In, The Pneumoconiosis, ed. by A. J. Lanza. New York, Grune & Stratton, 1963, pp. 73-101.
57. VanOrdstrand, H. S., DeNardi, J. M., and Zielinski, J. F.: Beryllium lung disease and its registry. Postgrad. Med., *36*:499-504, 1964.
58. VanOrdstrand, H. S., Hughes, R., DeNardi, J. M., and Cardmody, M. G.: Beryllium poisoning. J.A.M.A., *129*:1084, 1945.
59. Vorwald, A. J., Delahart, A. B., and Dworski, M.: Silicosis and Type III pneumoccus pneumonia, J. Indust. Hyg. & Toxicol., *22*:64-78, 1940.
60. Williams, R., and Hugh-Jones, P.: The significance of lung function changes in asbestosis. Thorax, *15*:109-119, 1960.
61. Wright, G. W., and Filley, G.: Pulmonary fibrosis and respiratory function. Am. J. Med., *10*:642, 1951.
62. Zohman, L. R., and Williams, M. H., Jr.: Cardiopulmonary function in pulmonary fibrosis. Am. Rev. Resp. Dis., *80*:700, 1959.

Chapter 43

Pneumoconioses: Pathologic Considerations

G. E. APONTE, M.D.

Pneumoconiosis refers to the effects on pulmonary function and structure of inhaled particulate matter (dusts), which may be of animal, vegetable, or mineral origin. Various mechanisms may be operative in their pathogenesis, and in many instances hypersensitivity plays an important role. Some mineral dusts may be inhaled as fumes. In general, however, the effects produced by the inhalation of noxious gases or fumes are not encompassed in the original concept of the pneumoconioses but fall more properly in the category of chemical pneumonias. Table 1 lists the better known disorders which may follow prolonged exposure to particulate matter.

Important occupational diseases, the pneumoconioses are the leading cause of workers' disability and compensation in many branches of industry. Chronic exposure often means more than pulmonary injury — particles of silica and carbon are frequently found in nonpulmonary tissues and urinary calculi containing silica have been described,[34] berylliosis is truly a disseminated disease, and there is evidence that chronic exposure to asbestos is associated with an increased incidence of neoplasms of the gastrointestinal tract.

Anthracosis is generally considered to be innocuous and a necessary consequence of urban life. However, under certain circumstances carbon dust can be pathogenic — 1) A condition similar to

TABLE I — THE PNEUMOCONIOSES

I — *Disorders due to mineral dusts or fumes**
1. Anthracosis
2. Silicosis
3. Coal-worker's pneumoconiosis
4. Asbestosis
5. Berylliosis

Others

6. Aluminum lung
7. Arc-welder's lung
8. Barium lung
9. Bauxite (Shaver's disease)
10. Cadmium pneumonia and pneumoconiosis
11. Carbon-electrode maker's lung
12. Fiberglas-plastic dust
13. Fuller-earth pneumoconiosis
14. Graphite lung
15 Hematite lung
16. Kaolinosis
17. Siderosis
18. Silver polisher's lung
19. Stannosis
20. Talcosis

II — *Disorders due to organic ducts of animal or vegetable origin*
1. Byssinosis
2. Bagassosis
3. Farmer's lung
4. Maple-bark stripper's lung
5. Pigeon-breeder's lung
6. Sequoiosis
7. Suberosis
8. Pulmonary lesions following the inhalation of pituary snuff
9. Mushroom-worker's lung

* Only the better known disorders have been listed.

coal-worker's lung has been found in persons occupationally exposed to carbon electrodes,[51] which do not contain silica. 2) The graphite pneumoconiosis of electrotypers is thought to develop from the additive effects of carbon dust and infection, the former acting by impeding pulmonary lymphatic drainage. 3) Coal dust appears to play a leading role in the production of the type of coal-worker's lung which is characterized roentgenographically by a pattern of fine pulmonary reticulation.

Silicosis

In Table 2 are listed factors known to be important in the pathogenesis of silicosis and certain other pneumoconioses.

Table 2 — Factors of Importance in the Pathogenesis of Silicosis

1. Size of particle
2. Concentration particle in air
3. Duration of exposure
4. Additive effects of dusts
5. Presence of other diseases
6. Individual susceptibility

In general, the particles which cause the greatest damage are smaller than 10μ. In the case of silicosis, they are usually smaller than 3μ and readily escape the clearing effect of epithelial ciliary activity. Particles smaller than 0.5 μ are probably exhaled as readily as they are inhaled. A concentration of 5 million particles of free silica per cubic foot of air has been defined as the maximal safe level of exposure. In the majority of cases, the duration of exposure has ranged from 10 to 15 years. In the infrequent cases of acute silicosis the duration of exposure is shorter, but seldom is it less than 2 years.[39] It has long been known that there exist individual variations in the susceptibility of individuals to the fibrogenic effects of silica dust. Indeed, knowledge of this fact lead to the concept that hypersensitivity is probably the mechanism whereby tissue damage takes place. Combination of the dust particles with tissue proteins is said to render the latter antigenic for the organism. The presence of alpha and beta globulins has been detected in the sclerotic nodules characteristic of the disease, and increases in the serum concentration of gamma globulins have been found. However, little work has been done during the past decade to elucidate further the nature and extent of this antigen-antibody reaction. Many questions remain and the question of pathogenesis is by no means fully answered. Previous theories of pathogenesis have included simple mechanical injury and chemical injury through the formation of silicic acids toxic for tissue proteins.

Some of the inhaled particles are expectorated but the smaller ones reach the alveoli where they promptly elicit an outpouring of histiocytes from the alveolar walls, and many are thus phagocytized. Although the tissue response is histiocytic, typical granulomas seldom develop. According to Gross *et al.*,[21, 22] the majority of the particles remain fixed at or near the sites of entrance where they begin to evoke the characteristic fibroblastic response. As fibrosis progresses, the number of histiocytes is reduced. The silica particles which are transported in the lymph are carried in the free state and are re-phagocytized upon reaching the regional lymph nodes. The highest concentrations of silica particles is found near the pulmonary hilum. The particles are more numerous in the upper two-thirds of the lung than at the base presumably because the greater mobility of the lower lobes prevents full penetration by the particulate matter. Silica particles tend to accumulate in the fixed portions of the lungs, in lymph spaces[19] around bronchi, bronchioles and blood vessels and beneath the pleura. Nodular fibrosis is characteristic of the disease, and is readily apparent in roentgenograms as well as histologically. The silicotic nodules are formed predominantly outside the walls of dividing respiratory bronchioles and consist of dense, avascular, concentric masses of reticular and collagenous fibers which are usually devoid of cells and contain free particles of silica, chiefly in the periphery. Silicotic nodules have been found to consist of about 40 per cent collagen protein and 20 per cent lipid, as well as alpha and beta globulins, and small amounts of carbohydrate. The prevailing ischemia tends to produce softening and cystic degeneration of the centers of the nodules. Although cavity formation can occur in silicosis uncomplicated by tuberculosis, the two disorders so frequently coexist that the presence of cavities in the roentgenograms of patients with silicosis should be taken to signify co-existing tuberculous disease until proved otherwise. The dust particles do not become permanently entrapped in the nodules but, being labile, are frequently transported to other portions of the lungs. This perpetuates tissue damage and also renders unreliable attempts to correlate the extent of nodular fibrosis with the concentration of silica particles in the nodules. Hemorrhage from tuberculous cavities which have developed in association with silicosis occurs infrequently because of the ischemic nature of the antecedent fibrotic pulmonary lesions. In some instances, severe diffuse pulmonary fibrosis may develop. It has been noted following exposure to such silica-containing substances as graphite, coal dust, hematite and kaolin. Some cases of diffuse massive pulmonary fibrosis are the result of the additive effects of silica dust and concomitant tuberculous infection.*

Vascular lesions tend to develop in the more advanced cases. The smaller branches of the pulmonary arteries and the pulmonary arterioles are predominantly involved, but when the fibrosis is massive and diffuse the entire arterial system may be affected. Although cor pulmonale is considered to be an infrequent clinical complication, at autopsy we have found hypertrophy of the right cardiac ventricle to be a common finding in cases of long-standing disease. As a rule, the histologic response to free silica in the lung is not typically granulomatous and consists for the most part of aggregates of histiocytes. A similar response has been noted following the injection of colloidal suspension of silica into the skin of volunteers.[14] Particles of free silica are best demonstrated histologically by examining acid-extracted and microincinerated preparations with the phase microscope. This method, however, does not permit cytologic localization of the material, which has been achieved by means of histochemical methods. Cytoplasmic particles of free silica stain metachromatically,[8] are P.A.S. – positive and resistant to diastase, and give a positive colloidal iron reaction.[14] They also have been found to emit a bluish-white autofluorescence.

Coal-worker's pneumoconiosis has been classified separately from true silicosis because of the modifying effect of coal dust on the tissue response. The

---

*An unusual type of tissue reaction to silica, without nodular fibrosis and resembling the lesion of pulmonary alveolar proteinosis, has been described in germ-free animals.[28]

changes produced depend primarily on the proportions of pure coal to silicotic dust and on the presence or absence of tuberculous infection. About 60% of the dust inhaled by coal workers is carbonaceous. Soft bituminous coal contains little silica or silicate but anthracite coal has a higher content. Three types of lesions have been noted: 1) Compound nodular lesions of silica and coal dust which resemble those already described for pure silicosis. 2) Massive pulmonary fibrosis, affecting chiefly the upper lobes and due to the combined effects of coal dust and coexisting tuberculous infection. 3) The so-called simple pneumoconiosis of coal workers, characterized by a roentgenographic pattern of fine reticulation involving mainly the upper two-thirds of the lungs and attributable almost entirely to the effects of coal dust alone.

Asbestosis

Asbestos bodies, which have been considered the histologic hallmark of asbestosis, are produced by the endogenous coating of asbestos fibers with an unusual protein gel rich in iron, presumably a protective mechanism. Uncoated asbestos fibers are difficult to find in routine sections since they remain unstained and often measure 0.5 μ or less in longest dimension. The number of asbestos bodies present in any given lung varies within a wide range and independently of the number of uncoated asbestos fibers present. Similar structures produced by other substances, such as spicules of coal, have been termed "curious bodies" or pseudo-asbestos bodies but are seen more frequently after digestion techniques than in routine sections. Impregnation of pulmonary elastic tissue with iron may also produce similar structures,[20] the so-called "elastosis bodies."[18] The latter are often clubbed and tend to provoke a giant-cell reaction. Stains for elastic tissue may reveal remnants of the latter, thus distinguishing them from asbestos bodies. They can also be distinguished by micro-incineration, after which the asbestos body still shows a yellow or orange coating which, upon treatment with HCl, reveals the bare asbestos fiber. Certain mammalian species, such as the rat and the dog, produce few asbestos bodies, the fibers remaining uncoated in the lung parenchyma. In the rabbit, on the other hand, asbestos bodies have been found within 7 days after the initial exposure.

The frequency with which asbestos bodies are found in the sputum has varied from 10-45% of cases in different reported series. Occasionally, they are found in the feces. The demonstration of uncoated asbestos fibers in sections of lung is clearly a more accurate indicator of exposure to asbestos than the demonstration of asbestos bodies. Two methods have been used:[3] 1) Tagging the asbestos fibers with a fluorochrome, such as berberine sulfate, for at least one month *in vivo,* and 2) Electronic ashing of tissue sections. Studies with the electron microscope have shown that the small asbestos fibers[29] are very important in the pathogenesis of the disease, which begins as an intracellular process.

The maximal damage in asbestosis is found in the lower lobes. The characteristic nodular fibrosis of silicosis does not occur and the fibrous tissue is much more cellular, not hyalinized and avascular. Bronchiectasis and cystic pulmonary lesions develop frequently, The cystic changes ("honeycombing") are bilateral and uniform in distribution and are considered to be a distinctive finding. They do not develop in the pneumoconioses due to particles of similar composition, such as talc and mica. Another frequent finding is pleural calcification which,[31, 32, 48] however, seldom develops sooner than 20 years after the initial exposure. It affects particularly the parietal pleura of the lower lobe and is bilateral in about half the cases. If trauma and infection can be ruled out as etiologic factors, bilateral pleural calcification of the lower lobes is considered to be virtually diagnostic of asbestosis. Pulmonary vascular changes do not develop as frequently as in silicosis. Dyspnea is the outstanding symptom, and frequently the only manifestation of the disease. Sputum is present in about 50 per cent of cases but cyanosis is not a frequent finding. The presence of rheumatoid factor[41] against human gamma globulins has been noted in the sera of some patients with asbestosis, particularly those whose disease is of grade 2 or 3 severity. Prolonged exposure to asbestos is associated with an increased incidence of certain malignant neoplasms.[6, 13, 23] In a study of 392 persons who had been exposed to asbestos for periods longer than 20 years, the incidence of bronchogenic carcinoma was found to be 7 times higher than in appropriate controls. A threefold rise in the incidence of cancer of the gastrointestinal tract was also noted. This series also included 10 cases of mesothelioma of the pleura and peritoneum. More recently, an increased incidence of ovarian tumors in exposed individuals has been suggested. Others have found a general increase in the incidence of death from non-neoplastic diseases.[13] The development of pulmonary carcinomas has not been limited to cases of exposure to a particular type of asbestos fiber, but the mesotheliomas seem to have occurred more often following exposure to crocidolite, the type of asbestos mineral prevalent in Australia and South Africa. In the United States, the predominant asbestos minerals are chrysolite and tremolite.

Berylliosis

The first report on berylliosis in the American medical literature appeared in 1945, thirteen years after it was originally described as a type of chemical bronchiolitis by Russian investigators. The term "berylliosis" was coined by Italian workers two years later and in 1936 reports of the disease, described as "metal-fume fever," appeared in the German literature. The only beryllium substance which does not produce disease in man is the ore itself, beryl. Beryllium metal, as well as beryllium oxides and certain beryllium salts have all been shown to be toxic for human tissues; the majority of cases having followed exposure to the oxide. *Acute* berylliosis is a chemical pneumonia characterized by pulmonary edema with the intra-alveolar accumulation of fibrin, erythrocytes and moderate numbers of leucocytes, but without the formation of granulomas. If the dose is sufficiently high, everyone exposed is affected to some extent. In a series of 170 cases of acute intoxication with beryllium reported by van Ordstrand and associates,[54] inflammation of the upper respiratory tract or tracheobronchitis was noted in 90 patients and pneumonia in 38. Five of the latter patients died. Other frequent manifestations include conjunctivitis, contact dermatitis and cutaneous ulcers. Individual susceptibility is a very important factor in the pathogenesis of *chronic* berylliosis since only about 1-2% of individuals chronically exposed develop clinical evidence of the disease. There may be a long latent period, as long as 15 years, between exposure and the clinical onset of disease. Chronic pulmonary berylliosis is an interstitial granulomatous pneumonia which may resemble sarcoidosis closely. Fibrosis is both diffuse and nodular. Conchoidal bodies may be seen in beryllium granulomas but are not specific for the disease. They are a protein complex impregnated with calcium and do not stain with stains for elastic tissue. The conchoidal bodies which may develop in the lesions of sarcoidosis can be stained with stains for elastic tissue. Crystals of beryllium may be seen as birefringent deposits within the conchoidal bodies. With time, the pulmonary granulomas of chronic berylliosis are converted into masses of hyalinized tissue. More accurate methods are needed for the determination of beryllium in tissue sections since excessive concentrations of the metal have been demonstrated in only about half the cases of berylliosis. The use of the laser beam looms promising in this respect.[42] Pulmonary emphysema is usually not very severe in chronic beryllium disease, although the occurrence of large subpleural blebs has been noted. Vascular damage is not pronounced and the development of cyanosis or cor pulmonale is infrequent. However, the prognosis in chronic beryllium disease is poor, death usually resulting from pulmonary insufficiency.

Chronic berylliosis is truly a systemic disease. Granulomatous lesions are found in the hilar pulmonary lymph nodes as well as in other tissues such as the liver. We have seen myocardial involvement at autopsy and others have noted the occurrence of myocarditis clinically,[25] and the occurrence of nephrocalcinosis as a result of beryllium poisoning has been noted.[16] The metal has also produced sarcomas of the tibia in experimental animals.[52] Increased concentrations of beryllium have been detected in every organ of the body except the brain.[25] Some patients develop indolent ulcers of the skin, particularly over the metacarpophalangeal joints, which are usually associated with a positive skin test. Chronic berylliosis may resemble sarcoidosis clinically as well as histologically. Important differences in the differential diagnosis include the rarity of axillary or cervical lymphadenitis and the lack of involvement of bones and salivary glands in beryllium disease. Also, the latter does not respond to steroid therapy. Toxic levels of beryllium in environmental air are also a health hazard for individuals who live in the vicinity of the main area of exposure. Hardy[25] refers to a total of 60 cases of "neighborhood beryllium disease" which have occurred in this country. The mortality rate in this group was 50%.

Other Mineral Dusts and Fumes[51]

The majority of reports of pulmonary disease following exposure to *aluminum* have appeared in the European medical literature. Most particles of aluminum metal powder are larger than 5 μ, but apparently smaller particles are present in sufficient concentration to become a health hazard in some instances. The pulmonary lesion is an interstitial fibrosis similar to that seen in bauxite disease, the most severe changes being noted near the pulmonary hila.

Arc-welder's lung, first described in 1936,[9] follows exposure to fumes containing mixtures of oxides, such as iron oxide, and traces of amorphous silica and silicates. Heavy deposits of iron are found in the alveolar septa and in the perivascular spaces. However, pulmonary fibrosis has been an infrequent finding and, when present, has been attributed to the silica and silicates in the inhaled air.

Most cases of *barium lung* follow the inhalation of dust particles containing barium salts. Exposure is followed by a brisk outpouring into the alveolar spaces of edema fluid rich in fibrinogen, but the inflammatory response is scant. Occasionally, barium sulfate used in diagnostic roentgenography escapes into the tissues and provokes a foreign-body reaction of variable intensity but which is associated with little or no fibrosis. However, some contrast media used in bronchograms have produced transient pneumonia.[44]

Bauxite lung, also known as Shaver's disease and corundum-smelter's lung, was first described 20 years ago.[49] It develops in persons who work with aluminum abrasives (Al_2O_3). The fumes contain about 7% silica but the typical silicotic nodules have not been found in the reported cases. The cause of the pulmonary injury is not known. Symptoms can develop as early as 3 months after the initial exposure and spontaneous pneumothorax is a frequent finding.

Cadmium, used in the manufacture of alloys, is released in the course of welding steel parts and is inhaled mainly as cadmium oxide. *Acute* exposures can produce severe pulmonary edema and a chemical pneumonia, which may be fatal. The pulmonary changes in cases of *chronic* exposure consist chiefly of moderately severe perivascular fibrosis and lymphocytic infiltration. Proteinuria is a common finding and the urine contains complexes of cadmium and protein.

Silica apparently plays no role in the pathogenesis of the massive pulmonary fibrosis which may develop in the pneumoconiosis of *carbon-electrode makers*. The pulmonary lesions are thought to result from the additive effects of carbon dust and low-grade tuberculous infection.

The inhalation of dust from *fiberglas-plastic* reportedly has produced pulmonary reactions in human beings. The irritant is calcium carbonate. Experimentally, this material has produced peribronchial and perivascular inflammation in monkeys and guinea pigs, without significant fibrosis.[46]

Fuller earth consists of about 90% aluminum silicate and also contains small amounts of quartz. The pulmonary changes resemble silicosis histologically and in their distribution in the lungs, but are much less severe. Clinical evidence of pulmonary involvement has developed only in a small per cent of individuals exposed and usually after a long latent period. Fatalities are rare.

Graphite consists of about 50% carbon and 10-20% silica, silicates being present in smaller concentrations. The roentgenographic changes in the lungs resemble the pneumoconiosis of coal workers. Pulmonary disease may develop in electrotypers from prolonged exposure to graphite and is thought to be the result of the combined effects of large concentrations of carbon and secondary infection.[17] Giant cells are often found in the lungs in cases of graphite pneumoconiosis and less frequently, asteroid bodies and structures resembling asbestos bodies have been found.[53]

Hematite (Fe_2O_3) is an ore of iron which contains about 10% silica. The pulmonary lesions are due to silica, modified by the presence of iron. It resembles the pneumoconiosis of coal workers and involves the upper halves of the lungs most severely. The color of the lungs is a striking brownish red. Although hematite itself is Prussian-blue negative, the lungs in these cases contain much hemosiderin, which gives a positive Prussian blue reaction. The serum concentration of iron has been found to be increased in some cases. The complications of hematite lung include emphysema, bronchiectasis and tuberculosis. Unlike the pneumoconiosis of coal workers, this disorder is associated with an increased incidence of bronchogenic cancer.

Kaolin,[30] also known as china clay, is a type of granite which contains aluminum oxide and silica, as well as mica and quartz. It can produce severe pulmonary disease, which is characterized by nodular lesions and vascular changes. The pathogenesis of the pulmonary changes may be related to the ability of kaolin to absorb antigenic proteins.[56] Pulmonary fibrosis is particularly severe in the presence of tuberculosis. This additive effect of concomitant tuberculous infection has also been demonstrated in experimental animals.[51]

Siderosis: The inhalation of pure iron oxide produces few pathologic changes in the lungs. However, when inhaled with other particles such as silica it can modify their effects to a significant extent. Such an action has been noted in the pneumoconioses of hematite workers, silver polishers and arc welders.

Silver polisher's lung[36] was originally described in 1945. The dust inhaled contains iron oxide and metallic silver. The latter combines with tissue proteins and stains the pulmonary elastic tissue black.

Stannosis develops from the prolonged inhalation of dust or fumes of tin oxide. The particles are deposited in the alveolar septa, around bronchioles and blood vessels, beneath the pleura, and in the hilar pulmonary lymph nodes, but do not elicit a very pronounced fibroblastic response.

Talcosis is an uncommon type of pneumoconiosis which may follow prolonged exposure to commercial talc (hydrated magnesium silicate). The fibrogenic agent is probably tremolite, a type of asbestos mineral. There develop small grayish pulmonary nodules, softer than the silicotic nodules and located chiefly in the lower lobes. The lesions are much more cellular than in silicosis or in coal-worker's lung and also contain much less carbon pigment. The nodular lesions in talcosis may coalesce to form larger masses, the centers of which tend to become excavated. In the walls of these cavities are often found basophilic bodies which stain positively for iron and probably represent fragments of asbestos fibers.

ORGANIC DUSTS OF ANIMAL OR VEGETABLE ORIGIN[33, 40, 43]

Byssinosis[1, 4, 5, 35]

Byssinosis is an occupational hazard in the textile industry. The disease affects persons who work with cotton, flax or hemp and is most prevalent in the cardroom workers. The acute symptoms consist of shortness of breath, cough and fever, characteristically developing on Monday upon return to work but gradually subsiding later in the week. The incidence of reactors among the exposed population is high and the acute manifestations occur independently of other environmental factors such as air pollution, climate and cigarette smoking. Continued exposure gradually leads to an impairment in ventilatory capacity and irreversible pulmonary changes. However, very few deaths have been recorded. Although antibodies to antigens of the cotton plant have been found in the sera of many of these patients, desensitization to these antigens has not been an effective form of therapy. It has not been shown conclusively that bysinnosis is primarily a reaction of hypersensitivity. A current view of pathogenesis is that some dusts of the textile industry contain a substance capable of inducing bronchial and bronchiolar spasm by the non-antigenic release of histamine. Unlike in cases of bronchial asthma, the patients with bysinnosis are not hypersensitive to inhaled histamine. Little is known about the pulmonary histopathologic changes in this disease.

Bagassosis[50, 57]

Bagasse is the fibrous residue of sugar cane after its juice has been extracted. The material is used to manufacture paper, cardboard, and other materials. The pathogenicity of bagasse was first demonstrated in 1937. Pulmonary changes develop following the inhalation of organic dust in the dry fibrous residue. Characteristically, dyspnea is severe and out of proportion to the physical findings. In the great majority of cases recovery is complete, but a few have developed chronic pulmonary disease with reduction in the maximal breathing capacity. The functional abnormalities resemble those found in farmer's lung. Relapses are frequent and are prone to occur at variable periods of time after re-exposure. Structural changes in the lungs have been noted only after prolonged exposure and have consisted chiefly of an interstitial pneumonia with the inflammatory cells predominantly mononuclear. Although the sera of affected persons frequently contain precipitins against extracts of bagasse, these are found almost as frequently in normal unexposed persons. Therapy with corticosteroids can be very effective, restoring pulmonary function practically to normal.

Farmer's Lung[12, 24, 47]

Farmer's lung develops after exposure to moldy organic dusts, such as are found in stale hay. Sensitive subjects develop shortness of breath, fever, cough and chills. Roentgenograms of the chest usually indicate the presence of an interstitial pneumonia. Frequently, there is evidence of a decrease in the vital capacity as well as signs of an alveolar-capillary block. The histopathologic changes in the lungs vary with the stage of the disease. In the early phases, there is interstitial infiltration with mononuclear cells, predominantly lymphocytes, but well-defined granulomas are noted in a minority of cases (9 of 24 cases in one reported series). Later, non-caseating granulomas develop and the changes resemble sarcoidosis or berylliosis. The presence of doubtly refractile bodies, probably particles of the inhaled material, has been noted in about half of the cases. Although the aforementioned changes are reversible, repeated or continued exposure tends to produce pulmonary fibrosis with permanent impairment in pulmonary function. The view that farmer's lung is the result of hypersensitivity is supported by more convincing data than in the case of bysinnosis or bagassosis. The sera of patients with farmer's lung contain precipitins against extracts of mold hay and against extracts of the mold Thermopolyspora polyspora, and inhalation of these extracts by susceptible individuals reproduces the disease.

Maple-bark Stripper's Lung[11, 33, 40]

Hypersensitivity to the spores of the fungus Coniosporium corticale (Cryptostroma corticale), which produces sooty-bark disease in maple trees, is probably the principal cause of maple-bark disease in man. The disorder resembles farmer's lung clinically and in the roentgenographic findings, as well as histologically. Fragments of the fungus can be found in the tissue. They have prominent, thick, brown walls and can be stained with the Grocott stain. Apparently, the organism does not grow in human tissues but persists as a foreign body. Inoculation of extracts of its spores into susceptible individuals elicits an immediate wheal reaction.

Pigeon-breeders Lung[15, 26]

Pigeon-breeder's, or pigeon-fancier's, disease is most frequently an acute disorder which follows within a few hours after contact with pigeons and tends to be accompanied by systemic manifestations. Subacute and chronic types of involvement have also been described. The chronic form may present clinically as progressive dyspnea without systemic manifestations. In affected subjects, manifestations of the disease can be induced by the cutaneous injection of extracts of dust from pigeon feathers or by the injection of sterile pigeon serum. Although the sera of these patients react with pigeon serum in a precipitin immunodiffusion reaction, these antibodies can be demonstrated in the absence of clinical disease. It has been suggested that an Arthus type of reaction underlies the pathogenesis of this disorder, a view supported by the occurrence of vasculitis and thrombosis at the cutaneous sites of antigenic challenge. However, the granulomatous type of pulmonary response is not in keeping with this hypothesis.

Sequoiosis[7] is a granulomatous pneumonia which develops upon the inhalation of sawdust from the redwood tree. Histologic examination reveals the presence of foreign material incrusted with iron and calcium as well as fibers resembling those seen in cases of farmer's lung. Michaels has described the development of pulmonary lesions in workers exposed to wood dust for many years.[38] The changes included fibrosis and centrilobular emphysema as well as the intra-alveolar accumulation of basophilic bodies associated with a foreign-body response. The sera of the affected individuals usually contain antibodies against antigens in the sawdust itself, or against molds or fungi in the sawdust.

Suberosis[2] affects workers in the cork industry. Clinically, the manifestations resemble bronchial asthma, and alveolitis as well as vasculitis have been found to be prominent histologic findings. This disorder is probably also the result of hypersensitivity.

The pulmonary lesions which may develop following the inhalation of pituitary snuff[43] probably represent hypersensitive reactions to bovine and porcine proteins in the extract. Although the offending antigen has not been identified, it is likely that hypersensitivity underlies the pathogenesis of mushroom worker's disease. Allergic pulmonary reactions to species of Aspergillus[27, 45] have been described. The aspiration of larger particles of vegetable matter can also produce, of course, a foreign-body granulomatous pneumonia.[37, 55]

REFERENCES

1. Arnoldsson, H., Bouhuys, A., and Lindell, S. E.: Byssinosis. Acta Med. Scand., *173*:761, 1963.
2. Avila, R., and Villar, T. G.: Suberosis. Lancet, *1*:620, 1968.
3. Berkley, C., Churg, J., and Selikoff, I. J.: The detection and localization of mineral fibers in tissue. Ann. N. Y. Acad. Sc., *132*:48, 1965.
4. Bouhuys, A.: Byssinosis in textile workers. Trans. N. Y. Acad. Sc., *28*:480, 1966.
5. Bouhuys, A., Heaphy, L. J., Jr., Schilling, R. S. F., and Welborn, J. W.: Byssinosis in the United States. N. Eng. J. Med., *277*:170, 1967.
6. Buchanan, W. D.: Asbestosis and primary intrathoracic neoplasms. Ann. N. Y. Acad. Sc., *132*: 507, 1965.
7. Cohen, H. I., Merigan, T. C., Kosek, J. C., and Eldridge, F.: Sequoiosis. A granulomatous pneumonitis associated with redwood sawdust inhalation. Am. J. Med., *43*:785, 1967.
8. Curran, R. C.: Observation on the formation of collagen in quartz lesions. J. Path. & Bact., *66*:271, 1953.
9. Doig, A. T., and McLaughlin, A. I. G.: X-ray appearances of lungs of electric arc welders. Lancet, *1*:771, 1936.
10. Duguid, J. B., and Lambert, M. W.: The pathogenesis of coal miner's pneumoconiosis. J. Path. & Bact., *88*:389, 1964.
11. Emanuel, D. A., Lawton, B. R., and Wenzel, F. J.: Maple-bark disease: Pneumonitis due to coniosporum corticale. N. Eng. J. Med., *266*: 7, 1962.
12. Emanuel, D. A., Wenzel, F. J., Bowerman, C. I., and Lawton, B. R.: Farmer's lung. Clinical, pathologic and immunologic study of 24 patients. Am. J. Med., *37*:392, 1964.
13. Enterline, P. E.: Mortality among asbestos products workers in the United States. Ann. N. Y. Acad. Sc., *132*:156, 1965.
14. Epstein, W. L., Skahen, J. R., and Kransnobrod, H.: The organized epithelioid cell granuloma: differentiation of allergic (zirconium) from colloidal (silica) types. Am. J. Path., *43*:391, 1963.
15. Fink, J. N., Sosman, A. J., Barboriak, J. J., Schlueter, D. P., and Holmes, R.A.: Pigeon breeder's disease. A clinical study of a hypersensitivity pneumonitis. Ann. Int. Med., *68*: 1205, 1968.
16. Fourman, P.: Investigation of nephrocalcinosis and nephrolithiasis. J. Clin. Path., *18*:568, 1965.
17. Gaensler, E. A., Cadigan, J. B., Sasahara, A. A., Fox, E. O., and Mac Mahon, H. E.: Graphite pneumoconiosis of electrotypers. Am. J. Med., *41*:864, 1966.
18. Gough, J.: Differential diagnosis in the pathology of a asbestosis. Ann. J. Y. Acad. Sc., *132*: 368, 1965.
19. Gross, P.: The perivascular spaces in the lung. Arch. Path., *66*:605, 1958.
20. Gross, P., de treville, T. P., Cralley, L. J. and Davis, J. M. G.: Pulmonary ferruginous bodies. Arch. Path., *85*:539, 1968.
21. Gross, P., Westrick, M. L., and McNerney, J. M.: Silicosis: the topographic relationship of mineral deposits to histologic structures. Am. J. Path., *32*:739, 1956.
22. ————: The pulmonary response to certain chronic irritants. Arch. Path., *68*:252, 1959.
23. Hammond, E. C., Selikoff, I. J., and Churg, J.: Neoplasia among insulation workers in the United States and special reference to intraabdominal neoplasia. Ann. J. Y. Acad. Sc., *132*: 519, 1965.
24. Hapke, E. J., Seal, R. M. E., and Thomas, G. O., with Hayes, M. and Meek, J. C.: Farmer's lung. A clinical, radiographic, functional and serological correlation of acute and chronic stages. Thorax, *23*:451, 1968.
25. Hardy, H. L.: Personal communication.
26. Hargreave, F. E. Pepys, J., Longbottom, J. L., and Wraith, D. G.: Bird breeder's (fancier's) lung. Lancet, *1*:445, 1966.
27. Henderson, A. H.: Allergic aspergillosis: review of 32 cases. Thorax, *23*:501, 1968.
28. Heppleston, A. G.: A typical reaction to inhaled silica. Nature, *213*:199, 1967.
29. Holt, P. F., Mills, J., and Young, D. K.: Experimental asbestosis with four types of fibers: importance of small particles. Ann. N. Y. Acad. Sc., *132*:87, 1965.
30. King, E. J., Harrison, C. V., Mohanty, G. P., and Nagelschmidt, G.: Effects of various forms of alumina on lungs of rats. J. Path. & Bact., *69*:81, 1955.
31. Kiviluoto, R.: Pleural plaques and asbestos: Further observations on endemic and other nonoccupational asbestosis. Ann. N. Y. Acad. Sc., *132*:235, 1965.
32. Kleinfeld, M.: Pleural calcification as a sign of silicatosis. Am. J. Med. Sc., *251*:215, 1966.
33. Liebow, A. A., and Carrington, C. B.: Hypersensitivity reactions involving the lung. Tr. & Studies Coll. Phys. Phila., *34*:47, 1966.
34. Lipworth, E., Bloomberg, B. M., and Reid, F. P.: Urinary calculi containing silica: a case report. South African M. J., *38*:50, 1964.
35. Massoud, A., and Taylor, G.: Byssinosis: antibody to cotton antigens in normal subjects and in cotton card-rom workers. Lancet, *2*:607, 1964.
36. McLaughlin, A. I. G., Grout, J. L. A., Barrie, H. J., and Harding, H. E.: Iron oxide dust and

the lungs of silver polishers. Lancet, *1:*337, 1945.

37. Merriam, J. C., Jr., Storrs, R. C., and Hoefnagel: Lung disease caused by aspirated timothy-grass heads. Am. Rev. Desp. Dis., *90:* 947, 1964.
38. Michaels, L.: Lung changes in woodworkers. Canad. M. A. J., *96:*1150, 1967.
39. Michel, R. D., and Morris, J. F.: Acute silicosis. Arch. Int. Med., *113:*850, 1964.
40. Pepys, J.: Pulmonary hypersensitivity diseases due to inhaled organic antigens. Ann. Int. Med., *64:*943, 1966.
41. Pernis, B., Vigliani, E. C. and Selikoff, I. J.: Rheumatoid factor in serum of individuals exposed to asbestos. Ann. N. Y. Acad. Sc., *132:* 112, 1965.
42. Prine, J. R., Brokeshoulder, S. F., McVean, D. E., and Robinson, F. R.: Demonstration of the presence of beryllium in pulmonary granulomas. Am. J. Clin. Path., *45:*448, 1966.
43. Rankin, J., Kobayashi, M., Barbee, R. A., and Dickie, H. A.: Pulmonary granulomatoses due to inhaled organic antigens. Med. Clin. N. A., *51:*459, 1967.
44. Dayl, D. F., and Spjut, H. J.: Pneumonic reaction induced by bronchogenic medium: clinical and experimental study. Am. Rev. Resp. Dis., *89:*503, 1964.
45. Riddle, H. F. V., Channell, S., Blyth, W., Weir, D. M., Lloyd, M., Amas, W. M. G., and Grant, I. W. B.: Allergic alveolitis in a malt worker. Thorax, *23:*271, 1968.
46. Schepers, G. W. H.: Pulmonary histologic reactions to inhaled fiberglas-plastic dust. Am. J. Path., *35:*1160, 1959.
47. Seal, R. M. E., Hapke, E. J., and Thomas, G. O., with Meek, J. C. and Hayes, M.: The pathology of the acute and chronic stages of farmer's lung. Thorax, *23:*469, 1968.
48. Selikoff, I. J.: The occurrence of pleural calcification among asbestos insulation workers. Ann. N. Y. Acad. Sc., *32:*359, 1965.
49. Shaver, C. G.: Pulmonary changes encountered in employees engaged in the manufacture of alumina abrasives. Occup. Med., *5:*718, 1948.
50. Smettana, H., Tandon, H. G., Viswanathan, R., Venkitasubramanian, T. A., Chandrasekhar, S., and Randhawa, H. S.: Experimental bagasse disease of the lung. Lab. Invest., *11:*868, 1962.
51. Spencer, H.: Pathology of the Lung. N. Y., The MacMillan Co., 1962.
52. Tapp, E.: Beryllium induced sarcomas of the rabbit tibia. Brit. J. Cancer, *20:*778, 1966.
53. Town, A. D.: Pseudoasbestos bodies and asteroid giant cells in a patient with graphite pneumoconiosis. Canad. M. A. J., *98:*100, 1968.
54. Van Ordstrand, H. S., Hughes, R., Denardi, J. M., and M. G. Carmody: Beryllium poisoning. J.A.M.A., *129:*1084, 1945.
55. Vidyarthi, S. C.: Diffuse military granulomatosis of the lungs due to aspirated vegetable cells. Arch. Path., *83:*215, 1967.
56. Vigliani, E. C., and Pernis, B.: Immunological factors in the pathogenesis of the hyaline tissue of silicosis. Brit. J. Indust. Med., *15:*8, 1958.
57. Weill, H., Buechner, H. A., González, E., Herbert, S. J., Aucoin, E., and Ziskind, M. M.: Bagassosis: A study of pulmonary function in 20 cases. Ann. Int. Med., *64:*737, 1966.

Chapter 44

Pulmonary Carcinogenesis from Exposure to Toxic Agents

F. WILLIAM SUNDERMAN, JR., M.D.

Ever since the Middle Ages, a pulmonary disease known as "Bergsucht" or "mountain consumption" has been known to be endemic among the miners of metallic ore in the vicinity of Schneeberg in Saxony.[1] The studies of Härting and Hesse in 1879 showed that "Bergsucht" actually represented pulmonary cancer, and provided the first recognition that pulmonary carcinogenesis might result from occupational exposures to toxic agents.[2] Subsequent investigations have demonstrated that inhalation of radioactive particles was the probable etiologic factor in pulmonary neoplasia among the Schneeberg miners.[3]

Knowledge of pulmonary carcinogenesis from inhalation of toxic agents has developed according to the customary sequence of elucidation of environmental and occupational carcinogens (Table 1). Clinical observations and epidemiological studies have generally furnished the stimulus for animal experiments, which in turn, have lead to the identification of the putative carcinogens. Investigations of the metabolism of the putative carcinogens have oftimes resulted in the isolation of more potent carcinogenic metabolites, (i.e. the proximate carcinogens). In some instances, synthesis of chemical congeners has lead to the discovery of compounds which are even more carcinogenic than the proximate carcinogens. As final steps in the typical sequence, it has frequently been possible to demonstrate carcinogen binding to nucleic acids and tissue proteins. In certain experimental systems, the carcinogens have been shown to induce acute alterations in the expression of genetic information.

TABLE 1 — CUSTOMARY SEQUENCE IN THE INVESTIGATION OF AN ENVIRONMENTAL OR OCCUPATIONAL CARCINOGEN

1. Clinical observation
2. Epidemiological substantiation
3. Carcinogenesis in experimental animals
4. Identification of putative carcinogen (s)
5. Elucidation of carcinogen metabolism
6. Isolation of active metabolites
7. Synthesis of carcinogenic analogs
8. Demonstration of:
   a. carcinogen binding to tissue proteins and nucleic acids
   b. Alteration of gene action system

In Table 2 are listed the chemical agents which have been shown by clinical and epidemiological studies to be associated with increased incidence of respiratory cancer,[3-5] and in Table 3 are listed the compounds which have been estabished as respiratory carcinogens by animal experimentation.[3-8] Selected references are cited in Table 3 to aid the

TABLE 2 — RESPIRATORY CARCINOGENS IMPLICATED BY EPIDEMIOLOGICAL STUDIES[3-6]

Organic Products and Compounds
Coal tar, coal gas and soot
Cigarette smoke and tar
Combustion products of petroleum
Crude isopropanol
Mineral oil
Mustard gas
Inorganic Substances
Minerals: asbestos
Metals: nickel, chromium, beryllium, arsenic, iron
Radioactive Particulates: uranium, plutonium, radium

reader who wishes further information regarding each of these carcinogens. For many of the compounds included in Table 3, the experimental evidence of carcinogenicity now includes the gamut of parameters which were cited in Table 1.

From a public health standpoint, principal attention has been focused upon the carcinogenic compounds which occur in urban atmospheres and in cigarette smoke[4, 57-60] (Table 4). The carcinogens which are present in urban atmospheres include polycyclic aromatic hydrocarbons, the epoxide and peroxide combustion products of petroleum, and metals such as nickel, chromium, and beryllium. Cigarette smoke contains carcinogenic polycyclic aromatic hydrocarbons, het-

TABLE 3 — RESPIRATORY CARCINOGENS IMPLICATED BY EXPERIMENTAL STUDIES

Compound	*Species**	*References*
Polycyclic Aromatic Hydrocarbons:		
3,4-benzpyrene	a, b, c	8-10
methylcholanthrene	a, b, f	11-15
dimethylbenzanthracene	a, b, c, g	8,16-20
Nitrosodialkylamines:		
dimethylnitrosamine	a, b	9,21-22
diethylnitrosamine	c, e	23,24
diamylnitrosamine	b	25
N-Nitroso Compounds:		
N-nitrosopiperidine	c	26
N-nitrosomorpholine	c	27
N-nitrosomethylurethan	b	28
Aromatic Amines:		
trifluoroacetamidofluorene	b	29
Dietary Factors:		
aflatoxin	b	30
cycasin	b	31,32
Other Organic Compounds:		
urethan	a	33-35
uracil mustard	a	36
4-nitroquinoline-N-oxide	a, b	37,38
Non-metallic Inorganic Compounds:		
diazomethane	b	39
hydrazine	b	40
Minerals:		
asbestos	b, f	41-43
Metals:		
nickel	a, b, d	44-48
chromium	a, b	49,50
beryllium	b, h	51,52
Radioactive Chemicals:		
^{90}Strontium	b	53
^{144}Cerium	b	54
^{239}Plutonium	g	55,56

*a = mouse e = rabbit
b = rat f = duck or fowl
c = hamster g = dog
d = guinea pig h = monkey

TABLE 4 — CARCINOGENS FOUND IN CIGARETTE SMOKE AND URBAN ATMOSPHERES

URBAN ATMOSPHERES[4,57]
Polycyclic Aromatic Hydrocarbons: 3,4-benzpyrene, benzofluoranthracene
Combustion Products of Petroleum: epoxides and peroxides
Metals: nickel, chromium, beryllium
CIGARETTE SMOKE[58-60]
Polycyclic Aromatic Hydrocarbons: 3,4-benzpyrene, dibenzpyrene benzanthracene, dibenzanthracene, benzophenanthracene
Heterocyclic Aromatic Hydrocarbons: dibenzacridine, dibenzcarbazol
Nitrosodiakylamines: methybutylnitrosamine
Metals: nickel, arsenic
Radioactive Compounds: ^{210}Polonium

erocyclic compounds, nitrosodialkylamines, nickel, arsenic, and traces of radioactivity, principally in the form of ^{210}polonium. In quantitative terms, 3,4-benzpyrene appears to be the principal carcinogen in both urban atmospheres and cigarette smoke.[57-60] A carcinogenic synergism among the constituents of cigarette tar has been postulated, inasmuch as the carcinogenic potency of cigarette tar is greater than the sum of its known carcinogenic ingredients.[58]

Epidemiological studies have furnished evidence that exposures to combinations of carcinogenic agents may be important in the development of pulmonary cancers. As a classic example, the age-specific male death rates for lung cancer in the U.S.A. in 1958 are listed in Table 5, categorized according to smoking habits and degree of urbanization.[5, 61] It may be seen that, according to Hammond and Horn,[61] the annual death rate from lung cancer was virtually nil among rural non-smokers, and that it reached 15 cases per 100,000 among urban non-smokers. The annual death rate from lung cancer among rural cigarette smokers was 65 per 100,000, and it increased to 85 per 100,000 among urban cigarette smokers.

TABLE 5 — DEATH RATE FROM LUNG CANCER BY PLACE OF RESIDENCE AND SMOKING HABITS[5, 61]

Locale	*Death Rate**
Rural Areas	
Never Smoked Regularly	0.0
Cigarette Smokers	65.2
Suburbs or Small Towns	
Never Smoked Regularly	4.7
Cigarette Smokers	71.7
Cities of 10,000-50,000	
Never Smoked Regularly	9.3
Cigarette Smokers	70.9
Cities of 50,000 or more	
Never Smoked Regularly	14.7
Cigarette Smokers	85.2

*Annual rate per 100,00 men age 50-69 years, standardized for age; cases with well-established diagnoses only, excluding adenocarcinoma.

An even more impressive illustration of the effect of combined exposures to carcinogenic factors is furnished by Selikoff and co-workers' recent study[62] of smoking habits in asbestos workers (Table 6) . Among 370 asbestos workers in the New York City area, no deaths from bronchogenic carcinoma were observed in 48 subjects who never smoked regularly, or 39 subjects who smoked only pipes or cigars. In contrast, 24 deaths from bronchogenic carcinoma were observed in 283 asbestos workers who regularly smoked cigarettes. The expected death rate from bronchogenic carcinoma among such cigarette smokers would have been 2.98, based upon the age-specific male death rates. Therefore, the proportionate mortality from bronchogenic carcinoma among the asbestos workers who smoked cigarettes was 8.1 times the mortality among men in other occupations who smoked cigarettes. Com-

TABLE 6 — EFFECT OF SMOKING HABITS UPON DEATHS FROM BRONCHOGENIC CARCINOMA IN ASBESTOS WORKERS[62]

Smoking Habits	*No. of Subjects*	*Expected Deaths*[a]	*Observed Deaths*	*Proportionate Mortalities*
Never smoked regularly	48	0.05	0	—
Pipe or cigar only	39	0.13	0	—
Regular cigarette smoking[b]	283	2.98	24	8.1[c]
All Subjects	370	3.16	24	7.6

[a]Based upon age-specific male death rates in U.S.A., adjusted according to smoking habits.
[b]Includes cigarette smokers who also smoked pipe or cigars.
[c]Proportionate mortality vs. C.S.A. non-smoking males = 92.

pared to non-smoking males in other occupations, the proportionate mortality associated with combined exposures to asbestos and cigarette smoke was 92 times.[62]

A relatively recent development in knowledge of pulmonary carcinogenesis has been the recognition that nickel and other trace metals may contribute to the carcinogenicity of tobacco smoke, asbestos fibers, and urban atmospheres. As listed in Table 7, measurements of the

TABLE 7 — IMPLICATION OF NICKEL AS A CARCINOGEN IN TOBACCO SMOKE

Author	*Date*	*Tobacco*	*No. of Brands Tested*	*Ni Content (μg Ni Per Cigarette)*
Cogbill + Hobbs[63]	1957	American		2.0
Voss + Nicol[64]	1960	Not stated	11	6.2 (3.6-11.0)
Sunderman + Sunderman[65]	1961	American	4	2.0[a] (1.6-2.5)
Fresh et al.[66]	1967	American	15	5.4 (0.2-11.6)
		Formosan	12	4.3 (1.1-14.0)

[a]20% of the Ni was recovered in the main-stream smoke. A heavy cigarette smoker (2 packs per day) would inhale approximately 5.8 mg Ni per year

average nickel content of cigarettes have ranged from 2.0 to 6.2 mg of nickel per cigarette.[63-66] Based upon the observation that 20 percent of nickel in cigarettes is released into the main-stream smoke, it is estimated that a smoker who inhales the main-stream smoke from 2 packs of cigarettes per day would be exposed to approximately 6 mg of nickel per year. The analyses given in Table 8 indicate that significant amounts of nickel are present in the crysotile variety of asbestos from Africa and Canada.[43, 67-71] Cralley and associates[69] have reported airborne levels of nickel in asbestos textile plants which are comparable to the levels of atmospheric nickel in nickel refineries. Measurements of nickel concentrations in urban atmospheres are summarized in Table 9.[72-74] The recent development of nickel additives for automobile gasoline may produce even greater atmospheric contamination with nickel. The importance of nickel as a pulmonary car-

TABLE 8 — IMPLICATION OF NICKEL AS A CARCINOGEN IN ASBESTOS

Author	*Date*	*Origin of Asbestos*	*Nickel Content of Asbestos (μg Ni/gm)*			
			Crocidolite	*Anthophylite*	*Amosite*	*Chrysotile*
Harington[67]	1965	Africa	< 10		80	5000
Gross *et al.*[43]	1967	Canada	<100		<100	135
Cralley *et al.*[68]	1967	Africa				1400
		Canada				1000
Jagatic *et al.*[69]	1967	Not Specified				4000
Dixon + Stokinger[70]	1968	Not Specified				1509
Cralley *et al.*[71]	1968	UICC Reference Samples (Particle size <10μ)	139	414	105	1676

cinogen, and current knowledge of nickel carcinogenesis have been discussed in a recent review article.[75]

Despite much speculation, there is presently little factual information regarding the mechanisms of the neoplastic transformation. Unknown steps link the carcinogen-induced acute alterations in expression of genetic information with the eventual development of neoplasms. Why is the control of cell replication impaired, and why is cellular differentiation altered in the neoplastic cell? How do cancer cells acquire their invasive and metastatic properties? Why is there a protracted latent period between the initial interaction of carcinogens with informational or regulatory macromolecules, and the ultimate development of clinically apparent cancer? Until answers are obtained to these fundamental questions in cancer biology, our understanding of pulmonary carcinogenesis from exposure to toxic agents will remain essentially empirical. Nonetheless, the identification of pulmonary carcinogens and the development of effective methods for safeguarding against exposure to these carcinogens will continue to contribute to the prevention and control of pulmonary cancer.

TABLE 9 — NICKEL CONCENTRATIONS IN URBAN ATMOSPHERES

Author	*Date*	*Location*	*μgNi/1000 cu meters*	
			Mean	*Range*
Tabor & Warren[72]	1958	20 cities in U.S.A.	26	8-47
Stocks[73]	1966	5 cities in Great Britain and Scandinavia	—	5-200
Sawicki[74]	1967	80 cities in U.S.A.	30	—

REFERENCES

1. Agricola, G.: De Re Metallica, Basel, 1597. Cited by Hueper, W. C.: Occupational and Environmental Cancers of the Respiratory System. New York, Springer-Verlag, 1966, p. 127.
2. Härting, F. H., and Hesse, M.: Der Lungenkrebs, die Bergkrankheit in den Schneeberger Gruben. Vjschr. Med. Gericht. K., *30*:296-309, 1879; *31*:102-132, 1879; *31*:313-337, 1879.
3. Hueper, W. C.: Occupational and Environmental Cancer of the Respiratory System. New York, Springer-Verlag, 1966, pp. 128-131.
4. Kotin, P.: Carcinogenesis of the lung: Environmental and host factors. *In,* The Lung (Eds.: Liebow, A. A. and Smith, D. E.). Baltimore, Williams and Wilkins, 1968, pp. 203-225.
5. Doll, R.: Preesnt knowledge of the causation of carcinoma of the lung. *In,* Carcinoma of the Lung (Ed.: Bignall, J. R.) Edinburgh, Livingstone, Ltd., 1958, pp. 43-114.
6. Kinosita, R.: Experimental lung tumors in animals. *In,* Lung Tumors in Animals (Ed.: Severi, L.). Perugia, Italy, Division of Cancer Research, 1966, pp. 59-84.
7. Stewart, H. L.: Comparison of histologic lung cancer types in captive wild mammals and birds and laboratory and domestic animals. *In,* Lung Tumors in Animals (Ed.: Severi, L.). Perugia, Italy, Division of Cancer Research, 1966, pp. 25-58.
8. Saffiotti, U.: Experimental respiratory tract carcinogenesis. Prog. Exp. Tumor Res., *11*:302-333, 1969.

9. Pylev, L. N.: Induction of lung cancer in rats by intratracheal insufflation of carcinogenic hydrocarbons. Acta Unio. Intern. Contra Cancrum, *19:*688-691, 1962.
10. Toth, B. and Shubik, P.: Carinogenesis in AKR mice injected at birth with benzo (a) pyrene and dimethylnitrosamine. Cancer Res., *27:* 43-47, 1967.
11. Rigdon, R. H.: Pulmonary neoplasms produced by methylcholanthrene in the white Pekin duck. Cancer Res., *21:*571-574, 1961.
12. Brown, C. E.: Carcinoma of rat lung from intrapleural methylcholanthrene. Arch. Path., *76:* 347-353, 1963.
13. Stanton, M. F., and Blackwell, R.: Induction of epidermoid carcinoma in lungs of rats: A "new" method based upon deposition of methylcholanthrene in areas of pulmonary infarction. J. Nat. Cancer. Inst., *27:*375-407, 1961.
14. Stevenson, J. L., and von Hamm, E.: Induction of pulmonary tumors in C57BL mice using strings impregnated with 20-methylcholanthrene. Acta Cytol., *7:*126-128, 1963.
15. Blenkinsopp, W. K., Relationship of injury to chemical carcinogenesis in the lungs of rats. J. Nat. Cancer Inst., *40:*651-661, 1968.
16. Howell, J. S.: Intranasal administration of 9, 10-dimethyl-1,2-benzanthracene to rats: The development of breast and lung tumors. Brit. J. Cancer, *15:*263-269, 1961.
17. Walters, M. A., and Roe, F. J. C.: The effect of dietary casein on the induction of lung tumors by the injection of 9,10-dimethyl-1,2-benzanthracene (DMBA) into new born mice. Brit. J. Cancer, *18:*312-316, 1964.
18. Della Porta, G., Kolb., L., and Shubik, P.: Induction of tracheobronchial carcinomas in the Syrian hamster. Cancer Res., *18:*592-597, 1958.
19. Beattie, E. J., Jr., Staub, E. W., Correll N., and Hass, G.: Bronchogenic carcinoma produced experimentally in the dog. J. Thoracic Cardiovasc. Surg., *42:*615-622, 1961.
20. Walters, M. A.: The induction of lung tumors by the injection of 9,10-dimethyl-1,2-benzanthracene (DMBA) into newborn suckling and young adult mice. Brit. J. Cancer, *20:*148-160, 1966.
21. Zak, F. G., Holzner, J. H., Singer, E. J., and Popper, H.: Renal and pulmonary tumors in rats fed dimethylnitrosamine. Cancer Res., *20:* 96-99, 1960.
22. Takayama, S., and Oota, K.: Malignant tumors induced in mice fed with N-nitrosodimethylamine. Gann, *54:*465-471, 1963.
23. Rapp, H. J., Carleton, J. H., Crisler, C., and Nadel, E. M.: Induction of malignant tumors in the rabbit by oral administration of diethylnitrosamine. J. Nat. Cancer Inst. *34:*453-458, 1965.
24. Dontenwill, W., and Mohr, U.: Carcinome des Respirationstructus nach Behandlung can Goldhamstern mit Diäthylnitrosamin. Z. Krebsforsch., *64:*305-312, 1961.
25. Druckrey, H., and Preussmann, R.: Erzeugung von Lungenkrebs durch subcutane Injektion von N,N-Diamylnitrosamin an Ratten. Naturwissenschaften, *49:*111-113, 1962.
26. Dontenwill, W., and Mohr, U.: Die organotrope Wirkung der Nitrosamine. Z. Krebsforsch., *65:*166-167, 1962.
27. Dontenwill, W., and Mohr, U.: Die Wirkung von Tabakrauch Kondensaten und Zigarettenrauch auf die Lunge des Goldhamsters. Z. Krebsforsch, *65:*62-71, 1962.
28. Druckrey, H., Preussmann, R., Afkham, J., and Blum, G.: Erzegung von Lungenkrebs durch Methylnitrosourenthan bei intravenöser Gabe an Ratten. Naturwissenschaften, *49:*451-452, 1962.
29. Morris, H. P., Wagner, B. P., Ray, F. E., Stewart, H. L., and Snell, K. C.: Carcinogenic effects of N,N[1],2,7-fluorenylenebis-2,2,2-trifluoroacetamide administered orally to Buffalo strain rats. J. Nat. Cancer Inst., *30:*143-162, 1963.
30. Butler, W. H., and Barnes, J. M.: Toxic effects of groundnut meal containing aflatoxin to rats and guinea pigs. Brit. J. Cancer, *17:*699-710, 1963.
31. Laqueur, G. L., Mickelsen, O., Whiting, M. G., and Kurland, L. T.: Carcinogenic properties of nuts from *Cycas Circinalis L.,* indigenous to Guam. J. Nat. Cancer Inst., *31:*919-952, 1963.
32. Hirono, I, Laqueur, G. L., and Spatz, M.: Tumor induction in Fischer and Osborne-Mendel rats by a single administration of cycasin. J. Nat. Cancer Inst., *40:*1003-1026, 1968.
33. De Benedictis, G., Malorano, G., Chilco-Bianchi, L., and Fiore-Donati, L.: Lung carcinogenesis by urethan in newborn suckling and adult Swiss mice. Brit. J. Cancer, *16:*686-689, 1962.
34. Lindop, P. J., and Rotblat, J.: Induction of lung tumors by action of radiation and urethan. Nature, *210:*1392-1393, 1966.
35. Kaye, A.M., and Trainin, N.: Urethan carcinogenesis and nucleic acid metabolism: factors influencing lung adenoma formation. Cancer Res., *26:*2206-2212, 1966.
36. Abell, C. W., Falk, H. L., Shimkin, M. B., Weisberger, E. K., Weisberger, J. H., and Gubareff, N.: Uracil nustard: A potent inducer of lung tumors in mice. Science, *147:*1443-1445, 1965.
37. Mori, K.: Preliminary note on adenocarcinoma of the lung in mice induced with 4-nitroquinoline-N-oxide. Gann, *52:*265-270, 1961.
38. Mori, K.: Induction of pulmonary tumors in

rats by subcutaneous injections of 4-nitroquinoline-N-oxide, Gann, *53:*303-308, 1962.

39. Schoental, R., and Magee, P. N.: Induction of squamous carcinoma of the lung and of the stomach and esophagus by diazomethane and N-methyl-N-nitrosourethane, resepctively. Brit. J. Cancer, *16:*92-100, 1962.
40. Bianchifiore, C., and Ribacchi, R.: Pulmonary tumors in mice induced by oral isoniazid and its metabolites. Nature, *194:*488-489, 1962.
41. Peacock, P. R., and Peacock, A.: Asbestos induced tumors in fowls. *In,* Lung Tumors in Animals (Ed.: Severi, L.). Perugia, Italy, Division of Cancer Research, 1966, pp. 558-571.
42. Wagner, J. C.: The induction of tumors by the intrapleural inoculations of various types of asbestos dust. *In,* Lung Tumors in Animals (Ed.: Severi, L.). Perugia, Italy, Division of Cancer Research, 1966, pp. 589-606.
43. Gross, P., De Treville, R. T. P., Tolker, E. G., Kaschak, M., and Babyak, M. A.: Experimental asbestosis: The development of lung cancer in rats with pulmonary deposits of chrysotile asbestos dust. Arch. Environ. Health, *15:*343-355, 1967.
44. Hueper, W. C.: Pulmonary lesions in guinea pigs and rats exposed to prolonged inhalation of powdered metallic nickel. Arch. Path., *65:* 600-607, 1958.
45. Toda, M.: Experimental studies of occupational lung cancer. Bull. Tokyo Med. Dent. U., *9*(3): 440, 1963.
46. Sunderman, F. W., Donnelly, A. J., West, B., and Kinkaid, J. F.: Carcinogenesis in rats exposed to nickel carbonyl. Arch. Industr. Health, *20:*36-41, 1959.
47. Sunderman, F. W., and Donnelly, A. J.: Studies of nickel carcinogenesis: Metastasizing pulmonary tumors in rats induced by the inhalation of nickel carbonyl. Amer. J. Path., *46:* 1027-1041, 1965.
48. Sunderman, F. W.: Metastasizing tumors in rats induced by the inhalation of nickel carbonyl. *In,* Lung Tumors in Animals (Ed.: Severi, L.) Perugia, Italy, Division of Cancer Res., 1966, pp. 551-564.
49. Payne, W. W.: Production of cancers in mice and rats by chromium compounds. Arch. Industr. Health, *21:*530-535, 1960.
50. Hueper, W. C., and Payne, W. W.: Experimental studies in metal cancerigenesis. Chromium Nickel, Iron, Arsenic. Arch. Environ. Health, *5:*445-462, 1962.
51. Schepers, G. W. H.: Biological action of beryllium: Reaction of the monkey to inhaled aerosols. Industr. Med. Surg., *33:*1-16, 1964.
52. Reeves, A. L., Deitch, D., and Vorwald, A. J.: Beryllium carcinogenesis: I. Inhalation exposure of rats to beryllium sulfate aerosol. Cancer Res., *27:*439-445, 1967.
53. Cember, H., and Watson, J. A.: Carcinogenic effects of strontium 90 beads implanted in the lungs of rats. Amer. Indust. Hyg. Assn. J. *19:* 36-42, 1958.
54. Cember, H., and Stemmer, K.: Lung cancer from radiactive cerium chloride Health Phys., *10:*43-48, 1964.
55. Clarke, W. J., Park, J. F., Palotay, J. L., and Bair, W. J.: Bronchoalveolar tumors of the canine lung following inhalation of plutonium particles. Amer. Rev. Resp. Dis., *90:*963-967, 1964.
56. Clarke, W. J., Park, J. F., and Bair, W. J.: Plutonium particle induced neoplasia of the canine lung. II. Histophathology and conclusions. *In,* Lung Tumors in Animals (Ed.: Severi, L.) Perugia, Italy, Division of Cancer Research, 1966, pp. 345-355.
57. Kotin, P., and Falk, H. L.: Atmospheric factors in pathogenesis of lung cancer. Advances Cancer Res., *7:*475-514, 1963.
58. Bayne-Jones, S., Burdette, W. J., Cochran, W. G., Farber, E., Fieser, L. F., Furth, J., Hickam, J. B., LeMaistre, C., Schuman, L. M., and Seevers, M. H.: Report of the Advisory Committee to the Surgeon General of the Public Health Service on Smoking and Health. U.S.P.H.S. Publication No. 1103, U. S. Government Printing Office, Washington, D. C., 1964, pp. 387.
59. Wynder, E. L., and Hofman, D.: Experimental tobacco carcinogenesis. Advances Cancer Res., *8:*249-453, 1964, Academic Press, New York.
60. Wynder, E. L., and Hofman, D.: Tobacco and Tobacco Smoke: Studies in Experimental Carcinogenesis. Academic Press, New York, 1966, pp. 317-494.
61. Hammond, E. C., and Horn, D.: Smoking and death rates. Report on 44 months of follow-up of 187,783 men. J.A.M.A., *166:*(10) 1159-1172, and *166:* (11) 1294-1308, 1958.
62. Selikoff, I. J., Hammond, and Churg, J.: Asbestos exposure, smoking and neoplasia. J.A.M.A., *204:*104-110, 1968.
63. Cogbill, E. C., and Hobbs, M. E.: Transfer of metallic constituents of cigarettes to the mainstream smoke. Tobacco Science, *1:*68-73, 1957.
64. Voss, R. C., and Nicol, H.: Metallic trace elements in tobacco. Lancet, *2:*435-436, 1960.
65. Sunderman, F. W., and Sunderman, F. W., Jr.: Nickel poisoning. II. Implication of nickel as a pulmonary carcinogen in tobacco smoke. Amer. J. Clin. Path., *35:*203-209, 1961.
66. Fresh, J. W., Sun, S. C., and Rampsch, J. W.: Nasopharyngeal carcinoma and environmental carcinogens. *In,* Cancer of the Nasopharynx

(Eds.: Mur, C. S. and Shanmugaratnam, D.). Unio Internat. Contra Cancrum Monograph No. 1, pp. 124-129, 1967, Munksgaard Press, Copenhagen.

67. Harington, J. S.: Chemical studies of asbestos. Ann. New York Acad. Sci., *132:*31-47, 1965.
68. Cralley, L. J., Keenan, R. G., and Lynch, J. R.: Exposure to metals in the manufacture of asbestos textile products. Amer. Indust. Hyg. Assn. J., *28:*452-461, 1967.
69. Jagatic, J., Rubnitz, M. E., Godwin, M. C., and Weiskopf, R. W.: Tissue response of intra-peritoneal asbestos with preliminary report of acute toxicity of heat treated asbestos in mice. Environ. Res., *1:*217-230, 1967.
70. Dixon, J. R., and Stokinger, H. E.: The role of trace metals in chemical carcinogenesis: The relation of trace metals to asbestos cancers. Prepublication manuscript presented at the Seventh Annual Meeting of the Society of Toxicology, Washington, D. C., March 1968.
71. Cralley, L. J., Keenan, R. G., Kupel, R. E., Kinser, R. E., and Lynch, J. R.: Characterization and solubility of metals associated with asbestos fibers. Amer. Indust. Hyg. Assn. J., *29:* 569-573, 1968.
72. Tabor, E. C., and Warren, W. V.: Distribution of certain metals in the atmosphere of some American cities. Arch. Industr. Health, *17:*145-151, 1958.
73. Stocks, P.: Recent epidemiological studies of lung cancer mortality, cigarette smoking and air pollution, with discussion of a new hypothesis of causation. Brit. J. Cancer, *20:*595-623, 1966.
74. Sawicki, E.: Airborne carcinogens and allied compounds. Arch. Environ. Health *14:*46-53, 1967.
75. Sunderman, F. W., Jr.: Nickel carcinogenesis. Dis. Chest., *54:*527-534, 1968.

Chapter 45

Hematologic Reactions to Drugs

FREDERICK I. VOLINI, M.D., DAVID RESK, M.D., and SHELDON E. KRASNOW, M.D.

INTRODUCTION

The adverse reactions of the hematopoietic system to drugs and chemicals can generally be described in terms of cytopenia, with but few exceptions. The cytopenia may involve one or more cell types. Thus one may observe a thrombocytopenia, leukopenia, or anemia, separately, or depression of all three major elements of the peripheral blood simultaneously, as in aplastic anemia. Myelofibrosis may be a later consequence in some cases of drug-induced aplasia. A leukemic reaction has also been attributed to the effect of drug or chemical exposure, especially in the case of benzene (1). The later type of hematologic reaction is unusual in that the predominate reaction appears to be a proliferative process but probably follows basic changes induced in chromosomes of the cell. A parallel to this may be found in the hyperplasia occasionally found in lymph nodes in some cases of Mesantoin exposure (2).

The mechanism of cytopenia with some drugs and chemicals has been established but in many cases, pathogenesis is unknown. The known mechanisms include: 1) Drug interference with DNA, RNA, or protein metabolism (3); 2) Immune injury in which the drug acts as an haptene, stimulating the production of antibody to the cell whether it be an erythrocyte, leukocyte (4) or platelet; 3) Aggravation of cellular enzyme deficiencies (5) whereby a cellular element has a shortened survival. This mechanism is well established for the erythrocyte deficient in glucose-6-phosphate dehydrogenase but the basic concept of enzyme deficiency may also apply to platelets, neutrophils and other more immature elements of the hematopoietic system; 4) Production of deficiency states such as those involving pyridoxine, folic acid and cyanocobalamin (6).

These four known mechanisms of drug toxicity all tend to produce cytopenia, whether it be thrombocytopenia, leukopenia, anemia or aplastic anemia. The various cytopenias resulting from drugs will be described according to the cell type affected, together with the clinical features of each condition.

I. THROMBOCYTOPENIA

Depression of platelets in the peripheral blood is a well-documented manifestation of drug toxicity and probably accounts for 15% of all reported drug reactions (7). Generally, thrombocytopenia is a relatively benign condition but if ignored, can result in serious bleeding diathesis with fatal outcome.

A. Predictable Drug-induced Thrombocytopenia

As with the other formed elements of the blood, platelets can be severely depressed when the patient is exposed to non-specific cell toxins. This kind of cytopenia is generally well-understood, being an extension of the basic therapeutic action of the drug or chemical. It occurs in almost all individuals exposed to an adequate dose of the agent. The actual severity of the syndrome is directly related to magnitude of the dose and usually many tissues show evidence of cell damage; platelet or blood cell depression being most obvious because of the high turnover rate of these elements. Examples of agents which can regularly induce thrombocytopenia include: 1) Alkylating agents such as nitrogen mustard and its analogues; Antimetabolites such as 6-mercaptopurine, methotrexate, etc.; Periwinkle alkoloids: Vincristine, vinblastine; and actinomycin; 2) Ionizing radiation; 3) Various organic compounds used in industry such as benzene and toluene, and heavy metals such as arsenic.

The mechanism of platelet and other cell depression in these cases varies but is generally found to result from interference with some basic cell function such as DNA or RNA synthesis, protein synthesis and maintenance of cell structure.

B. Unpredictable Drug-induced Thrombocytopenias

The second type of thrombocytopenia is less well-understood, although platelet antibodies have been demonstrated in many instances (8, 9, 10). A typical history with this type of reaction would include: A. A symptom-free period of drug exposure varying from a week to many months, B. Sudden onset of thrombocytopenia with its attendant bleeding diathesis, C. Usually, a rapid return of platelet levels to normal after withdrawal of the offending agent, D. Recurrence of severe thrombocytopenia after "challenge" with the agent. Other features which distinguish this idiosyncratic response include the sporadic appearance of this syndrome (the overwhelming number of patients exposed to the agent never developing platelet depression) and a lack of relationship between the dose of drug and the development of thrombocytopenia.

Many drugs have been implicated as a cause of idiosyncratic platelet depression. Some of these have produced this syndrome many times, as for example quinidine (Fig. 1). Purpura may appear after years of intermittent exposure to the drug. Other important drugs producing the same syndrome (7, 11) include: quinine, antibacterial sulfonamides, such as sulfamethoxpyridazine (Kynex), sulfisoxazole (Gantrisin), sulfonamide derivatives, such as tolbutamide (Orinase), carbutamide, chlorpropamide (Diabinese), acetazolamide (Diamox), thiazide diuretics, such as chlorothiazide (Diuril), hydrochlorothiazide (Hydrodiuril), sedatives and tranquilizers, such as allylisopropylacetylurea (Sedormid), meprobamate (Miltown, Equanil) and miscellaneous agents, such as diphenylhydantoin sodium (Dilantin), phenylbutazone, and digitoxin. Numerous other drugs have been implicated in the occasional case of thrombocytopenia. Some of these drugs have been given together with other medications which renders a clear-cut etiologic relationship very difficult to establish with certainty.

As seen from the length and diversity of the list, idiosyncratic drug thrombocy-

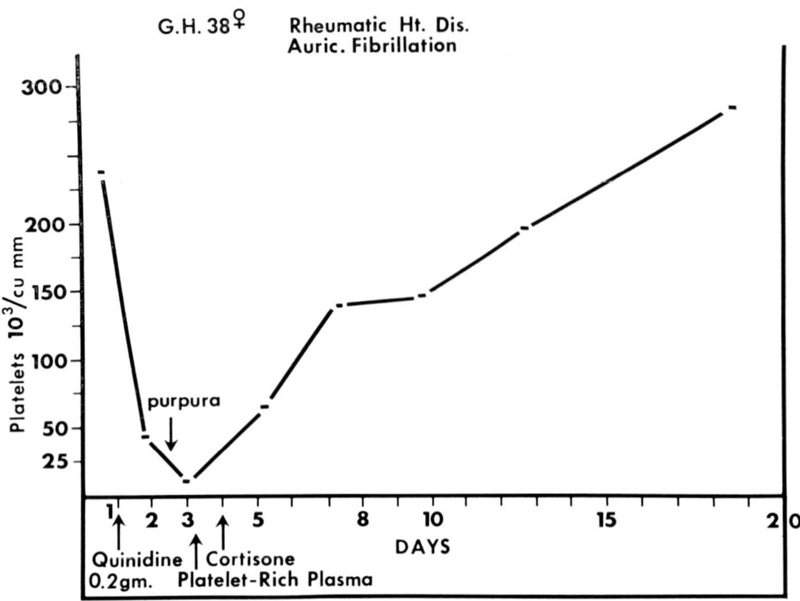

Figure 1. A case of quinidine-induced thrombocytopenia in a 38-year-old female with rheumatic mitral stenosis. The thrombocytopenia developed after 2 years of intermittent use of the drug. The same phenomena was inadvertently induced after a single dose of quinidine three months later.

topenia is not related to a single or small class of biochemical compounds. The clue to this problem resides in the rare "hypersensitive" individual and the nature of his "hypersensitivity."

As previously mentioned, it has been clearly shown that this type of thrombocytopenic purpura is the result of an immune mechanism. Serum factors from affected patients have been shown to cause platelet agglutination in the presence of the offending drug (Fig. 2) and when complement is added, platelet lysis occurs (7). Platelet antibodies have been demonstrated by a variety of other procedures including: A) Inhibition of clot retraction when patient plasma is added to normal blood in the presence of the drug (19); B) Complement fixation during the combination between antibody, platelet, and drug (20, 21); Indirect antiglobulin consumption (22).

The actual mechanism of platelet-drug-antibody interaction is still not entirely clear. Earlier workers in this field considered that the administered drug combined with intact platelets and acted as an haptene to induce platelet antibody formation. Subsequent reaction between the antibody and drug-platelet complex resulted in platelet agglutination and lysis. More recent studies indicate that the administered drug combines with a soluble serum macromolecule and this complex then serves to induce antibody formation. Subsequent antibody reacts with the macromolecule-drug combination to form soluble antigen-antibody complexes. Platelet damage occurs when these antigen-antibody complexes are passively adsorbed onto platelet surfaces (13, 16).

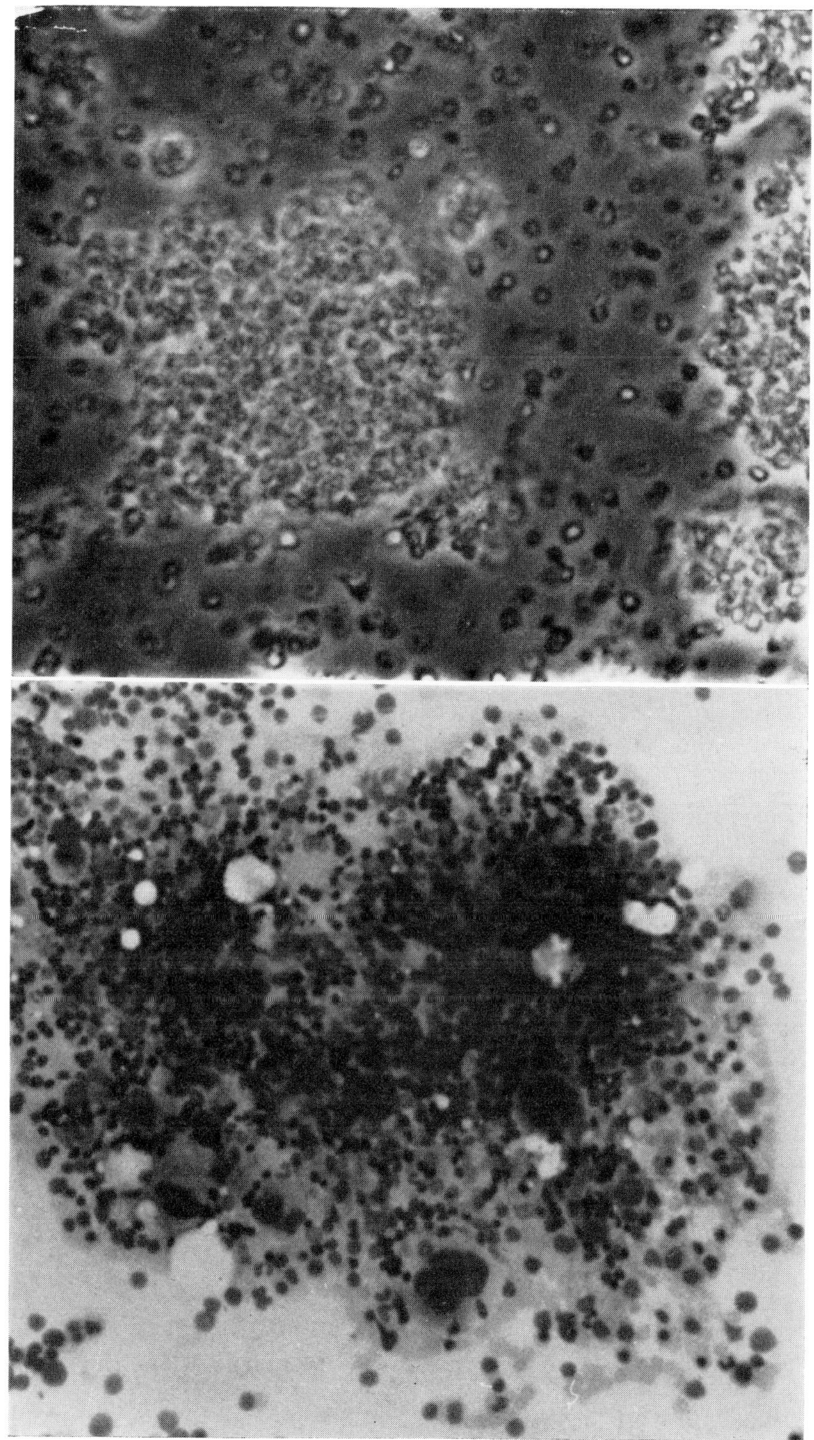

Figure 2. Clumping of platelets observed after incubation of patient's serum with normal donor platelets and quinidine. Controls with normal serum failed to agglutinate platelets.

Figure 3. Marrow particles from a 38-year-old female who developed severe thrombocytopenia following quinidine exposure. Megakaryocytes were markedly increased throughout most particles.

C. Symptomatology and Clinical Course

As expected, symptoms and signs are those of a bleeding diathesis. This may range from a few scattered cutaneous petechiae to fatal intra-cranial hemorrhage (23). More serious hemorrhagic problems are usually limited to those patients who continue to receive the offending drug in the face of manifest thrombocytopenia.

Routine laboratory studies generally are of limited value in pinpointing a specific etiology. Complete blood counts are usually unremarkable except for thrombocytopenia. Bone marrow preparations usually show normal cellularity and composition. There is seldom any morphological abnormality of the megakaryocytes, although they have been described as being increased in some cases (Fig. 3). A fairly simple and rapid method of demonstrating drug-induced anti-platelet antibodies is that which depends on inhibition of clot retraction (19). This procedure probably can be performed in most clinical laboratories and would be of great help in establishing the diagnosis.

D. Treatment

Effective treatment lies in early recognition of the etiology and immediate cessation of the offending agent. Corticosteroids are indicated and should be given in adequate dosage (25, 26). For immediate control of troublesome bleeding, platelet concentrates and fresh whole blood are helpful. Prognosis is excellent, usually with complete disappearance of symptoms and a return of platelet counts to normal within a week to ten days. Serious complications are usually limited to patients who continue to be exposed to the offending agent.

Prevention of the individual attack is at present impossible since there is no way of predicting which individual will develop this type of idiosyncratic response. Serious complications and death in an established case can be prevented by awareness of this syndrome and immediate cessation of the causative drug.

II. AGRANULOCYTOSIS

Agranulocytosis represents one of the most common hematologic reactions to drugs and accounts for approximately 40% of the cases reported to the Registry on Blood Dyscrasias (27). Various types are recognized: 1) The insidious mild neutropenia with little evidence of overall reduction in the total leukocyte count; 2) The acute fulminant agranulocytosis with almost complete absence of granulocytes and marked leukopenia; 3) The chronic granulocytopenia with mild to moderate reduction in neutrophils.

Of greatest importance is the second variety of acute granulocytosis which is an often fatal disease characterized by insidious development of infection, usually of the pharynx associated with fever and prostration. Occasionally, a toxic hepatitis and skin rash may be associated (28). Numerous drugs have been responsible for this type of reaction. Of those reported to the Registry (830 cases), the phenothiazines such as promazine, mepazine, prochlorperazine and imipramine account for approximately 45% of the total. The group of anlgesics together accounted for almost 18%, while sulfonamides, as a group, accounted for 12%. In 7% of cases, chloramphenicol was involved (28). Anti-thyroid drugs such as thiouracil, propylthiouracil and methimazole account for almost 7% of the cases of agranulocytosis.

This syndrome may occur after a single dose of a drug but more commonly it occurs in patients who have received continuous therapy for periods of 1 to 6 weeks or more. It may occur following a single dose of a drug which has been given intermittently over a period of months. In some cases of agranulocytosis, antibodies have been demonstrated by immuno-fluorescence with fluorescein labeled anti-human globulin (29). Also, leukocyte agglutination tests involving a combination of normal donor leukocytes with patient serum have demonstrated drug-dependent antibodies. The intradermal leukocyte skin test may also be positive (30).

Of greatest importance is the prevention of these reactions by means of regular monitoring of the peripheral blood at frequent intervals during the course of therapy. The patient must be apprised of the possibility of drug reaction and report any unusual symptoms such as fever, sore throat, skin rash or jaundice. The drug must be stopped promptly after such symptoms develop and preferably earlier, as indicated, by milder reduction of granulocytes in the peripheral blood.

III. ANEMIA

The anemias induced by drugs may be classified according to the following:

1. Anemia due to depression of red cell precursors in the marrow.
   - A. Isolated erythroid aplasia.
   - B. Aplastic anemia.
2. Anemia due to destruction of erythrocytes.
   - A. Immune hemolytic anemia.
   - B. Oxidant drug-induced hemolytic anemia.
3. Anemia due to interference with nutrients required in erythropoiesis (megaloblastic anemias).

The anemia associated with marrow depression may exhibit a relatively pure form of erythroid aplasia. This has been noted many times and with a variety of drugs. The drug most frequently involved is chloramphenicol (31). Less often the sulfonamides and benzene have been incriminated. The syndrome of erythroid aplasia bears similarity to that found in cases of thymoma. The aplasia may be temporary but in some cases is prolonged, with the development of chronic aplastic anemia. Panhypoplasia of marrow may follow exposure to the cytotoxic drugs with the development of severe anemia. This is usually overshadowed, however, by the associated thrombocytopenia and leukopenia with development of the more serious complications such as bleeding and infection.

Aplastic anemia, a term coined by Ehrlich in 1888, is applied to those clinical states in which the bone marrow is functionally unable to produce red blood cells in the usual number and in which there is usually an associated leukopenia and thrombocytopenia. The marrow is often hypocellular (Fig. 4) but may be hypercellular. As the number of causes for aplastic anemia has increased, the terms applied to this conditon have multiplied so that this syndrome has also been called hypoplastic anemia, aregenerative anemia, and primary refractory anemia. C. Moore has suggested that a better term might be "bone marrow failure."

Classification of aplastic anemias is difficult because of a number of conditions that resemble it, as for example:

1. The megaloblastic states which may cause a pancytopenia but which are

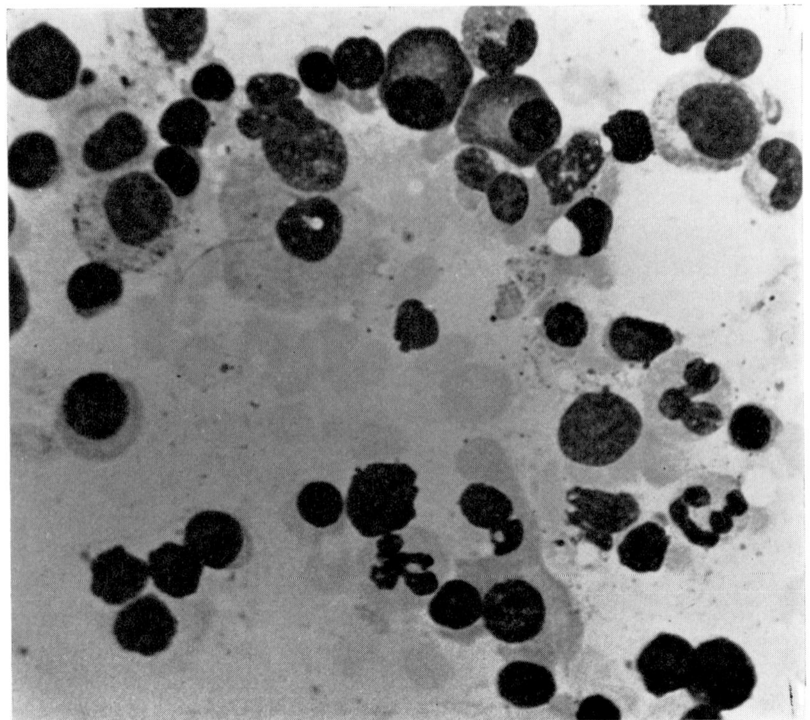

Figure 4. Hypocellular marrow showing depletion of normal myeloid elements. Lymphocytes and plasma cells were the main components of the marrow in this case which followed exposure to sulfonamides.

differentiated by morphology of the marrow.

2. Hypersplenism, which may be differentiated by the presence of a large spleen usually due to a specific etiology. Special studies demonstrating the increased destruction of cells by the spleen or marrow inhibition may be necessary.
3. Lymphoma and the myeloproliferative disorders which may on occasion be difficult to separate from aplastic anemia.

Some uncommon causes of aplastic anemia include:

1. Those associated with thymoma.
2. The refractory sideroblastic anemias.
3. Paroxysmal nocturnal hemoglobinuria (PNH) which can masquerade as an aplastic anemia for years before PNH is finally diagnosed. Some of these cases appear to be drug-related.
4. Congenital and familial pancytopenia (Fanconi syndrome).

The term aplastic anemia tends to be more specifically applied to the cases of bone marrow failure secondary to drugs and chemical agents. These can be classified as follows: Type 1. Agents which regularly produce aplastic anemia if a sufficient dose is given, viz., Roentgen rays, radium, chemotherapeutic agents for cancer, lymphoma or leukemia and benzene; Type 2. Those agents which are uncommonly associated with bone marrow failure.

For those drugs and agents that regularly produce aplastic anemia, the close relationship and time sequence of blood and marow change is well established. The drugs most frequently incriminated in aplastic anemia in the Type 2 category are to be found in the report of Erslev derived from data in the Registry on Adverse Reactions of the Council on Drugs of the AMA in 1964 (32). In the order of frequency, this would include: Chloramphenicol, antibacterial sulfonamides, phenylbutazone, anticonvulsants especially mephenytoin, benzene and other organic solvents, insecticides, especially chlorophenothane and the gold salts (Fig. 5). Bone sections may exhibit a fatty marrow (Fig. 6) and after years of exposure, myelofibrosis (Fig. 7) and myeloid metaplasia (Fig. 8) may be found.

The hemolytic anemias induced by drugs occur in 2 broad categories: 1) Those associated with exposure to oxidant drugs; 2) Those in which an antibody to the erythrocyte is demonstrable. The oxidant drug reactions may be induced by a wide variety of drugs. This includes the antimalarials such as primaquine, pamaquine, pentaquine and quinacrine. Analgesic preparations containing phenacetin, antipyrine, acitonalide and aminopyrine may induce the same type of hemolytic process. The sulfonamides and related compounds are not infrequently involved and a variety of antibacterial agents such as furadantin, paraaminosalicylic acid and chloromycetin may also produce shortened survival of the erythrocyte.

The anemia associated with oxidant drugs has been known for many years but only recently (33) has the mechanism of hemolysis been clarified. The erythrocyte depends for its energy primarily upon the formation of ATP regenerated through the Embden-Myerhof pathway. The main source of reduced ATP arises out of the initial reactions in the pentose phosphate pathway, namely, the conversion of glucose-6-phosphate to 6-phosphogluconate and the subse-

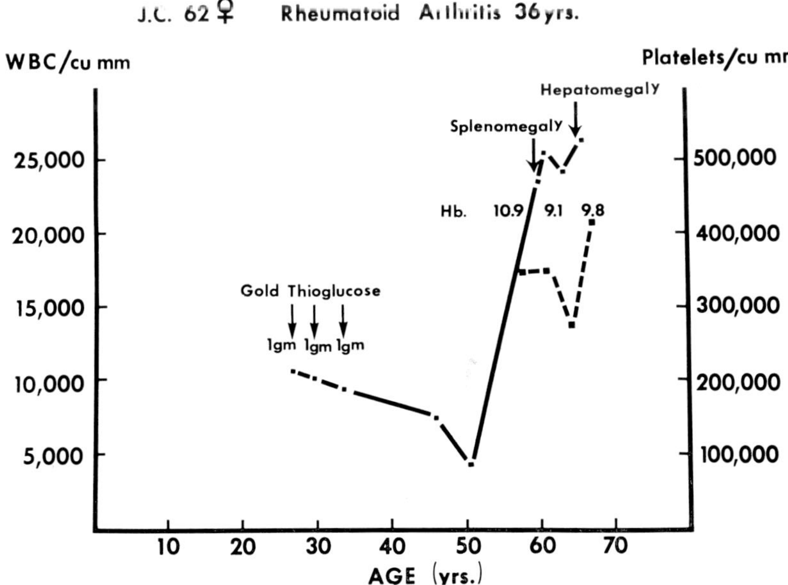

Figure 5. Aplastic anemia and myelofibrosis developing in a 62 year old female who received gold salts for rheumatoid arthritis.

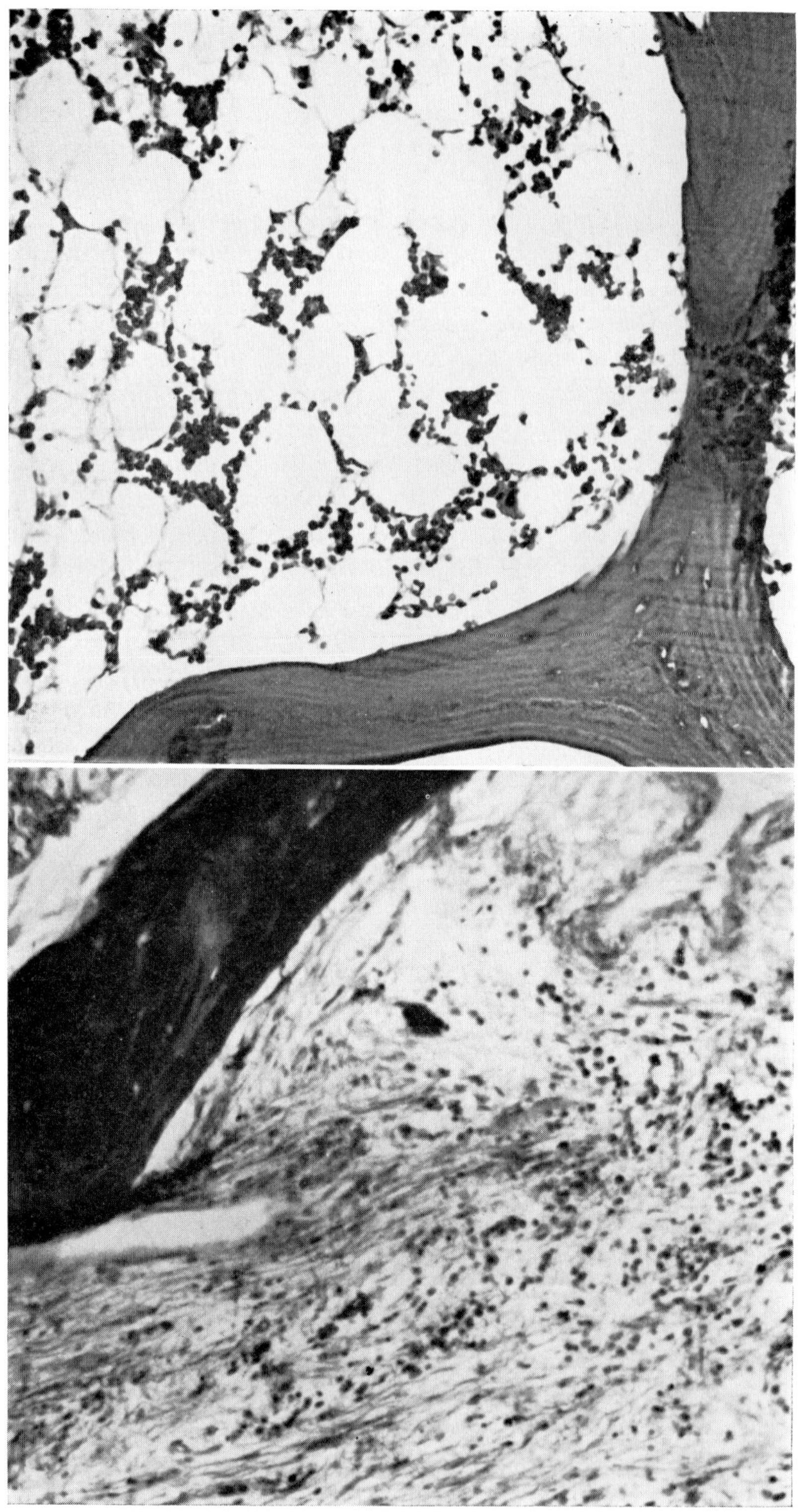

Figure 6. Sections of marrow which display panhypoplasia prior to phase of myelofibrosis in case illustrated in Figure 5.

Figure 7. Reticulum stain of marrow showing early phase of myelofibrosis following aplasia induced by gold salts.

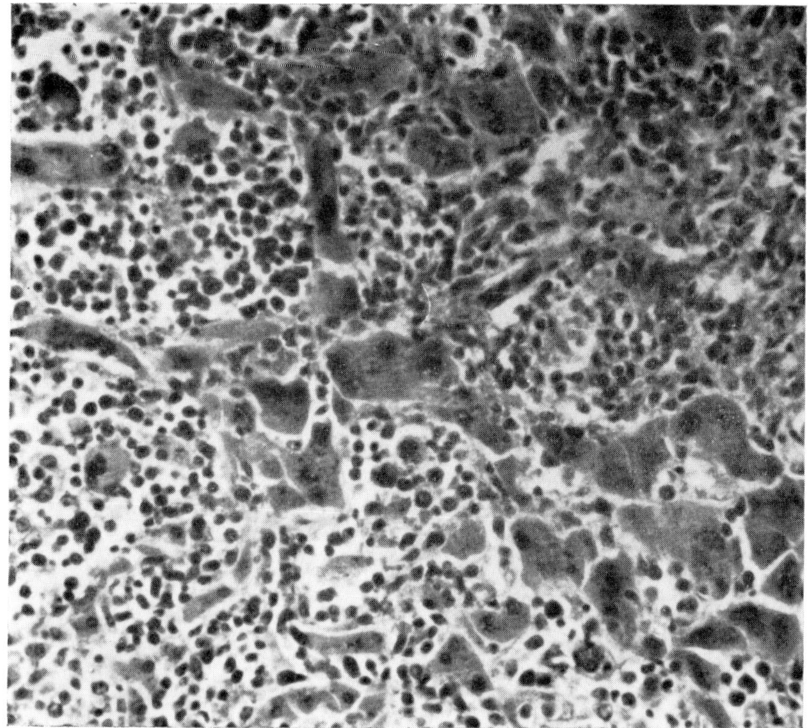

Figure 8. Liver biopsy displaying extensive myeloid metaplasia in hepatic sinusoids, in case illustrated in Figure 5.

quent conversion to ribulose-5-phosphate. The first step in this reaction is regulated by the enzyme glucose 6 phosphate dehydrogenase. It is the latter enzyme which is deficient in individuals (Fig. 9) susceptible to the oxidant agents. The cell which is deficient in G-6-PD is unable to form sufficient TPNH to overcome the oxidative effect of the drug. Hemoglobin is oxidized to methemoglobin with formation of Heinz bodies (Fig. 10, 11) and destruction of the cell. Other deficiencies which predispose the cell to the destructive effects of oxidant drugs include glutathione reductase, reduced glutathione deficiency and the presence of hemoglobin Zurich (34). The clinical effects of oxidant drug-induced hemolytic anemia vary considerably in severity. The G-6-PD deficiency has been found in approximately 13% of American Negro males and a somewhat greater incidence in American Negro females, although the hemolytic process is far less frequent in the female.

The hematologic reactions to chloramphenicol may be quite varied. Anemia, leukopenia and aplastic anemia have all been reported many times. The anemia following chloramphenicol may be a selective feature or may be associated with pancytopenia. When the anemia occurs alone, it may be due to the oxidant activity of the drug in a cell deficient in glucose-6-phosphate dehydrogenase.

Alternately, chloramphenicol may produce red cell aplasia of marrow or finally, it may produce only a reticulocytopenia with essentially normal marrow cellularity and associated vacuolization of erythroblasts (Fig. 12).

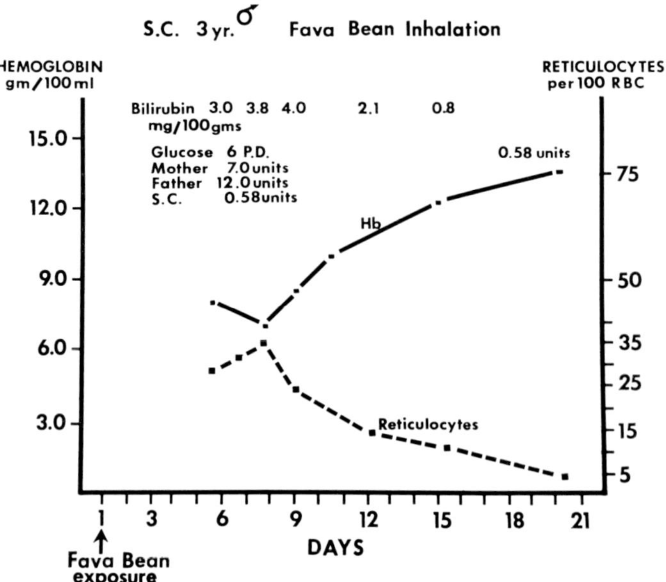

Figure 9. Hemolytic anemia developing in 3-year-old male of Italian parents after exposure to fava beans. The patient displayed a marked reduction in erythrocyte G-6-PD.

The immune hemolytic anemias induced by drugs may involve a wide variety of substances such as quinine, quinidine, phenacetin, penicillin and methyldopa (35). In such cases the indirect Combs test is positive when the specific drug is added to patient serum and normal erythrocytes (36).

The anemias associated with drug-induced deficiency states result in a megaloblastic type of process. This has been found with the folic acid deficiency following Dilantin therapy, the vitamin B_{12} deficiency following barbiturate therapy and the pyridoxine deficiency following isonicotinic acid hydrazide therapy. This type of anemia was first described by Mannheimer following weeks of Dilantin treatment for epilepsy in a young patient. A number of other drugs have been responsible for the same type of megaloblastic response and these include primidone, phenobarbital, amobarbital, secobarbital and more recently with nitrofuration (37). In its most typical form the anemia occurs in an individual past middle age, more often in the female (Fig. 13) who develops ulcerative lesions of the mouth and neurologic symptoms, especially paresthesia. Usually the patient has been receiving the drug continuously for months before anemia is noted. The condition is essentially dose-related. Initially, slight macrocytosis is noted, which progresses to a more severe anemia with development of a characteristic megaloblastic hyperplasia in the marrow (Fig. 14). The response to folic acid is rapid and uniform and it is generally unnecessary to discontinue the drug so long as folic acid therapy is maintained.

IV. LEUKEMIA

Various drugs have been implicated in the etiology of leukemia. Most prominent among these are benzene and phenylbutazone. In at least 4 reports in-

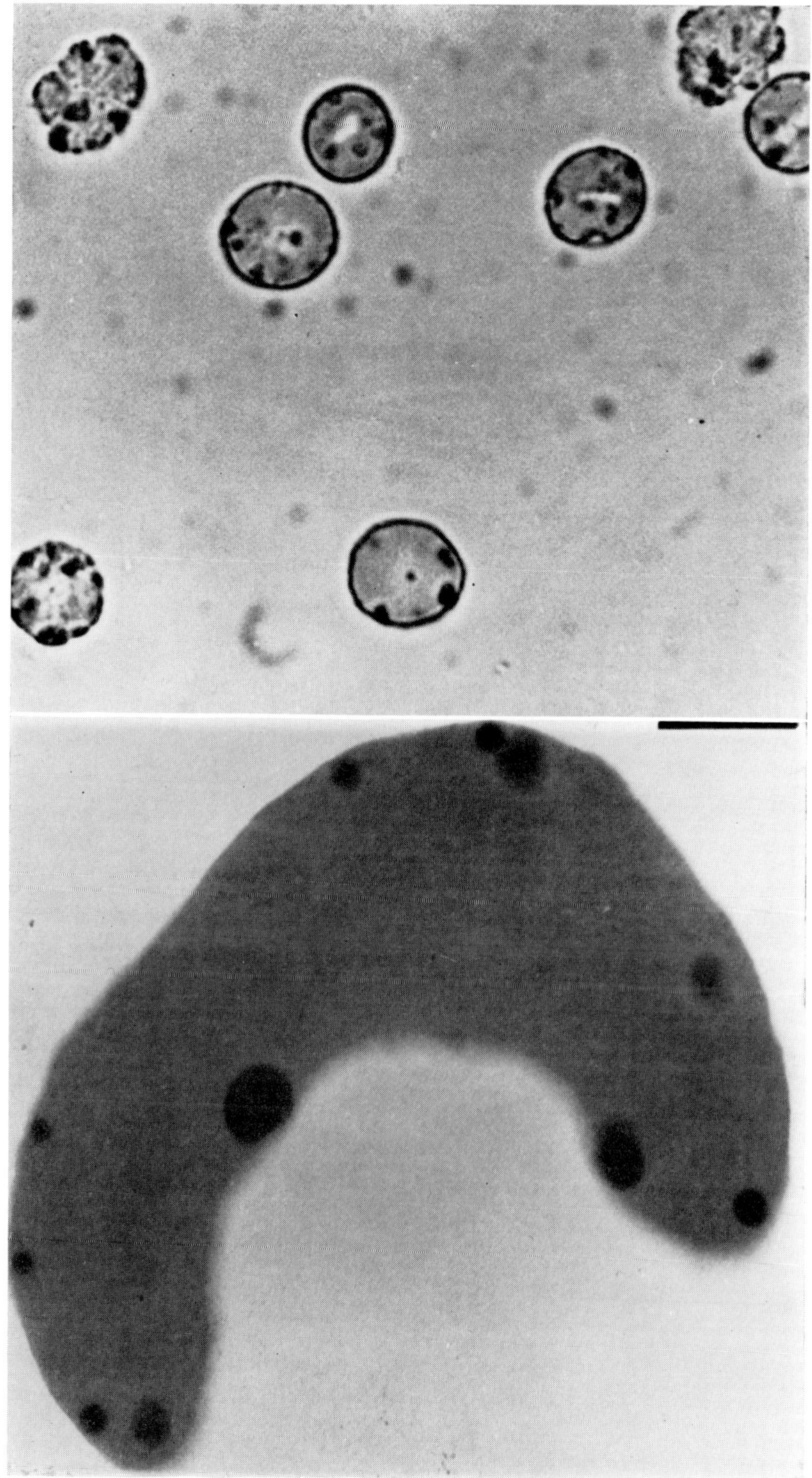

Figure 10. Heinz bodies observed by phase microscopy in erythrocytes in case illustrated in Figure 9.

Figure 11. Electron-dense material beneath erythrocyte membrane representing denatured hemoglobin (Heinz bodies) in case illustrated in Figure 9.

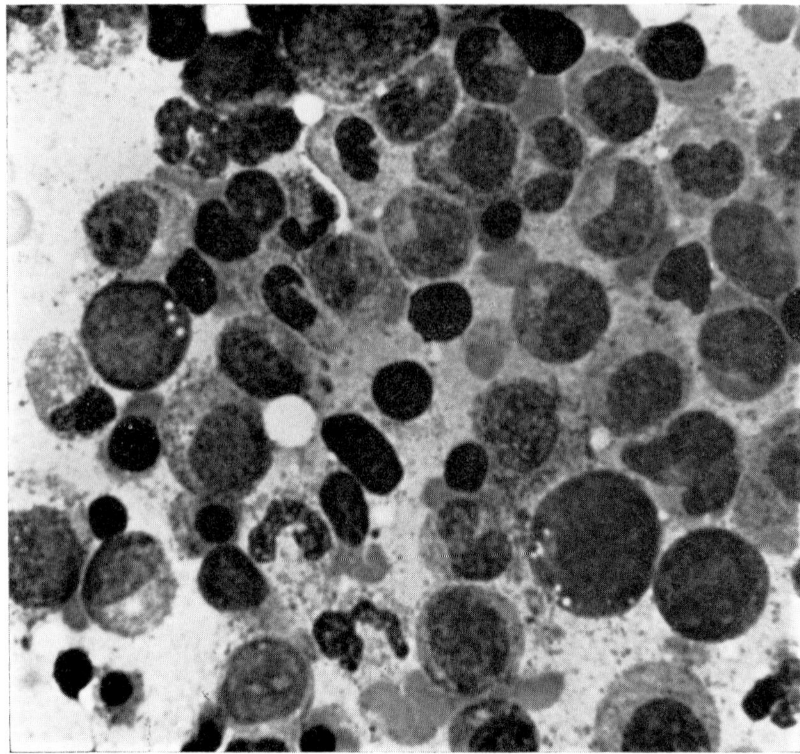

Figure 12. Vacuolization of basophilic normoblasts in marrow from case of acute hemolytic anemia following chloramphenicol treatment for pneumonia in a 54-year-old diabetic.

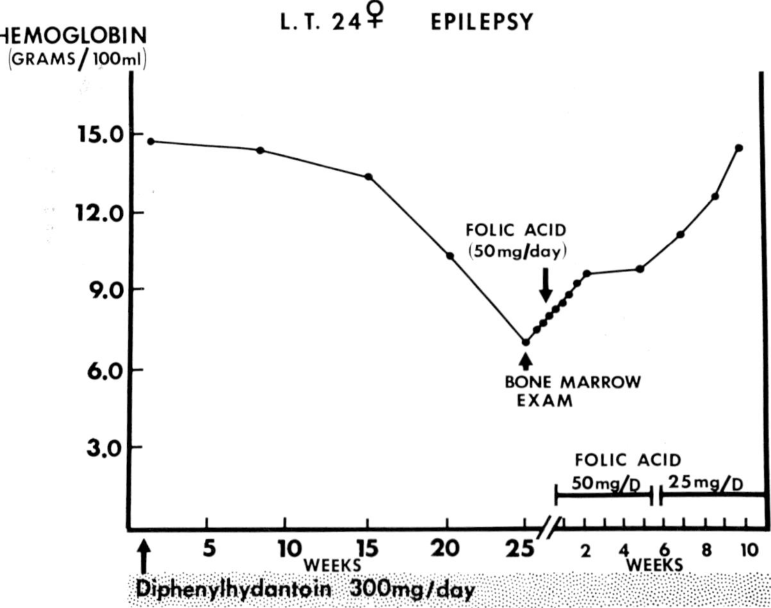

Figure 13. A 24-year-old female developed anemia during 6 months of therapy with diphenylhydantoin. The anemia was reversed by folic acid therapy despite continuation of drug.

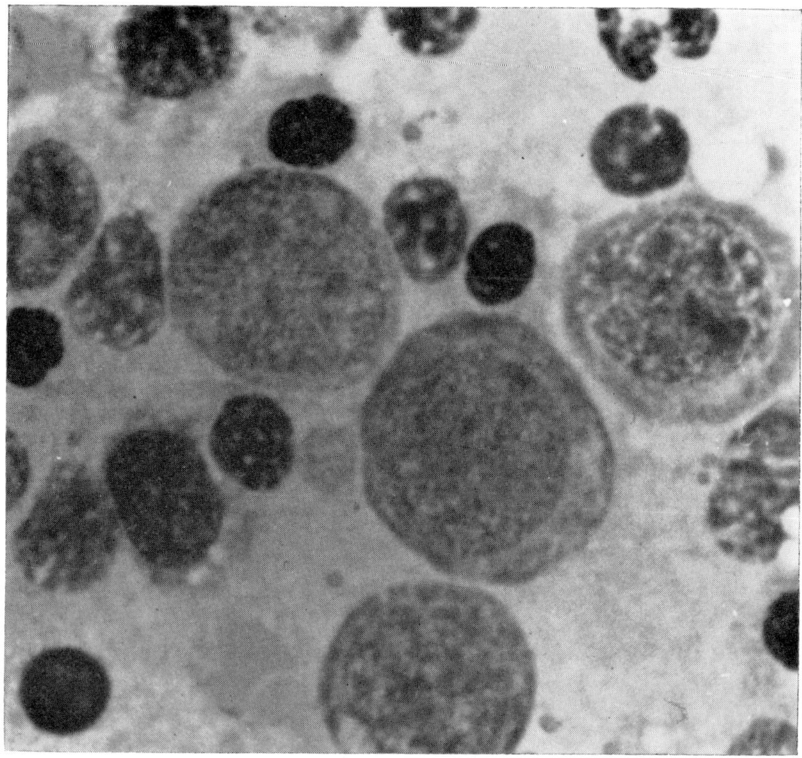

Figure 14. Megaloblastic hyperplasia of marrow which followed diphenylhydantoin therapy in case illustrated in Figure 13.

volving large numbers of patients exposed to benzene, there were frequent hematologic complications of which 10% were leukemia. The evidence for leukemia as a manifestation of drug reaction is admittedly only circumstantial, but rather compelling. The incidence is said to be approximately 20 times higher than that expected in the general population (38), and far greater than that with exposure to any other agent except perhaps irradiation. Most often, the type of leukemia that develops is the acute myeloblastic form which follows a period of leukopenia after many months or years of benzene exposure. In this respect, the leukemia following benzene exposure is very much like radiation-induced leukemia. Both may be preceded by an episode of aplastic anemia and in both there have been demonstrated various abnormalities in chromosomes (39). These chromosomal changes are probably important in leukemogenesis with both agents.

Phenylbutazone has also been incriminated in a number of cases where this drug was administered and followed by acute myeloblastic leukemia. When compared to control series with other drugs the incidence is admittedly much greater and suggests a possible role of phenylbutazone in leukomogenesis.

SUMMARY

The predominant type of hematologic reaction to drugs is cytopenia which may involve the leukocytes, erythrocytes or platelets. Pathogenetic mechanisms include direct cytotoxicity, immune injury, oxidant injury to the enzyme-poor cell and induction of deficiency states; but with many drugs the pathogenesis is unknown. The cytopenia often involves only one cell type and is self limited when the drug is withdrawn. Multiple cytopenias and aplasia are the more serious reactions and here the use of the known responsible drugs becomes a calculated risk. To a certain extent the reactions may be dose-related and in such cases, close monitoring with blood counts may identify a reaction before irreversible complications take place.

BIBLIOGRAPHY

1. Erf, L., and Rhoads, C. P.: The hematological effects of Benzene (Benzol) poisoning. J. Indust. Hyg. & Toxicol., *21:*421-435, 1939.
2. Saltzstein, S., and Ackerman, L.: Lymphadenopathy induced by anticonvulsant drugs and mimicking clinically and pathologically malignant lymphomas. Cancer, *12:*164-172, 1959.
3. Karnofsky, D. A.: Mechanisms of action of anticancer drugs at a cellular level. Cancer J. Clin., *18:*233-234, 1968.
4. Miescher, P. A., and Pepper, J. J.: Drug-induced allergic blood dyscrasias. *In,* Textbook of Immunopathology. 1968, pp. 277-281.
5. Beutler, E.: Drug-induced blood dyscrasias — III. Hemolytic anemia. J.A.M.A., *189:*143-144, 1964.
6. Heinivaara, O., and Palva, I.P.: Malabsorption and deficiency of vitamin B_{12} caused treatment with paraaminosalicylic acid. Acta Med. Scand., *177:*337-341, 1965.
7. Huguley, C. M.: Drug-induced blood dyscrasias. In, Disease-a-Month. 1963, 1-52, 1963.
8. Ackroyd, J. R.: The cause of thrombocytopenia in Sedormid purpura. Clin. Sci., *8:*269-290, 1949.
9. Ackroyd, J. F.: Allergic purpura, including purpura due to foods, drugs and infections. Amer. J. Med., *14:*605-632, 1953.
10. Bolton, F. B.: Thrombocytopenic purpura due to quinidine; serologic mechanisms. Blood, *11:* 547-564, 1956.
11. Wintrobe, M.: Clinical Hematology, 6th Ed. Philadelphia, Lea & Febiger, 1967, pp. 898-899.
12. Huguley, C. M., *et al.:* Adverse hematologic reactions to drugs. Progress in hematology, Vol. V. New York, Grune & Stratton, 1966, p. 118.
13. Horowitz, H. E., and Nachman, R. L.: Drug purpura. In, Seminars in Hematology, Vol. II, No. 4. New York, Grune & Stratton, 1965, pp. 289-290.
14. Crosby, W. H., *et al.:* Drug-induced blood dycrasias — IV. Thrombocytopenia. J.A.M.A., *189:*417-418, 1964.
15. Best, W. R.: Drug-associated blood dyscrasias. J.A.M.A., *185:*286-290, 1963.
16. Young, R. C., *et al.*: Thrombocytopenia due to digitoxin. Amer. J. Med., *41:*605-14, 1966.
17. Report from Council on Drugs, A.M.A., Registry on adverse reactions. April-May, 1965.
18. Report from Council on Drugs, A.M.A., Registry of adverse reactions. June, 1967.
19. Weintraub, R. M., *et .al.:* Rapid diagnosis of drug-induced thrombocytopenic purpura. J. A. M. A., *180:*528-532, 1962.
20. Kabat, E. A., and Mayer, M. M.: Experimental Immunochemistry, 2nd ed., Springfield, Thomas, 1961, pp. 133-240.
21. Shulman, N. R.: Immunoreactions involving platelets. I. A steric and kinetic model for formation of a complex from a human antibody, quinidine as a haptene and plates; and for fixation of complement by the complex. J. Exp. Med., *107:*665, 1968.
22. Dausset, J., and Colombani, J.: Detection of anti-leukocyte and anti-platelet antibodies by the antiglobulin consumption test. In, Immunological Methods. Ackroyd, J. F., Ed. Philadelphia, F. A. Davis Co., 1964, pp. 575-595.
23. Ratnoff, O. D.: Bleeding Syndromes. Springfield, Thomas, 1969, pp. 128-132, 136-139.
24. Schen, R. J., and Rabinowitz, B. A.: Thrombocytopenic purpura due to quinidine. Brit. Med. J., :1502-1505, 1958.
25. Rosenthal, M. C.: Bleeding disorders secondary to platelet anomalies. In, Conn, F. (Ed.) : Current Therapy. 1967. Philadelphia, W. B. Saunders, 1967, pp. 219-223.
26. Adelson, E.: Bleeding disorders secondary to platelet anomalies. In, Conn, H. F. (Ed.) : Current Therapy, 1968. Philadelphia, W. B. Saunders Co., 1968, pp. 237-242.
27. Huguley, C. M., Jr.: Hematological reactions. J.A.M.A., *196:*408, 1966.
28. Huguley, C. M., Jr.: Drug-induced blood dyscrasias II,. Agranulocytosis. J.A.M.A., *188:*817-818, 1964.
29. Walzer, R. A., and Einbinder, J.: Immunoleukopenia as an aspect of hypersensitivity to propylthiouracil. J.A.M.A., *184:*743-746, 1963.
30. Friedman, E. A., *et al.:* Delayed cutaneous hypersensitivity to leukocytes in disseminated Lupus Erythematosus. New Eng. J. Med., *262:* 486, 1960.
31. Huguley, C., Jr., Lea, J., Jr., and Butts, J.: Adverse hematologic reactions to drugs. In, Progress in Hematology. New York, Grune and Stratton, 1964.

32. Dern, R. J., Weinstein, I. M., LeRoy, G. V., Talmage, D. W., and Alving, A. S.: The hematolytic effect of primaquine. I. The localization of the drug-induced hemolytic defect in primaquine-sensitive individuals. J. Lab. Clin. Med., *43:*303, 1954.
33. Beutler, E.: Glucose-6-phosphate dehydrogenase deficiency in non-spherocytic congenital hemolytic anemia. Seminars Hemat., *2:*91-138, 1965.
34. Frick, P. G., Hizig, W. H., and Betke, K.: Hemoglobin Zurich. I. A new hemoglobin anomaly associated with acute hemolytic episodes with inclusion bodies after sulfonamide therapy. Blood, *20:*261-271, 1962.
35. Levine, B.B.: Immunochemical mechanisms of drug allergy. In, Textbook of Immunopathology. New York, Grune & Stratton, 1968, pp. 260-276.
36. Harris, J. W.: Studies on the mechanism of a drug-induced hemolytic anemia. J. Lab. Clin. Med., *47:*760-775, 1956.
37. Bass, B. H.: Megaloblastic anemia due to nitrofurantoin. Lancet, *1:*530, 1963.
38. DeGowin, R. L.: Benzene exposure and aplastic anemia followed by leukemia 15 years later. J.A.M.A., *185:*748, 1963.
39. Pollini, G., and Colombi, R.:Il danno cromosomico midollare nell'anemia aplastica benzolica. Med. Lavoro., *55:*241, 1964.

Chapter 46

Monitoring Cytotoxic Immunosuppression in Man

JOHN W. REBUCK, M.D., PH.D., JOSEPH M. BEALS, M.D., and DEAN A. LESHER, M.D. PHD.

PRINCIPLE OF TEST

A small test lesion scarified on the volar surface of the forearm is coated with antigen and covered with a cover-slip which is changed at timed intervals so that responding exudative leukocytes can be identified as to number and type in a sequential fashion. The cover-slips are stained like blood smears and afford a permanent record of the monitored reaction. The sequence of leukocytic migrations correlates directly with the patient's blood-forming, leukocytic transport, immunologic and leukocytic functional capabilities.[4-6] A base-line test lesion is studied prior to therapy and at any desired interval during or after immunosuppressive therapy and/or organ transplant status. The procedure is inexpensive, harmless and almost painless.

MATERIALS REQUIRED

1. Safety razor and blades to remove hair from skin surface.
2. Seventy percent alcohol swabs to prepare test sites. (Preparation should avoid leaving a residuum of any material that might be harmful to leukocytes.)
3. Sterile Bard-Parker scalpel blade #22. (Large rounded surface to avoid cutting.)
4. 15mm square clean glass cover-slips. #1½ thickness.
5. Wax-marking pencil.
6. File cards to be cut into 15mm squares.
7. Household aluminum foil.
8. Petri dishes.
9. Disposable needles and syringes for application of antigen.
10. Open flame source for sterilization of forceps.
11. Cover-slip forceps for changing cover-slips.
12. Micropore surgical tape 2″ roll No. 1535 3M Co.
13. Diphtheria toxoid (Parke-Davis) to serve as antigen.
14. Glassine envelopes for skin-window cover-slips.
15. Blood stain (the authors prefer Leishman's stain).
16. Glass slides for mounting cover-slips.
17. Rubber cement, for temporarily mounting cover-slips after staining.
18. Permount for permanent mounting of cover-slips after staining.

PREPARATION OF MATERIALS

Chemically clean cover-slips are marked with the letter "R" on one side. Together with the small cardboard square cut from the file cards one marked cover-slip is wrapped in aluminum foil. Fifty or so of these individually wrapped, foil covered kits are placed in a Petri dish and sterilized in the autoclave. For subsequent "life-island" use, several outerwrappings are sterilized with the Petri dishes. Otherwise, even after opening the Petri dish, each cover-slip is still sterile until use within its own wrapping of foil.

PROCEDURE FOR APPLICATION OF THE SKIN-WINDOW TEST

Any plane surface of the skin may be utilized, usually the volar surface of the forearm or the anterior surface of the thigh are suitable. The excess hair is shaved for two square inches and the area swabbed with 70% alcohol. A small (3 to 4 mm diameter) circular area is slowly scraped with the scalpel blade until the oozing dermal papillae are reached. Since the rete pegs are intact residual scarring almost never occurs. A drop (0.05 ml) of diphtheria toxoid is applied to the surface of the lesion, *not* injected intradermally. Sterile forceps are used to select the cover-slip from the opened kit and the cover-slip is placed over the antigen-coated lesion with the "R" reading true (Fig. 13). If the "R" is reversed wax will be placed into the lesion. Next the sterile forceps are used to cover the glass with the sterile cardboard which not only prevents breakage but prevents adherence of the glass to the surmounting two inch square of surgical tape which is next applied over the entire area. The time of scarification marks the beginning of the test inflammatory reaction. In controls, leukocytes responding to the combination of trauma, antigen and glass migrate to the undersurface of the cover-slip within 30 minutes to an hour. Ordinarily, cover-slips are removed first at 3 hours, and another cover-slip put into place in the same manner. The cover-slip with the responding leukocytes is air-dried immediately after removal and placed in the appropriately labelled glassine envelope or it can be stained immediately like a blood smear. Best staining of small cover-slips has been achieved by mounting the cover-slip with cell-side up or with the "R" in reverse with a small drop of rubber cement on an ordinary glass slide. The entire slide is then flooded with stain and buffer as required. After staining, the cover-slip is mounted with permount cell-side down and cleaned. The responding leukocytes are similarly monitored at 6, 9, 12, 14, 24, and 30 hours, although the test may be abbreviated to only the 9 and 12 hour or 12 and 14 changes if deemed necessary (immunologically competent lymphocytes peak at from 8 to 14 hours in normal controls, see discussion below).[4]

INTERPRETATION

In normal controls at 3 hours of inflammation, a moderate exudate is composed of numerous neutrophilic leukocytes together with a few migrated blood monocytes and local tissue macrophages (histiocytes or large mononuclears).[4-6] At 6 hours of inflammation, an abundant exudate equivalent to the area of the test lesion will be found on the cover slip. The leukocytes will again be largely neutrophilic leukocytes, although a few migrated blood lymphocytes and monocytes together with the sparse large macrophages (histiocytes) of the region will be observed. At 9 hours, the abundant exudate persists and although neutrophilic leukocytes still predominate, an appreciable number, perhaps 25% of the cells will be migrated small and medium-sized lymphocytes, a few monocytes and histiocytes comprise the remainder of the cell types. At 12 hours of human inflammation, the test site area is filled with the exudative response (Fig. 1). Al-

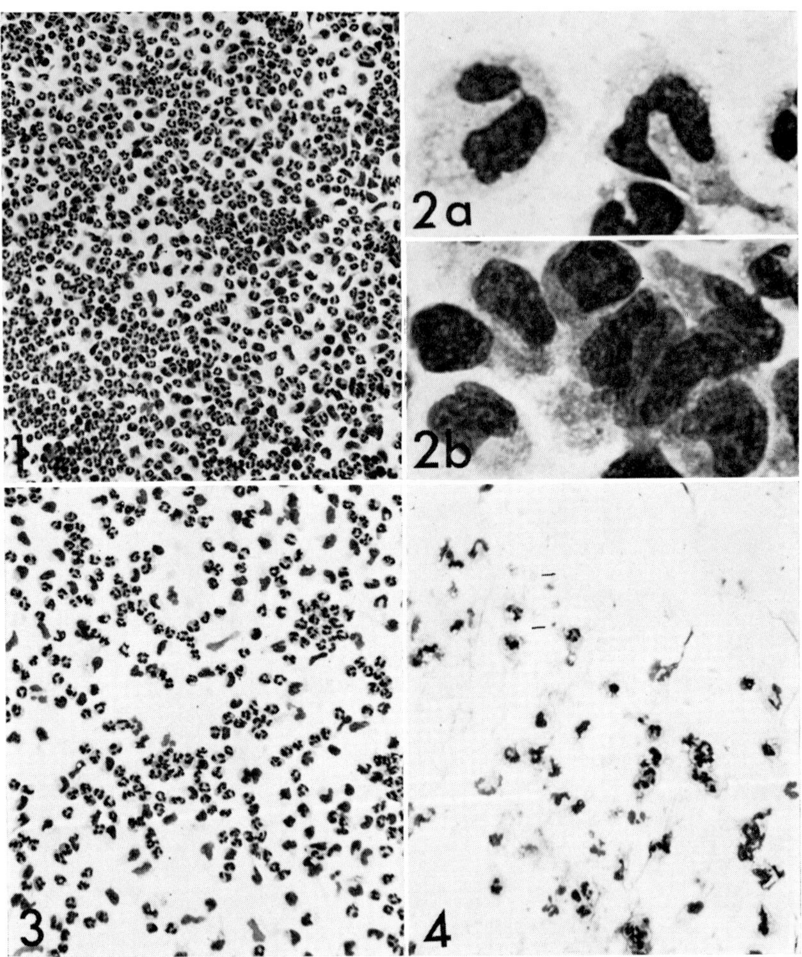

Figure 1. Low power view of normal leukocytic response to antigen. Full cellularity. Compare with Figures 3, 4, 7, 8, 9 and 10. Leishman's stain, X150.

Figure 2a. Monocytes in the exudative response at 12 hours of inflammation in a patient with a marked peripheral blood monocytosis. Leishman's stain, X1100.

Figure 2b. Lymphocytes in the normal exudative response to antigen in controls at 12 hours of inflammation. Leishman's stain, X1100.

Figure 3. Low power view of slightly diminished response to antigen in base line lesion of patient A with renal impairment due to chronic glomerulonephritis. Twelve hours of inflammation. Leishman's stain, X150.

Figure 4. Low power view of further diminished response to antigen in patient A after renal transplant. Twelve hours of inflammation. Immunosuppression with prednisone and imuran. Leishman's stain, X150.

though quantitation can be achieved by direct counting, in actual practice, such a low power photomicrograph furnishes an equally significant record of the amount of responding exudate. Lymphocytes from the blood approach the neutrophils in number. The lymphocytes measure 8 to 12 μm in diameter (Fig. 2b) far below the size measurements of the less numerous migrating monocytes (Fig. 2a). The lymphocytes, however, caught in ameboid motion and flattened against the glass may show irregularity of nuclear outline and the customary nuclear indentation usually masked in their globular condition in the blood. Monocytes migrate in numbers proportional to their numbers in the blood stream, in man with few exceptions this is in the 3 to 10 hour range. At 14 hours of inflammation, neutrophils have lost much of their cytoplasm peripheral to their nuclear lobes and are much smaller in diameter than their blood counterparts. Lymphocytes have enlarged their cell bodies by a μm or two as they begin their transformation to macrophages or large mononuclears. Monocytes also enlarge their cell bodies, accentuate their large horse-shoe-shaped nuclear outlines and lose their dust-like azurophilic granulation. They remain 6 μm larger than the transforming lymphocytes however. Both lymphocytes and monocytes show a histiocytic transformation of their nuclear chromatin patterns. The coarse heavy chromatin pieces of the lymphocytic nucleus are dispersed into the fine angular pieces of the histiocytic nuclear pattern as nucleoprotein activation takes place, similarly the thready chromatin strands of the human monocytic nuclear chromatin patterns are also dispersed in to the fine angular pieces of the histiocytic nucleus. For a description of the gradual transformation of the blood lymphocytes and monocytes into histiocytes (large mononuclears), the reader is referred to our earlier papers in which the 16, 18, and 21 hours of human inflammation neutrophils have largely degenerated and the trilineaged macrophages or large mononuclears predominate in the abundant exudate.[4-6]

Abnormal responses may be accurately quantitated if the test lesion has been made with a small diameter of 3 to 4 mm so that the entire exudative sample appears as a spot of the same diameter in the center of the removed cover-slip. Low power photomicrography (Figs. 1, 3, 4, 7, 8, 9, 10) serves as a permanent record of the quantitative response and can be inserted in the patient's history. Several examples of abnormal responses will be described and illustrated as follows.

In patient A suffering from renal impairment due to chronic glomerulonephritis, the exudative response in the base-line study was somewhat diminished (Fig. 3) at 12 hours of inflammation in contrast to the normal full leukocytic outpouring to be found at the same time in normal controls responding to similar antigenic stimulation (Fig. 1). The leukocytic response was further decreased (Fig. 4) in the same patient after immunosuppressive therapy with prednisone and imuran. The patient had received a renal transplant at the time of this study. Cellular examination of the nature of the responses reveals that prior to therapy (Fig. 5) the patient was still capable of a lymphocytic response at 12 hours of inflammation although the number of lymphocytes was reduced. With immunosuppressive therapy lymphocytes were almost completely deleted from the exudate (Fig. 6) which consisted predominantly of neutrophilic granulocytes.

In patient B, renal impairment was due to chronic pyelonephritis. The base-line exudative response (Fig. 7) was sparser than that of the above patient and significantly diminished when compared to that of the normal control (see Fig. 1). Cellular analysis of the base-line response (not illustrated) revealed some retention of lymphocytic participation in the leukocytic outpourings about the an-

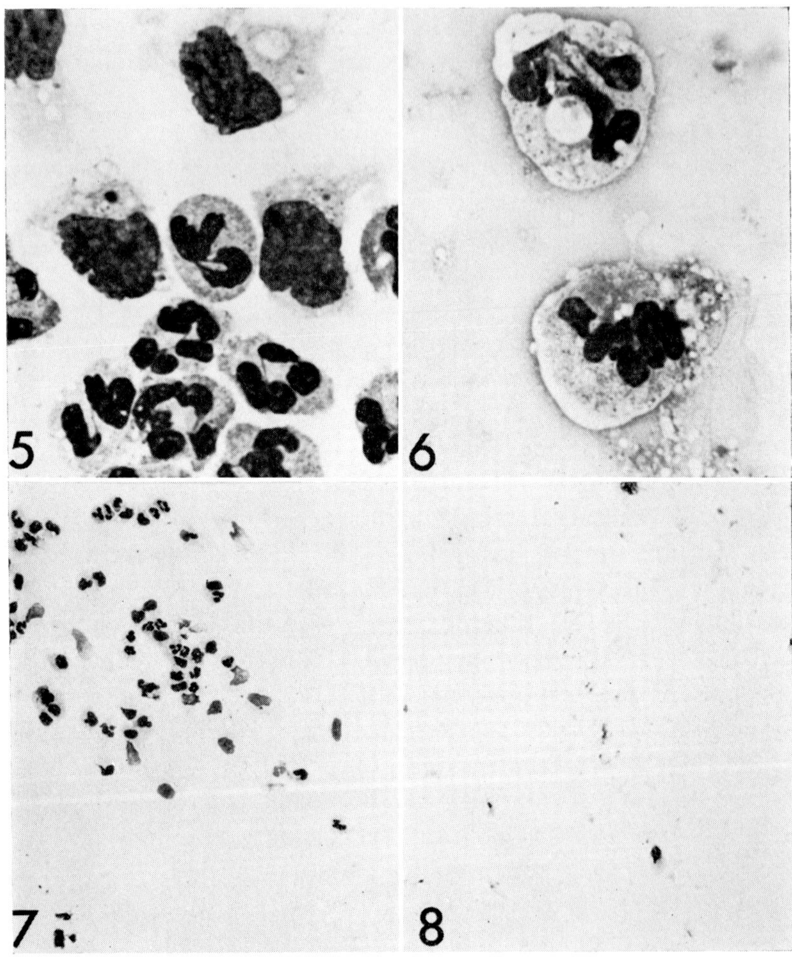

Figure 5. Transforming lymphocytes and neutrophils in base line lesion of patient A with renal impairment due to chronic glomerulonephritis. Twelve hours of inflammation. Leishman's stain, X1100.

Figure 6. Edematous neutrophils in diminished response of patient A after renal transplant. Immunosuppression with prednisone and imuran. Leishman's stain, X1100.

Figure 7. Low power view of diminished response to antigen in base line study of patient B with renal impairment due to chronic pyelonephritis. Twelve hours of inflammation. Leishman's stain, X150.

Figure 8. Absence of leukocytic response to antigen in patient B after renal transplant. Immunosuppression with prednisone and imuran. Twelve hours of inflammation. Leishman's stain, X150.

tigen. With immunosuppression effected by prednisone and imuran, study of a test lesion in the postoperative period after renal transplantation revealed a complete absence of leukocytic response (Fig. 8) concurrent with a terminal septicemic state.

Conversely, in patient C the base-line response (Fig. 9), with renal impairment due to chronic glomerulonephritis, was diminished quantitatively although some meager lymphocytic migrations (Fig. 11) were still capable of being mounted. After renal transplantation,

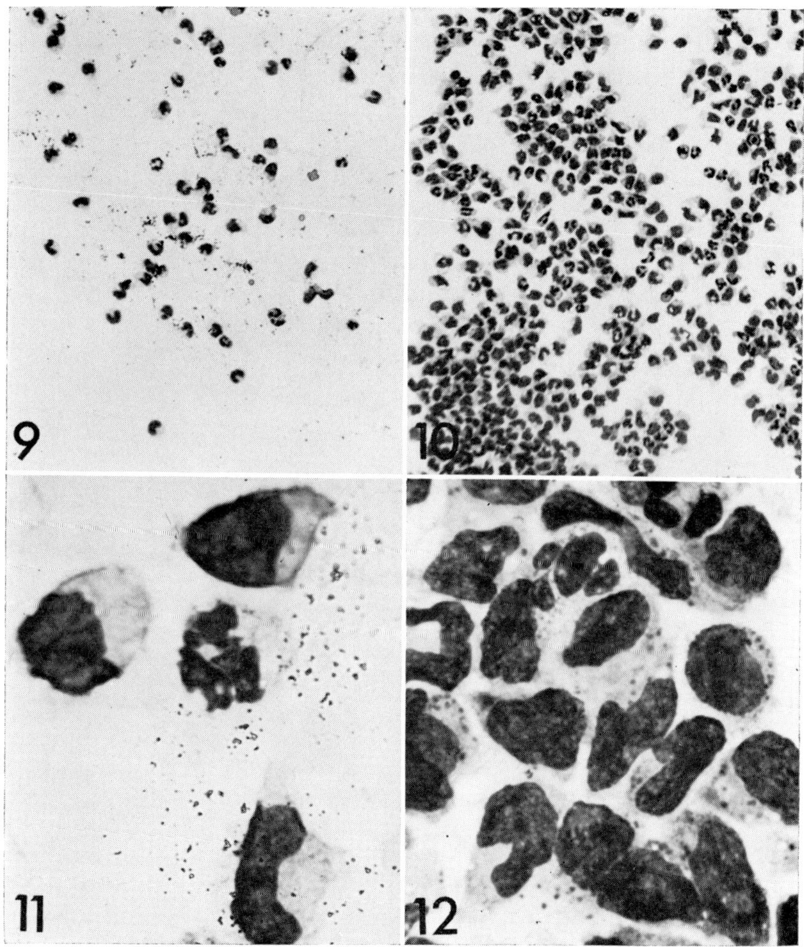

Figure 9. Low power view of diminished response to antigen in base line study of patient C with renal impairment due to chronic glomerulonephritis. Nine hours of inflammation. Leishman's stain, X150.

Figure 10. Low power view of increased response to antigen in patient C. after renal transplant. Immunosuppression with medrol and imuran. Ten hours of inflammation. Leishman's stain, X150.

Figure 11. Transforming lymphocytes and a neutrophil in base line lesion of patient C with renal impairment due to chronic golmerulonephritis. Nine hours of inflammation. Leishman's stain, X1100.

Figure 12. Increased lymphocytes in patient C after renal transplant. Immunosuppression with medrol and imuran. Ten hours of inflammation. Leishman's stain, X1100.

and in spite of immunosuppressive therapy with medrol and imuran, a marked increase of responding leukocytes was observed (Fig. 10) approaching the numbers to be found in Fig. 1. Furthermore, the cellular type at a precocious 10 hours of inflammation (Fig. 12) was predominantly lymphocytic in nature.

Other abnormal leukocytic migrations which we have observed concurrent with homograft rejection in man[5] have shown:

A. Increased fibrin deposition.

B. Increased eosinophilic granulocyte migrations.

C. Increased basophilic granulocyte migrations.

D. Increased foreign-body giant cell formations.

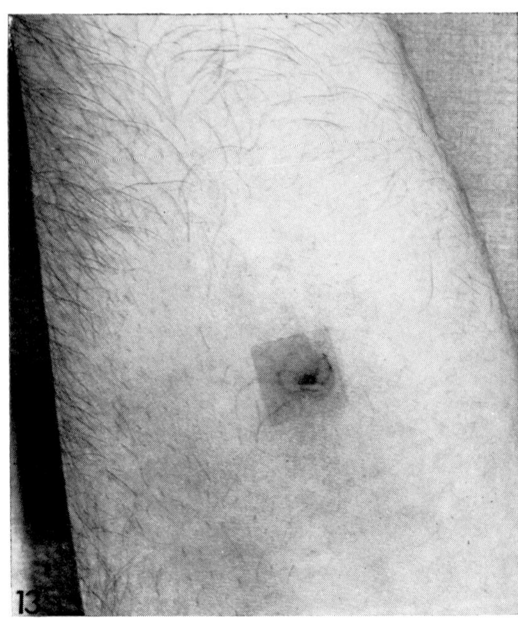

Figure 13. Application of sterile cover-slip to small (3 mm di.) scarified test lesion underlying, volar surface of forearm.

DISCUSSION

With increased use of the skin window technic for monitoring patients with organ transplantation as well as monitoring patients with definitive disease processes, the abnormalities of leukocytic responses to antigenic stimulation in such patients will continue to cast further light both upon leukocytic functions in themselves as well as the mechanisms of the diseases so studied.

The first use of the skin window for monitoring human reaction to antigen demonstrated that volunteers carrying antibodies to the stimulating antigen responded with precocious and enhanced lymphocytic migrations to the antigen in the test lesions. Similarly, if the human volunteer lacked circulating antibodies to the test antigen, an identical precocious and enhanced lymphocytic migration to the antigen in the test lesions could be produced by simple addition of specific exogenous antibody to the test lesion at the time of primary antigen application. Conversely, either lack of globulin in general (hypogammaglobulinemia) or lack of specific antibody to the stimulating antigen in the test lesion led to failure of lymphocytic migrations. Furthermore, patients with Hogkins disease with its accompanying immunologic paralysis presented significantly diminished lymphocytic migrations in response to antigenic stimulation.

The initial use of the skin window for monitoring immunosuppression consisted in the now widely confirmed observations that excess corticotrophic hormone of the pituitary or cortisol of the adrenal led to diminished leukocytic responses to antigen marked by diminished or absent lymphocytic responses, diminished neutrophilic responses and diminished phagocytic capabilities of all responding leukocytic types. Evidence has now been submitted above that the technic is equally as effective in monitoring other chemotherapeutically induced modes of immunosuppression.

Attention has been focused on monitoring lymphocytic participation in the response to antigen in the patient under care because of the known immunologic competency of the lymphocyte and its transformational products in initiating and effecting the graft versus host reaction[3] and effecting graft rejection.[1] However, the skin window method monitors as well the nature and degree of neutrophilic responses especially in regard to fractions of complement,[2] which latter have been invoked by some workers as an important component of graft rejection. Furthermore, there is abundant evidence that the lymphocytes and other responding leukocytes in the skin window test lesions function in close correlation with circulating antibody parameters and reflect any important changes in this area, even if a quantitatively minor but qualitatively avid antibody against the graft, as yet unrecognized, should subsequently be found.

It is proposed that this simple, painless and inexpensive test will prove useful in monitoring the immunologic defenses of man in a long list of useful tools altering these defenses such as radiation and antilymphocyte serum which are already at hand or in that armamentarium which lies in the future.

As a result of the above work, the importance of following the absolute lymphocyte count in the peripheral blood of the patient subjected to elective immunosuppression as an ancillary monitoring device has become apparent.

REFERENCES

1. Dammin, G.: The pathology of human renal transplantation. In, Human Transportation. Ed. by F. T. Rappaport and J. Dausset. New York, Grune and Stratton, 1968. pp. 170-200.
2. Gewurz, H., Page, A. R., Pickering, R. J., and Good, R. A.: Complement activity and inflammatory. Neutrophil exudation in man. Int. Arch. Allergy, *32:*64-90, 1967.
3. Gowans, J. L., McGregor, D. D., and Cowan, D. M.: The role of small lymphocytes in the rejection of homografts of skin. In, The Immunologically Competent Cell. Ed. by G. E. W. Wolstenhome and K. Knight. Boston, Little Brown and Co., 1963, pp. 20-29.
4. Rebuck, J. ., Coffman, H. I. Bluhm, G. B., and Barth, C. B.: A structural study of reticulum cell and monocyte production with quantitation of lymphocytic modulation of nonmultiplication type to histiocytes. Ann. N. Y. Acad. Sci., *113:*595-611, 1964.
5. Rebuck, J. W., Jenny H., and Kelly, A. P.: A new method for the study of leukocytic responses to miniature homografts in man. Federation Proc., *27:*441, 1968.
6. Rebuck, J. W., Whitehouse, F. W., and Noonan, S. M.: Energization of lymphocytes transforming to macrophages in human inflammation. Biochem. Pharmacol. Suppl. March, 1968. Chemical biology of inflammation, pp. 159-170.

Chapter 47

Vasculitis from the Use of Antibiotics, Drugs and Toxic Agents

JACOB CHURG, M.D.

Among the more serious but fortunately uncommon effects of exposure to chemical substances such as antibiotics, drugs, insecticides, etc., is generalized inflammation and necrosis of blood vessels. Some of these substances may exert direct toxic effect on the vascular wall, though they seldom do so in the usual dosages and concentrations. Much more often, vasculitis is the result of sensitization of the indivdual to a particular chemical or a related group of chemicals. These compounds act as haptens, presumably combining with the individual's own proteins and inducing formation of appropriate antibodies. It is believed that complexes of the antigen and antibody are deposited in and cause damage to the vascular wall.

The true incidence of vasculitis, that is the "attack rate" among all patients who receive or come in contact with any given substance is very difficult to determine. Considering the widespread use of antibiotics, drugs, pesticides, weed-killers and petroleum chemicals, the incidence must be very low. It is not even possible to count accurately the number of published cases. The majority of publications deal with a single offending substance and a single case, but some report upon a number of cases of various etiologies, and others mention in passing a number of substances purportedly causing vasculitis. A rough idea of relative frequency can be gleaned from the perusal of the Index Medicus for the past twenty years. The frequency with any given substance was mentioned in a sample of 50 papers is given in the Table. The most frequent offenders were penicillin, sulfonamides, thiouracils, iodides and hydantoin derivatives. Only the first three are considered by

TABLE — RELATIVE FREQUENCY OF ETIOLOGIC AGENTS IN "ALLERGIC" VASCULITIS DUE TO CHEMICALS
(Based on 50 Reports)

Penicillin	12	Aspirin	1
Chloramphenicole	2	Stilbamidine	1
Tetracyclines	2	p-Naphthylamine	1
Streptomycin	2	Guanethidine	1
Griseofulvin	1	Chlorpromazine	1
Sulfonamides	9	Barbiturates	1
Iodides	6	Hydralazine	1
Thiouracils	5	Organic arsenicals	1
Hydantoins	3	Heavy metals	
Phenacetin	2	(gold, mercury,	
Isoniazids	2	bismuth) each	1
p-Aminosalicylic acid	2	Estrogen	1
Phenylbutazone	2	Myleran	1
Quinidine	2	DDT	1
		Weed killers	1
		Petroleum products	1

Symmers in 1962 study as being of any practical importance (1). However, all are known sensitizers which produce a variety of reactions in addition to vasculitis. Rostenberg in reviewing 58 cases of life threatening skin eruptions due to drugs, found sulfonamides to be most frequently responsible, with hydantoins in the second place (2).

PATHOLOGY

McComb (3) employed the term "allergic" vasculitis to cover a variety of clinical and pathological syndromes whose common denominator is inflammation of vascular wall. Large or small arteries, arterioles, veins or capillaries may be involved in any segment of the greater and sometimes also the lesser circulation. The lesions may be necrotizing or nonnecrotizing, few or many, disseminated or limited to one organ. Inflammation may assume granulomatous character and extra-vascular granulomata may be present in the surrounding tissue (4, 5). Depending upon the particular combination of features, the disease is called classical periarteritis nodosa, hypersensitivity angiitis, allergic angiitis and granulomatosis, Wegener's granulomatosis, cutaneous arteriolitis, nodular vasculitis, anaphylactoid purpura or temporal arteritis (4). In many instances, the disease does not fit into any of these categories.

According to Winkelmann and Ditto (7), drug reaction produces a fairly typical pattern in the skin, with widespread involvement of vessels in the upper corium, perivascular homogenization and necrosis of the connective tissue and vascular and perivascular infiltration largely with polymorphonuclear neutrophils and eosinophils. The inflammatory cells tend to undergo nuclear fragmentation (leukocytoclastic angiitis). In some of their patients, autopsy revealed in addition periarteritis nodosa in the internal organs while others died without such involvement. However, renal disease was present in all of their fatal cases, in the form of diffuse or focal "embolic" glomerulonephritis.

ETIOLOGY

Allergic etiology of vasculitis was first proposed by Gruber (8) who postulated sensitization to bacterial products in the course of infection. It is now generally accepted that vasculitis can be caused not only by bacterial products (e.g., vaccines) (9) but by protein antigens in general. In man, vasculitis has been observed in serum sickness (10, 11) and it has been produced in animals by injection of foreign protein (12). However, no clear-cut allergic etiology can be demonstrated in the majority of cases. In every instance where vasculitis occurs during or after contact with a chemical, causal relationship must be weighed against coincidence. The proof of relationship is generally much more circumstantial than in the case of protein antigens.

Development of haptenic allergy depends to a great extent upon individual predisposition and occurs only in a minority, generally a small minority of all people exposed to the usual dosages or concentrations. While it is possible to sensitize animals with haptens, so far no clear-cut evidence has been given that vasculitis can be produced in this manner. To establish even a tentative etiologic relationship in any given instance, several conditions must be fulfilled: (1) Proper time relation, that is appearance of vasculitis shortly after exposure to the chemical; (2) Evidence of current or past sensitization, e.g., in the form of a skin rash which appears after contact or ingestion of the chemical and disappears after the latter is discontinued. However, severe, even fatal skin manifestations can occur without development of vasculities, and conversely periarteritis nodosa may be present without skin manifestations. (3) The presence in patient's serum of specific antibodies which react with the chemical. Such antibodies can be demonstrated by skin testing or by passive transfer to another person and challenging the site of transfer with the chemical in question (Prausnitz-Küstner reaction). The presence of antibodies is manifested by an inflammatory response which may include vasculitis (13). Unfortunately, vasculitis may exist in the patient without demonstrable antibodies and may be absent despite the presence of antibodies (14). All too often, one has to fall back on the statistical evidence. It is much easier to accept, though not to prove, the etiological role if the chemical has been associated with onset of vasculitis in a number of cases. The problem is further complicated by the frequent simultaneous administration of several antibiotics or drugs, and by the presence of infection. Indeed, some authors have proposed a synergistic effect of infection and the drug (15), the former acting as a sensitizing and the latter as a provoking agent.

A brief mention must be made of steroids as a possible cause of vasculitis, nearly always in patients with rheumatoid arthritis. This is a surprising possibility in view of the inhibitory effects of steroids upon inflammatory processes. However, it is now known that vasculitis occurs as often in treated as in untreated rheumatoid arthritis (16). It would appear that steroids do not cause inflammation of blood vessels, though they possibly may aggravate it. Furthermore, vasculitis in rheumatoid arthritis does not carry the same serious implication as "allergic" vasculitis.

CLINICAL MANIFESTATIONS

As is well known, vasculitis manifests itself by constitutional symptoms, such as fever, weakness and weight loss, and by local symptoms due to variable multisystemic involvement including the heart, lungs, kidneys, gastrointestinal tract, central and peripheral nervous system, musculoskeletal system and skin. Occasionally, only one system such as skin is predominantly or exclusively involved. Symptomatology of vasculitis is treated in standard textbooks and has been excellently reviewed a few years ago by McComb (3). Only a few pertinent points will be mentioned here.

The organ most frequently involved is the *skin*. Erythematosus and purpuric rash is found in the majority of patients, and in more severe cases may be bullous and necrotizing. The rash is not necessarily due to vasculitis, but may be only an evidence of sensitization. If the offending agent is discontinued or removed from contact with the patient, the rash fades, only to reappear if the contact is resumed. However, second administration or continuous administration may lead to the development of vasculitis. Biopsy of a purpuric spot may show inflammation of very small vessels, on the order of capillaries or precapillaries. Biopsy of nodules, if present, (and they are uncommon) may reveal a more diagnostic involvement of large vessels perhaps with necrosis of the wall. Sometimes extra-vascular necrotizing and granulomatous lesions are found which are also specific.

Heart

Myocarditis is not common, but has been reported especially with sulfonamides. It manifests itself by arrhythmia, electrocardiographic changes or cardiac failure. Endocarditis occurs very seldom, mainly in cases of Wegener's granulomatosis.

Respiratory System

Sinusitis is often seen in patients with allergic background. Severe destructive inflammation is typically present in Wegener's granulomatosis; it may involve nose, sinuses, mouth, larynx or pharynx. Inflammatory infiltrates in the lungs are common; some of these are migratory as in Loeffler's pneumonia. Destructive lesions simulating neoplasms are seen almost exclusively in Wegener's granulomatosis. Asthma, either of recent onset, or long-standing, has been noted in 10-20% of patients.

Genito-Urinary Tract

Focal glomerulonephritis is one of the more common manifestations of vasculitis. In McCombs series, it was present in 1/3 of cases and manifested itself by hematuria, moderate albuminuria, cylindruria. Occasionally, glomerulonephritis was severe enough to lead to renal failure. Interestingly enough focal glomerulonephritis may accompany cutaneous eruption or localized necrotizing lesions of the upper respiratory tract, without the presence of generalized arteritis.

Blood

Markedly elevated sedimentation rate, anemia and leukocytosis are common findings. Marked eosinophilia (over 15-20%) is almost invariably associated with a background of allergy, such as asthma, hay fever or drug hypersensitivity, but slight eosinophilia (5-10%) may occur without such a background.

Muscles

Skeletal muscles are quite frequently involved and are conveniently used for diagnostic biopsies. However, only those muscles should be biopsied which show pain, tenderness or weakness, or which show electromygraphic changes (17).

PROGNOSIS AND THERAPY

Prognosis of vasculitis depends, at least to a degree, upon the size of vessels involved as well as upon extent and character of the lesions. If only capillaries and precapillaries show inflammation, as in anaphylactoid purpura, spontaneous recovery is usual. If larger size vessels are affected by inflammation and especially if they show necrosis, chances for recovery are much smaller though somewhat better if arteritis or arteriolitis is limited to the skin.

Steroid therapy has greatly improved the outlook. Of the 72 cases of McComb's, (3) only 6 of the 17 untreated but 37 of the 55 treated patients were alive after 1 year and of the treated patients who died, nearly half died of causes unrelated to vasculitis, such as leukemia and cancer. In the Mayo Clinic series of periarteritis nodosa, 48% of the 110 steroid treated patients survived 5 years, but only 13% of the 20 untreated patients (17). Prognosis was best when the therapy was started early with sufficiently large doses and continued for a long time. Such therapy was effective in preventing serious complications such as hypertension and renal disease. On the other hand, in advanced cases, rapid healing and scarring of vascular lesions may lead to renal failure and to malignant hypertension (18).

SUMMARY

Vasculitis is a rare but serious complication of ingestion or contact of chemical substances of rather small molecular weight such as antibiotics, drugs, pesticides and weed-killers. The most important of these appear to be penicillin, sulfonamides and hydantoins. Skin rash is an important warning sign. It is assumed that the offending substances act as haptens, combining with proteins of the body to produce sensitizing antigens. The pathological changes and clinical manifestations are similar to those of vasculitis due to sensitization with protein antigens and of vasculitis of unknown origin. Early and energetic administration of steroids has considerably reduced, but has not completely eliminated serious morbidity and mortality.

REFERENCES

1. Symmers, W.St.C.: The occurrence of angiitis and of other generalized diseases of connective tissues as a consequence of the administration of drugs. Proc. Roy. Soc. Med., *55:*20-28, 1962.
2. Rostenberg, A., Jr., and Fagelson, H. J.: Life-threatening drug eruptions. JAMA, *194:*660-662, 1965.
3. McCombs, R. P.: Systemic "'allergic" vasculitis. JAMA, *194:*1059-1064, 1965.
4. More, R. H., McMillan, G. C., and Duff, G. L.: The pathology of sulfonamide allergy in man. Amer. J. Path., *22:*703-735, 1946.
5. Waugh, D.: Myocarditis, arterities, and focal hepatic, splenic, and renal granulomas apparently due to penicillin sensitivity. Amer. J. Path., *28:*437-447, 1952.
6. Lee, D. K. and Andrews, J. M.: Temporl arteritis developing in the course of sulfonamide therapy. JAMA, *200:*720-721, 1967.
7. Winkelmann, R. K., and Ditto, W. B.: Cutaneous and visceral syndromes of necrotizing or "allergic" angiitis: a study of 38 cases. Medicine, *43:*59-89, 1964.
8. Gruber, G. B.: Zur Frage der Periarteritis nodosa mit besonderer Berucksichtigung der Gallenblasen — und der Nieren — Beteiligung. Virchows Arch., *258:*441-501, 1925.
9. Bishop, W. B., Carlton, R. F., and Sanders, L.L.: Diffuse vasculitis and death after hyperimmunization with pertussis vaccine. Report of a case. New Eng. J. Med., *274:*616-619, 1966.
10. Clark, E., and Kaplan, B. I. Endocardial, arterial and other mesenchymal alterations associated with serum disease in man. Arch. Path., *24:*458-475, 1937.
11. Rich, A. R.: The role of hypersensitivity in periarteritis nodosa as indicated by seven cases developing during serum sickness and sulfonamide therapy. Bull. Johns Hopkins Hosp., *71:* 123-140, 1942.
12. Rich, A. R., and Gregory, J. E.: The experimental demonstration that periarteritis nodosa is a manifestation of hypersensitivity. Bull. Johns Hopkins Hosp., *72:*65-88, 1943.
13. McLetchie, N. G. B., MacDonald, R. M., and Cutts, J. H.: Polyarteritis nodosa; report of a case with proof of a drug allergy (penicillin). Canad. M. A. J., *76* (3):213-216, 1957.
14. Winton, S. S., and Nora E. D. Immunologic aspects of penicillin reactions. Amer. J. Med., *18:*66-73, 1955.
15. Groth, O., Lindemark, C. O., and Sjoberg, S. G.: Necrotizing angiitis with multiple widespread hemorrhagic infarctive lesions of the skin. Acta Med. Scand., *180:*565-570, 1966.
16. Gardner, D. L.: Pathology of the Connective Tissue Diseases. Baltimore, Williams and Wilkins Co., 1965.
17. Frohnert, P. P., and Sheps, S. G.: Long-term follow-up study of periarteritis nodosa. Amer. J. Med., *43:*8-14, 1967.
18. Ehrenreich, T., and Olmstead, E. V.: Malignant hypertension following the administration of cortisone in periarteritis nodosa. A.M.A. Arch. Path., *52:*145-154, 1951.

Chapter 48

Dermatologic Manifestations to Toxic Agents

PETER N. HORVATH, M.D.

With its large surface area in direct contact with the environment, the skin is frequently exposed to toxic substances. This is readily reflected by the high incidence of cutaneous reactions under conditions of exposure. Anatomically, the organ complex that we call the skin consists of the epidermis, dermis, and the subcutaneous fat. This complex is capable only of limited morphological responses which through the years have been well described as primary and secondary lesions.

TABLE I: BASIC REACTIVE MORPHOLOGIC PATTERN OF THE SKIN

Macule	Scales
Wheal	Excoriations
Papule (plaque)	Fissures
Nodule	Crusts
Vesicle (bulba)	Ulcers
Pustule	Scars
	Pigmentation

Skin reactions to toxic agents encompass the entire spectrum of these basic lesions. Such conditions represent a significant proportion of the ordinary clinical practice and also are an important problem in occupational or industrial medicine. In many instances, the principle underlying a particular skin reaction is poorly understood. This chapter will emphasize those mechanisms which are generally accepted as important factors in the production of cutaneous lesions.

The application of irritating substances to the skin will produce a variety of lesions ranging from burns and ulcers to a mild dermatitis. The term "primary irritant dermatitis" is used to describe this group of reactions, which are nonspecific in nature and are reproducible in most individuals under appropriate circumstances. The cutaneous lesions depend on the concentration of the offending agent and the length of exposure. For example, high concentration of strong acids, alkalis, and phenol will always produce extensive changes. This response is nonallergic and consists of direct damage to the cells of the skin.

A much more common form of primary irritant dermatitis is produced by repeated exposure to low concentrations of "mild" irritants, such as soap, detergents and solvents. In this situation, direct cell damage is not a major factor, but the physico-chemical protective mechanisms of the skin are impaired. The more obvious changes consist of the depletion of the surface lipid film, a shift of the pH of the skin to the alkaline side, and mild damage to the cells in the horny layer.

Table II: Classes of Allergic Reactions Occurring Within the Skin

	Anaphylaxis	*Arthus Reaction*	*Delayed Sensitivity*
Active antibody	Reagin	Precipitating antibody	Cell mediated
Test response	Intradermal scratch test Immediate response	Arthus reaction. Intermediate response	Delayed tubercvulin type response
Clynical cutaneous pattern	Erythema Urticaria Angioneurotic edema	Serum sickness Cutaneous vasculitis	Allergic contact dermatitis Homograft rejection

The clinical picture may vary from minimal skin changes to severe and disabling dermatitis, which appears to be irritated by the mildest of substances. "Housewives eczema" is a good example of this type of reaction pattern. There is no distinguishing hallmark of primary irritant dermatitis and it may predispose to the development of allergic eczematous dermatitis (9). In same eruptions, both primary irritancy and allergic contact sensitization may be implicated.

While the exact details of allergic reactions in the skin are not well understood, Table II summarizes our knowledge of the various allergic reaction pattern.

Anaphylaxis is mediated by a circulating skin sensitizing antibody called reagin. Although its exact composition is controversial, at least part of the IgA globulin fraction has reaginic activity (6). Fortunately, anaphylaxis is a relatively rare condition in man. The cutaneous symptoms consists of erythema, urticaria and angioneurotic edema. The systemic manifestations include bronchial spasm, edema of the larynx, diarrhea, vomiting, and shock. In humans, it occurs after insect bites and administration of drugs, but in the milder cutaneous forms no cause may be found. In fact, in many patients with urticaria and angio-neurotic edema, the existence of an allergic mechanism cannot be confirmed.

The Arthus reaction consists of interaction of a circulating precipitating antibody and an injected antigen. It takes place within the lumen of blood and lymphatic vessels and surrounding tissue spaces. This interaction results in antigen-antibody aggregates which lead to formation of intravascular leukocyte-platelet thrombi, and massive local inflammatory reaction. The cutaneous lesions are localized and may appear within 2-4 hours after injection of the antigen. In appearance, there is a great diversity from small infiltrated erythematous papules and purpura, to marked local necrosis due to vascular occlusion· The Arthur phenomenon offers a very suitable explanation for the mechanism involved in the production of cutaneous vasculitis on a true allergic basis (8). Clinically, such localized reactions are often seen after repeated injections of foreign protein, such as anti-sera.

Delayed hypersensitivity implies a delay in clinical response to the antigen-antibody interaction, which may average 48-72 hours. This reaction is cell-mediated and involves the lymphocyte system, including the lymph nodes (10). Circulating antibodies have not been implicated in this reaction pattern. This type of response occurs in bacterial and my-

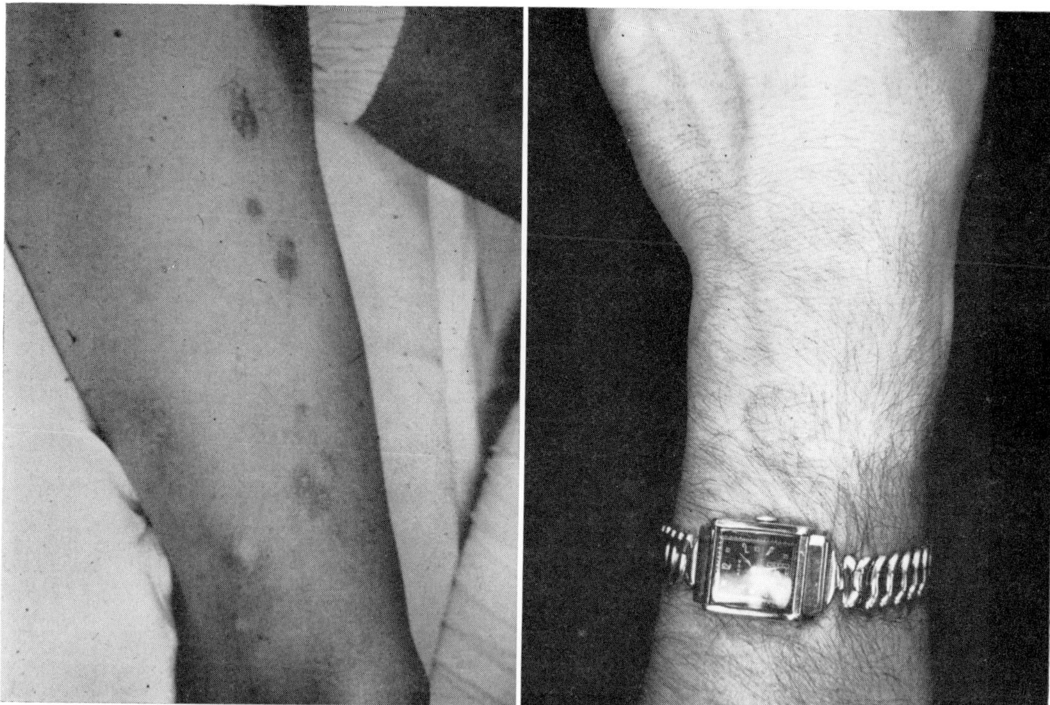

Figure 1. Local reaction to injections of protamide-zinc insulin, a clinical manifestation of the Arthus phenomenon.

Figure 2. Typical delayed hypersensitivity of the eczematous contact type due to nickel in the stainless steel watch case. Note that the gold metal band did not produce any cutaneous reaction.

cotic infections, allergic contact dermatitis, and homograft rejection response (2).

Cutaneous lesions due to drugs are produced through various theoretical mechanisms, most of which are controversial and do not account for all the clinical findings in any particular reaction. Table III lists better understood reactive patterns said to be involved in drug eruptions.

In general, any type of basic skin lesion can be produced by drugs and a single drug can produce more than one type of response. For example, penicillin has been reported to produce anaphylactic shock, urticaria, angioneurotic edema, serum sickness, fixed eruptions, exfoliative dermatitis, and allergic contact dermatitis.

TABLE III: POSSIBLE MECHANISMS INVOLVED IN DRUG ERUPTIONS

1. True allergy
2. Shwartzman phenomenon
3. Enzymatic differences
4. Toxic response (over-dosage)
5. Cumulative effects
6. Ecological inbalance
7. Light induced dermatoses
   Photo-toxic
   Photo-allergic

All facets of the allergic mechanism can be implicated in the production of drug eruptions. Anaphylactic or urticarial reactions occur after the administration of penicillin, salicylates, and morphine derivatives. Arthus reactions are seen subsequent to repeated injections of foreign protein such as anti-sera and some types of insulin. Delayed hypersensitivity reactions manifest themselves as allergic contact dermatitis to topical medications. Notable offenders are benzocaine, sulfonamides and penicillin.

The Shwartzman phenomenon is advanced by some as a theoretical explanation for hemorrhagic drug eruptions (11). This explanation assumes the existence of a pre-existing infection which "prepares" the skin and the drug then acts as an "eliciting agent." While not yet proven, this explanation may account for some instances of drug-induced vasculitis. Enzymatic differences offer the brightest future promise for the explanation of normal and abnormal drug responses. Most of the known enzymatic differences are on a genetic basis, as for example, primaquine induced hemolytic anemia (7). Although such explanations have not been applied to drug eruptions as yet, the precipitation of clinical manifestations of porphyria by hepato-toxic agents, such as barbiturates and estrogens, can be explained in this manner (14).

A toxic response ensues when the therapeutic requirements are close to the toxic level. Methotrexate in therapeutic doses may produce toxic alopecia.

Cumulative effects occur when the drug is deposited in the tissues during prolonged administration. Arsenical de-

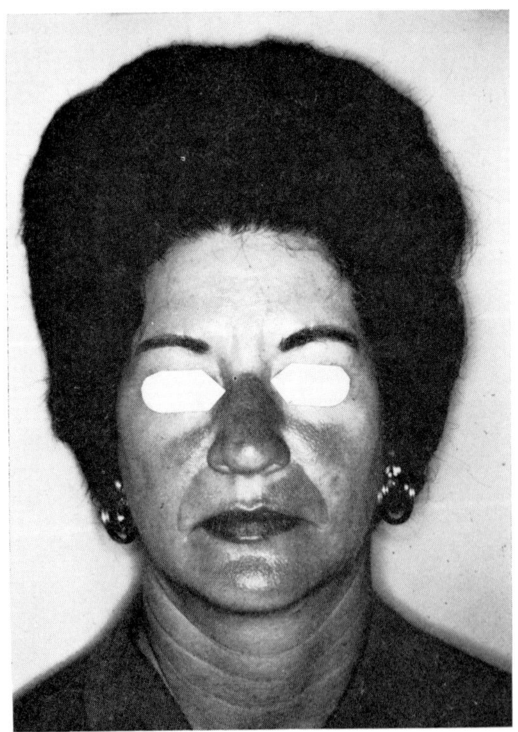

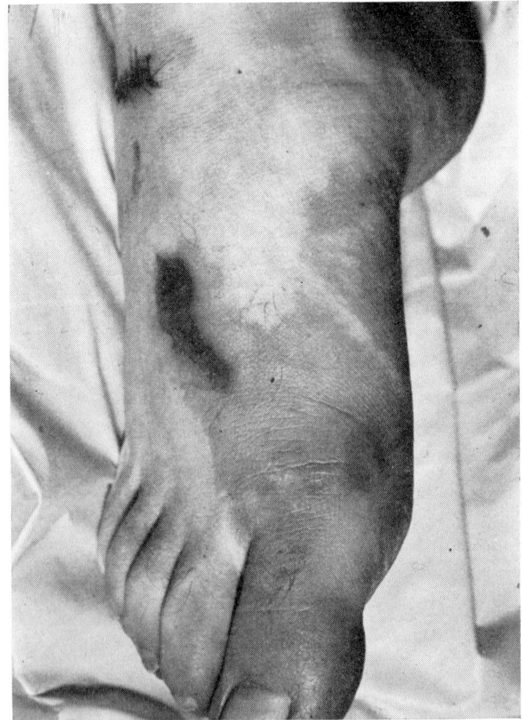

Figure 3. Hemorrhagic lesions in a patient with chronic ulcerative colitis, appearing after the administration of oral sulfonamide. This possibly can be explained as a type of Schwartzman phenomenon. Note: This is former figure 4.

Figure 4. Phototoxic reaction due to oral demethylchlortetracycline (Declomycin) and sunlight. Note: This is former figure 3.

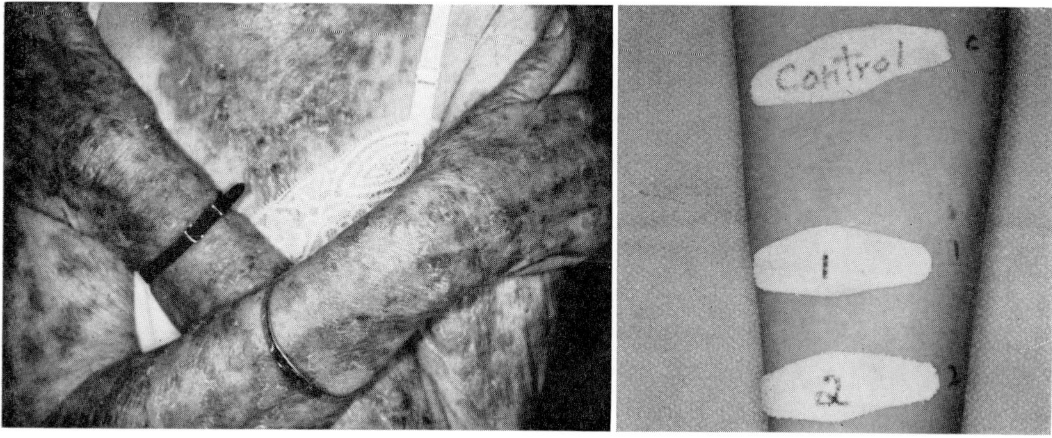

Figure 5. Photo-allergic dermatitis produced by sunlight and a thiazide diuretic.

Figure 6. Demonstration of patch testing technique on forearm. Control represents tape without allergen.

posits in the skin producing hyperpigmentation, keratosis or malignancy are a prime example of this type of reaction.

Ecological imbalance develops when a drug changes the natural balance of the patient's microorganisms. Tetracycline alters the normal flora of the gastrointestinal tract resulting in diarrhea and monilial vulvo-vaginitis.

Certain drugs are changed by light and produce cutaneous lesions under these circumstances. These drugs are able to absorb energy from light and are altered by this process of absorption. This altered substance then either affects the skin directly by a so-called photo-toxic reaction or becomes an allergen and initiates a photo-allergic reaction (12). The photo-toxic response clinically resembles sunburn, while the lesions of photo-allergic dermatitis are similar to other dermatoses of allergic origin (3).

The active drug in light sensitive eruptions may be administered systemically or applied topically. Dimethylchlortetracycline orally in sufficient dosage produces photo-toxic eruptions. Sulfonamides and phenothiazines orally may produce both photo-toxic and photo-allergic reactions. Topical application of coal tar products results in a phototoxic reaction, while antiseptics used in toilet soaps, such as bithionol and tribrom-salicylanilide, produce a photoallergic response.

TESTING PROCEDURES

Unfortunately, only a few routine diagnostic procedures are of value for lesions of the skin:

1. *Biopsy.* As the microscopic picture of cutaneous response to toxic agents is not specific, this procedure, even in the hands of a skilled dermatopathologist, does not yield useful data. Often its value is that of excluding other possibilities. Under some circumstances, deposits of heavy metals, such as gold, silver, or arsenic, may be identified, either in the skin or the hair and nails.

2. *Intradermal or Scratch Tests.* Intradermal or scratch tests are used for the detection of reagins in the skin, which appear to be implicated in the production of immediate type of hypersensitivity, such as anaphylactic drug reaction,

some types of urticaria, hay fever and asthma. In the diagnosis and management of routine clinical dermatologic problems, such tests have been of little practical value.

3. *Patch Test.* This test consists of application of substances to the skin to detect the possibility of cutaneous sensitivity. (13) This sensitivity usually is specific and is of the delayed type. The mechanism consists of cell-mediated response produced by the lymphocytes. In essence, the patch test reproduces the allergic sensitivity in a miniature form. The procedure consists of applying the test material in intimate contact with the skin for 48 hours, after which the patch is removed and the skin reaction evaluated. The tests should be applied to nonhairy skin that is completely normal. In the presence of a widespread eruption, testing should be postponed until the condition subsides. Owing to rare complications, such as scarring or depigmentation, normally uncovered areas of the body should be avoided. While special patch-testing tapes are commercially available (Elastopatch, Duke Laboratories), the square plastic Bandaid (Johnson & Johnson) is adequate for most purposes. If such Bandaids are irritating, patches can be made of Dermicel (Johnson & Johnson).

The evaluation of the cutaneous reaction is graded, according to its intensity, from +1 to +4:

0 — no reaction
1+ — erythema only
2+ — erythema and palpable infiltration
3+ — erythema, papules and vesiculation
4+ — erythema, vesciles, bullae and erosions

Nonspecific irritation from tape and pressure may be excluded by delaying the evaluation about 20 to 30 minutes. Also, a control patch test should be performed with the adhesive tape alone. While any material may be used for testing, it is essential to employ it in the proper concentration and a suitable vehicle. Embodying years of experience, extensive lists are available for proper patch testing (5). Generally speaking, a primary irritant reaction will subside quickly, but a true allergic one will persist for several days and occasionally will develop as late as 72 hours or more. The systemic administration of corticosteroids or antihistamines will not interfere with the performance of patch testing as only the weakly positive test responses are affected (5).

Under some conditions, variants of the patch test are employed. The "open" patch test consists of application of the suspected material without the adhesive patch. This is employed when the substance in question, such as a spray or a vapor, may be irritant when occluded. It is often employed in testing cosmetics. Another specialized form is the photopatch test (4). Here, the routine patch test is applied in duplicate for 24 to 48 hours. Then one of the patch test sites is irradiated by a standardized source of ultraviolet light. The skin reaction here can consist of erythema, wheals, papules and vesicles. The sites are evaluated at intervals of 24 hours, 72 hours, and one week.

Usage and immersion tests are useful when prolonged exposure to mild primary irritants is suspected in the production of skin lesions. Such technique requires a prior clearing of the eruption and close personal observation of the skin during the test period. It involves either the deliberate re-exposure of the patient to the conditions that are under suspicion or the repeated immersion of the hands into the test solutions. Such usage or reexposure tests are useful, es-

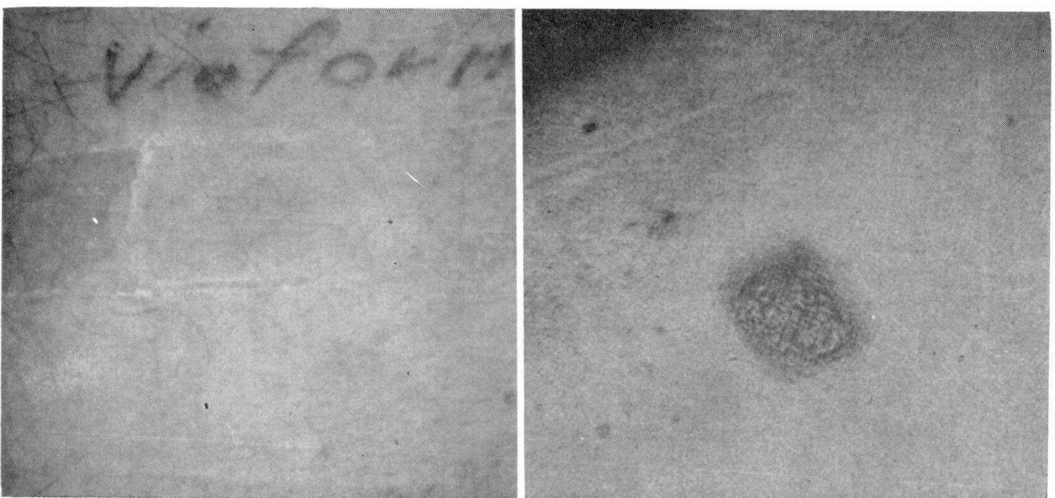

Figure 7. Positive patch test due to Vioform, graded as one plus.

Figure 8. Positive patch test due to 5% nickel sulfate, graded as 3 plus.

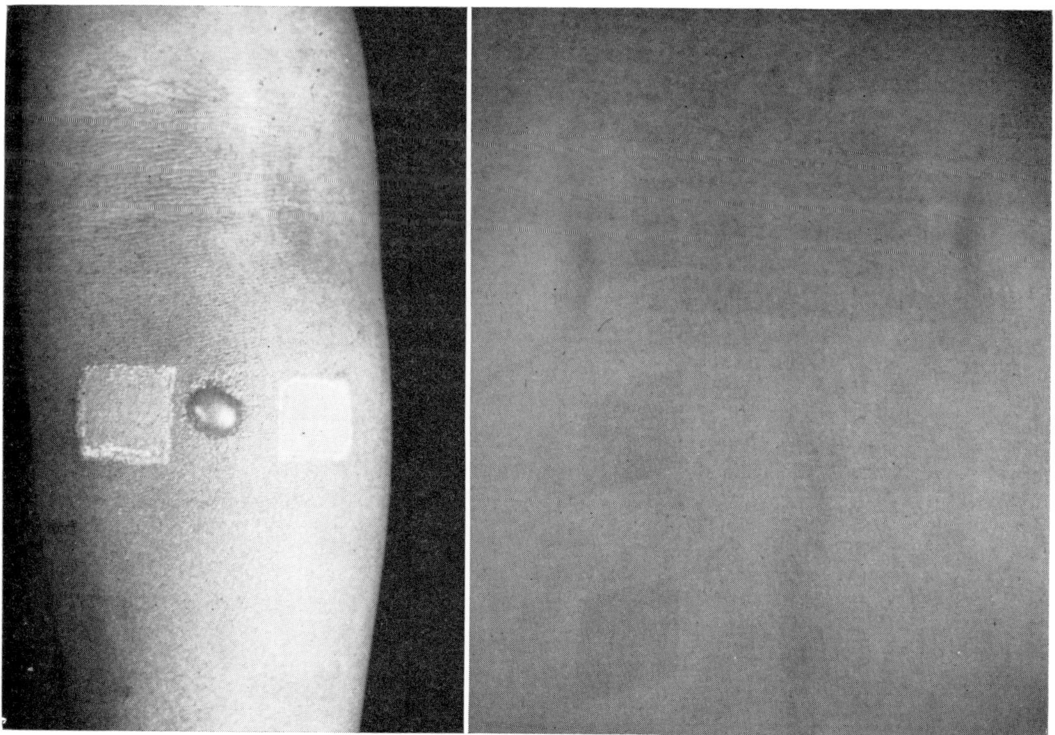

Figure 9. Positive patch test due to poison ivy, oleoresin 0.1% in acetone, graded as 4 plus.

Figure 10. Positive photo-patch tests in a patient receiving 450 mg per day of demethychlortetracycline (Declomycin). Lowest patch test represents longest exposure.

pecially when the patch test results may be equivocal. When properly performed, this test often provides the decisive information for the management of cutaneaus problems due to external substances.

Test procedures for evaluating eruptions, presumably due to drugs, are of little practical value in clinical practice. An occasional patch test or microscopic examination may be of some use. The practitioner depends on a high index of suspicion and a thorough knowledge of the eruptions produced by drugs for the management of such problems.

The latest advances in skin testing employ the patch test to measure the immunologic competence of the lymphocyte system, which mediates the delayed type of response. Experimental sensitization can be reliably achieved in most individuals by the application of 2,4-dinitrochlorobenzene to the skin. In Hodgkin's disease, especially of the more extensive variety, a significant number of patients were unable to develop contact sensitization to dinitrochlorbenzene. (1) Thus, the capability to develop contact allergy may be used as another reliable test in evaluating patients with diseases involving the lymphocytes.

REFERENCES

1. Brown, R. S., Haynes, H. A., Foley, T. H., Godwin, H. A., Berard, C. W., and Carbona, P.: Hodgkin's disease, immunological clinical and histological features in 50 untreated patients. Ann. Int. Med., *67:*291, 1967.
2. Chase, M. W.: Delayed hypersensitivity. Med. Clin. N. America., *49:*1613, 1965.
3. Epstein, S.: Photoallergy vs phototoxicity. In, Dermatoses Due to Environmental and Physical Factors. Ed., Rees, R. B. Springfield, Thomas, 1962, p. 119.
4. Epstein, S.: Simplified photopatch testing. Arch. Derm., *93:*216, 1966.
5. Fisher, A. A.: Contact Dermatitis. Philadelphia, Lea J. Febiger, 1967, pp. 257-307.
6. Heremans, J. F., and Vaerman, J. P.: Beta 2A globulin as a possible carrier and allergic reaginic activity. Nature, *193:*1091, 1962.
7. Kalow, W.: Pharmacogenetics. Philadelphia, W. B. Saunders, 1962.
8. Parish, W. E., and Rhodes, E. L.: Bacterial antigens and aggregated gamma globulin in the lesions of nodular vasculitis. Brit. J. Derm., *79:*131, 1967.
9. Rostenberg, H., Jr.: Primary irritant dermatitis vs. allergic eczematous contact dermatitis. In Dermatoses Due to Environmental and Physical Factors, (Ed.) Rees, R. E. Springfield, Thomas, 1962, p. 15.
10. Rostenberg, A. J.: The pathogenesis of eczematous sensitization. Acta derm.-venereal., *45:*1-8, 1965.
11. Rostenberg, A. J.: The Shwartzman phenomenon. A review with a consideration of some possible dermatological manifestations Brit. J. Derm., *65:*389, 1953.
12. Shelly, W. B.: Photosensitizers. In, Dermatoses Due to Environmental and Physical Factors. (Ed.) Rees, R. B. Springfield, Thomas, 1962, p. 88.
13. Shelley, W. B.: The patch test J.A.M.A., *200:* 170, 1967.
14. Vail, J. T., Jr.: Porphyria cutanea tarda and estogens. J.A.M.A., *201:*671, 1967.

Chapter 49A

Envenomation by the Arachnida

PAUL N. MORGAN, PH.D.

A wide variety of natural biological products such as bacterial toxins, plant poisons and animal venoms are among the most potent of known toxic agents. Because of their dramatic pharmacological actions, these substances play primary roles in the etiology of certain pathological conditions; and yet, in the majority of these conditions, especially those produced by animal venoms, diagnostic clinical laboratories are unable to identify the specific biological substances producing the toxic manifestations. In such cases it is necessary for the clinician to recognize classic symptomatology and relate this information to the case history of the patient. It is equally important for those in research laboratories to study and learn more about these natural biological poisons.

Of all natural biological toxic materials, venoms are perhaps the most dramatic. Shortly after a patient has been bitten or stung by a venomous animal, serious clinical manifestations normally develop which can be severe and ultimately lethal. A wide variety of animals, invertebrate and vertebrate, possess venomous capacities. In this chapter only a relatively small group will be considered. These are well known and feared by the general public but they represent a group which has been poorly characterized in research laboratories.

The taxonomic phylum Arthropoda von Siebold and Stannius, 1845, contains about four-fifths of all the known animals in the world. Its members are invertebrates which are bilaterally symmetrical and have hard exoskeletons and jointed appendages arranged in pairs. In smaller taxonomic subgroups, there are several classes which contain animals with great medical significance since they can affect man in many ways. One of these, Class Arachnida, contains many related animals which have no venomous capacities. These include ticks and mites which are very important in the transmission of certain infectious diseases but the Class Arachnida also contains other related animals which are less readily recognized by those interested in medical aspects of entomology. Also included in this class are two orders of venomous animals, the scorpions and the spiders, some species of which are of significant medical importance since envenomation of man does occur in many geographical areas and can be fatal. It is these groups, the scorpions and the spiders, that will be considered in this chapter.

Scorpions (Fig. 1) are certainly among the most primitive animals. It is thought that these were among the first forms of organized life to abandon the seas and successfully adapt to a terrestrial environ-

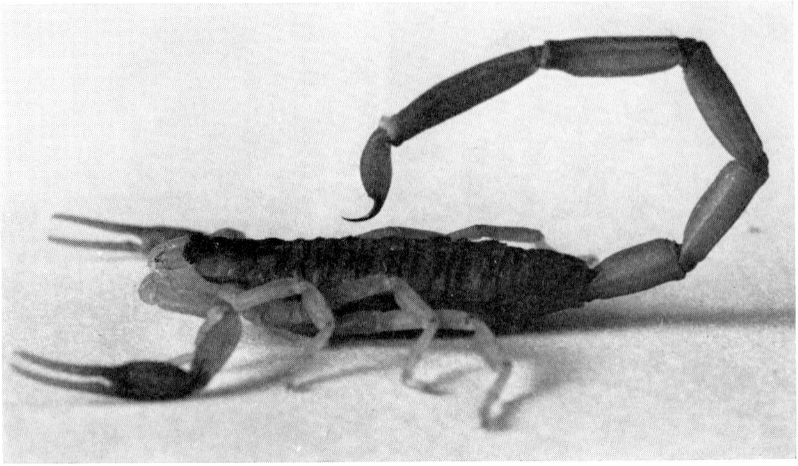

Figure 1. A common scorpion.

ment. Extremely conspicuous and menacing with their crab-like appendages and a long, segmented tail ending in a bulbous sac containing a prominent stinger, scorpions have been noted and feared since the dawn of civilization. They have been included in the oldest myths and they have been granted a celestial place in the zodiac.

Throughout the world, between 600 and 700 species of scorpions have been described; in the United States, only about 30 species have been found. Having nocturnal habits, they remain well hidden in cracks and small openings during daylight hours. At night and in the darkness, they venture out of seclusion and search for food and water. They normally prefer to avoid direct contact with man but when trapped in loose clothing or when disturbed abruptly, scorpions can strike rapidly and accurately with their long flexible tails to inflict a very deep and painful sting. All species possess venom glands associated with the stinger and venom is normally introduced by the stinging process. Fortunately, most species of scorpions have a venom which is non-lethal for man but it does produce localized reactions which can be painful and uncomfortable. Such cases are characterized by sharp burning sensations at the site of the sting, swelling and discoloration. Anaphylactic reactions have been reported following scorpions' stings but fortunately they appear to be rare.

In restricted areas of the United States, that is, the arid regions of the southwest, and in other parts of the world, there are highly poisonous varieties of scorpions whose stings produce much more dramatic and frequently, fatal reactions. In North Africa, South America and Mexico, scorpion stings are responsible for more deaths than snake bites. The venoms from these scorpions possess potent convulsant neurotoxic properties and may or may not possess the properties of producing localized swelling and discoloration. In such instances, the pain produced by the initial sting is rapidly followed by peculiar, sharply painful sensations which extend from the area of the sting. As venom is disseminated, the patient may develop itching sensations in the nose, mouth and throat. Speech becomes impaired and symptoms continue to develop which indicate generalized involvement of the central nervous system. Convulsive episodes come in waves, each increases in severity. Death, when and if it occurs, is closely associated with respiratory and circulatory failure, although exhaustion from the repeated convulsive seizures could also contribute to the lethal effects of this venom. Normally, if the patient survives the first six hours, recovery usually occurs within 2 or 3 days without any residual effects.

Known primarily as spinners of silk threads, spiders are invariably associated with the weaving of elaborate, ingenious and beautiful webs. More than 30,000 species have been characterized so that spiders are certainly the most dominant group of the Arachnids. With such variety, it is easy to understand that these animals show great variations in anatomical features and habits. Most are solitary but play an important role in the control of certain insect populations. Although all spiders have venom glands and a biting apparatus which are used for securing food, very few are capable of harming man. Their venoms show little toxicity for the tissues of man and few have a biting apparatus capable of penetrating his skin.

Most notorious of venomous spiders is *Latrodectus mactans,* commonly referred to as the black widow. Jet black and distinctively characterized by a red hourglass design on her abdomen (Fig. 2), this spider lives her life in an inverted position while clinging to a web which she uses as a home, a nursery and an effective food trap. Her eyesight is poor despite four pairs of eyes, but her reflexes are remarkably responsive to any vibrations on her web. Any gentle movements immediately attract her attention and she reacts accordingly. She prefers a dark, cool, moist area to spin her web and one which abounds with insects. Today such environments are found around such places as porch steps, rubbish heaps, lumber piles and

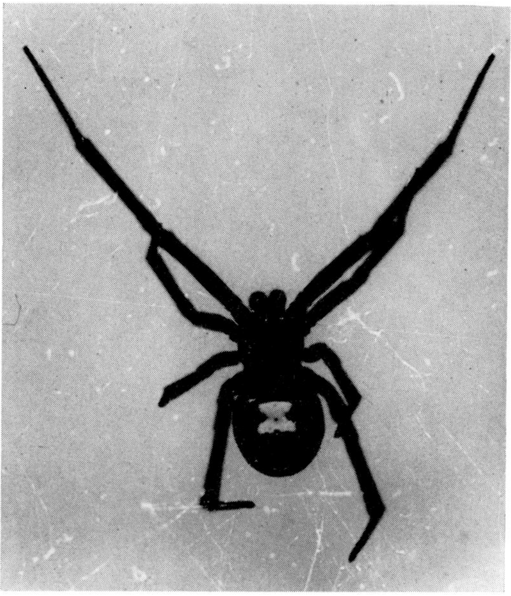

Figure 2. The black widow spider, **Latrodectus mactans.**

in gardens and vineyards. In such areas, man rarely comes in intimate and prolonged association with the black widow and her web. Bites in man are certainly not as numerous as they were when outdoor privies were so common to our society. A few years ago, the underside of the "one- or two-holers" offered an optimal environment for this spider and her web. In this area, man frequently came in intimate and prolonged contact with the web, and envenomation frequently occurred.

Symptoms of the bite invariably include an instant burning pain at the site even though the spider is rarely seen. The local pain intensifies up to three hours or so during which time severe cramps, rigidity and spasms of large muscle groups always develop. Most frequently, abdominal muscles are involved so that the "board-like" rigidity and tenderness may suggest an abdominal emergency. Systemic reactions continue to develop and may include nausea, vomiting, visual difficulties, profuse cold sweating and shock. In severe cases, convulsions, paralysis, delerium, urinary retention and cynosis may terminate in death of the patient within two or three days. These manifestations are uncommon however, and normally symptoms diminish and recovery is complete.

Within the last decade, it has been recognized that the bite of another spider, *Loxosceles reclusa,* was capable of producing serious clinical manifestations in man. The brown recluse spider is extremely common in certain geographical areas of the United States and increasingly large numbers of cases are being reported. Several deaths have also been documented in southwestern and central United States.

As the name implies, this spider is a recluse and it lives a nocturnal life in close association with man and his habitation. It is inconspicuous but can be recognized by the presence of the dark violin-shaped design which extends over its cephalothorax (Fig. 3). Being a poor web builder, this spider hunts its food only at night. Man is bitten only when the spider is pressed to the bare skin. Such instances arise when the spider is hidden in clothing being donned or when man unintentionally rolls on a wanderer in his bed.

Man may be unaware of envenomation since little early pain is associated with the bite. Within three to six hours, however, a characteristic lesion begins to develop around the site of the bite. After a transient erythema, a small bleb or blister develops which seems to give rise to a zone of hemorrhage and discoloration. This area is very well demarcated and appears to spread in a bizarre gravitational manner. The central area of this lesion shows ischemia and over a period of several days or weeks, it turns dark in color and firm to the touch. Within the first few days, this lesion may be surrounded by a petechial rash. After the first week, the central area of this lesion becomes dark, mummified and a tough, leatherly eschar eventually covers the central area of the lesion. Several weeks or even months may be ensue before this eschar separates and is lost. The resulting open ulcer may require several additional weeks or months for healing. In many instances, skin grafting is necessary to close this ulcer, and even then, grafts may take poorly. In rare instances, the bite of this spider may evoke more severe systemic reactions during the first week. These include fever, chills, malaise, weakness, nausea, vomiting and joint pain. A severe vascular crisis may develop, leading to anemia, hemoglobinuria, thrombocytopenia, the consequences of which seem to be the prin-

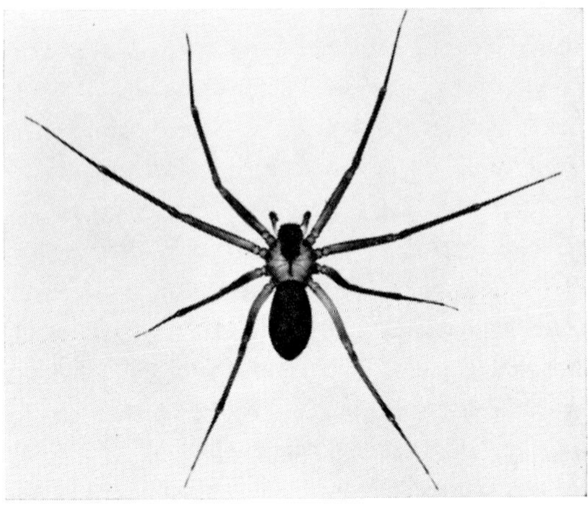

Figure 3. The brown recluse spider, **Loxosceles reclusa.**

ciple factors associated with the fatalities which have been reported.

In those geographical areas where the brown recluse spider is in abundance, the bite of this arthropod probably represents a greater hazard to man than any other. The spider lives with man and as such more intimate contact will result. Although fatalities are rare, the lesion and its management over a long period of time represent important problems for the clinician.

SUMMARY

Of the innumerable species contained in the class Arachnida, only the scorpions and spiders have venomous capacities. In specific geographical areas, these may play important roles in disease since envenomation of man may be rather common. Most scorpions are rather innocuous; however, in specific areas of the world, their stings do produce a significant number of fatalities. Of the tremendous number of spiders, only a few are capable of inflicting serious damage. Two species, the black widow and the brown recluse, do have such capacities, since they have potent venoms and biting apparatuses which can produce envenomation of man, the results of which can be most severe.

Addendum: A Method for Extracting Pure Venom from Spiders

PAUL N. MORGAN, PH.D.

INTRODUCTION

At least two species of spiders, the black widow and the brown recluse, have been shown to have significant medical importance in certain geographical areas of the United States.[1] The venoms from these spiders have not been studied as extensively as venoms from other animals because of several factors. Certain problems, such as the minuteness of venom volumes and the complexity of venom apparatuses, have made it extremely difficult to obtain satisfactory preparations for study. Without a relatively pure preparation, few definitive characterizations of such complex biological poisons can be undertaken.

The method presented has been highly successful in obtaining satisfactory venom preparations from one species of spider, *Loxosceles reclusa*. Several spiders can be processed in a relatively short period of time so that adequate amounts of reasonably pure venom are available as needed.

PRINCIPLE

A spider is placed in a holding device so that the anterior portion of the cephalothorax is free and accessible. Electrical impulses of high voltage and low amperage are applied locally to an area of the cephalothorax just over the venom glands. The process apparently produces contractions of the glands without producing coagulation damage since a small drop of venom slowly accumulates on the anterior portion of the fangs. This venom, relatively free from contaminating tissues and fluids, is readily collected in capillary tubes and can be accurately quantitated by volumetric and gravimetric methods.

SPECIAL EQUIPMENT

The apparatus shown in Figure 4 is used for holding spiders and for the delivery of electrical charges. It consists of a six-volt Eveready battery #773 (or equivalent) (A) wired to a six-volt automobile ignition coil (B) and a flat metal plate (F) so that when the microswitch (D) is closed and opened, a high voltage direct current is discharged through the center wire of the ignition coil to the heavily insulated electrode which is tipped with a small gage inoculating needle (C). A spider is immobilized on the flat metal plate (F) by an adjustable arm (E) made from a kymograph arm and tipped with soft sponge. The entire system is mounted on a ringstand so that it is compact and mobile.

PROCEDURE

1. An unanesthetized spider is grasped with forceps by the distal segment of a foreleg and carefully led onto the flat metal plate (F) (see Fig. 4). It is held in place while the metal arm (E) tipped with soft sponge is lowered to immobilize the spider. In a satisfactory position, the abdomen of the spider is pressed to the plate by the sponge and the cephalothorax is projecting slightly over the edge of the plate.

2. The point of the needle (C) is touched to an area of the cephalothorax just posterior to the eyes. Closing and opening the microswitch (D) produces an electrical charge which can be seen as a spark. Three or four such charges are normally sufficient to produce maximum contractions of the venom glands.

3. Within a few seconds a small drop of fluid accumulates on the fangs (see Fig. 5). This drop is collected by capillary action in a microcapillary tube (Aloe

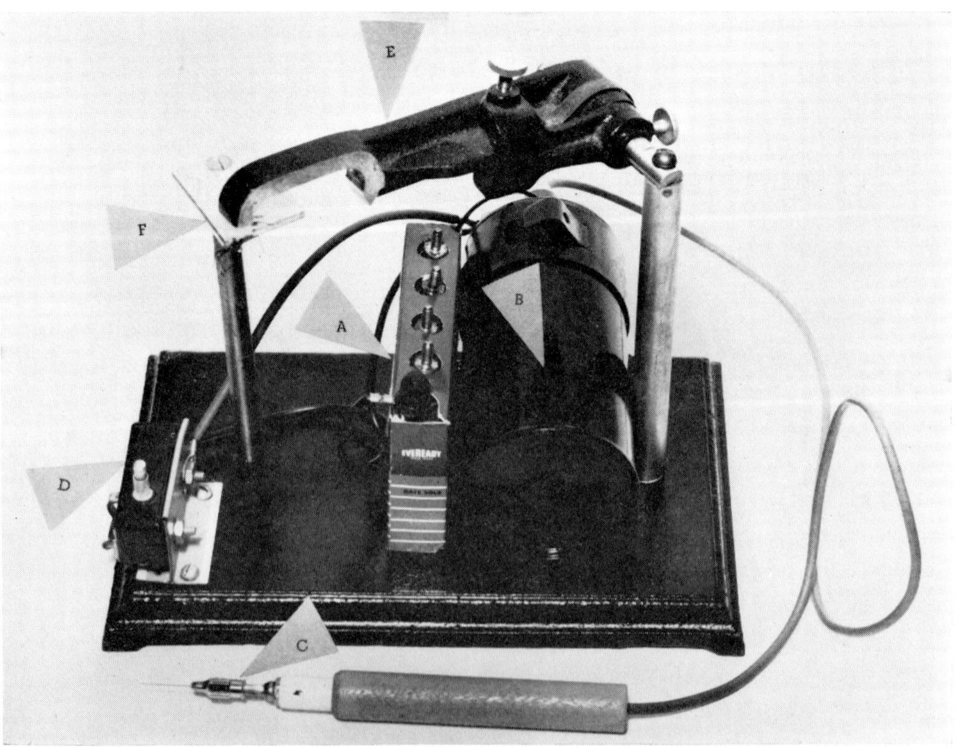

Figure 4. An apparatus for extracting venom from spiders.

Scientific Co., St. Louis, Mo., No. 23919P) which previously was weighed and calibrated for total volume content. Quantitation can include measurement of volume and wet weight while venom is in the capillary tube.

4. After quantitation, this reasonably pure drop of venom can be used successfully for any of a wide variety of studies. Normally, it is expressed from the capillary tube into a measured volume of a suitable diluent.

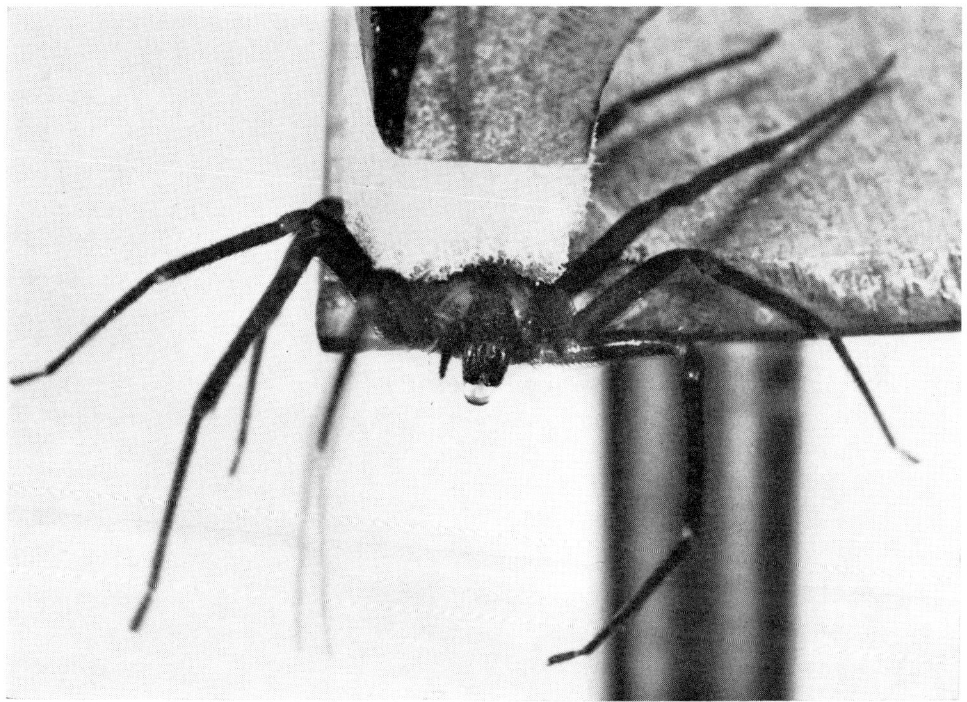

Figure 5. Pure venom from a brown recluse spider.

Discussion

As shown in Figure 5, venom from brown recluse spiders can be extracted in reasonably pure form by the method described. Preliminary studies[2] have shown that the method is reproducible and has provided data which indicates that the venom from *Loxosceles reclusa* is a very potent and interesting biological poison. Since other species of the Genus *Loxoseles* occur in the United States as well as members of the Genus *Latrodecutus* (the widow spiders), it would seem that many more definitive studies should be devoted to venoms of these and other venomous spiders. The use of extraction methods, such as the one described above, can provide a convenient material for such studies.

REFERENCES

1. Wingo, C. W.: Poisonous Spiders and Other Venomous Arthropods in Missouri. Agricultural Experiment Station Bulletin 738, University of Missouri, 1967.
2. Morgan, P. N.: Preliminary studies on venom from the brown recluse spider, *Loxosceles reclusa*. Toxicon. *6*:161-165, 1969.

Chapter 49B

Bee Venom and Snake Venom: Clinical Contrasts

HALLA BROWN, M.D.

A patient usually knows whether he has been stung by a bee or bitten by a snake. However, there are occasions when a patient presents an enormous swelling which developed a short time after walking in the dark or through dense brush or woods. Sometimes only a prick was felt and the patient was unaware of anything unusual until swelling and/or fever developed. Such cases have occurred in the Washington area and they usually pose a serious problem to the physician.

Table I shows a summary of the contrasting effects of bee sting and snakebite in humans. The snakes referred to are indigenous to North America — rattlesnakes, copperheads, water mocassins, and coral snakes. Maine, Alaska, and Hawaii are the only states free of poisonous land snakes. The Hymenoptera, bees, hornets, wasps, and yellow jackets, are found throughout the country. Every year during the past decade more people have died from bee stings than from bites of poisonous snakes.[1] Bee stings occur more often in suburbia than on the farm, snake bites more often in the wilds. Snake bites usually are single, but bee stings may be single or multiple. When multiple, the patient may suffer the toxic symptoms of envenomation rather than the allergic symptoms of anaphylaxis. However, most patients who die from a bee sting, die from a single sting.

Fifty per cent of stings occur on the head or the hand.[2] Most snake bites occur on the lower limbs.

The honeybee leaves one mark per sting (insect), the venom being extruded from a sac at the posterior end of the abdomen, whereas the snake usually leaves two fang marks. The fangs are canalized teeth through which venom from the salivary glands is injected. A light strike may leave only one fang mark. At times, the snake's venom will have been used up by a previous bite so that envenomation does not occur. In one series, 24 of 161 consecutive bites were dry.[3] The amount of venom injected by a bee is minute (0.0005 ml); that injected by a snake varies from 0.5 ml to several mls depending on the size of the snake.

Pain usually is marked during a sting or bite but occasionally is insignificant. The onset of symptoms is rapid, within minutes following a sting, but after a snakebite, symptoms may be delayed several hours, especially after a coral snake bite. In such cases, respiratory paralysis may set in after a totally symptom-free period of 6-8 hours.

The severity of symptoms may range from almost nil to death. Mild symptoms usually consist of local swelling only. Generalized swelling, urticaria, dyspnea, asthma, cyanosis, collapse in anaphylactic shock usually precede death by a sting. Most poisonous snake bites are followed by the onset of local swelling. With considerable envenomation, swelling may spread to contigous areas of the trunk followed by fever, loss of consciousness, hemolysis, renal shut down, or respiratory paralysis, depending on the type of toxin. Death from a sting usually is rapid, within 10-60 minutes (4). Death from a snakebite occurs days or weeks later.

Stings rarely are followed by complications, but bacterial infection (including tetanus) and necrosis necessitating amputation of a limb are common sequelae of snakebite.

Most patients recover within 2 hours of the effects of a sting so that hospitalization only occasionally is necessary. For snakebite patients, hospitalization is

TABLE I: CONTRASTS BETWEEN BEE STINGS AND POISONOUS SNAKE BITE IN HUMANS

	Bee (Hymenoptera)	*Snake (USA)*
Prevalence	All states	All states except Maine, Alaska, Hawaii
Incidence of fatality	More frequent	Less frequent
Geography	Suburbia	Wild country
Size of patient	Unimportant (adults)	Important (children)
Number of stings or bites	Single or multiple	Single usually
Site	Head and hand	Extremity, lower
Puncture sites	1 per insect	2 (or 1) fang marks
Venom extruded from	Sac in post part of of abdomen	Salivary glands through fangs
Amount of venom	Minute (.0005 ml)	Greater (.5 to several ml., depending on size of snake)
Pain	Always	Usually excruciating (depending on species)
Onset of symptoms	Rapid, within minutes	Slower, within minutes to hours.
Severity	Whole gamut	Whole gamut
Symptoms	1. Local swelling 2. Generalized swelling, urticaria, dyspnea, asthma, cyanosis, collapse, anaphylactic shock 3. Death	1. Local swelling 2. Entire limb and contiguous trunk, fever, loss of consciousness, hemolysis, renal shut down, respiratory paralysis 3. Death
Fatality	Rapid, within minutes	Within days — slow
Complications	Few	Common
Secondary infection	Uncommon	Common
Necrosis (amputation)	Never	Common
Recovery	Fast (minutes to hours)	Slow (days-weeks-months)
Hospitalization	Infrequent	Usual
Mechanism	Allergic (antibodies)	Toxic (hemo-, neuro-, proteolytic enzymes)
Immediate treatment	Epinephrine, etc.	Supportive, antivenin, prevention of infection.

mandatory since recovery is slow, and even after discharge a limb may remain exquisitely painful for months.

Death from a sting is attributed to an allergic mechanism. The patient in response to a previous sting (or stings) has developed circulating antibodies. Upon reintroduction of the antigen (bee venom), the antibodies combine with it, causing cell damage with the release of histamine and with symptoms typical of allergic shock.

In contrast, death from envenomation occurs from poisoning, the exact mechanism and sequence of action of toxins and enzymes remaining unclear.

The treatment of stings is that for any severe allergy, epinephrine being the drug of choice. For snakebite, intravenous injection of antivenin, prevention of infection, and supportive treatment are necessary.

REFERENCES

1. Parrish, H. M.: Am. J. Med. Sci., *245:*129, 1960.
2. Brown, H., and Bernton, H. S.: Allergy to the Hymenoptera. V. Clinical study of 400 Cases. Presented at AMA Meeting, San Francisco, June 1968.
3. Conn, J.: Current Therapy
4. Barnard, J. H.: Severe hidden delayed reactions from insect stings. N. Y. State J. Med., *66:*1206, 1966.

Chapter 50

Laboratory Diagnosis of Drowning

WERNER U. SPITZ, M.D.

Drowning is notoriously known as a difficult and often unreliable postmortem diagnosis. In spite of a considerable effort spent in an attempt to establish objective and dependable criteria for the laboratory diagnosis of drowning, there is today more controversy associated with this diagnosis than with any other single cause of death.

The gross and microscopic appearance of the lungs in drowning is nonspecific and closely resembles that in severe pulmonary edema as seen in deaths associated with circulatory failure. This similarity is often so striking that in the presence of advanced coronary artery disease, or a well documented history of epilepsy in a body recovered from water the distinction between drowning and such other natural causes of death may be a matter of considerable speculation. Asphyxia may equally resemble drowning very intimately, and many text books refer to drowning as asphyxia due to obstruction of the airway by the drowning fluid. This situation may perhaps be best exemplified in the inability to distinguish between a case of strangulation thrown into water after death and drowning. It is believed, however, that only 10-15% of all drowning victims die of actual asphyxia, resulting from reflex closure of the glottis or laryngospasm. In the vast majority of cases, death by drowning results from complex patho-physiological events which differ profoundly according to the chemical composition of the submersion fluid. Drowning in fresh water and sea water must therefore be considered as distinctly separate entities.

DROWNING IN FRESH WATER

Water enters the lungs and due to its hypotonicity, is rapidly absorbed into the circulating blood stream. Hemodilution and an increase of the blood volume result. Hemodilution is associated with hemolysis and upset of the normal balance of the blood's constituents.

DROWNING IN SEA WATER

Sea water is strongly hypertonic (usually over 3.0% salt concentration). There occurs a rapid diffusion of salts into the blood stream, while water moves from the circulation into the pulmonary alveoli. Hemoconcentration and pulmonary edema are prominent features. No hemolysis occurs.

It is usually considered that fresh and sea water drowning are indistinguishable from each other grossly and microscopically, and as alluded to earlier, both conditions are indistinguishable from certain other causes of death. Because of this, and the chemical and physical alterations believed to occur in the body fluids, pathologists engaged in forensic work have turned to the laboratory for the diagnosis of death by drowning.

Numerous criteria, some believed to be more dependable than others, have been reported since the turn of the century. Practically each of these was accepted by forensic pathologists until experience showed their questionable value.

Carrara,[1] in 1902, established disproportionate dilution of left heart blood in fresh versus salt water drowning on the basis of specific gravity, freezing point and electrical conductivity determinations. Revenstorf,[9] also in 1902, stressed the diagnostic value of the cryoscopic examination, particularly in borderline cases. In 1903, Placzek[8] emphasized the diagnostic value of the specific gravity method and in 1921 Gettler[3] published a test for drowning involving the micro-chemical determination of chlorides in blood from the right and left heart chambers. A difference in the sodium chloride concentration of the two sides of the heart in excess of 25 mg/100 ml of blood indicated drowning. In salt water drowning the chloride level is higher in left heart blood, while the reverse occurs in drowning in fresh water. Gettler's observations have since been challenged repeatedly and there exists considerable diversity of opinion regarding the merits of this test. In 1944, Moritz[5] suggested magnesium as being more reliable than chlorides, particularly for the determination of sea water drowning, and in 1955 Freimuth *et al.*[2] using specific gravity values of heart plasma concluded that negative differences between the left and the right side may be obtained in either drowning or nondrowning cases, while positive values usually indicate that death was caused by means other than drowning.

Now as before, there persists discrepancy and uncertainty with respect to all chemical tests used for the diagnosis of drowning.

Perhaps the major obstacle to the reliability of chemical drowning tests is the rapidity of onset of post mortem changes in both blood and tissues. The publication therefore by Incze[4] in 1941 of the finding of diatoms in the lungs and the systemic circulation of individuals recovered from water as a diagnostic test for drowning, even after advanced decomposition, was a widely acclaimed event, particulary in Europe. The finding of diatoms in the lungs was considered indicative of the inhalation of water in which these silica coated algae find their natural habitat.

The portal of entry of diatoms into the blood stream was believed to be via the lungs through microscopic tears of alveolar walls which occur in the process of forceful water inhalation.[6] It was after the diatom method for the diagnosis of drowning was well established in Europe that it began to spread to several North American medico-legal departments, but in 1963 shadow was cast on this method by the recovery of diatoms in the liver and in other organs of individuals who had died of causes other than drowning.[10] Diatoms were also shown to be present in significant numbers in the air. The ubiquity of diatoms has been known to metereologists for many years, but has never been considered by forensic pathologists.

Whether these algae present in the organs are resorbed through the gastro intestinal tract[11] or are inhaled during life,[6,7] or whether they represent a contaminant, has neither been clarified by us nor is the literature quite clear on this point.

This discrepancy has since given rise to a large volume of literature of pros and cons with respect to the validity of diatoms in the diagnosis of death by drowning and there is hardly a medicolegal journal which has not taken part in the "war of diatoms" in one way or another.

In the past year lungs have been examined from experimental animals after fresh and salt water drowning, asphyxia and experimental edema, selectively stained for peroxidase.[13] Differences in the histologic picture were detected, such as pronounced acute nonspecific perivasculitis, particularly in salt water drowning which persisted for at least 5 hrs. after death. This has notably been overlooked by those using conventional staining methods. Quantitative assays of peroxidase in these lungs showed levels of about 800 Units in fresh water drowning, 6400 in salt water drowning; asphyxia and pulmonary edema showed levels of intermediate order between these two drowning groups, but approaching the salt water series (3700 and 5100 Units respectively). Anesthetized-decapitated animals served as controls and the level of peroxidase in their lungs was close to 1500 Units.

These findings or similar enzyme studies may one day be refined and find applicability in the determination of drowning deaths.

In conclusion: No single reliable chemical or physical test is yet available for diagnosing drowning. Only a conscientious scrutiny of all possible criteria, particularly the findings at autopsy and the consideration of the exact circumstances in each case together corroborate the diagnosis.

REFERENCES

1. Carrara, M.: Untersuchungen über den osmotischen Druck and die specifische elektrische Leitfähigkeit des Blutes bei der Fäulnis. Vierteljahrsschr. gerichtl. Med., *24:*236, 1902.
2. Freimuth, H. C., and H. E. Swann: Plasma specific gravity changes in sudden deaths. A.M.A. Arch. Path., *59:*214-218, 1955.
3. Gettler, A. O.: A method for the determination of death by drowning. JAMA, *77:*1650, 1921.
4. Incze, Gy: Fremdkörper im Blutkreislauf Ertrunkener. (Verh. d. Ges. ungarischer Pathologen 1940/41) cit. in: Zbl. allg. Path., path. Anat., *79:*176, 1942.
5. Moritz. A. R.: Chemical methods for the determination of death by drowning. Physiol. Rev. Baltimore, *24:*70-88, 1944.
6. Mueller, B, and D. Gorgs: Studien über das Eindringen von corpusculären Wasserbestandteilen aus den Lungenalveolen in den Kreislauf während des Ertrinkungsvorganges. Dtsch. Z. gerichtl. Med., *39:*715-725, 1949.
7. Otto, H.: Über den Nachweis von Diatomeen in menschlichen Lungenstauben. Frankf. Z. Path., *71:*176-181, 1961.
8. Placzek, M.. Die Blutdichte als Zeichen des Ertrinkungsvorganges. Vierteljahrsschr. gerichlt., Med., *25:*3, 1903.
9. Revenstorf: O. Über den Wert der Kryoskopie zur Diagnose des Todes durch Ertrinken. Münch. med. Wschr. *2:*1880, 1902.
10. Spitz, W. U.: Diagnose des Ertrinkungsvorganges durch den Diatomeen Nachweis in Organen. Dtsch, Z. gerichtl. Med., *54:*42-45, 1963.
11. Spitz, W. U., and H. Schmidt: Weitere Untersuchungen zur Diagnostik des Ertrinkungsvorganges durch Diatomeen-Nachweis. Dtsch. Z. gerichtl. Med., *58:*195-204, 1966.
12. Spitz, W. U., Hebel, R., and Michaelis, M.: Enzymatic changes in asphyxia, experimental pulmonary edema and drowning. Am. J. Clin. Path., *51:*102-106, 1969.
13. Spitz, W. U., Silverman, B. A. and Michaelis, M.: Histochemical changes in experimental drowning, pulmonary edema and asphyxia — J. Forens. Med., *16:*79-85, 1969.

Chapter 5

Toxicity from Electrical and Chemical Burns

RUSSELL S. FISHER, M.D.

ELECTRICAL INJURY

The occurrence of humoral toxic agents following electrical injury is unknown except for those associated with thermal burning as a component of the electrical injury. There are, in addition to the local burn, however, certain pathologic findings at a distance from the contact points which are worthy of mention.

The physiological effects of electrical current which may result fatally, impinge upon the heart or the central nervous system depending upon the nature of the circuit, that is to say arm-to-arm, or head to right arm — left arm, etc. In the case of a circuit involving the heart, ventricular fibrillation occurs most frequently with AC current; cardiac arrest without fibrillation apparently occurs with rare DC current exposures. The amount of electricity necessary to cause fibrillation is variable, but it would appear that as little as 50 to 70 milliamperes can cause fatal fibrillation where the exposure is through skin surfaces. Some cases have been reported in which as little as 1/10th of a milliamp was claimed to have produced fibrillation in accidents where internal electrodes such as pacemakers inadvertently became "shorted." It has now been confirmed repeatedly that the onset of fatal fibrillation may occur from electrical shock prior to onset of coma. Thus, the Maryland Medical Examiner's Office has documented two cases of fatal electrical contact wherein the victim was able to talk and/or walk for seconds after he was free of electrical contact, but thereafter collapsed and died a cardiac death within minutes.

In addition to the cardiac effect and caused by even lesser amounts of current flow than 50 milliamps, there is an associated spasm of skeletal muscle which may produce clenching of the hands and inability to release one's self from the contact. This may be associated with such violent spasm of the respiratory muscles that they are paralyzed leading to asphyxia. The serious central nervous system effect is apparently one of paralysis of respiratory center due to current passage through the area and fatal delay in recovery of the nerve cell function upset by the current passage.

The local injurious effects of electrical discharge are due to thermal burning and in some cases the burning cannot be recognized as due to electricity versus some other localized hyperthermic agent. However, in most cases the electrical burn produces such high local temperatures that there is dense condensation of the collagen, vesiculation or splitting of the epidermis or subepidermal areas and a peculiar elongation of the basal nuclei of the epidermis and sweat glands producing spindle shaped nuclei. This characteristic has been called "streaming of the nuclei." The collagen denaturation due to the high temperature characteristically causes the collagen to stain with a bluish tint with H & E and while this also accompanies thermal burning the localization and extent of this tinctorial alteration is frequently sufficient to make one reasonably confident that the burn in question is from an electrical source. A further alteration in the nuclei of endothelial cells in the blood vessels and some of the fibroblasts of the media of blood vessels has been described by Jellinek. In this effect, the nuclei of the vascular media tend to be twisted to resemble spirals. The changes may occur at quite distant points from the site of contact and are apparently localized in the arterial and venous walls because the blood is such an excellent conductor of electricity that current passage within the body is largely through the vascular tree. In addition to this, there is a tendency to localized necrosis or splitting of the intima, occasionally with fracturing of the internal elastic lamella and splitting of the media. These arterial changes are obviously prone to be followed by thrombosis and not infrequently this complication necessitates amputation of an extremity even though the local burn at some distal location might have been treated with much less drastic surgical procedures. Jellinek has described a case which might be labelled "generalized toxemia following electrocution" in which an individual made contact with a 25,000 volt alternating current source with one contact in the right hand and the other in the occipital region of the scalp. Artificial respiration resulted in effective resuscitation and several hours after the accident the patient seemed to be recovering. He then developed generalized shivering, hyperthermia, extreme pain in the right hand and forearm with absence of arterial pulsation and 18 hours later amputation of the right upper extremity was required. By this time, there had developed hemoglobinuria and loss of consciousness with cardio-respiratory dysfunction. It is assumed that the myoglobinuria or hemoglobinuria in such cases is related to muscle degeneration associated with nuclear injury similar in character to that which occurred in the arterial tree although it is also believed that passage of electrical current through blood leads to hemolysis. The observations are isolated and further study is indicated. Schnetz has reported gangrene 3 or 4 years following electrical shock to an extremity but this observer believes this finding needs further critical evaluation.

Lightning represents a specialized form of electricity wherein extremely high voltage differentials occur with a condensor like discharge and occasionally a person may act as an electrode in connecting cloud and ground. In such cases, about one fourth of those hit are killed. The fatal mechanism would appear to be physiologic derangement as by any current flow through the body in fatal circuits although secondary burns due to clothing ignition or blast effect due to massive atmospheric pressure fluctuations must also be considered in some cases. The peculiar arborescent skin erythema seen in victims of "lightning strike" is regarded as evidence of coincident vascular paralysis rather than a fatal effect. Intense local edema has also been described following high voltage injury and this is most reasonably explained by local nervous, capillary and lymphatic paralysis as an effect of current passage.

TOXEMIA FOLLOWING CHEMICAL BURNS

There is little to distinguish the systemic after effects of chemical burns from purely thermal burns. True there may be absorption of chemical or metallic substances from burns from such agents as sulphurous acid, chromium or nickel salts and some systemic effects due to the specific agent may be visualized but these do not differ from poisoning by the chemical compound absorbed by other routes. Meanwhile the picture of toxemia due to burns should be differentiated from the "shock phase" of burn effect· Walker *et al.* have commented on this and their summary is worthy of quotation:

> "The shock phase is marked by hemoconcentration, fall in blood pressure, rapid pulse and cold extremities. The patient usually recovers from shock within twenty-four hours unless death has supervened. The phase of toxemia, on the other hand, produces headache, vomiting, drowsiness, fever and oliguria and usually makes its appearance on the second day, lasting three or four days. Patients dying in phase of toxemia show changes in the parenchymatous viscera, liver, kidneys and adrenal glands and also in the intestine and the central nervous system that are not seen in patients dying of shock within the first day or so. The changes observed in patients dying during toxemia are not, however, considered pathogomonic, since somewhat similar changes have been produced in experimental animals by prolonged low blood pressure and by hyperthermia."

The changes in the liver are accompanied by elevated bilirubin, BSP retention and altered cephalin flocculation. Renal function impairment leading to increased nitrogen retention is also a prominent component of the toxemia picture. The pathologic picture associated with these biochemical alterations may take one of three forms (1) irregular necrosis of the liver indistinguishable from that occurring in shock from any cause; (2) a non-specific diffuse or periportal inflammatory infiltrate probably responsive to sepsis complicating the infection of burned areas, and (3) fatty infiltration, again probably a part of the systemic response to deranged metabolism. Likewise, the renal changes of toxic nephrosis with "swollen" kidneys and extensive microscopic epithelial degeneration throughout the entire tubule is regarded as a toxic phenomenon associated with many severe burns. Other variants of renal changes frequently seen with burns are lower nephron nephrosis and osmotic nephrosis. Adrenal degeneration especially in the inner third of the cortex has also been described frequently in burns and provides rationale for treatment of burn victims with replacement adrenal cortical extract. Gastrointestinal ulcers known as Curling's ulcers also are a part of the systemic effects of burns although it is not known whether their etiologic mechanism is gastric hyperacidity or via neural or humoral mechanisms.

REFERENCES

1. Fischer/Spann: Pathologie des Trauma. München, 1967, p. 173-178.
2. Gonzales, T. A., Vance, M., Helpern, M., and Umberger, C. J.: Legal Medicine Pathology and Toxicology. New York, Appleton-Century-Crofts, Inc., 2nd Ed., 1954, pp.534-547.
3. Jellinek, S.: Spezifisch elektrische Zellveränderungen in Geometrischer Gestaltung. Virch. Arch., *301*:28-48, 1938.
4. Mueller, B.: Gerichtliche Sedizin Springer. Berlin-Göttingen-Heidelberg pp. 498-503, 1953.
5. Ponsold, A.: Lehrbuch der Gerichtlichen Medizen. Stuttgart, G. Thieme, 1967, 3rd Ed., pp. 391-394.
6. Walker, J. Jr., Saltonstall, H., Rhoads, H. E., and Lee, W. E.: Toxemia syndrome after burns. Arch. Surg., *52*:177-186, 1946.

Chapter 52

Suicide in Relation to Toxic Agents

EARL B. WERT, M.D.

INTRODUCTION

Self-imposed mortality is viewed as a "final common pathway," a symptom, resulting from diverse influences. The forensic pathologist plays a vital part in the complete elucidation of such cases, and a "multiple disciplinary approach" is necessary, combining all technics which have bearing on the emotional and technical aspects of such cases.

Suicide has been among the twelve leading causes of death in the United States for the past fifteen years. There are good reasons to suspect the actual rate to be two to four times that reported. Although there are no national statistics on unsuccessful attempts at self destruction, the data from the Suicide Prevention Center at Los Angeles, Cal., suggest the incidence to be eight times the actual suicidal rate. About a fourth of self-imposed mortality (26.9% in 1964) is caused by toxic agents.

Interesting data on global suicide rates are provided by the World Health Organizations. For example, some countries (Hungary, Austria, West Germany, Japan) have at least twice the suicide rate of the U.S.A., while others (Mexico, Jordan) have only half the rate reported in the U.S.A. However, these comparisons are rendered less meaningful by variations in compiling and reporting data.

In the interest of providing comparable data, the international classification of suicide as employed by the World Health Organization is recommended for all forensic agencies (see Table 1).

TABLE 1: SUICIDAL DEATHS: INTERNATIONAL CLASSIFICATION

E 970	Analgesics and soporifics
E 971	Other liquids and solids, including
	Strychnine
	Phenol and cresol compounds
	Lye and potash
	Mercury
	Arsenic
	Fluorides
E 972	Domestic gas
E 973	Other gas, including:
	Motor vehicle exhaust gas
	Carbon Monoxide
	Carbon Dioxide
E 974	Hanging
E 975	Submersion
E 976	Firearms
E 977	Cutting
E 978	Jumping
E 979	Other

That the problem is predominantly one of white males, increasing markedly with age, beginning at about 25, is shown in Table II, indicating the large differences existing between the black and white races as well, which is almost certainly much greater than indicated. The author's data from the deep South show black suicides less than 1% of the white. The tendency for white people to oppose vigorously the decision of suicide by local authorities, not met among the black, suggests the disparity to be even greater than that presented in Table II.

TABLE II: SUICIDE RATES (PER 100,000) BY RACE, SEX, AND AGE, U.S.A. (1964)

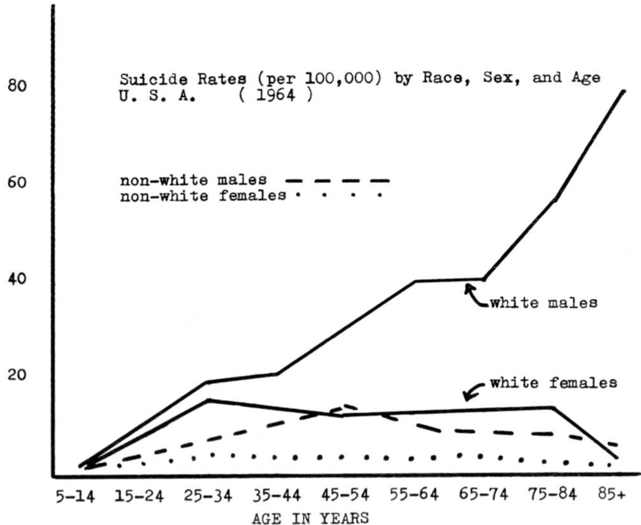

The relationship of death as caused by toxic agents to suicides in general is presented in Table III. It is noted that the rate of death due to poisonous substances generally remains rather steady at about one fourth of the total due to all forms of injury. Table IV indicates the important role played by barbiturates and by other analgesic and soporific substances.

The data are further presented in Table V, where the sharp contrast between barbiturates and other analgesics is seen, and the place of the tranquilizing drugs (meprobamates). Table VI presents data from the U.S. Department of Health, Education, and Welfare depicting the inter-relationship of the chief agents employed in death due to toxic drugs.

TABLE III: PERCENTAGE DISTRIBUTION OF SUICIDE BY MEANS OF INJURY (13)

Int. Code	*Means of Injury*	*1950*	*1960*	*1964*
E 970	By analgesic and soporific	4.7	8.5	12.4
E 971	By solids and liquids — other	5.8	3.9	3.3
E 972	By gases in domestic use	6.5	1.0	0.4
E 973	By gases — other	*6.2*	*9.4*	*10.8*
E 974	By hanging, strangulation	21.0	17.7	14.6
E 975	By submersion (drowning)	3.9	3.2	2.6
E 976	By firearms, explosions	43.0	47.4	47.6
E 977	By cutting, piercing	3.1	2.6	1.9
E 978	By jumping from high places	3.7	3.7	3.7
E 979	By other and unspecified	2.1	2.7	2.7
	By poisonous substances, generally	23.2	22.8	26.9

TABLE IV: NUMBER OF SUICIDAL DEATHS BY SPECIFIC CAUSE IN INTERNATIONAL CLASSIFICATION E 970 (13)

Class	*Drugs*	*1963*	*1960*	*1957*	*1954*
A	Morphine and other opium derivatives	7	12	12	16
B	Barbituric acid and derivatives	1,997	1,290	817	721
C,D,E.F.G.	Salicylates, anti-pyretic and bromides	76	57	29	23
H	Other analgesic and soporific substances	488	226	123	87
M	Unspecified drugs	98	31	12	9
	Total	2,666	1,616	993	856
	Total suicides	20,819	19,031	16,629	16,348

TABLE V: NUMBER OF SUICIDES DUE TO BARBITURATES, OTHER ANALGESIC AND SOPORIFIC SUBSTANCES AND MEPROBAMATE (1954-1963) (13)

Year	*Suicide by Barbiturates*	*By Other Analgesics*	*By Meprobamate*
1954	721	86	—
1955	781	94	1
1956	765	95	3
1957	817	122	1
1958	912	167	1
1959	1073	178	1
1960	1290	226	0
1961	1341	250	2
1962	1738	360	2
1963	1997	484	1
Total =	11,435	2,062	12

(From: U.S. Dept. of H.E.W., published lit. and from the Wallace Laboratories.)

THE INVESTIGATION

Few problems facing the forensic pathologist are comparable in magnitude to those involving the elucidation of suicide — a term now outmoded and replaced by "self-imposed mortality, intentional (or not intentional)." Often in practice the forensic pathologist is charged with the decision as to the mode, or intent, involved in the demise. This decision involves a "multi-disciplined" approach to the events, including a knowledge of the "psyche in its social setting," as well as the conventional disciplines of forensic pathologist, including gross and microscopic pathology,

TABLE VI: NUMBER OF SUICIDES BY ANALGESIC AND SOPORIFIC SUBSTANCES

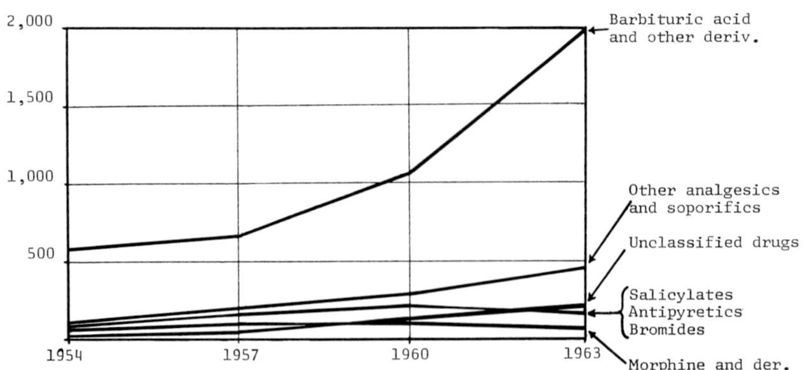

morbid physiology, the toxicologic action of poisons, etc. Thus not only must the investigator demonstrate the causative agent, but if possible establish the intent of the subject.

The investigation must begin at the earliest moment, and be carried out by those interested in these matters. The study must include the inspection of the sites inhabited by the deceased, and the interrogation of family and associated persons including clergy and physicians. Meticulous search of the premises may produce fragments of destroyed suicidal notes, sometimes in waste-baskets at some distance from the subject's usual environment. One may find evidence of other methods of self-destruction having been tried or considered — the author has studied cases where guns have been fired into the bed before barbiturates were ingested, and where the subject cut the inside of his thigh with a razor blade, apparently testing his pain tolerance before taking soporific drugs as a second choice.

Ancillary evidence of self-imposed mortality, intentional, may be found in the form of insurance policies recently obtained or reinstated and the policies mailed to beneficiaries. Multiple policies of small value are suspect — in the author's experience an accountant who died from an overdose of multiple soporifics had obtained twenty policies of less than $10,000 each, perhaps with the thought that each would be too small to be contested by the insuring agency. Unfortunately, data of this type are not usually decisive, but in the interest of impartial adjudication must be part of the forensic pathologist's records to be presented before the court.

THE AUTOPSY

Certain aspects of the examination should be stressed when the cause of death is unknown. The proper collection of materials for definitive toxicology study is paramount.

The examiner should have the advantage of studying the body fully clothed and unembalmed. The clothing may reveal bottles, prescriptions, notes, as well as stains, odors, scratches, or particulate trace matter indicating the recent whereabouts of the individual.

On those occasions when arterial injections have been performed in the embalming process prior to autopsy, serious limitations are presented. While the forensic pathologist may satisfy his personal convictions as to the agent producing death by the analysis of the embalming fluid, compared with that found in the organs, this evidence could be presented in a court of law only with the greatest difficulty, if at all. Variations in the fluid, contamination of the tubing and metal fixtures, competence of the morticians . . . all present variables which are legally quite insurmountable. Further, formaldehyde interferes with the identification of cyanides, chloral hydrate, methyl alcohol, some alkaloids, and makes all poison extractions difficult due to the hardness of the tissues. Certain substances may still be determined — salicylates, barbiturates and strychnine, for example.

Maintaining additional aliquots of blood, urine, tissue, and stomach contents in an anaerobic, frozen state is mandatory as a routine in all forensic work. Frequently a reference laboratory will be called on to re-evaluate the initial findings.

Preservatives should not be added, with the exception of blood maintained for alcohol levels. Here 0.4 grams of sodium fluoride per ounce of blood will preserve the alcohol level indefinitely, especially if refrigerated.

The conventional complete autopsy method is followed with emphasis on certain details.

Following the primary incision into the peritoneal cavity and routine observations, the iliac arteries and veins are firmly ligated to insure blood remaining in the lower extremities. No hazard of diffusion of drugs from the viscera into this blood is possible and the samples of blood from the legs thus cannot be impeached due to the possibility of diffusion, as is the case of heart blood and its proximity to the stomach and lungs.

The bladder is next fixed by a towel clamp or suitable instrument and held while a puncture is made to admit a chemically clean pipette, with bulb for aspiration; or a syringe and needle may be used. In any event the urine must be placed immediately in 20 ml aliquots in small plastic bags, sealed, and frozen. The urine is collected in its entirety.

As with all postmortem examinations, the complete evisceration technic en bloc is recommended. The author has found no other modification completely satisfactory. The initial skin incision is made at the lowest caudal margin of the neck in males at about the suprasternal notch, a point easily covered by the collar at viewing. In females, more consideration is given to the exigencies of the viewing garments. In any event, employing a long narrow blade with a sharp point, one is able to remove tongue and larynx intact by cutting across the floor of the mouth at the attachment of the frenulum, then cutting alongside the tongue and dorsally until the tongue is delivered through the neck, attached to the laryngeal and esophageal structures, with epiglottis intact. The mouth need not be opened by this maneuver, but the inside of the mouth cleared by the examining finger. Caudad the incision is made distal to the prostate and at the most distal point of the rectum close to the anus. The entire viscera are then removed from the body cavity.

After removal of viscera, samples are taken anaerobically from each iliac vein by the following technic. As stated above, samples are removed from the leg veins to obviate the effects of diffusion to and from the lungs and sites of high concentration of drugs such as the liver and stomach (16). Further, a technic designed to obtain and store the blood under rather strict anaerobic conditions is mandatory to prevent the escape of highly volatile gases such as halogenated hydrocarbons and of carbon dioxide (18).

A 20 cc syringe and a 13 gauge needle with multiple points of perforation in the shaft — perhaps 8 or 10 are used. (These perforations can readily be made with a suitably small high speed drill.) The perforations obviate the matter of clots impeding the flow of blood into the needle. Small "Whirl-Packs" or similar plastic bags capable of being sealed are employed, samples are introduced with the plastic bags collapsed, to prevent contamination by air.

The legs are elevated to insure a good flow of blood, and all blood from the legs, harvested in 20 cc aliquots, is frozen without preservative.

The early recognition of the effect of poison at the autopsy may save time in identification of the causative agent. Table VII lists the more important physical findings associated with poisons.

INTERPRETATION AND DECISIONS

Deliberate delay by the forensic pathologist in his decision as to the nature of the demise, and especially in communicating these decisions to the press, and to the family will obviate much stress and confusion. One must not be forced into signing the death certificate prematurely, or into making arbitrary decisions, regardless of the pressures from the family, clergy, press, lawyers, or the State Health Department. Not only may such arbitrary decisions be unfair to interested parties, but such "fictitious accuracy" causes loss of confidence in the forensic pathologist and his methods among the agencies of the community. In fact, the quality of the medicolegal office may be gauged in part by the number of cases signed as "cause and mode of death unestablished." By delay, one enhances the probability of an objective decision. Frequently evidence continues to be obtained even weeks after the demise. Ultimately, the decision may very properly rest with a court of law.

The matter of establishing the mode (intent) is especially difficult in death due to soporifics. The chief drugs employed are barbiturates which account for some 75% of suicidal deaths by drugs in 1963. Here, a state of "automation" or confusion may occur after non-lethal doses, and the additional lethal quantities may indeed have been taken unintentionally. The problem is further complicated by the synergistic effect of many drugs, of which alcohol is the most common. Quantitative relationships existing among combinations of drugs have yet to be delineated, due to the many variables. Further, one should distinguish between the compulsive, impulsive act of a young mother who swallows a handful of sleeping capsules, or aspirin tablets following a series of arguments with her husband over money, drinking, etc. . . . These sudden, unreasoned acts are not to be compared with the 55-year-old woman described by Havens in *The Anatomy of a Suicide* (2) where the problems were deeply seated in the personality of the victim, with their untoward development over a lifetime, culminating in her jumping from a cliff as her last attachments to life were taken from her through the loss of her daughter and the inept psychiatric support of the moment.

Certain predisposing factors are known to be related to self-destruction, chief among these are depression, schizophrenia, and alcoholism. Less commonly associated are a history of downward or unstable work, physical illness, financial reverses, and social or psychological isolation, including disappointment in love. One must be prepared for the "Richard Cory Syndrome" taken from the poem of E. A. Robinson in which the handsome young man, with a good station in life, one calm summer night went home and took his life. Statements from the associates of the deceased to the effect that "Yes, he had been depressed, but in the past few days had seemed to have solved all his problems, and taken a new lease on life," must be considered with circumspection. Of course the victim may indeed have solved his problems by electing suicide as his escape. Finally, serious students of the problem of self-imposed mortality will wish to be familiar with the work of the French sociologist Emil Durkheim, who offers a statistical approach to the matter of suicide using sociologic data. The first English translation of "Le Suicide" became available in 1951 (1).

TABLE VII: PHYSICAL FINDINGS AT AUTOPSY ASSOCIATED WITH POISONING

I. AGENTS PRODUCING ABNORMAL COLORING OF THE SKIN

a. Stains in scars, about the lips, on the face and hands.

COLOR	AGENT SUSPECTED
brown-black	iodine; silver nitrate
dark brown	bromine
yellow	Atabrine; picric acid; nitric acid; oxalic acid
bleached white	phenols and derivatives; lysol
ashen gray	mercuric chloride

b. Generalized coloring, especially in dependent portions.

COLOR	AGENT SUSPECTED
cherry pink, red	carbon monoxide; cyanides; nitrites; nitrates (sodium and potassium)
blue, slate blue, blue-gray	silver salts
yellow	Atabrine; picric acid
bluish-brown	nitrobenzene; chlorates; acetanilids; also all those listed under cyanosis

c. Abnormal coloring of the gums.

COLOR	AGENT SUSPECTED
blue-black gum line	lead; mercury; bismuth (usually chronic); silver

	AGENT SUSPECTED
d. Abnormal texture of skin, rash.	bromides, arsenic; sufonamide drugs; coal-tar derivatives such as acetanalid; phenacetin; amidopyrine; antipyrine; methenamine; antimony; belladonna; opium, turpentine; chloral barbiturates; iodines; gold; Atabrine; phenolphthalein; quinine; Tridione; propylthiouracil; borates; Dilantin and many others,.. including drug allergies

	AGENT SUSPECTED
e. Skin cyanotic	hydrocyanic acid phenol; nitro-benzol; carbon dioxide; silver nitrate

	AGENT SUSPECTED
f. Skin hemorrhagic	phosphorus; mushroom poisoning

II. ODORS ON BODY, VOMITUS, BODY FLUIDS

ODOR	AGENT SUSPECTED
phenolic (like disinfectants, pungent)	phenols, creosote
sweet (ether like)	ether
sweet (penetrating)	chloroform; acetone
bitter almonds	cyanides
violets	turpentine in urine
stale tobacco	nicotine
pears	chloral hydrate
alcoholic (fruit like)	alcohols
garlic	phosphorus, tellurium, arsenic
shoe polish	nitrobenzene

Many other aromatic substances may be recognized, with experience, such as carbon tetrachloride, hydrogen sulphide, mercaptans, aniline, naptha, gasoline, carbon disulfide, benzene, xylene, pyridine, methyl salicylate, camphor, chlorine compounds, formaldehyde, acetone, paraldehyde, and many others.

III. AGENTS PRODUCING MISCELLANEOUS FINDINGS

FINDING	*AGENT SUSPECTED*
a. Pupils contracted	atropine, stramonium, henbane, scopalmine, gelsemium
b. Putrefaction markedly delayed	alcohol, arsenic, mercury
c. Dry gangrene of extremities	ergot
d. Blood chocolate colored	potassium chlorate

IV. AGENTS PRODUCING COLORED MATERIALS

FINDING	*AGENT SUSPECTED*
Purple, pink color	arsenpotassium permanganate, cobalt salts
blue, blue-green	copper salts, Paris green
green	nickel salts
yellow, red-yellow	picric acid, nitric acid, acriflavine selenium, pyridium, potassium or lead chromate
bright red	mercurochrome
black or brown, granular, "coffee-grounds"	sulfuric acid, oxalic acid, HCL
white deposits or granules on mucosa of stomach, with red center of inflammation or ulceration	arsenic, antimony
particles luminous in dark	phosphorus
green shining particles	cantharides

INTERPRETATION OF TOXICOLOGIC DATA

Many problems beset the forensic pathologist in evaluating the results of toxicologic study. First, is the matter of accuracy. Rarely will the prosecutor have carried out the analysis himself. He must therefore have established the reliability of his chemist by various quality control measures, for both common and rarely encountered agents, and be assured of the competence of this laboratory. Secondly, even with confidence in the values obtained, the interpretation is difficult. Since minimal lethal quantities have yet to be established with certainty for most poisons. Is the amount reported lethal? Did the agent cause death, or was it incidental, death being due to other causes? Would this amount be expected to cause death in a healthy individual, or only in one debilitated, chronically ill? Should the matter of synergistic effect be considered? Does the value indicate an acute phase, or has the drug been administered over a prolonged period, with tolerance to the substance having been acquired (e.g. arsenic, where hair, bone, nails would be valuable)? Could the agent have been administered medicinally in sublethal quantities? Was the poison actually taken by the subject during life? Is the substance present in the form to be found after it has been metabolized? In cases associated with fire, with carbon monoxide in the blood, was death due to the poison or to the carbon monoxide? Could other agents have been present, now decomposed? Obviously, many questions are unanswerable, but the forensic pathologist will resolve many problems by retaining in the frozen state suitable aliquots in replicate of all tissues, including blood.

When more than one drug is found the problem is especially difficult, particularly when the synergistic effects are known, as with alcohol and barbiturates. If the patient presents a significant alcohol level at death, and had been unconscious some hours prior to death, it may be helpful to establish the maximal blood alcohol level. This may be done albeit roughly by calculation — alcohol is metabolized in the blood of the comatose patient at the rate of 0.02% per hour. By exterpolation back to the time the patient may have imbibed the last drink the maximal level may be guessed at.

In gauging the intent, or mode, of the demise the forensic pathologist must be aware of the tendency for certain drugs, especially the rauwolfia compounds to induce or enhance suicidal trends. Depressions are known to be associated with these drugs, and suicidal impulses are reported in some 20% of these patients, accompanied by lethargy, unhappiness, withdrawal, anxiety, anorexia, and weight loss. Usually, these symptoms are seen in patients with a tendency to depression, in whom the drug has been given in relatively large doses for at least a month, and the pattern is not always reversible on withdrawal of the drug.

Phenobarbital, as well, has been reported to enhance suicidal trends in depressed patients.

The role of alcohol in this regard is less certain. The Maryland (13) studies during a five-year period included 1,455

TABLE VIII: GUIDE FOR MATERIALS TO BE SUBMITTED FOR ANALYSIS

Note: Multiple aliquots of amounts indicated in Table are placed in plastic bags and sealed, then frozen. Frequently questionable results require confirmation by a reference laboratory.

SPECIMEN	AMOUNTS	NOTES ON TOXIC AGENTS
URINE	All available, save in 50 ml aliquots.	Suitable for most types of poisoning, especially morphine. Small drops should be obtained with Pasteur pipette even when bladder seems empty.
BLOOD	200 ml aliquots.	Barbiturates, cyanide, methemaglobin, carbon monoxide, sulfonamides, bromides, alcohols, metals. Morphine not found in blood.
STOMACH	Isolate solid materials. Isolate liquid in 3 - 5 aliquots according to volume. Entire stomach wall.	Stomach wall must be examined for corrosion; note odor. See Table VII.
INTESTINE	Entire small and large intestine, leave intact submitting 24" long segments, labeled, from large and small bowel.	Heavy metals excreted through wall of large intestine; note ulceration.
BRAIN	200 gram aliquots, entire brain.	Volatiles, barbiturates, alkaloids, alcohols.
LIVER	300 gram aliquots, entire liver.	Heavy metals, barbiturates, fluorides, Oxalates, sulfonal.
KIDNEY	Each kidney, separately.	Heavy metals, especially mercury, sulfonamides.
BONE	200 gram aliquots. Sternum, 6 ribs separately are easily obtained; femur, tibia.	Useful in evaluating duration of lead, arsenic poisoning; levels vary according to bone.
LUNG	Each lung, separately.	For identification of inhaled poisons.
HAIR, FINGERNAILS	10 gram aliquots.	Chronic arsenic poisoning, useful in evaluating the duration of the poisoning. Pull out, do not cut, to aid orientation.
MUSCLE	200 gram aliquots	Confirmation of all poisons, especially in advenced decomposition.
BILE	15 ml aliquots, all available.	Morphine and derivatives concentrated.
FAT	200 gram aliquots.	DDT and related compounds. Include deep fatty subcutaneous tissue and muscle; especially valuable for morphine and derivatives.
SKIN	Needle puncture sites and scars, 4 cm X 6 cm.	Attempts may have been made to obscure the needle puncture site. The umbilicus and perineum are known to have been used.

suicides, in 617 of which the blood alcohol was determined and levels of 0.05% found in 35%. Thus, about one-third of suicide victims have significant blood alcohol levels. Alcohol intensified the existing or latent mood. Studies indicate the danger of suicide is appreciable only in chronic alcoholism of some 15 years or longer.

Meprobamates, on the other hand, are specific anti-anxiety agents producing no significant behavioral impairment at clinical doses, no confusion, no suicidal tendency. A study by Bell (17) indicates a lessening of the tendency to suicide in patients on meprobamate therapy.

The matter of barbiturate-alcohol synergism remains unexplained, and unquantitated. Increasing the difficulty of such studies are the variables of individual sensitivity, body weight, habituation, food in the stomach, and the type of barbiturate.

Although the exact amount of poison

TABLE IX: LETHAL DOSE (FOR 150 LB. HUMAN) OF COMMON POISONS
(Data collected from literature)

Agent		*Agent*	
Barbiturates	1.0 - 5.0 g	Metrazol	2.0 g
Boric acid	10.0 g	Morphine	0.25 g
Bromides	unknown	"Moth balls"	15.0 g
Canthariden	0.03 g	Muscarine	0.05 g
Camphor	2.0 g	Nicotine	0.06 g
Carbon monoxide	40% saturation	Nitrates	8.0 g
Chloral hydrate	7.0 g	Nitric acid	5.0 ml
Chlorates	2.0 g	Nitrites	8.0 g
Chlorodane	8.0 g	Nitrobenzine	2.0 ml
Carbon tetrachloride	4.0 ml	Oxalates	5.0 g
Chloroform	25.0 ml	Paraldehyde	100.0 ml (2.0 g)
Cocaine	0.5 g (p.o.)	Parathion	0.015 g
Codeine	0.8 g	Permanganate	5.0 g
Croton oil	1.0 ml	Phenacetin	5.0 g
D.D.T.	15.0 g	Phenols	10.0 ml
Demoral	1.0 g	Phenothiazines	1.0 - 5.0 g
Digitalis	2.0 g	Phosphates, org.	0.015 g
Dilantin	2.0 g	Phosphoric acid	8.0 ml
Dinitroortho-cresol	2.0 g	Physostigmine	0.06 g
Doriden	10.0 g	Picrotoxin	0.10 g
Emetine	0.2 g	Pilocarpine	0.130 g
Ephedrine	0.6 g	Plasmochin	0.5 g
Epinephrine	0.05 g	Procaine	10.0 g
Ergot	1.0 g	Pyrethrum	low toxicity
Oils, essent.	unknown	Pyribenzamine	1.0 g
Ether	25.0 ml	Quinine	20.0 g
Ethyl alcohol	0.5 to 1.0 L.	Rotenone	low toxicity
Ethyl bromide	100.0 ml	Santonin	1.0 g
Ferrous sulfate	30.0 g	Silver	2.0 g
Fluoracetate sodium	0.05 g	Solanine	0.2 g
Fluorides	4.0 g	Strychnine	0.075 g
Formaldehyde	30.0 ml	Sulfa drugs	varies with drug
Gold, salts	unknown	Sulfides	200 ppm (H_2S gas)
Heroin	0.2 g	Sulfuric acid	5.0 ml
Hydrochloric acid	5.0 ml	Sulfonal	10.0 g
Hypochlorite	15.0 ml	Thallium	0.3 g
Insulin	variable	Thiocyanate	15.0 g
Iodides	50.0 g	Thiourea	10.0 g
Iodine	2.0 g	Toxalbumins	? (very toxic)
Kerosene	100.0 ml	Toxaphene	3.0 g
Lead	10.0 g	Tridione	6.0 g
Marihuana	0.5 g (?)	Turpentine	30.0 ml
Mercury comp.	0.5 g	Warfarin	low toxicity
Methyl alcohol	75.0 ml	Zinc	15 g
Methyl salicylate	30.0 ml		

taken by the victim is seldom known, the amount in the body may be roughly estimated from stomach contents, blood and organ levels, or from ancillary data (prescriptions, vials, etc.). In Table IX are listed the approximate quantities that have been reported to be lethal for a 150 lb. human. It must be noted that these values are only approximate due to variations imposed by speed of absorption, habituation, individual sensitivity, drug combinations, etc. The role of alcohol acting synergistically with chloral hydrate, paraldehyde, anti-convulsants, anti-histamines, tranquilizers, and other depressants must be considered in this regard.

The time interval between ingesting a fatal dose of drug or poison and death is often of value in the interpretation of the case, Watanbe (8) furnishes data on this point, employing the term LT 50 for the time within which 50% of the population will die following such a dose. See Table X, from Watanbe.[8]

TABLE X: TIME INTERVAL BEFORE DEATH AFTER ACUTE INGESTION OF POISON
(Minimum lethal time forms left part of solid bar; LT-50 forms right part of bar)

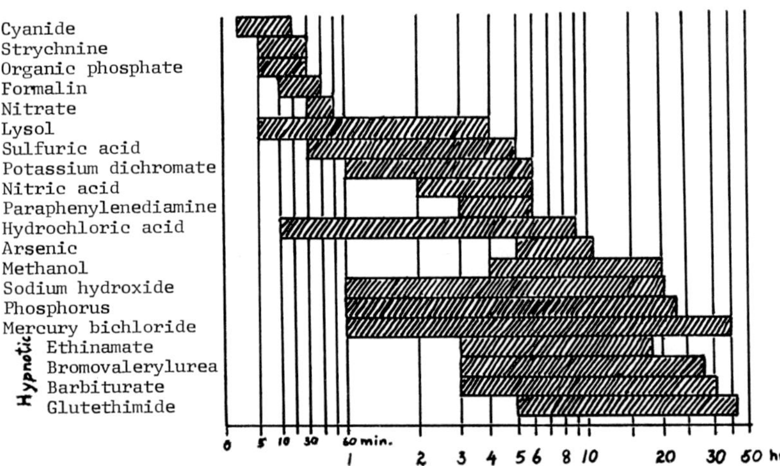

Watanbe (8) calls attention to the fact that undissolved tablets may remain undissolved in the stomach of the comatose patient for considerable periods, in some cases up to a week. Thus, lavage may be helpful in the clinical management of such cases even after several days. Further, interpretation of the time intervals must be made with some caution in view of these findings (Table XI). Certain drugs may have exerted their effect by a curious phenomenon illustrated by the case of meprobamate poisoning reported by Jenis (3). Here the meprobamate lay relatively inert in the stomach of the comatose patient, and resisted lavage. Clinically, the patient recovered, temporarily, death following this lucid interval, presumably when vital activity returned to the stomach with absorption of a truly lethal amount of meprobamate which was unrecognized since the lavage had been ineffectual.

Data establishing the toxic and lethal

TABLE XI: PHYSICAL STATE OF DRUG TAKEN IN TABLET FORM IN STOMACH AT TIME OF AUTOPSY: 210 CASES IN WHICH PERSON LIVED MORE THAN 6 HOURS DURING 10-YEAR PERIOD

State of Tablet	*6-24 Hour*	*1-3 Day*	*4-7 Day*	*Per Cent*
Undissolved	15	7	1	11.0
Granules	47	40	1	41.9
Qualitative exam. Positive	39	41		38.1
Qualitative exam. Negative	7	7	3	9.0
Total	108	97	5	100.0

levels of drugs and other poisons in the blood and vital organs are difficult to obtain in humans. Levels are subject to interpretation in the individual case. In Table XII data on the more common agents have been collected (6).

TABLE XII: INTERPRETATION OF CHEMICAL FINDINGS IN BLOOD AND INTERNAL ORGANS

Agent	*Concentration*	*Comments*
Arsenic	1.0 mgm per 100 ml liver	Significant of poisoning, not necessarily lethal.
Alcohol, ethyl	0.5 mgm per 100 ml blood	Lethal level. If death is delayed lower values may be found, since alcohol is metabolized at the rate of about 0.02%/hour.
Alcohol, methyl	0.05 mgm per 100 ml liver	May be found in higher levels before metabolism to formaldehyde.
Barbiturates	1.0 mgm to 5.0 mgm per 100 ml blood	Low values significant in the slower acting forms, while higher values are significant in more rapid acting drugs. All are more important in the presence of other soporific drugs or alcohol.
Carbon monoxide	30% sat. blood	Significant in elderly as a cause of death.
	40%-50% "	This level will cause death if victims exposed to lower concentration over a prolonged period.
	60%-80% "	These high values found in victims having breathed in environments of high concentrations.
	10% "	Saturation, or less, usually found in smokers or city dwellers.
Chlordiazepoxide (Librium)	1.9 mgm per 100 ml blood	Found in a fatal case, following an overdose of 500 mgm.
Codeine	any amout in blood	May be found in the blood only if a massive dose has been given.
Cyanide	1.0 mgm per 100 ml blood	Approximate fatal level.
Demoral	any amount in blood	May be found in blood only after a massive dose.
Glutethimide (Doriden)	1.0 mgm per 100 ml. blood	This level indicates poisoning, lethal level uncertain. Ingestion of 1.0 gm. produces level of 0.7 mgm/100 ml of blood. Lethal dose is about 10.0 grams. Altho lethal level may have been exceeded death may be delayed and lower levels found due to metabolism of drug.
Imipramine (Tofranil)	10.0 mgm per 100 ml liver	Value reported in some fatal cases

Lead	0.5 mgm per 100 ml liver	Significant of poisoning, but lead an ubiquitous substances, and not a lethal level.
Meprobamate	16.5 mgm per 100 ml blood	(High therapeutic level is 1.0 mgm) Lethal level reported in fatal case after massive dose, gavage, etc.
Mercury	any amount in blood or tissue	Any amount considered toxic not an ubiquitous substance like lead.
Methapyrilene	1.2 and 3.0 mgm per 100 ml blood	Found in two fatal cases.
Morphine	1.0 mgm per 100 ml urine fatal level	Not found in blood, but concentrated in bile, urine, and may be found in tissues at injection site; heroin is metabolized to morphine in body.
Nicotine	0.03 mgm (blood) 1.0 mgm per 100 ml blood	Level in heavy smokers. Level reported in fatal cases.
Phenothyazines (Tranquilizers)	0.1 mgm (blood) 0.2 mgm (blood) 12.0 mgm (liver) 0.2, 12.0 mgm per 100 ml	Expected value after 1.0 gram dose Reported in fatal case Reported in fatal case Blood and liver level resp. after repeated 4.0 gram dose daily, fatal case.
Paraldehyde	50.0 mgm per 100 ml blood	Reported as total acetaldehyde.
Propoxyphene (Darvon)	5.7, 10.0 mgm per 100 ml blood	Reported in two fatal cases.
Salicylates	30.00 mgm blood 100.00 mgm " 25.0 mgm " (all per 100 mgm blood)	Toxic levels, not lethal Lethal, but variable May be found in arthritic patients on high doses.
Thallium	1.0 mgm per 100 ml urine	Level reported in fatal cases.

CONCLUSIONS

The complete elucidation of self destruction due to toxic agents requires a multi-disciplinary approach on the part of the forensic pathologist, beginning with a detailed investigation of the scene for clues as to the behavior and intent of the subject, a consideration of the psyche of the individual in its "social setting," and a complete autopsy. The postmortem examination is highly specialized requiring inquiry into ordinary morbid processes as well as those of forensic implication. Here special technics are required, the most important of which are those for collecting in replicate under anaerobic conditions suitable aliquots for chemical analysis, and maintaining these in a frozen state until the chemical nature of the problem is completely elucidated. Finally, the forensic pathologist must attempt to equate the findings with the real intent, or mode, of the demise, with due consideration to the interaction of drugs, and especially to the basic true motives of the subject. Should the decision of the pathologist wish to be contested in a court of law, the observations and data must be suitable for presentation before such a body.

BIBLIOGRAPHY

1. Durkheim, Emile: Suicide; A Study in Sociology, 1897. Translated by Spaulding, John A., and Simpson, George. New York, The Free Press, 1951.
2. Havens, Leston L.: The anatomy of a suicide. New Eng. J. Med., *272*:401-406, 1965.
3. Jenis, E. H., *et al.:* Acute meprobamate poisoning: A fatal case following a lucid interval. J.A.M.A., *207*:361-362, 1969.
4. Kaye, Sidney: Handbook of Emergency Toxicology. Springfield, Thomas, 1961.

5. Litman, R. E., *et al.*: Investigations of equivocal suicides. J.A.M.A., *184:*923-929, 1963.
6. McBay, A. J.: Chemical findings in poisonings. New Eng. J. Med., *274:*1257-1258, 1966.
7. Soencer, A. E., and Green, Nicholas M.: Suicide by ingestion of halothane. J.A.M.A., *205:*702-703. 1968.
8. Watanbe, Tomio: Atlas of Legal Medicine. J. B. Lippincott., 1968.
9. Bulletin of Suicidology. Publisher by the National Clearinghouse for Mental Health Information. Superintendent of Documents, U. S. Government Printing Office, Washington, D. C. 20402.
10. The Change in Mortality Trend in the United States. Public Health Service Publication No. 1000 — Series 3 — No. 1. Superintendent of Documents, U. S. Government Printing Office, Washington, D. C. 20402.
11. Mortality Trends in the United States 1954 - 1963. Public Health Service Publication No. 1000 — Series 20 — No. 2. Superintendent of Documents, U. S. Government Printing Office, Washington, D. C. 20402.
12. Suicide in the United States 1950 - 1964. Public Health Service Publication No. 1000 — Series 20 — No. 5. Superintendent of Documents, U. S. Government Printing Office, Washrington, D. C. 20402.
13. Symposium on Suicide — Oct. 14, 1965. The George Washington University School of Medicine. Yochelson, Leon. Ed. 1967.
14. World Health Statistics Report — 11 Special Subjects — Suicide. World Health Organization, Geneva, Switz. *21:* No. 6, 1968.
15. Kaye, Sidney, and Hagg, Harvey B.: Terminal blood alcohol concentrations in ninety-four fatal cases of acute alcoholism. J.A.M.A., *165:* 451-452, 1957.
16. Turkel, H. W., and Gifford, H. Erroneous blood alcohol findings at autopsy. J.A.M.A., *164:*1077-1079, 1957.
17. Bell, J. L., Tauber, H., Santy, A., and Pulito, F.: Treatment of depressive states in office practice. Dis. Nerv. Syst., *20:*263, 1959.
18. Spencer, J. A. E., and Green, N. M.: Suicide by ingestion of halothane. J.A.M.A., *205:*702-3, 1968.

INDEX

B

C

E

F

G

H

M

N

S

T